SICHER'S
ORAL ANATOMY

SICHER'S

ORAL ANATOMY

E. LLOYD DuBRUL, D.D.S., M.S., Ph.D.

Founder and former Head of the Department of Oral Anatomy,
University of Illinois, College of Dentistry;
Professor Emeritus, Department of Oral Anatomy,
University of Illinois, College of Dentistry;
Professor Emeritus, Department of Anatomy,
University of Illinois, College of Medicine, Chicago, Illinois

SEVENTH EDITION

with **501** illustrations, including **24** in color

The C. V. Mosby Company

ST. LOUIS • TORONTO • LONDON   1980

SEVENTH EDITION

Previous editions copyrighted 1949, 1952, 1960, 1965, 1970, 1975

Printed in the United States of America

The C. V. Mosby Company
11830 Westline Industrial Drive, St. Louis, Missouri 63141

Library of Congress Cataloging in Publication Data

DuBrul, E   Lloyd.
  Sicher's oral anatomy.

  Previous editions entitled Oral anatomy; editions
1-4 by H. Sicher and editions 5-6 by H. Sicher and
E. L. DuBrul.
  Bibliography: p.
  Includes index.
  1. Head.   2. Neck.   3. Teeth.   I. Sicher,
Harry, 1889-   Oral anatomy.   II. Title.   III. Title:
Oral anatomy.   [DNLM: 1. Head—Anatomy and histology.
2. Neck—Anatomy and histology.   3. Tooth—Anatomy
and histology. WU101 S565o]
QM535.S52 1980   611'.91   80-15943
ISBN 0-8016-4605-7

TS/CB/B 9 8 7 6 5 4 3 2 1   02/A/284

Preface

Oral anatomy is a special anatomy of the head and neck. Its special emphasis is the oropharyngeal continuum, dominated by a functional complex called the oral apparatus. Its subject matter deals in detail with distinctive components that make up the complex and the ensemble the components play in the performance of the apparatus. It is completely clear, therefore, that this textbook is *not* a "dental anatomy." The dentition is but one component of the intricately integrated oral apparatus.

It is now 52 years since the original book on this subject was published, written in German; it is over 30 years since its first modified version was published, written in English. During this time the use of the book by students and teachers of anatomy has gradually increased; lately this increase has come with quickened crescendo, as evidenced by the last edition, which was translated into Portuguese and Spanish.

Through the fifth and sixth editions of this classic work I have tried to direct the development of the text toward a more comprehensive and modern treatise. I hope the present text approximates this goal. It accents a logical basis for anatomic structure such that its function can be inferred, tested, and analyzed. Apart from the great intellectual appeal of such a slant, it has the additional virtue of making anatomy genuinely interesting to the beginning student, thus permitting its factual content to be more readily retained.

To all those familiar with earlier editions it will be apparent at once that this, the seventh edition, has been extensively rewritten. It has been attempted in a style as simple and succinct as possible without loss of functionally or clinically significant detail.

Many older concepts, especially those concerning growth, function, and neural mechanisms and so forth, have either been replaced or expanded, based on the most recent relevant research. The text has been reset to accommodate certain illuminating and instructive innovations. The more conspicuous of these are as follows.

Special sections on the basic biology of the major components of the oral apparatus have been developed to *explain* (rather than merely to describe) the functional form of a construct. For example:

1. Chapter 2 "The Skull," opens with a section on general features, which presents the phylogenetic explanation for the present form of the human skull.

A section on architectural analysis clarifies the biomechanics of skull structure in terms of simplified engineering models.

2. Chapter 3, "The Musculature," opens with an explanation of the mechanisms of contractile structures, followed by a discussion of the architecture of skeletal muscles to make more understandable the section on the specific action of muscles.

3. Chapter 4, "The Craniomandibular Articulation," opens with the structural design of the jaw joint, which is developed in depth by an overview of the biologic engineering of synovial joints in general. The section on movements is based on the classical laws of motion and their relevance in clarifying the movements of biologic structures. The chapter is climaxed by the most recent concepts of the intriguing neural mechanisms that control oral movements.

Careful analyses of the underlying designs of certain complicated entities have brought out functional facts that were previously obscure. The deftness of tongue manipulation, the valve actions of oropharyngeal and nasopharyngeal sphincters, the double valve action of the larynx, and the surprising biomechanics of the dentition as a unit are demonstrated and illustrated by simplified models.

In the second part of the book, which concerns applied anatomy, Chapter 14, "Propagation of Dental Infections," contains an entirely new section, entitled "Basic Plan of the Neck." It defines the triangles of the neck and points out their importance as clinical landmarks and surgical guides. But to make the section more instructive, the confusing descriptions of the cervical fasciae found in most textbooks are reduced to a simple basic arrangement. The functional and surgical significance of these fasciae and the fascial "clefts" they enclose are pointed out. The procedures for surgical access to the so-called fascial spaces emerge as a logical consequence of the basic plan of the cervical fasciae. This plan is illustrated by simple drawings.

Twenty-six new "figures" (some are composites of several illustrations) have been incorporated into the text. Some replace older, unsatisfactory illustrations; some are entirely new, and these include simple line drawings by the author to accentuate basic biomechanical ideas.

Comment on the new title of the book seems apropos. In all accuracy it should read *Sicher and Tandler's Oral Anatomy*. But this would be awkward, and since the first English version was rewritten by Professor Harry Sicher as *Oral Anatomy*, the present title seems a fitting dedication to the memory of my old friend and colleague.

I remain, as ever, indebted to the entire faculty and staff of the Department of Oral Anatomy in the College of Dentistry of the University of Illinois. The stimulating research of the faculty members, the tedious typing and retyping of the manuscript by Phillip Conrad and Paulette Ligon of the secretarial staff, and the photographic assistance of William Winn of the technical staff, all made this edition of *Oral Anatomy* possible.

E. Lloyd DuBrul

Contents

Figures in color

CHAPTER 1

Introduction

EVOLUTION OF ORAL ANATOMY

Any history, however cursory, will at least record the sequence of events flowing through the span of existence of some particular subject. In a discipline such as anatomy, the historic sequence points the direction of development of the science. In a book about a special anatomy, the book's history will reveal its evolving aim.

The first edition of this book under the title *Oral Anatomy*, by Harry Sicher (1949), emerged from a modified translation of the original classical text on the subject entitled *Anatomie für Zahnärzte*, by Harry Sicher and Julius Tandler (1928). Both authors were then at the University of Vienna. Tandler, a dominant figure in European medicine, was head of one of the two departments of anatomy at the University. Sicher was his student. The German edition defined, for the first time, the scope and some of the significance of the anatomy of the human oral complex. Among other innovations, it established the anatomic basis and technical procedure for systematic block anesthesia of the area of distribution of the fifth cranial nerve, to which surprisingly little has been added since that time. The preface to the first edition of *Oral Anatomy* pointed out that the book "tries to bridge the gap between theory and practice." But since no scientific discipline can advance without the persistent elaboration of theory, anatomists must persist in uncovering the substrate of principles responsible for the structure of living things. In the specific field of oral anatomy this means the continuing investigation of feeding behaviors in general, along with the elaboration of biomechanics of vertebrate oral systems in particular.

Thus the continuing aim of this work is clear. It is to present those maturing concepts of form and function that give an increasingly reliable picture of the working anatomy of the oral apparatus in its integration with the total organism. This, then, is the present stage of anatomic evolution in the tradition of a sequence of most distinguished Viennese anatomists—Hyrtl, Zuckerkandl, Tandler, and Sicher.

Although the present treatment of head and neck anatomy is basic to general dentistry, it has distinct bearing on a number of related clinical areas, including orthodontics, oral, maxillofacial, and plastic surgery, otolaryngology, and speech pathology. Furthermore, physical anthropologists, primatologists, comparative anatomists, and linguists should find the work useful. It offers a definitive basis for comparison and evaluation of biomechanical adaptation both in fossil hominids and in different extant forms.

1

At present, courses in anatomy are often ineffectual for dental students. They are taught by anatomy departments whose major charge is to present a general introduction to human anatomy for the future medical practitioner. Emphasis is on the body cavities and their contents as a basis for general medicine. The logical assumption is that those students who develop interest in the various specialties will pursue the anatomy of their special fields later on.

But dentistry is already a specialty of medicine, perhaps more clearly defined as "orthopedics of the oral apparatus." Therefore the dental student must be given the anatomy of his specialty in some depth right from the beginning, when the anatomic material is at hand. This textbook is an attempt to fulfill such a need. Thus the book is "not intended to replace but to supplement textbooks on . . . human anatomy," which "are at the same time too broad and not deep enough"* for this specialty.

SUBJECT MATTER OF ORAL ANATOMY

The realm of oral anatomy is the head and neck; its theme is the structural basis underlying the biomechanics of all the activity of the oral apparatus, which includes its functional extensions. And so it must be understood that not only major bodily readjustments, but also the development of speech, with its shifts in neural feedback control circuits, have impinged on the local feeding adaptations. All of these phylogenetic influences have, in some way, contributed to the specific kinds of movements man now makes with his oral apparatus. Evidence gleaned from such sources becomes essential for a modern textbook on human oral anatomy. It is only by tacit dependence on this total background influence that a presentation in depth of the workings of the oral apparatus can be developed, even though discussion in detail of this background is not essential to the text.

The subject matter of oral anatomy is most clearly exposed by means of a convenient analytical model. Thus the oral apparatus is a functional unit that can be defined in terms of nine structural components:

1. *Basal bones.* This component is represented by the upper and lower jaws and their buttressing extensions in the skull. It involves their specific form and relations to the biomechanics of the skeletal framework of the head and neck (Chapter 2).

2. *Masticatory musculature.* This component comprises the major muscles that move the jaw in chewing. They represent the effort forces involved in a complicated jaw-lever system (Chapter 3).

3. *Craniomandibular articulation.* This is the fulcrum of the lever system. It is made up of a pair of peculiar roving bases from which moments of force can be exerted (Chapter 4).

4. *Dentition.* This is itself a working unit, made up of individual components. The structure of each component is functionally related to its distance from the fulcrum and the effort force. Each tooth, therefore, provides a special working

---

*From the preface to the first English edition (1949).

area on which the load is applied in chewing, and all exhibit structural features for protection of their supporting structures (Chapter 5).

5. *Supporting structures.* These exactingly engineered constructs support the units of the dentition. They contain slings of ligaments in intricately buttressed sockets wired with neural circuits signaling special information; these ligaments are firmly fitted with a sturdy covering mucosa that seals off the roots of the teeth like tight gaskets at their necks (Chapter 5).

6. *Limiting structures.* These are special muscular boundaries that wall off the oral cavity and limit the flow of contents in the mouth. The outer limiting structures are the lips and cheeks formed by the facial muscles, lined by skin outside and by mucosa inside, and the oral floor. These structures form a continuous tube with the pharynx, which extends past the larynx and leads into the esophagus at the cricopharyngeal sphincter. The inner limiting structures are the tongue and its attachments. Functioning in intimate coordination, they limit and control food masses moving into and speech pulses moving out of the oral cavity (Chapters 3, 5, and 6).

7. *Salivary glands.* These, with their secretions, are essentially adjustable lubricating devices. They also provide some antibacterial and preliminary digestive action. The fluids keep the oral mucosa flexible and slippery, and they are essential in food processing as the tongue molds and packs the bolus into a pliable, streamlined form for smooth passage through the pharynx and esophagus (Chapter 5).

8. *Blood and lymph supply.* The entire system of vessels is essentially an energy input–waste output device, which is complicated by the conduction of defense, stabilizing, and reparative materials. In effect, the intricately laced transport channels keep the working parts refueled, protected, viable, and in continuous operation (Chapters 7 and 8).

9. *Neural control system.* From the biomechanical aspect, discriminative selection and summation of an enormous variety of exteroceptive inputs from the special sense organs—smell, sight, and taste—and from touch and pressure organs in the skin and oral mucosa alert and initiate activity of the oral apparatus for feeding. Once in motion, proprioceptive feedback circuits continually monitor the movements that produce the precise rhythms of jaw positioning, tooth contact, and cheek-tongue cadences seen in chewing and molding the bolus. In speaking, this system monitors the movements made in molding resonated speech sounds. These are closely correlated with neural inputs from the vibrating larynx and are further monitored by corrective feedback from the auditory system. (Chapters 6 and 9).

It must be distinctly understood that although the designation of separate functional components may be biologically meaningless out of context of the total working unit called the oral apparatus, the device affords a focus on local structural detail that has direct impact on appropriate clinical procedure.

The device, then, serves several purposes. It prepares a bridge to the section on regional and applied anatomy. In so doing it not only makes it easier to assimilate a mass of complicated anatomic structure by breaking this down into functional components to be grasped one at a time, but it also tends to define major areas of clinical specialties. Thus basal bones (the maxillae, mandible, and their connections) and the limiting structures (the facial muscles, etc.) state clearly the realm of maxillofacial surgery. Growth of basal bones integrated with the eruption of the dentition defines the specialty of orthodontics. The dentition is the area of concentration of operative dentistry. The supporting structures are the concern of periodontology. The craniomandibular joint and the masticatory masculature lie at the core of prosthodontics. The neural control systems form the basis for diagnosis and block anesthesia. Obviously, all the components as a unified totality are the concern of all. Resting firmly on this basic anatomic science, the section on regional and applied anatomy points up important, specific, common examples of the application of anatomic knowledge, but the absolute necessity of ever wider application is implicit and is pointed out here and there throughout the text.

PART I

Descriptive and functional anatomy

CHAPTER 2

The skull

GENERAL FEATURES

The human head is a tightly fitted composite of special organ complexes—the brain, olfactory organ (nose), eyes, ears, and oral apparatus. The skull is the consolidating framework that holds these components together. But phylogenetically the skeleton of the head arose from two distinct supporting frameworks in early vertebrates, the viscerocranium (or splanchnocranium) and the neurocranium. In mammals the parts have fused to a relatively solid cranium and movable mandible. Here the prevailing design is a fore-and-aft lineup of segments, with the viscerocranium forming antechambers for the respiratory and digestive tracts at the front, the neurocranium housing the brain and special sense organs at the back, and the whole lying in line with the horizontal body layout behind. With the development of the secondary palate, respiratory and digestive tracts are completely separate, so that the nose is now not only an organ of smell but also the beginning of the respiratory tract.

It is now quite clear that three major influences were responsible for the gross remodeling of the human skull: (1) development of erect bipedalism, (2) expansion of the brain, and (3) modification of the oral apparatus. Predominant among these was cranial adaptation to erect bipedal posture.

It is obvious that reorienting a large vertebrate animal through 90 degrees in the gravitational field, from a habitually horizontal posture to a habitually vertical posture, must be compensated for by drastic renovation throughout the body. The outstanding effect on the skull was a sharp bending between its neural and visceral segments. Thus the facial complex was rotated down in front while the neural component was rotated down in back. In this way the enlarged brain came to lie on the top (cranial) end of the body, but the cranial base was severely compressed. The general effect can be likened to bending a bar of taffy; it becomes domed on top and buckled up on the bottom. This accounts for the acute buckling up of the cranial base at the sella turcica (pituitary fossa) with the sharply slanting clivus, which is clearly demonstrated in a midsagittal section of the head (Fig. 2-1). As consequences of these extraordinary readjustments, the linear continuity between brain and spinal cord is minimally disturbed, the organ complexes retain their functional orientation to the environment, the skull is well balanced atop a vertical spinal column, and the head is now adjusted for horizontal rotation to scan the environmental surround. But, as will

7

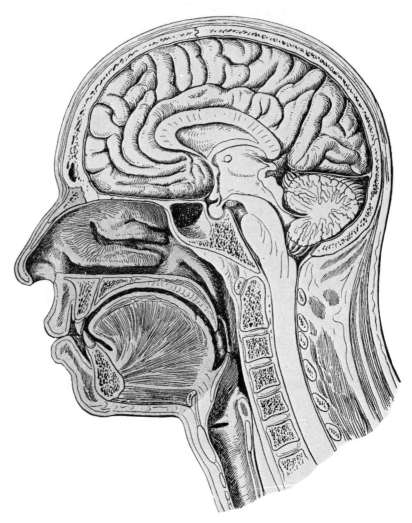

Fig. 2-1. Semidiagrammatic median section through the head and neck; relation of neural to visceral part of the head. Visceral area is shaded. Note bent skull base at the pituitary fossa (sella turcica). (Sicher and Tandler; Anatomie für Zahnärzte.)

be pointed out later, this has put certain restrictions on the biomechanical adaptations of the oral apparatus.

It is revealing to note that, in overall form, phylogenetic changes are not paralleled by ontogenetic changes in the human skull. Primitive forms of man like *Homo erectus** and *Homo sapiens neanderthaliensis* (Neanderthal man) had low cranial vaults and large, powerful, projecting masticatory skeletons that gradually became *reduced* in their successors. But the newborn human does not have a primitive-

---

*Priceless fossils of *Homo erectus* from China, formerly known as *Sinanthropus* (Peking man) were lost during World War II. Their ultimate fate is still being sought by anthropologists.

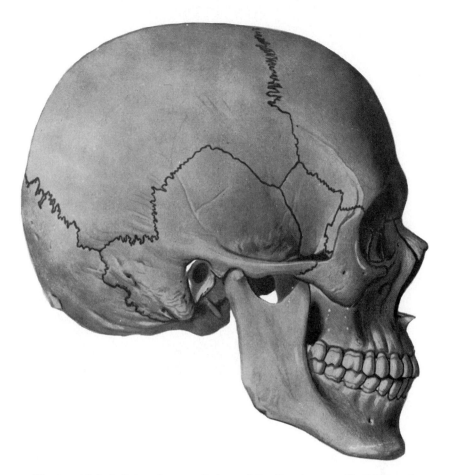

Fig. 2-2. Adult skull, lateral aspect. (Sicher and Tandler: Anatomie für Zahnärzte.)

looking skull. On the contrary, its skull is characterized by the enormous predomi-
nance of the neurocranium over the masticatory skeleton, which is almost hidden
below the bulging forehead. As the child grows, the masticatory skeleton becomes
increased in size, power, and projection. It is the reverse of phylogeny.

Although it is assumed that the ancestors of vertebrates had a segmental arrangement of the skeleton of the head, such a segmentation is obscured in mammals. The
only exception seems to be in the occipital region, where traces of segmentation can
be detected during early development.

The human skull is thus most easily described as having neural and facial parts,
although there is no distinct demarcation between the two (Figs. 2-2 and 2-3). The
neural part of the skull itself is made up of the cranial base and the cranial vault
(calvaria). The occipital region of the cranial base mediates the movable connection
with the vertebral column. Anteriorly and superiorly the parietal region follows,
connecting laterally with the temporal region. The anterior end of the neurocranium

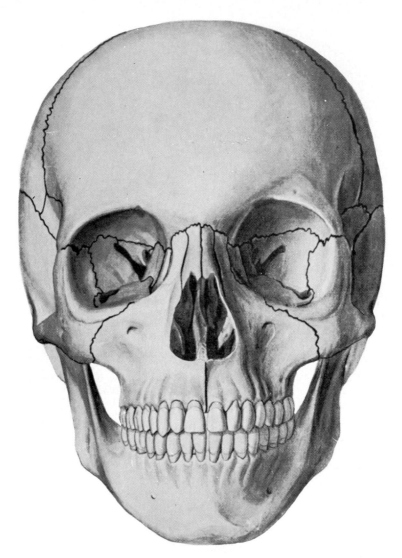

Fig. 2-3. Adult skull, anterior aspect. (Sicher and Tandler: Anatomie für Zahnärzte.)

is the frontal region, which is generally considered a part of the face because it forms the skeleton of the forehead.

The facial skeleton is situated below the anterior part of the cranial base. In it we find the orbits housing the eyeballs and their accessory organs. The nasal cavities are placed with their upper part between the orbits, whereas their lower part is flanked by the maxillary sinus on either side. Below the nasal region we see the maxillary region. Finally, the mandibular region forms the lowermost part of the facial skeleton.

In a mechanical sense the skull is composed of two parts: cranium and mandible. The bones of the skull are, for the greater part, flat bones. In the region of the cranial

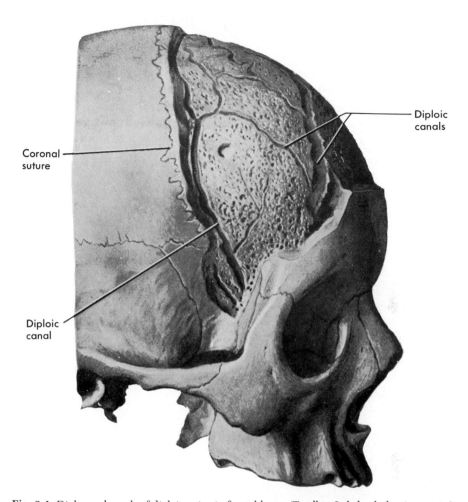

Coronal
suture

Diploic
canals

Diploic
canal

Fig. 2-4. Diploe and canals of diploic veins in frontal bone. (Tandler: Lehrbuch der Anatomie.)

vault they are almost evenly thick. In the cranial base and facial skeleton the bones are far more irregular in their dimensions, partly because they form the capsules of sense organs and partly because of mechanical influences. Where they are regular, the bones of the skull consist of two compact plates, the external and internal laminae. These are separated from each other by a thin layer of spongy bone which, in the skull, is called a diploe. In some places the diploe may be lacking so that the two plates fuse to a uniformly compact bone, whereas other bones contain a great amount of spongy bone. The spongy bone is not developed in some bones of the facial skeleton, for instance, in the nasal bones and lacrimal bones. In some bones of the cranial base and in the mandible the spongy bone is well developed.

The diploe of the bones on the convexity of the skull contains wide branching diploic canals (Fig. 2-4), which house thin-walled veins, the diploic veins of Breschet. These veins start in the region of the vertex of the skull and lead radially to the circumference of the skull in the frontal, parietal, and occipital bones. The diploic canals open on the outer surface of the skull, where the diploic veins empty into neighboring extracranial veins.

The internal plate of the flat bones of the skull has often been called lamina vitrea, or glassy plate, and was considered to be more brittle and fragile than the outer plate. This contention was founded on observations of injuries of the skull (for instance, by a blunt instrument) in which the inner lamina was much more extensively splintered than the outer. Cases are known in which the outer lamina in persons falling from considerable height did not show any injury, whereas a star-shaped fracture was

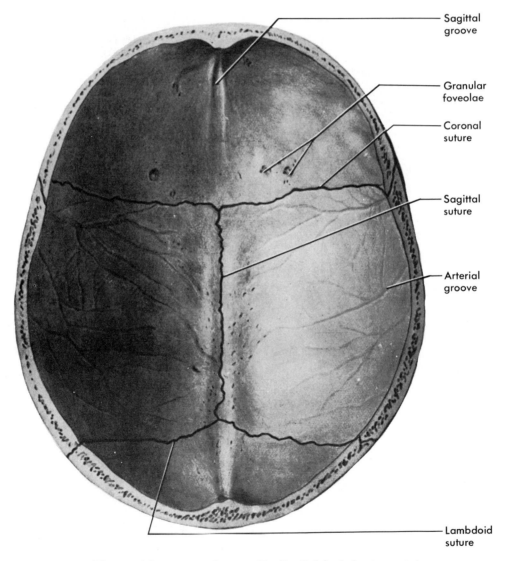

Fig. 2-5. Calvaria, internal aspect. (Tandler: Lehrbuch der Anatomie.)

observed in the inner lamina. Fractures of the internal lamina are often dangerous, causing ruptures of some arteries of the dura mater of the brain, because the dura is fused to the inner periosteum of the bones of the skull. Such a fracture is difficult to diagnose if the outer lamina does not show any injury.

A different and more plausible explanation has been found for the greater susceptibility of the inner lamina to injuries. A deforming impact on the convexity of the skull compresses the outer lamina and severely stretches the inner lamina. A break of continuity always occurs first on the side of tension, as in an attempt to break a stick over one's knee. This contention is borne out by penetrating shot wounds of the head which, at the exit of the bullet, may damage the inner lamina less severely than the outer lamina, since the mechanical conditions are here reversed.

On the inner surface of the brain capsule several peculiarities of the surface can be observed that are not confined to any one bone and, therefore, merit a more general description. Because of the correlation between growth of the brain and its bony capsule, the cerebral convolutions cause impressions in the bone, the digitated impressions. These irregular grooves were thus designated because they resemble impressions made with the fingertips in soft wax or clay. The grooves are, as a rule, rather wide, shallow, irregular, and often branching and are separated from each other by more or less sharp irregular and branching ridges, the cerebral juga. In the adult, digitated impressions and cerebral juga are more fully developed on the base of the skull with the exception of the occipital bone, which is in relation to the cerebellum and not to the convoluted cerebrum.*

The veins and arteries of the dura mater also are situated in grooves of the bones of the neurocranium (Fig. 2-5). The venous grooves, which contain the venous sinuses of the dura mater, are wide and shallow and are bounded by blunt, not prominent, elevations. They do not branch. In contrast to the venous grooves, those which house arteries are narrow and relatively deep and are bounded by sharp, bony borders. They branch frequently. By studying the venous and arterial sulci a good picture may be gained of the arteries and veins of the dura mater. Such information is, for instance, important in the evaluation of fossil human remains.

Especially on either side of the midline of the cranial vault, one finds circular or oval depressions, which are beset with small secondary pits (Fig. 2-5). They are called granular foveolae because they contain the arachnoid granulations of the brain, which drain the cerebrospinal fluid.

BONES OF THE SKULL
Occipital bone

The occipital bone (Figs. 2-6 to 2-8) develops by the fusion of four endochondral elements and one membranous element. The four cartilaginous bones are the unpaired portion of the squama called the planum nuchale, the paired lateral parts,

---

*It must be made clear that the detail of sulci and gyri of the *brain* is not reflected in the brain *capsule*, so that intracranial casts must be evaluated with great care.

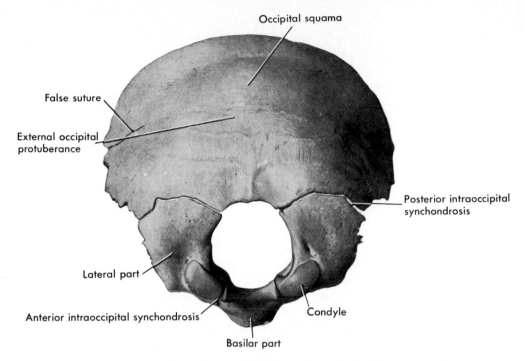

Fig. 2-6. Occipital bone of 2-year-old child. (Tandler: Lehrbuch der Anatomie.)

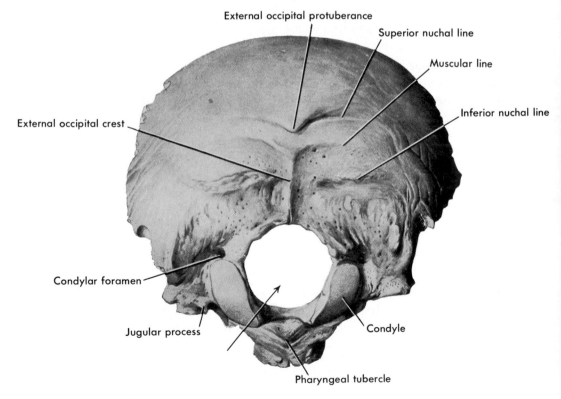

Fig. 2-7. Occipital bone, external aspect. Arrow points into occipital foramen. (Sicher and Tandler: Anatomie für Zahnärzte.)

and the unpaired basilar part (Fig. 2-6). These parts surround a large elliptical opening, the foramen occipitale magnum, which is the communication between the cranial
cavity and the vertebral canal. Through this foramen magnum the continuity between
brain and spinal cord is established, and the vertebral arteries and spinal accessory
nerves enter the cranial cavity. Above the planum nuchale the membranous part of
the squama is added and is called the interparietal bone.

The basilar segment is a strong wedge-shaped bone with a square anterior surface,
which is joined to the basisphenoid by the spheno-occipital synchondrosis. This cartilaginous junction, an important site of cranial growth, ossifies between the sixteenth
and twentieth year of life. The posterior sharp edge of the basilar part is concave and
forms the anterior rim of the occipital foramen. The inferior surface is elevated by a
small tubercle at its center, the pharyngeal tubercle, to which the pharyngeal raphe is
attached; otherwise the inferior surface is rough and serves for the insertion of muscles. The upper surface is slightly hollowed, ascending steeply anteriorly to join with
the body of the sphenoid. It is part of the basal slope, the clivus, which supports the
medulla oblongata and cerebral pons. The lateral borders are rough and are connected with the temporal bone in the petro-occipital fissure. A shallow groove follows the
lateral border on the upper surface; it contains a venous sinus, the inferior petrosal
sinus (see Fig. 2-49).

The lateral part consists, on either side, of a posterior flat and thin portion and an
anterior plump part, which carries, on its inferior surface, the greater part of the
occipital condyle, an elliptical articulating facet by which the skull articulates with the
first cervical vertebra, the atlas. The most anterior part of the condyle is contributed
by the basilar part. A shallow depression behind the occipital condyle is, in most
cases, perforated by a variably wide canal, the condylar canal. Through it runs a vein
connecting intracranial with extracranial veins, the condylar emissarium. Above the
condyle where the bone slopes steeply to the rim of the occipital foramen, the pars
lateralis of the occipital bone is perforated by a horizontal canal that is directed laterally and anteriorly and that is frequently divided by a horizontal bar of bone. This is
the hypoglossal canal, through which passes the hypoglossal nerve. The lateral border
of the pars lateralis is deeply notched behind a slight prominence, the jugular tubercle, which marks on the cerebral surface the fusion of the basilar and lateral parts. The
notch itself, the jugular notch, forms with an opposing notch of the temporal bone,
the jugular foramen. Behind this notch a strong, irregular process, the jugular process, juts upward, medially surrounded by a wide but relatively shallow groove containing the sigmoid sinus. The groove is rarely symmetrical, and in most skulls the
right groove is wider than the left. The condylar canal opens into the anterior end of
the sigmoid sulcus.

The occipital squama participates in bounding the occipital foramen posteriorly.
The squama forms an irregular triangle, the lateral sides of which are joined in sutures
to the parietal bones above and to the mastoid plate of the temporal bone below (Fig.
2-2). The outer surface is divided into a larger upper and a smaller lower field by a
rough line, the superior nuchal line. The upper part is generally smooth and forms

part of the cranial vault. The lower part serves for the attachment of the muscles of the neck and is part of the cranial base. The superior nuchal line itself starts in the midline at a bony prominence of variable strength, the external occipital protuberance. From here the nuchal line forms an arch on each side, the convexity of which is directed upward. Above this line there is, sometimes, a fine bony ridge, the supreme nuchal line. It is faintly marked and serves as the origin of the occipital muscles. The area below the superior nuchal line is rough and divided into a right and left half by the external occipital crest, which runs from the external occipital protuberance to the border of the occipital foramen. An inferior nuchal line runs parallel to the superior nuchal line, crossing the occipital crest. The development of the nuchal lines, occipital crest, and especially the external occipital protuberance is dependent on the development of the musculature of the neck. All these markings are, therefore, generally much stronger in the skulls of men than in those of women.

The inner surface of the squama is divided into four shallow fossae by a cross-shaped system of ridges, the cruciate eminence. Where horizontal and vertical bars cross, the bone is elevated to form the internal occipital protuberance. The upper part of the vertical crest and the horizontal crests are hollowed out by shallow grooves

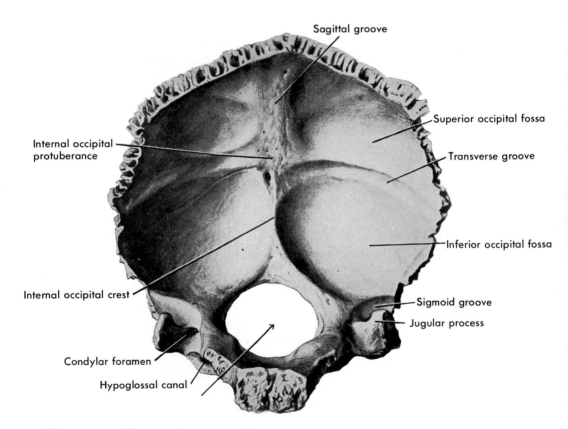

Fig. 2-8. Occipital bone, internal aspect. Arrow points into occipital foramen. (Sicher and Tandler: Anatomie für Zahnärzte.)

containing sinuses of the dura mater. Along the upper half of the vertical crest runs the posterior end of the superior sagittal sinus; the horizontal furrows contain the transverse sinuses. The sagittal sulcus continues, in the majority of cases, into the right transverse sulcus. The lower part of the vertical ridge, the internal occipital crest, is sharp and splits near the occipital foramen into two branches that surround the opening. These lines indicate the course of occipital and marginal sinuses. Of the four fossae on the inner side of the occipital squama, the two lower ones are smooth. They contain the hemispheres of the cerebellum and are part of the posterior cranial fossa. The superior occipital fossae contain the occipital lobes of the cerebrum and may show some cerebral juga and digitated impressions (Fig. 2-8).

Sphenoid bone

The sphenoid bone of the adult (Figs. 2-9 to 2-12) consists of a body and three paired processes. The body continues forward from the basilar part of the occipital bone and reaches anteriorly into the nasal cavity. Embryologically, the body consists of an anterior part, the presphenoid, and a posterior part, the basisphenoid, which are connected by a synchondrosis. Before birth or soon afterward, these two parts of the body fuse. Of the processes of the sphenoid bone, the lesser wings jut laterally from the upper edge of the body. They are attached to the presphenoid and form part of the floor of the anterior cranial fossa. The greater wings, attached to the basisphenoid, bound the anterior part of the middle cranial fossa. The pterygoid laminae develop as separate bones and form the most posterior part of the lateral nasal wall.

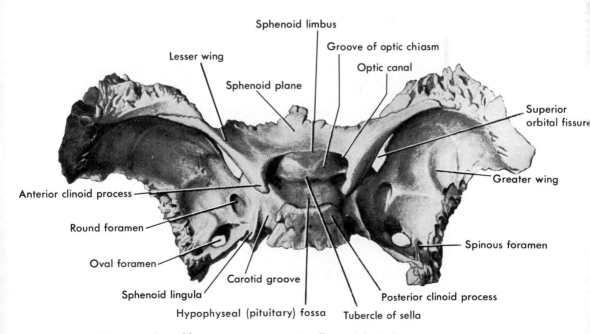

Fig. 2-9. Sphenoid bone, superior aspect. (Tandler: Lehrbuch der Anatomie.)

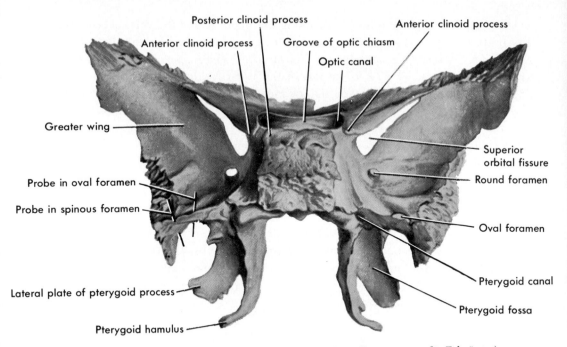

Fig. 2-10. Sphenoid bone, posterior aspect. (Sicher and Tandler: Anatomie für Zahnärzte.)

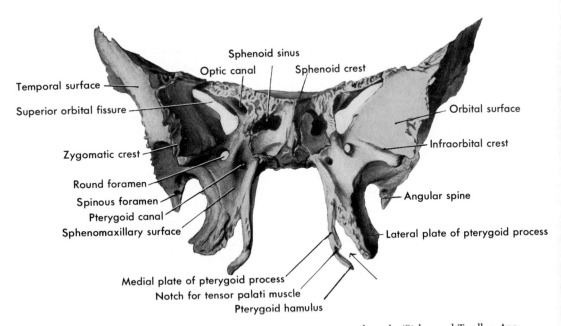

Fig. 2-11. Sphenoid bone, anterior aspect. Arrow points to pterygoid notch. (Sicher and Tandler: Anatomie für Zahnärzte.)

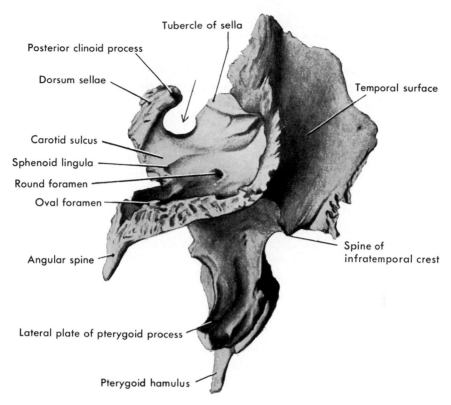

Tubercle of sella

Posterior clinoid process

Dorsum sellae

Temporal surface

Carotid sulcus

Sphenoid lingula

Round foramen

Oval foramen

Spine of
infratemporal crest

Angular spine

Lateral plate of pterygoid process

Pterygoid hamulus

Fig. 2-12. Sphenoid bone, right lateral aspect. Arrow points to sella turcica. (Sicher and Tandler: Anatomie für Zahnärzte.)

The square posterior surface of the body of the sphenoid bone is joned to the anterior surface of the occipital bone by the spheno-occipital synchondrosis. As was previously mentioned, occipital and sphenoid bones fuse between the sixteenth and twentieth year of life by ossification of the cartilage. The upper, or cranial, surface of the sphenoid body ascends steeply anteriorly in continuation of the occipital clivus. Widening slightly, it ends abruptly, undercut by a deep fossa, the hypophyseal or pituitary fossa, or the Turkish saddle, sella turcica. The anterior border of the ascending part of the body, dorsum sellae, is elongated on either side and ends in a small knob, the posterior clinoid process.

The anterior border of the hypophyseal fossa is marked by a blunt transverse ridge, tuberculum sellae, the lateral ends of which sometimes are elevated to form the middle clinoid processes. In front of the tuberculum sellae, a transverse groove is known as the sulcus chiasmatis, although the optic chiasm is not contained in this groove. The anterior border of the sulcus chiasmatis is formed by a fine but sharp crest, the sphenoid limbus, in front of which the horizontal sphenoid plane extends, projecting in the midline as the ethmoid spine.

The inferior surface of the sphenoid body is elevated in the midline in a low ridge, the sphenoid rostrum, which is linked to the vomer, the plowshare bone. The sphenoid rostrum is continuous with the sphenoid crest, marking the midline on the anterior surface of the sphenoid body. The crest joins the perpendicular plate of the ethmoid bone which, together with the vomer, forms the bony part of the nasal septum. To the anterior surface of the sphenoid body are fused two small bones, the sphenoid conchae, in which the pneumatization of the sphenoid bone starts. In this process the sphenoid body is hollowed out by two air-filled cavities that communicate with the nasal cavity and remain separated from each other by the asymmetrical sphenoid septum. Above the aperture of the sphenoid sinuses, shallow depressions are often found that owe their development to the expansion of posterior ethmoid cells into the sphenoid bone.

The lateral surfaces of the sphenoid body are, for the most part, fused to the lesser and greater wings. Above the root of the greater wing a sulcus cuts into the lateral surface of the bone on either side of the dorsum sellae; it contains the internal carotid artery and is called the carotid sulcus. Laterally the sulcus is bounded by a sharp, tonguelike projection, the sphenoid lingula.

The lesser wings of the sphenoid bone are narrow, triangular plates of bone arising from the sphenoid body by two roots. The optic nerve, accompanied by the ophthalmic artery, passes into the orbit through the optic canal between the two roots. The anterior border of the lesser wing is rough and serrated and joins the frontal bone in a suture. The posterior smooth border is concave, thickens medially, and ends in a rounded projection, the anterior clinoid process. Anterior and posterior clinoid processes may be linked by a bony bridge developing as an ossification in the dura mater. Anterior and middle clinoid processes are, normally, linked by a ligament; if this ligament ossifies, a foramen is formed through which the internal carotid artery passes (foramen clinoideo-caroticum). The superior surface of the lesser wing is a lateral extension of the sphenoid plane and forms part of the anterior cranial fossa. The inferior surface forms the most posterior part of the orbital roof and is perforated by the optic canal.

The greater wing arises in a rather wide area from the lateral aspect of the posterior part of the sphenoid body. Viewed from the cranial surface, the greater wing is a concave, irregularly triangular plate of bone. The anterior border can be divided into two parts, a medial half that is smooth and a lateral half that is rough. The smooth part, with the lesser wing, borders the superior orbital fissure. Through the fissure, which is wide in its medial and narrow in its lateral part, pass the oculomotor, trochlear, and abducent nerves, the ophthalmic nerve (the first division of the trigeminal nerve), and the ophthalmic veins. The rough lateral portion of the anterior border of the greater wing is widened into a triangular surface that joins the frontal bone. The lateral border of the greater wing is concave and extends posteriorly to a sharp bony angle. From this angle a sharp bony projection, the angular spine, juts downward. Its medial surface is often horizontally grooved by the chorda tympani nerve. The upper corner of the greater wing connects with the parietal bone; the concavity of the lateral border joins the squama of the temporal bone. The posteromedial border of the greater wing reaches from the region of the sphenoid lingula to the angular spine and is connected with the petrous part of the temporal bone in the sphenopetrosal fissure. The angular spine itself is perforated by a relatively narrow canal, the foramen spinosum, for the entrance of the middle meningeal artery into the cranial cavity. In front of and medial to the foramen spinosum, a larger opening is found, the *foramen ovale* (oval foramen). It transmits the mandibular nerve (third division of the trigeminal, or fifth cranial nerve). On the inner (cranial) surface in front of the foramen ovale, the foramen rotundum (round foramen) is found. It lies immediately below the medial end of the superior orbital fissure and transmits the maxillary nerve (second division of the trigeminal nerve). Between the two a small, variable foramen, the foramen of Vesalius, transmits an emissary vein (p. 515). The cranial surface of the greater wing shows digitated impressions and cerebral juga. Its lateral part is traversed by a narrow, sharp groove containing a branch of the middle meningeal artery.

The outer surface of the greater sphenoidal wing participates in bounding four cavities, or spaces, of the skull: the orbit and temporal fossa above, and the pterygopalatine and infratemporal fossae below. The upper part of the wing is divided by a vertical rough crest into a medial and a lateral part. The crest itself connects with the zygomatic bone and is, therefore, termed the zygomatic crest. Medial to the crest a smooth, approximately square surface, facing inward and forward, forms the posterior part of the lateral orbital wall. This orbital surface is bordered below by a smooth ridge, the infraorbital crest. Lateral to the zygomatic crest, the surface of the greater wing, facing laterally, is slightly concave in an anteroposterior direction and is part of the temporal fossa. Its lower end is marked by a sharp but irregular bony crest that projects at its anterior end as a bony spine, infratemporal crest, and infratemporal spine. (Fig. 2-12). The lower part of the greater wing below the infraorbital crest, the sphenomaxillary surface, faces anteriorly toward the pterygopalatine fossa and continues downward on the pterygoid process. Near its upper border it is perforated by the round foramen. The part of the greater wing below the infratemporal crest, the infratemporal surface, is in a horizontal position and forms the roof of the infratemporal fossa.

The pterygoid process arises at the connection between the greater wing and the body of the sphenoid bone. On the inner border of its root the pterygoid process curves medially as a thin, short lamella of bone, the vaginal process, which is closely applied to the lower surface of the sphenoid body. The root of the pterygoid process itself is perforated by the pterygoid or Vidian canal, which runs a sagittal and horizontal course (Fig. 2-11). Its posterior opening is seen just below the carotid sulcus; its anterior opening is found in the inferior and medial corner of the sphenomaxillary surface of the greater wing. The canal contains the pterygoid nerve and artery.

The pterygoid process is split into a wider and shorter lateral and a narrower and longer medial plate. The upper parts of the two plates are fused at their anterior edges. Below, they are separated by the pterygoid notch, into which fits the pyramidal process of the palatine bone. The two pterygoid plates are, in a posterior view, separated by a deep fossa, the pterygoid fossa. Above this fossa, at the posterior

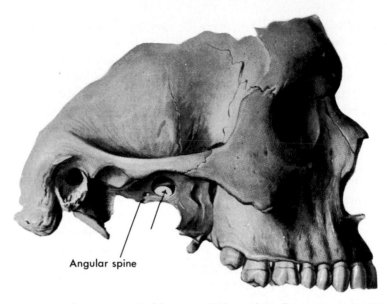

Angular spine

Fig. 2-13. Pterygospinous foramen is marked by arrow. (Sicher and Tandler: Anatomie für Zahnärzte.)

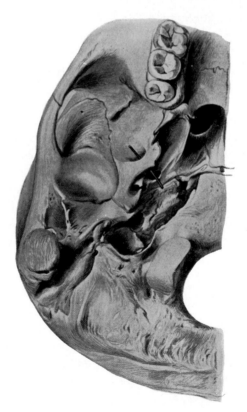

Fig. 2-14. Temporobuccal foramen is marked by a probe. (Sicher and Tandler: Anatomie für Zahnärzte.)

aspect of the root of the medial pterygoid process, a second shallow fossa, the scaphoid fossa, gives origin to the tensor palati muscle. The inferior end of the lateral plate is wide and rounded and continued by the lateral surface of the pyramidal process of the palatine bone. The inferior end of the medial plate ends in a thin, curved, hooklike process, the pterygoid hamulus, which turns laterally and posteriorly. The hamulus is separated from the medial plate itself by a deep notch, through which the tendon of the tensor palati muscle passes.

Two variations that develop by the ossification of normally ligamentous structures must be mentioned. The posterior border of the lateral pterygoid plate is linked to the angular spine by a thin plate of dense connective tissue. Ossification of this tissue forms a bony bridge that connects the spine with the lower surface of the greater wing to form the pterygospinous foramen (Fig. 2-13). On the anterolateral border of the oval foramen a shallow sulcus can be observed, which is bridged by a short ligament. Between bone and ligament runs the anterior branch of the mandibular nerve. Because it splits into the buccal nerve and one of the motor nerves for the temporal muscle, the anterior branch was once called temporobuccal nerve or nervus crotaphiticobuccinatorius. If the ligament ossifies, it bounds a foramen, the temporobuccal foramen or porus crotaphiticobuccinatorius of Hyrtl (Fig. 2-14). The ossification between the pterygoid process and the angular spine may not be of clinical importance, whereas the bony bar bordering the temporobuccal foramen may be an obstacle to an injection of the third division of the trigeminal nerve at the oval foramen.

Frontal bone

The squama of the frontal bone (Figs. 2-15 and 2-16) forms the vertical, anterior wall of the cranial vault; the paired, horizontal, orbital portions form the greater part of the roofs of the orbits. The latter are separated from each other by the ethmoid notch, the anterior boundary of which is formed by a jagged field, extending forward and downward as the nasal spine. The nasal bones are joined to this area. On the anterior surface, the squama and orbital parts are separated from each other by the smooth supraorbital rim, which is continued laterally as a strong, downwardly curved process, the zygomatic process of the frontal bone, which connects with the frontal process of the zygomatic bone. The medial third of the supraorbital rim is full and rounded. Close to its nasal end a shallow groove is found in which the frontal branch of the frontal nerve leaves the orbit and turns to the forehead. At the junction of medial and sharper lateral two thirds of the rim a deeper, lateral notch is found for the supraorbital branch of the frontal nerve. The ligament that normally connects the ends of the supraorbital notch may ossify and transform the notch into a supraorbital foramen.

Above the supraorbital rim the bone is elevated to a blunt ridge, which, as a rule, is better developed in men. Because of its relation to the eyebrows, this ridge is termed the superciliary arch. The most prominent regions of the frontal squama, the frontal eminences above the superciliary arches, correspond to the point at which the

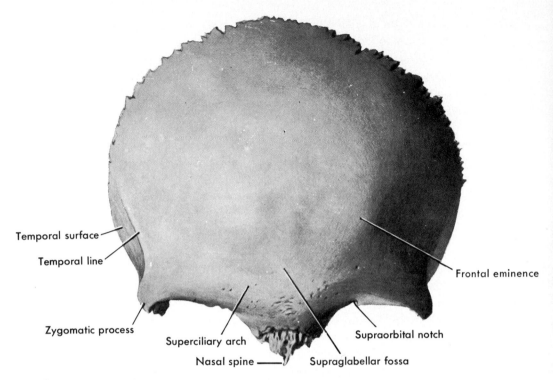

Temporal surface

Temporal line

Zygomatic process

Superciliary arch

Nasal spine

Supraglabellar fossa

Frontal eminence

Supraorbital notch

Fig. 2-15. Frontal bone, anterior aspect. (Sicher and Tandler: Anatomie für Zahnärzte.)

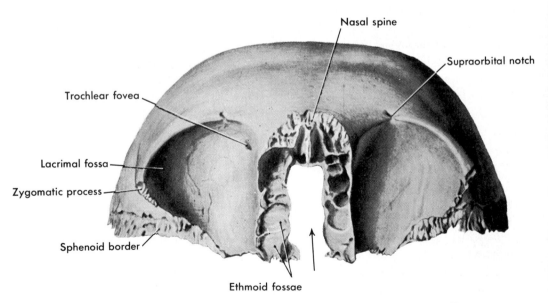

Nasal spine

Supraorbital notch

Trochlear fovea

Lacrimal fossa

Zygomatic process

Sphenoid border

Ethmoid fossae

Fig. 2-16. Frontal bone, inferior aspect. Arrow points into ethmoid notch. (Sicher and Tandler: Anatomie für Zahnärzte.)

ossification of the frontal bones started on either side. The slight elevation that is observed on most skulls above the root of the nose is the glabella.

On the lateral surface of the squama a rough crest commences at the zygomatic process and turns upward and backward. It is the temporal line, which often divides into a superior and inferior branch close to the posterior border of the frontal bone. This line marks the boundary between the greater frontal and the much smaller temporal surfaces of the frontal bone.

The orbital, or lower, surface of the orbital part of the frontal bone is generally in a horizontal position. It is a triangular field that is concave in a mediolateral direction. The concavity is deepest in the lateral area of the orbital part at the root of the zygomatic process. The lacrimal gland is situated in this concavity; hence the term lacrimal fossa. Close to the anteromedial corner of the orbital surface, the pulley for the superior oblique muscle of the eyeball is fastened to a shallow groove, the trochlear fovea, which is sometimes walled posteriorly by a sharp bony process, the trochlear spine.

The cranial surface of the frontal bone shows a gradual transition between the squamous and orbital parts. This is in contrast to the sharp and angular limitation of these two surfaces at the outer aspect of the bone. The difference is caused by a divergence, in the supraorbital region, of the outer and inner plates of the frontal bone between which the frontal sinus extends. A sharp crest, the frontal crest, begins at the inner surface immediately in front of the ethmoid notch and continues upward in the midline. After a variably long course, the crest widens and flattens and is grooved for the superior sagittal sinus, a venous space of the dura mater. On both sides of the crest and sagittal groove, irregular fossae containing the granulations of the arachnoid membrane of the brain are found. In the lateral areas of the cranial surface, furrows containing branches of the middle meningeal artery may be seen. The cranial surface of the orbital roof itself is slightly convex toward the cranial space and always shows distinct cerebral juga and digitated impressions.

Starting from a point in the midline, the posterior border of the squama curves downward and slightly forward and then inward to a triangular sutural field that ends anteriorly at the zygomatic process. The triangular field itself serves as the junction with the greater wing of the sphenoid bone (Fig. 2-16). In front of it the zygomatic bone links with the zygomatic process. Above the triangular area the posterior border of the frontal squama joins the parietal bone on either side in the coronal suture. This suture is complicated by the presence of toothlike processes of the two bones, which partly interdigitate and partly fit into sockets of the other bone. In its inferior third the suture changes its type, insofar as here the frontal bone is beveled to receive the overlapping lower anterior edge of the parietal bone. Medial to the triangular sphenoid surface the posterior border of the frontal bone is rather sharp where it connects with the lesser wing of the sphenoid bone. At the ethmoid notch the border turns sharply forward. Lateral to the ethmoid notch the inner and outer lamellae of the orbital part of the frontal bone separate, the outer lamella ending farther laterally than the inner. Between the sharp edges of these lamellae are found fossae, separated from each other by transverse ridges. These fossae form the roofs of the upper cells of the ethmoid bone. The most anterior fossa is considerably deeper and extends far anteriorly and superiorly as the frontal sinus. The two frontal sinuses are separated from each other by an irregularly bent septum. The edge of the external plate is, in its greater posterior part, linked to the lamina papyracea of the ethmoid bone; its smaller anterior part is in contact with the lacrimal bone. In the suture between ethmoid bone and the outer plate of the orbital part of the frontal bone are the anterior and posterior ethmoid foramina (see Fig. 2-51). The ethmoid notch is closed by the cribriform plate of the ethmoid bone, which is joined to the edges of the inner orbital plate. The horseshoe-shaped rough and pitted surface in front of the entrance to the frontal sinuses joins with the nasal bones and the frontal processes of the maxillae. The perpendicular plate of the ethmoid bone is connected to the inner surface of the nasal spine of the frontal bone.

The frontal bone develops as a paired bone, the two halves of which are separated by the frontal suture, which is still present at birth. Normally the suture closes during the second year of life but may persist in a small percentage of individuals as the metopic suture.

Ethmoid bone

The unpaired ethmoid bone (Figs. 2-17 to 2-19) fits into the ethmoid notch of the frontal bone so that its cribriform plate forms the middle part of the floor of the anterior cranial fossa. The cribriform plate itself is perforated on either side by two rows of small openings, through which olfactory nerves enter the cranial cavity.

The rather intricate structure of the ethmoid bone is most easily understood if it is studied at first in a diagrammatic frontal section (Fig. 2-17). Such a diagram reveals that in the midline a perpendicular plate joins the horizontal cribriform plates. Part of the vertical plate reaches into the cranial cavity as the crista galli, or cock's comb. The greater part of the vertical plate below the cribriform plate is part of the nasal septum. Another vertical plate is fastened, on either side, to the lateral edges of the cribriform plate, thus forming the middle and the upper nasal conchae. The conchal plates of the ethmoid bone are linked by irregular bony platelets to a second lateral pair of vertical plates, forming part of the medial wall of the orbit. Because of their extreme thinness these plates have been termed paper plates, laminae papyraceae. Between the conchal plate and the paper plate extends the ethmoid labyrinth. It consists of a number of ethmoid cells that communicate with the nasal cavity. The cells of the ethmoid labyrinth are partly open at the borders of the ethmoid bone and reach into neighboring bones, which then complete their walls. The frontal bone forms the roof of the upper ethmoid cells; posterior cells may reach into the sphenoid bone; inferior cells may reach into maxilla and palatine bones. Anterior cells are laterally closed by the thin plate of the lacrimal bone.

The conchal plate of the ethmoid bone is incompletely divided by a horizontal slit into an upper and a lower part (see Fig. 2-53). This slit cuts into the plate from behind for about two thirds of its anteroposterior extent. The inferior margins of the two parts

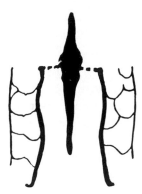

Fig. 2-17. Diagrammatic frontal section through ethmoid bone. (Modified from Sicher and Tandler: Anatomie für Zahnärzte.)

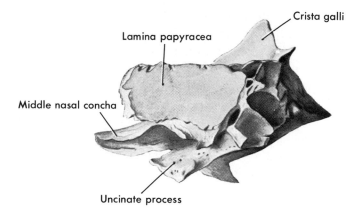

Fig. 2-18. Ethmoid bone, right lateral aspect. (Sicher and Tandler: Anatomie für Zahnärzte.)

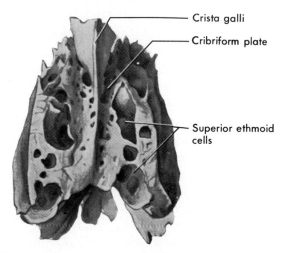

Fig. 2-19. Ethmoid bone, superior aspect. (Sicher and Tandler: Anatomie für Zahnärzte.)

of this plate, representing the upper and middle nasal conchae, are slightly thickened and rolled in; their free surface is irregularly pitted. The gap between them is the upper nasal passage or meatus. The space below and lateral to the edge of the middle nasal concha is the middle nasal meatus. Its lateral wall is cut by a sickle-shaped slit with its concavity facing upward and backward (see Fig. 2-54). This slit, the ethmoid (semilunar) hiatus, is bounded anteriorly and inferiorly by a thin swordlike plate of bone, the uncinate process, and is bounded superiorly and posteriorly by a rounded protruding ethmoid cell, the ethmoid bulla. The ethmoid hiatus leads upward into the ethmoid infundibulum and through it into the frontal sinus. The aperture of the maxillary sinus is found at its posterior inferior end.

The lateral borders of the cribriform plate connect with the inner plate of the orbital parts of the frontal bone. The posterior border of the cribriform plate is linked to, and partly covered by, the ethmoid spine of the sphenoid bone. The upper border of the lamina papyracea forms a suture with the external lamina of the orbital part of the frontal bone. Its anterior border joins the lacrimal bone; its inferior border joins the maxilla and, near the posterior corner, the palatine bone. The posterior border of the lamina papyracea is connected to the sphenoid bone.

The intracranial part of the vertical plate of the ethmoid bone, the crista galli, is lower in its posterior part and higher in its anterior part. Anteriorly two winglike extensions join the sagittal crest of the frontal bone. The nasal part of the perpendicular plate is connected posteriorly to the sphenoid crest, anteriorly to the nasal spine of the frontal bone. The posteroinferior border joins the vomer, and the anteroinferior border joins the cartilage of the nasal septum (see Fig. 2-55).

Temporal bone

The temporal bone (Figs. 2-20 to 2-23) develops by the fusion of three elements that can still be separated from each other at birth (Fig. 2-20). The petrosal bone forms the capsule of the inner ear; its mastoid surface is exposed at the lateral aspect of the skull. The temporal squama forms part of the lateral wall of the skull and contains the articulating surface for the mandible. The tympanic bone gives attachment to the eardrum or tympanic membrane. To these is later added the styloid process, a part of the visceral skeleton. Early in life the petrosal bone, squama, and tympanic bone fuse with one another, whereas the styloid process may remain independent for some time. Although the boundaries between the different elements of the temporal bone have partly disappeared in the adult, it is helpful to describe them separately.

The petrosal bone can be likened to a four-sided pyramid, the base of which forms the mastoid area behind the external auditory meatus. The axis of the pyramid is directed anteriorly and medially; its apex is linked to the posterior corner of the sphenoid body. The mastoid surface is roughly quadrangular and projects downward as a strong conic bony process, the mastoid process, which is, to a variable degree, hollowed out by air spaces communicating with the cavities of the middle ear. The mastoid process is separated from the inferior surface of the pyramid by a deep notch, the mastoid notch, from which the posterior belly of the digastric muscle takes its origin. A sharp groove medial to the mastoid notch contains the occipital artery. Anteriorly, the mastoid portion continues without a sharp boundary into the squamosal portion, which is above the external acoustic meatus. Farther down, the base of the mastoid process is, even in the adult, sharply demarcated from the tympanic bone by the tympanomastoid fissure. The upper border of the mastoid part forms a deep

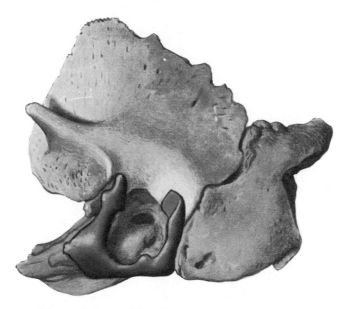

Fig. 2-20. Left temporal bone of a 1-year-old child. Petrosal part, yellow; squama, gray; tympanic ring, dark gray. (Sicher and Tandler: Anatomie für Zahnärzte.)

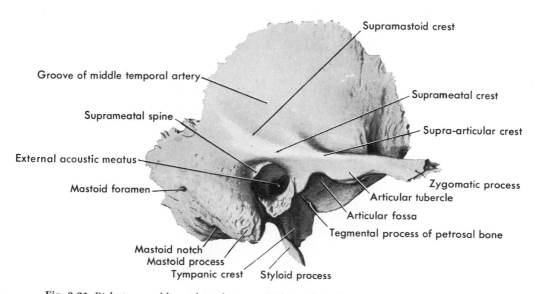

Fig. 2-21. Right temporal bone, lateral aspect. (Sicher and Tandler: Anatomie für Zahnärzte.)

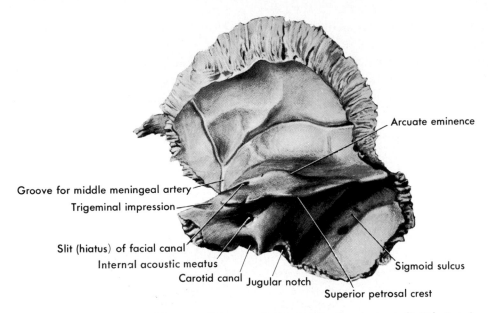

Arcuate eminence

Groove for middle meningeal artery

Trigeminal impression

Slit (hiatus) of facial canal

Internal acoustic meatus

Carotid canal

Jugular notch

Sigmoid sulcus

Superior petrosal crest

Fig. 2-22. Right temporal bone, medial aspect. (Sicher and Tandler: Anatomie für Zahnärzte.)

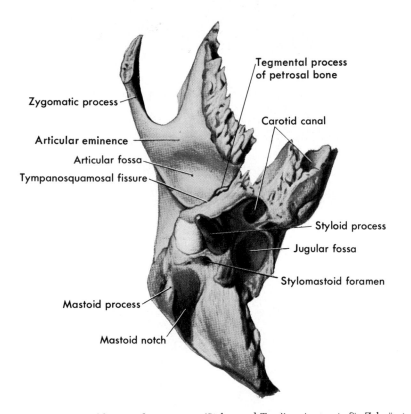

Tegmental process of petrosal bone

Zygomatic process

Carotid canal

Articular eminence

Articular fossa

Tympanosquamosal fissure

Styloid process

Jugular fossa

Stylomastoid foramen

Mastoid process

Mastoid notch

Fig. 2-23. Right temporal bone, inferior aspect. (Sicher and Tandler: Anatomie für Zahnärzte.)

angle with the posterior border of the squama, the parietal notch, into which the posteroinferior corner of the parietal bone fits. The posterior border of the mastoid part is joined to the occipital bone. Through the temporo-occipital suture, or through the bone in front of the suture, runs a variably wide canal, the mastoid foramen, which contains an emissary vein.

Of the four surfaces of the pyramid, the anteroinferior surface is hidden from view by the tympanic bone and forms the medial wall of the middle ear. The inferoposterior surface is visible at the base of the skull (see Fig. 2-50). It is bounded posteriorly by a sharp edge, which is joined to the occipital bone in the petro-occipital fissure. In about the middle of its course this edge is interrupted by the variably deep jugular notch, which, together with the corresponding jugular notch of the occipital bone, surrounds the jugular foramen. In many skulls the notch and the foramen are subdivided by bony spines into a smaller anteromedial nervous part and a larger posterolateral venous part. The former serves for the exit of the glossopharyngeal, vagus, and accessory nerves and, in some individuals, the deep petrosal sinus; the latter contains the internal jugular vein. In most skulls the inferior petrosal sinus passes through a separate opening in front of the nervous part of the jugular foramen.

Laterally and in front of the jugular notch the posteroinferior surface of the pyramid is hollowed out to a variably deep, round, and smooth fossa, the jugular fossa, which contains the enlarged cranial part of the internal jugular vein. Laterally to the fossa the styloid process is attached to the pyramid. Its base is partly surrounded by bone, the vaginal process, and from here the base projects anteriorly and inferiorly to a variable distance. Between the styloid process and the base of the mastoid process is situated the stylomastoid foramen, through which the facial nerve leaves the skull. In front of the jugular fossa and separated from it by a sharp bony crest lies the entrance into the carotid canal, which courses upward and then bends sharply into a horizontal plane and continues anteriorly and medially. The canal, containing the internal carotid artery and the sympathetic carotid plexus, surrounded by a cushioning venous plexus, opens at the apex of the pyramid. Between the jugular fossa and the carotid canal a shallow depression contains the superior ganglion of the glossopharyngeal nerve. The narrow tympanic canal, which leads the tympanic nerve into the tympanic cavity, begins in the petrosal fossula. Medially and to the front of the petrosal fossula and on the posterior edge of the pyramid one encounters a funnel-shaped fossa at which the cochlear aqueduct opens.

The two surfaces of the pyramid that face toward the cranial cavity are separated from each other by a sharp edge that begins at the parietal notch of the mastoid part and can be followed anteriorly and medially to the apex of the pyramid. Close to the apex the edge is interrupted by a shallow groove over which the root of the trigeminal nerve passes from the posterior to the middle cranial fossa. The trigeminal groove leads into a shallow depression on the anterosuperior surface of the pyramid, the trigeminal impression, which contains part of the semilunar or Casserian ganglion of the trigeminal nerve. Lateral to the trigeminal groove, the upper edge of the pyramid is furrowed by a narrow channel that contains the superior petrosal sinus.

A smooth prominence anterior to the middle of the superior pyramidal crest is caused by the superior semicircular canal of the labyrinth and is called the arcuate eminence. At a slit or hiatus of the facial canal in front of the arcuate eminence a furrow begins and extends medially and anteriorly. The furrow is named after the greater (superficial) petrosal nerve, which is contained in it. Parallel to and close to this sulcus a lateral narrower sulcus harbors the lesser (superficial) petrosal nerve. The anterior boundary of the anterosuperior surface of the pyramid is short and is linked by fibrous tissue to the posterior border of the greater wing of the sphenoid bone at the sphenopetrosal fissure. The anterior border of the pyramid and the anterior border of the squama form an angle that receives the angular spine of the sphenoid bone. A canal that begins in the cavity of the middle ear opens in this angle. The canal is divided by a horizontal bony plate into an upper compartment, containing the tensor tympani muscle, and a lower compartment, which forms the bony part of the auditory or Eustachian tube. The lateral part of the anterosuperior surface of the pyramid forms the roof of the middle ear and is therefore called the tegmen tympani. This plate of bone continues in the direction of the slope of the tympanic roof anteriorly and inferiorly into a tonguelike bony process that is situated between the squama and the tympanic bone. Its edge is visible at the inferior aspect of the temporal bone in the fissure that bounds the articular fossa posteriorly (Figs. 2-21 and 2-23).

The fourth surface of the pyramid faces posteriorly, superiorly, and medially toward the posterior cranial fossa. It is separated from the inner surface of the mastoid part by a deep groove that traverses the mastoid part in an anteriorly convex course. It is the sigmoid sulcus, containing part of the sigmoid sinus. Near the center of the posterior surface of the pyramid the internal auditory meatus starts with a well-rounded opening, the internal auditory porus. The facial nerve, acoustic nerve, and internal auditory artery enter here. Behind and lateral to this opening, a fine slit leads into a canal, the vestibular aqueduct, which is connected with the cavities of the labyrinth.

In the adult the temporal squama consists of two parts bent at a right angle. The zygomatic process arises from the boundary between the two parts. The larger, vertical, or temporal, portion of the squama forms part of the lateral wall of the cranial cavity; the horizontal, or basal, portion is visible from the cranial base and forms the articulating surface for the mandible. The lateral surface of the vertical squama is generally smooth and, in its posterior part, is often traversed by a vertical groove containing the middle temporal artery. The upper convex semicircular border of the squama is beveled on its inner side and beset by parallel ridges. It joins and overlaps the parietal bone in the squamosal suture.

The zygomatic process is a narrow horizontal bar of bone compressed mediolaterally. It juts laterally then curves forward to join the temporal process of the zygomatic bone in a suture that slants down and back, to complete the zygomatic arch. The process arises from the temporal squama by two strong roots, an anterior root that runs anterolaterally as the articular eminence and a posterior, or lateral, root that extends forward from the supramastoid crest. Thus the lateral root can be divided into three parts, the supra-articular crest in front, the suprameatal crest next, and the supramastoid crest behind.

The supra-articular crest is deeply notched on its inferior surface, which forms the articular fossa. This is thus called the articular notch, which ends posteriorly in the postglenoid process. The articular notch is an important surgical landmark in exposure of the craniomandibular articulation (Fig. 2-21).

The suprameatal crest forms the upper side of the suprameatal triangle. The lower side of the triangle is formed by the sharp posterosuperior edge of the acoustic meatus often made prominent by a suprameatal spine. The triangle is completed by a line joining the ends of the first two sides. The upper arm of the triangle (suprameatal crest) marks the level of the floor of the middle cerebral fossa and the edge of the dura. The triangle bounds the suprameatal fossa, which overlies the mastoid antrum. These also have been used as important landmarks in surgery of the ear and mastoid regions (Fig. 2-21).

It is important to note that the articular eminence has no anterior slope. Instead the eminence continues anteriorly into the flat infratemporal surface of the squama (preglenoid plane). Behind the eminence the bone is excavated to a variably deep fossa that is bounded posteriorly by the concavity of the tympanic bone, the mandibular fossa. However, only the squamosal part of this fossa, the articular fossa, is part of the mandibular articulation. The posterior border of the articular fossa is elevated, in its lateral part, to a variably high process, the postglenoid process. It is but rarely missing and, if well developed, it is cone-shaped in lateral view and sharply demarcated from the tympanic bone, which lies behind it. In such cases it becomes obvious at once that the articular fossa is confined to the squama of the temporal bone.

The tympanic bone is a strongly curved plate that forms the anterior, inferior, and posterior walls of the external auditory meatus. Posteriorly it remains demarcated from the mastoid part by the tympanomastoid fissure, whereas in the adult a boundary line with the pyramid is no longer visible, although its former position is marked by the implantation of the styloid process. In front of the styloid process and partly covering its root, the tympanic bone is elevated to a sharp crest, the tympanic crest, which can be followed to the anterior boundary of the carotid canal. The tympanic bone in front of the tympanic crest is slightly concave and takes part in forming the mandibular fossa. This portion of the tympanic bone is sometimes perforated by a variably wide opening that is a remnant of a defect normal in children from 2 to 5 years of age and should not be confused with pathologic erosions. In the mandibular fossa the boundary between the tympanic bone and the squama is marked by a deep fissure that is simple in its lateral part and is here called the tympanosquamosal fissure. In its medial part, however, the inferior process of the tegmen tympani is wedged between the tympanic bone and the squama and protrudes between these bones like the tip of the tongue between the lips. Thus the fissure is divided medially into an anterior part, petrosquamosal fissure, and a posterior part, petrotympanic fissure, or Glaserian fissure. Through the lateral part of the latter the chorda tympani emerges from the tympanic cavity to continue its course deep in the medial part of the fissure.

The temporal bone of the newborn infant is shaped radically differently from that of the adult. Of great practical importance is the lack of a mastoid process and, furthermore, the fact that temporal and basal parts of the squama are situated almost in one vertical plane. Consequently, the stylomastoid foramen lies unprotected on the lateral surface of the skull. This entails an exposure of the facial nerve to injuries, as for instance, in child delivery by forceps. Moreover, the articular surface is not in a horizontal position but faces outward and downward. The articular tubercle is almost nonexistent. The tympanic bone is represented by a thin, C-shaped bony ring that gives attachment to the tympanic membrane. The changes that occur in the early years of postnatal life will be described in the section on cranial growth.

Parietal bone

The parietal bone (Figs. 2-24 and 2-25) is a quadrangular cup-shaped bone. The serrated medial border joins the parietal bone of the other side at the sagittal suture. The anterior border, which is at a right angle to the sagittal border, is in contact with the frontal bone in the coronal suture. The posterior border, almost parallel to the anterior border, forms the lambdoid suture with the occipital squama. The lateral or inferior border is in contact with three bones. Its middle part, concave and beveled from without, is joined to, and overlapped by, the squama of the temporal bone. In front of the squamous border the parietal bone is in contact with the greater wing of the sphenoid bone; behind the squamous border the parietal bone is united with the mastoid notch of the temporal bone.

The outer surface of the parietal bone is smooth and has its highest convexity slightly below its center. The parietal tuber corresponds to the first center of ossification. Below the eminence a rough line, the inferior temporal line, can be traced from the lower part of the coronal border in a convex course to the mastoid border of the parietal bone. It can be followed anteriorly on the frontal bone to its zygomatic process and posteriorly on the temporal bone as the supramastoid crest. The inferior temporal line limits the area of origin of the temporal muscle. Above this line a second but less distinct line, the superior temporal line, passes through the parietal eminence. It is the superior boundary of the temporal fossa. The space between the temporal lines is the area of attachment of the temporal fascia.

At or behind the level of the boundary between the posterior third and the middle third of the sagittal border, and close to it, the parietal bone is perforated by an opening through which an emissary vein connects intracranial and extracranial veins. This foramen, the parietal foramen, is often lacking on one or both sides. The concave inner surface of the bone shows, as its most prominent feature, narrow, deep, branching arterial grooves, which contain branches of the middle meningeal artery. One groove starts at the squamosal part of the lower border, another one in front of it close to the anteroinferior corner. Along the midline a shallow and wide depression runs the entire length of the parietal bone and forms, together with the corresponding semisulcus of the other parietal bone, the sagittal sulcus for the superior sagittal sinus. At the posteroinferior corner another sinus, the sigmoid sinus, grooves the parietal bone and causes a wide and shallow depression, the sigmoid sulcus. Variably deep irregular depressions along the sagittal sulcus contain arachnoid granulations.

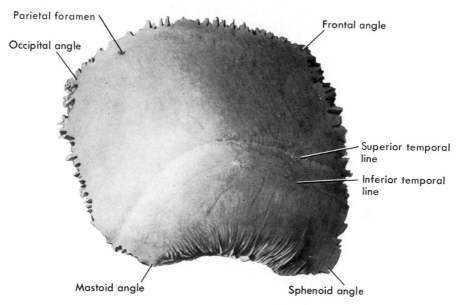

Fig. 2-24. Right parietal bone, external aspect. (Sicher and Tandler: Anatomie für Zahnärzte.)

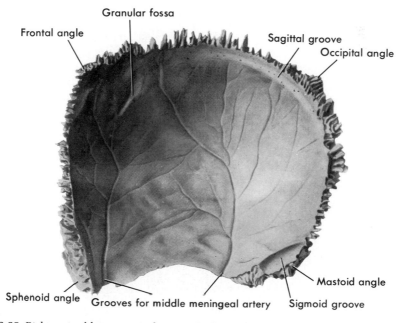

Fig. 2-25. Right parietal bone, internal aspect. (Sicher and Tandler: Anatomie für Zahnärzte.)

Maxilla

The maxilla (Figs. 2-26 to 2-31) consists of a central body, which is hollowed out by the maxillary sinus, and four processes. One of these, the frontal process, ascending from the anteromedial corner of the body, serves as the connection with the frontal bone. A second, forming the lateral corner of the body, connects with the zygomatic bone and is, therefore, called the zygomatic process. The horizontal palatine process arising from the lower edge of the medial surface of the body forms, with the process of the other maxilla, the major anterior part of the skeleton of the hard palate. Finally, the curved alveolar process, extending downward, carries the sockets for the maxillary teeth.

The body of the maxilla can be described as a three-sided pyramid with its base facing the nasal cavity. It lies in an almost horizontal axis, the apex being elongated into the zygomatic process. The three sides of the pyramid are a superior, or orbital, surface forming the greater part of the orbital floor; an anterolateral, or malar, surface forming part of the skeleton of the cheek and face; and a posterolateral, or infratemporal, surface turned toward the infratemporal fossa. The base is rimmed on its inferior edge by the alveolar process housing the tooth row.

The medial, or nasal, surface of the maxillary body contains, in its posterior part, the large irregular maxillary hiatus leading into the maxillary sinus. Behind this opening the bone is roughened for its junction with the vertical plate of the palatine bone. Beginning above the middle of the posterior border, a shallow sulcus, the pterygopalatine groove, descends obliquely downward and forward. It terminates at the angle formed by the posterior border of the palatine process and the medial surface of

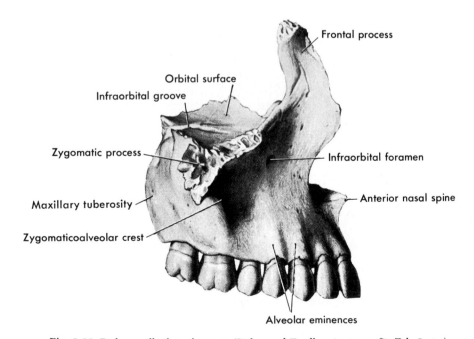

Fig. 2-26. Right maxilla, lateral aspect. (Sicher and Tandler: Anatomie für Zahnärzte.)

the body. The upper edge of the nasal surface contains, in its posterior part, one or two shallow depressions that complete and close some ethmoid cells. Farther forward a rather deep vertical groove that flattens out inferiorly, the lacrimal sulcus, can be seen. This sulcus is bordered in front by the continuation of the posterior border of the frontal process and in the back by a prominent bony spine that projects from the

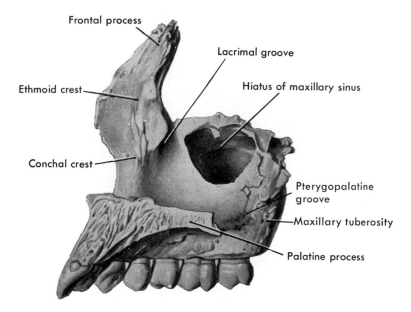

Fig. 2-27. Right maxilla, medial aspect. (Sicher and Tandler: Anatomie für Zahnärzte.)

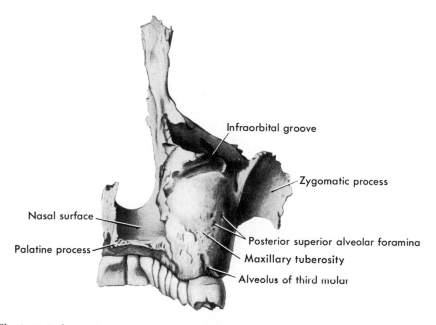

Fig. 2-28. Right maxilla, posterior aspect. (Sicher and Tandler: Anatomie für Zahnärzte.)

anterior edge of the maxillary opening. The remainder of the anterior half of the nasal surface of the maxillary body is slightly concave and terminates anteriorly at the sharp border of the piriform or anterior nasal aperture. In front of the lacrimal sulcus and at its lower end a horizontal rough crest, the conchal crest, serves for the attachment of the inferior nasal concha.

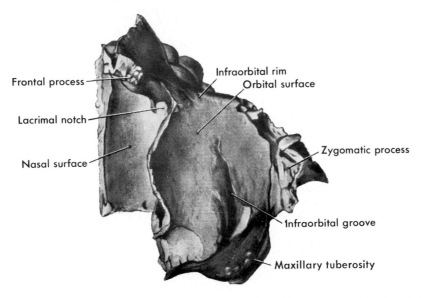

Fig. 2-29. Right maxilla, superior aspect. (Sicher and Tandler: Anatomie für Zahnärzte.)

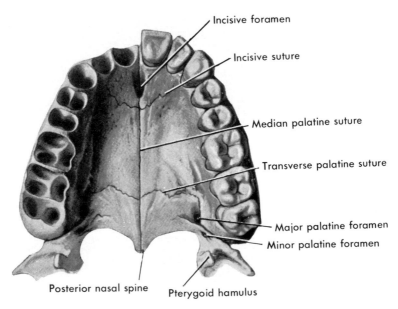

Fig. 2-30. Hard palate. On right side, empty sockets of alveolar process. (Sicher and Tandler: Anatomie für Zahnärzte.)

The orbital surface is triangular and slightly sloping laterally and anteriorly. Its medial edge is sharp and joins, in its anterior part, the lacrimal bone, and in its posterior part, the lamina papyracea of the ethmoid bone. At its posterior corner the palatine bone completes the orbital floor with its triangular orbital process. The anterior border of the orbital surface is smooth in its medial half. This part is thickened and forms a portion of the infraorbital rim. The lateral part of the anterior border of the orbital surface is rough and continues laterally onto the triangular sutural surface of the zygomatic process. This entire area serves as the junction with the zygomatic bone. Posteriorly the orbital surface is separated from the infratemporal surface by a blunt border that forms the inferior boundary of the inferior orbital fissure. From approximately the middle of this border a groove courses anteriorly on the floor of the orbit. This groove, the infraorbital sulcus, contains the infraorbital nerve and vessels. The lateral edge of the sulcus is rather sharp and bends tonguelike over the lateral part of the sulcus. Farther forward this thin bony process completely covers the infraorbital sulcus and transforms it into the infraorbital canal. Anteriorly the bony roof of the canal, known as the orbital plate, thickens considerably. Thus the canal descends in its most anterior part and turns slightly inward at the same time. If one were to extend the axes of the two infraorbital canals, they would converge downward and would cross each other at a point 1 to 2 cm. in front of the upper central incisors. Frequently a suture line can be seen extending from the infraorbital foramen upward to the infraorbital rim. This is the line at which the orbital plate, overgrowing the infraorbital sulcus, joins the maxillary body.

A characteristic, although rare, anomaly of the infraorbital canal should be mentioned. The infraorbital canal and foramen are sometimes shifted laterally, and the

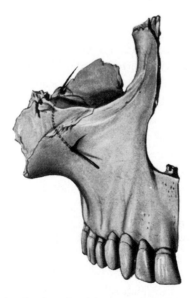

Fig. 2-31. Variation of infraorbital canal and foramen, marked by a probe. (Sicher and Tandler: Anatomie für Zahnärzte.)

canal follows a laterally convex arch through the base of the zygomatic process, which may be of clinical importance in anesthesia of the infraorbital nerve (Fig. 2-31).

The anterolateral surface of the maxillary body forms the skeleton of the anterior part of the cheek and is, therefore, called the malar surface. It is bounded posteriorly by a bony crest that begins at the tip of the zygomatic process and continues in an arc, concave laterally and inferiorly, in the direction of the socket of the first molar, to disappear at the base of the alveolar process. This bony crest is the zygomaticoalveolar crest, or jugal ridge. Medially the malar surface extends to the edge of the border of the piriform aperture; in the midline the bone projects at the lower border of the aperture as a sharp spine that forms, with the corresponding projection of the contralateral bone, the anterior nasal spine. The lateral part of the anterior surface that continues onto the zygomatic process is concave. The concavity, the canine fossa, is variably deep and contains near its upper and inner corner the opening of the infraorbital canal, the infraorbital foramen. This foramen is found exactly below the boundary between the smooth and roughened parts of the anterior border of the orbital surface, that is, below the most medial point of the zygomaticomaxillary suture. The border of the infraorbital foramen is sharp in its upper and lateral circumference and blunt below and medially, because of the oblique course of the infraorbital canal.

The posterior or posterolateral surface of the maxillary body, the infratemporal surface, is part of the anterior wall of the infratemporal fossa. This surface is convex in its greater medial part; the lateral part continues into the posterior concave surface of the zygomatic process. The posterior convexity of the maxillary body is called the maxillary tuberosity or tuber. The posterior superior alveolar nerves enter the bone in the center of this surface through two or three fine openings, the posterior superior alveolar foramina. They lead into narrow canals that run downward and forward in the thin wall of the maxillary sinus. In older individuals the canals are usually open toward the sinus for a shorter or longer distance. They converge with the most posterior of the anterior superior alveolar canals. These take their origin from the infraorbital canal, 4 to 6 mm. behind the infraorbital foramen. They begin either as one common canal, which soon branches, or they take their origin independently from the infraorbital canal. They are contained first in the roof and then in the anterior wall of the maxillary sinus from which they fan out, the posterior canal to communicate with one of the posterior superior alveolar canals and the most anterior canal to travel medially and downward into the alveolar process of the incisor teeth. The anterior alveolar canals also are partly open toward the maxillary sinus, especially in older individuals in whom the maxillary body is gradually and increasingly hollowed out by the expanding maxillary sinus.

The infraorbital canal itself juts into the maxillary sinus at the border between its roof and anterior wall. The wall between the infraorbital canal and the maxillary sinus can be defective in persons with a large maxillary sinus.

The zygomatic process of the maxilla is the elongated apex of the pyramidal body. Its triangular superior surface is inclined laterally and is irregularly rough. It serves as the suture with the zygomatic bone. The anterior surface of the zygomatic process is an extension of the anterolateral surface of the maxillary body; the posterior surface is concave and continues into the convex infratemporal surface of the body of the maxilla.

The frontal process is a bony bar which, in the Caucasian race, lies in an almost sagittal plane. Its anterior border takes part in forming the upper border of the piriform aperture and then extends upward in a straight edge, to which the nasal bone is joined. The posterior border of the frontal process arises approximately at the anteromedial corner of the orbital surface; it is in contact with the lacrimal bone. The upper border of the frontal process is thickened and abuts the frontal bone. Parallel to and close to the posterior border, a blunt vertical crest (the anterior lacrimal crest) runs up the lateral surface of the frontal process. Behind this crest the frontal process forms part of the lacrimal groove. In front of the lacrimal crest the lateral surface of the frontal process is smooth and fairly flat. The inner surface of the frontal process is, near its lower end, crossed by a horizontal fine ridge, the ethmoid crest, to which the middle concha of the ethmoid bone is attached.

From the lower surface of the body of the maxilla arises the alveolar process. It consists of two roughly parallel plates of bone that unite behind the last tooth to form a small, rough prominence, the alveolar tubercle, which often contains a single large marrow space. The lateral or external alveolar plate continues upward into the anterolateral and posterolateral surfaces of the maxillary body; the internal alveolar plate continues into the palatine process and behind the posterior end of the latter into the nasal surface of the maxillary body. The deep furrow between the two alveolar plates is divided by radial bony plates into the sockets of the individual teeth (Fig. 2-30). These interalveolar or interdental septa connect the outer and inner alveolar plates. The sockets for multirooted teeth are, in turn, divided by intra-alveolar, or interradicular, septa. In the socket for the first premolar the intraalveolar septum is parallel to the alveolar plates; in the sockets of the molars a sagittal septum divides the socket of the lingual root from those of the buccal roots, which themselves are separated by a secondary frontal septum.

The palatine process arises as a horizontal plate from the body of the maxilla at the boundary between the body and the alveolar process. The palatine process is, in anteroposterior direction, shorter than the body of the maxilla and terminates posteriorly with a rough beveled border, to which the horizontal plate of the palatine bone is joined in the transverse palatine suture; thus the skeleton of the hard palate is completed. At the corner between the posterior edge of the palatine process and the medial wall of the maxilla the bone is notched where the pterygopalatine sulcus ends. The palatine bone closes this notch to form the major palatine foramen. From this notch the palatine groove extends anteriorly at the border between the palatine and alveolar processes. The groove houses the anterior palatine nerve and vessels.

The border between the palatine and alveolar processes is sharp only in its posterior part, where the two processes join at almost right angles. Anteriorly the angle between these processes is not so sharply defined, and in the region of the canine and incisors the inner plate of the alveolar process continues in a smooth curve into the palatine process.

The lower, or oral, surface of the palatine process is rough and irregular. The nasal surface is smooth and transversely concave. Along the midline the bone is elevated to the sharp nasal crest, which serves as the attachment of the nasal septum. The nasal crest is divided into an anterior high part, the incisive crest, and a posterior lower part. The transition between the two parts is abrupt. The low posterior part connects with the bony skeleton of the nasal septum; the high anterior part connects with the cartilaginous skeleton of the nasal septum. At the boundary between these two portions of the nasal crest a canal commences in the nasal floor close to the midline and continues downward, anteriorly, and medially, to unite with the canal of the other side in a common opening. The canal is called the incisive or nasopalatine canal; the common opening is the incisive fossa, or anterior palatine foramen. The canals transmit the nasopalatine (Scarpa's) nerves and vessels and also contain remnants of the nasopalatine ducts, the organ of Stensen. The nasopalatine nerves are sometimes contained in narrow partitions of the incisive canal. These small canals are known as Scarpa's canals. The left canal of Scarpa opens at the anterior circumference of the incisive foramen, and the right opens at the posterior circumference, which may be of importance in anesthesia.

The incisive canal marks the boundary between the two constituent parts of the maxillary bone that unite early in embryonic life, the premaxilla and the maxilla proper. From the nasal opening of the incisive canal a remnant of the line of fusion between the premaxillary and maxillary palatine processes can sometimes be traced; more often, however, the remnant of the incisive suture is observed at the oral surface of the palatine process. Here it begins at the incisive foramen and extends toward the mesial border of the canine socket.

Palatine bone

The palatine bone (Figs. 2-32 to 2-34) supplements the maxilla and furnishes the link between the maxilla and the sphenoid bone. In the main it consists of a horizontal plate and a vertical plate joined at right angles. The horizontal plate, with its smooth superior, or nasal, surface and its rough inferior, or oral, surface, forms the posterior part of the hard palate. Its anterior beveled border overlaps the palatine process of the maxilla in the transverse palatine suture. The medial border connects with the palatine bone of the other side in the median or interpalatine suture, which is a continuation of the intermaxillary suture. At its nasal surface the medial border is elevated to a sharp crest that continues with that of the other side, the nasal crest of the maxillary bones. The posterior border of the horizontal plate is concave and terminates medially in a sharp spine that forms, in conjunction with that of the contralateral bone, the posterior nasal spine. In front of its posterior border, the oral surface of the horizontal plate is often elevated as a sharp transverse ridge, the palatine crest. The lateral border, between the horizontal and vertical plates, is connected to the medial surface of the maxilla at the level between the body and the alveolar process. This border is cut near its anterior end by a notch that completes a similar notch in the maxilla to form the major palatine foramen.

The vertical plate of the palatine bone is almost twice as high as it is wide. Its

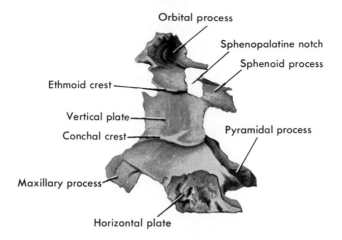

Fig. 2-32. Right palatine bone, medial aspect. (Sicher and Tandler: Anatomie für Zahnärzte.)

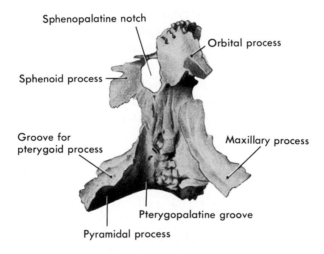

Fig. 2-33. Right palatine bone, lateral aspect. (Sicher and Tandler: Anatomie für Zahnärzte.)

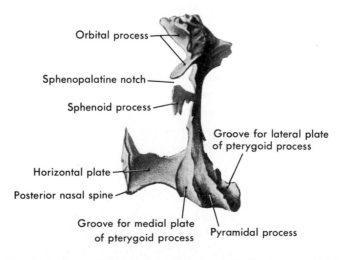

Fig. 2-34. Right palatine bone, posterior aspect. (Sicher and Tandler: Anatomie für Zahnärzte.)

upper border is divided by the deep sphenopalatine notch into two processes, a larger anterior orbital process and a smaller posterior sphenoid process. The greater part of the vertical lamella is in contact with the inner surface of the maxillary body posterior to the opening of the maxillary sinus. A tonguelike maxillary process of the vertical lamella, arising in the inferior part of its anterior border, closes the posteroinferior part of the maxillary hiatus, thus narrowing it considerably. On the outer surface of the vertical plate a sulcus begins below the sphenopalatine notch and ends at the notch of the major palatine foramen. This sulcus, the pterygopalatine groove, fits to the pterygopalatine groove of the maxilla and thus completes the walls of the ptery-gopalatine canal. Above this sulcus and around the palatine notch the lateral surface of the vertical plate of the palatine bone is smooth and forms the inner wall of the pterygopalatine fossa.

The sphenoid process behind the sphenopalatine notch joins the sphenoid body. The orbital process fits onto the posterosuperior corner of the maxillary body, where its orbital, infratemporal, and nasal surfaces meet. It completes the orbital surface of the maxilla at its posterior corner. The orbital process is often hollowed out by a shallow fovea that closes a posteroinferior ethmoid cell. Behind this fovea the orbital process is connected to the anterior surface of the sphenoid body. Since both the orbital and sphenoid processes are joined to the sphenoid bone above, the notch between these processes is closed by the body of the sphenoid to form the sphenopal-atine foramen, a communication between pterygopalatine fossa and nasal cavity.

The medial, or nasal, surface of the vertical plate is generally smooth. At the border between the inferior third and middle third it is traversed by a sharp hori-zontal ridge, the conchal crest, which serves as the attachment of the inferior concha. Near its base the orbital process is crossed by another horizontal rough line, the ethmoid crest, to which the posterior end of the middle nasal concha of the ethmoid bone is joined.

From the junction of vertical and horizontal plates at the posterolateral corner of the palatine bone, the short, stout pyramidal process arises. It serves as the firm anchorage of the maxillopalatine complex to the lower end of the pterygoid process of the sphenoid bone. The pyramidal process fills the pterygoid notch between the medial and lateral pterygoid plates, which themselves fit into grooves at the posterior surface of the pyramidal process. The lower surface of the pyramidal process contin-ues the oral surface of the horizontal palatine plate at the posterolateral corner just behind the greater palatine foramen. Medially and behind this foramen the process carries a variably developed sharp crest. Behind the greater palatine foramen are one or two, sometimes even three, smaller openings (the lesser palatine foramina) at which narrow canals open that branch from the pterygopalatine canal and perforate the pyramidal process.

Zygomatic bone

The zygomatic bone (Fig. 2-35) consists of a diamond-shaped body or basal plate with its longer diagonal lying in an almost horizontal plane. Thus it has four angles and four borders. The upper angle is drawn out superiorly and inwardly as a strong process, triangular in cross section, which connects with the frontal and sphenoid bones, the frontal or frontosphenoidal process. The posterior angle is elongated into the temporal process, which joins the zygomatic process of the temporal bone to complete the zygomatic arch. The whole anteroinferior border is sutured to the maxillary bone. The posteroinferior border is free and continues the zygomaticoalveolar crest laterally and posteriorly. It is called the masseteric border because it serves as the origin of the masseter muscle. The anterosuperior border of the plate is smooth, concave, and thickened to form the lateral portion of the lower orbital rim. The posterosuperior border ascends from the zygomatic arch behind the orbit and borders the temporal fossa anteriorly. A strong vertical crest, the sphenoid crest, juts medially from the frontal process to join with the zygomatic crest of the greater wing of the sphenoid bone.

The frontal process extends as a continuation of the superior corner of the basal plate and is, in cross section, triangular. Its outer surface faces anteriorly and laterally and continues the malar or external surface of the zygomatic plate. Its anterior border forms the lateral circumference of the orbital entrance; its posterior border ascends from the zygomatic arch behind the orbital entrance and borders the temporal fossa anteriorly. A strong crest, the sphenoid crest, juts medially and posteriorly to join the zygomatic crest of the greater wing of the sphenoid bone. This crest separates an anteromedial from a posterolateral surface of the frontal process. The anteromedial surface is smooth and slightly concave and forms the anterior part of the lateral orbital wall. The posterolateral surface, strongly concave, forms the anterior incomplete wall of the temporal fossa. At the orbital surface of the zygomatic bone, approximately at the border between its horizontal and vertical parts, an opening leads into the zygomatic canal, which divides within the bone into two branches. One branch opens at the malar surface of the basal plate, approximately at the base of the frontal process, as the zygomaticofacial foramen. The second opens near the upper end of the temporal surface of the frontal process as the zygomaticotemporal foramen. Through these canals run the zygomatic nerve and its two branches, the zygomaticofacial and the zygomaticotemporal nerves.

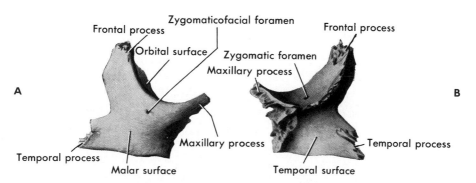

Fig. 2-35. Right zygomatic bone. **A,** Lateral aspect. **B,** Medial aspect. (Sicher and Tandler: Anatomie für Zahnärzte.)

Nasal bone

The nasal bones (Fig. 2-36) fit between the two frontal processes of the maxillae and form the upper part of the bridge of the nose. Each bone is irregularly quadrilateral. The short upper border is thickened and joins the frontal bone. The lower border is sharp and forms the upper part of the circumference of the piriform aperture. The posterolateral border joins the frontal process of the maxilla; the shorter anteromedial border serves as the junction to the nasal bone of the opposite side. The outer surface of the nasal bone is slightly convex, and the inner surface is concave. A narrow groove on the inner surface carries the external branch of the lateral ethmoid nerve down to a notch at the lower border or to a small foramen above it.

The nasal bones show great variations in length, width, curvature, and in their position; these variations influence the external shape of the nose and face. Racial differences are prominent. There is, in most skulls, a marked asymmetry between the two bones.

Lacrimal bone

The lacrimal bone (Fig. 2-37) is an irregularly rectangular thin plate of bone that joins the frontal process of the maxilla anteriorly, the lamina papyracea of the ethmoid bone posteriorly, the frontal bone superiorly, and the body of the maxilla inferiorly. The outer surface is divided by a sharp vertical crest, which, at its inferior end, is elongated into a sharp anteriorly bent hook-shaped process, the lacrimal crest and lacrimal hamulus. The larger part of the lateral surface of the bone, behind the lacrimal crest, is part of the medial wall of the orbit. The concave portion in front of the lacrimal crest, together with the posterior part of the frontal process of the maxilla, forms the lacrimal sulcus, which houses the lacrimal sac. The inner surface of the lacrimal bone closes the anterior ethmoid cells like a lid.

The lower border behind the hamulus joins the inner border of the orbital surface of the maxilla; the part of the inferior border in front of the hamulus extends downward as the maxillary process and bridges the lacrimal sulcus of the maxilla, thus closing the upper part of the nasolacrimal canal. The lower end of this process joins the lacrimal process of the inferior nasal concha.

Inferior nasal concha

The inferior nasal concha (Fig. 2-38) consists of an oval plate that is blunt at its anterior end and more sharply pointed at its posterior end; its free convex inferior border is somewhat thickened and often slightly rolled in. The medial surface is irregularly pitted and convex; the lateral surface is more nearly smooth and concave. The convex surface is turned toward the common nasal cavity, and the concave surface is turned toward the inferior nasal passage. The upper border serves as the attachment of the concha to the maxillopalatine complex. Its anterior part is joined to the conchal crest of the maxilla, and its posterior part is joined to the conchal crest on the vertical plate of the palatine bone. The middle part is elongated into the roughly

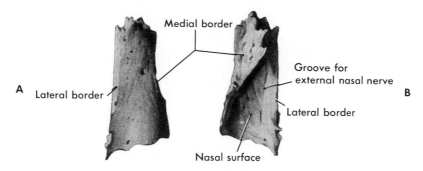

Fig. 2-36. Right nasal bone. **A,** External surface. **B,** Internal surface. (Sicher and Tandler: Anatomie für Zahnärzte.)

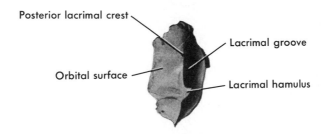

Fig. 2-37. Right lacrimal bone, lateral surface. (Sicher and Tandler: Anatomie für Zahnärzte.)

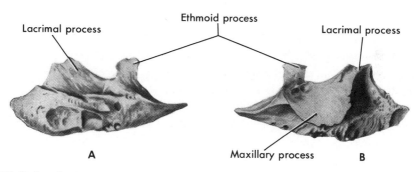

Fig. 2-38. Right inferior concha. **A,** Medial (nasal) surface. **B,** Lateral surface. (Sicher and Tandler: Anatomie für Zahnärzte.)

triangular maxillary process, which projects downward and fits into the lower corner of the maxillary hiatus to narrow this opening. Two other smaller processes arise from the upper border, both extending upward. The anterior of these two, the lacrimal process, located approximately between the anterior and middle third of the superior border of the concha, bridges the lower part of the lacrimal sulcus on the inner surface of the maxillary body and reaches upward to join the descending process of the lacrimal bone. In this way the lacrimal sulcus is, in its entire length, transformed into a canal that opens below the line of attachment of the lower concha into the inferior

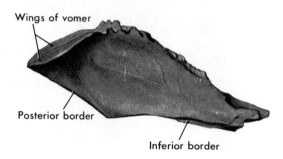

Fig. 2-39. Vomer, right surface. (Sicher and Tandler: Anatomie für Zahnärzte.)

nasal passage. The posterior of the two superior processes, the ethmoid process, extends across the hiatus of the maxillary sinus upward to join the uncinate process of the ethmoid bone.

Vomer

The vomer, or plowshare bone (Fig. 2-39), forms the posterior part of the nasal septum. It is a thin pentagonal plate of bone, normally situated in the midsagittal plane. The posterosuperior border is the thickest and is split into two winglike processes, which are attached to the lower surface of the sphenoid body; the sphenoid rostrum is received into the furrow between the two processes, the wings, or alae, of the vomer. The posterior free border, slightly concave, smooth, and sharp, forms the posterior border of the nasal septum and separates the choanae, the posterior nasal apertures. The inferior border fits to the nasal crest of the palatine and maxillary bones, the anterior shortest border to the posterior slope of the incisive crest of the maxilla. The anterosuperior border joins the perpendicular plate of the ethmoid bone in its posterior part and the cartilaginous nasal septum in its anterior part. Along the plate of the vomer, the sulcus for the nasopalatine nerve courses diagonally downward and forward from above and behind. Behind and below this sulcus, the vomer consists of one thin plate of bone; above and in front of the sulcus, a right and left plate are separated by a deep, narrow cleft into which the cartilage of the nasal septum fits. This cleft is extremely variable. Its variability is partly caused by the irregularities of the nasal septum, which is but rarely straight; in most individuals it is bent toward one or the other nasal cavity. At the height of the bend a sharp bony crest frequently develops from the convex surface of the bone.

Mandible

The mandible (Figs. 2-40 to 2-44) consists of a horseshoe-shaped body continuous upward and backward on either side with the mandibular rami. The body is thick, has a rounded lower border, and carries the alveolar process on its upper border. It extends backward from the chin at the midline symphysis to the anterior limit of the ramus. The ramus is, for the most part, a thin quadrilateral plate. It extends backward from the groove for the facial artery (antegonial notch) to include the region called the

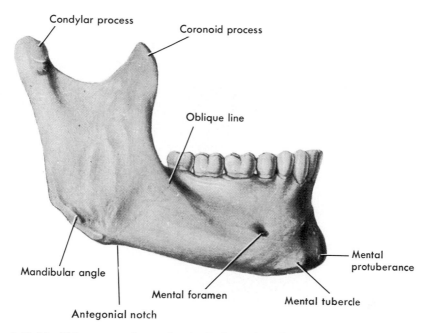

Condylar process

Coronoid process

Oblique line

Mental protuberance

Mandibular angle

Mental foramen

Mental tubercle

Antegonial notch

Fig. 2-40. Mandible, outer surface, right side. (Sicher and Tandler: Anatomie für Zahnärzte.)

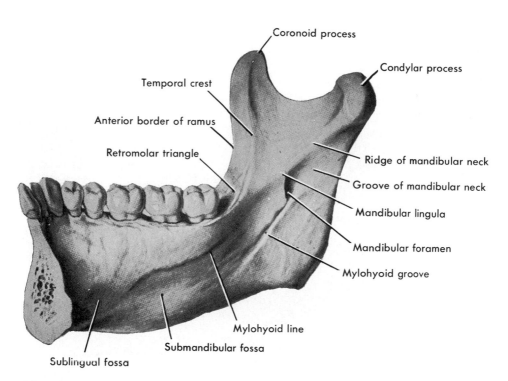

Coronoid process

Condylar process

Temporal crest

Anterior border of ramus

Retromolar triangle

Ridge of mandibular neck

Groove of mandibular neck

Mandibular lingula

Mandibular foramen

Mylohyoid groove

Mylohyoid line

Submandibular fossa

Sublingual fossa

Fig. 2-41. Right mandibular half, medial surface. (Sicher and Tandler: Anatomie für Zahnärzte.)

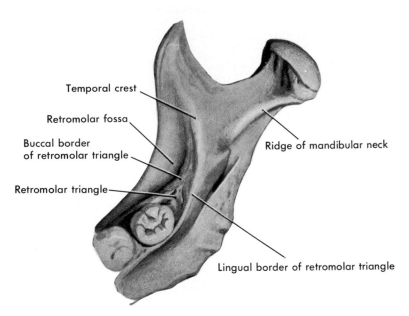

Fig. 2-42. Right mandibular ramus, superomedial aspect. (Sicher and Tandler: Anatomie für Zahnärzte.)

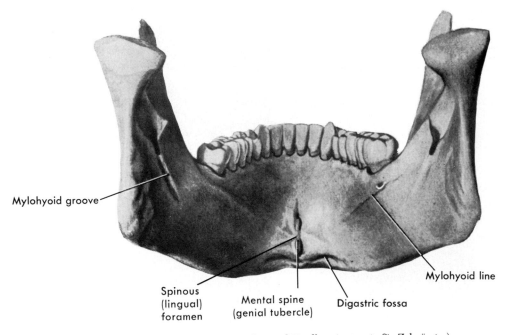

Fig. 2-43. Mandible, posterior aspect. (Sicher and Tandler: Anatomie für Zahnärzte.)

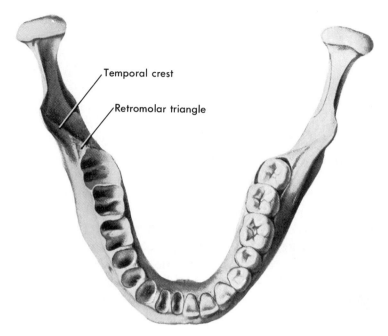

Temporal crest

Retromolar triangle

Fig. 2-44. Mandible, superior aspect. On right side are empty sockets of alveolar process. (Sicher and Tandler: Anatomie für Zahnärzte.)

mandibular angle. It reaches upward to end in two processes, the anterior muscular coronoid process and the posterior articular condylar process.

In and adjacent to the midline the anterior surface of the body projects to form a triangular prominence, the mental protuberance or bony chin. The base of this triangle coincides with the lower border of the body and is extended on either side as a small tubercle, the mental tubercle. A depression, the mental fossa, lies laterally on either side of the triangular chin. Two or three tiny openings through which small blood vessels pass are fairly constant in this fossa. Also, a small, raised oval area for the origin of the mentalis muscle can be found in the fossa.

The mental foramen, through which the mental nerve and blood vessels pass, is located on the lateral surface of the body between the roots of the first and second premolars (sometimes below the second premolar). In the vertical dimension, the foramen lies halfway between the lower border of the mandible and the alveolar margin. Sometimes, especially in younger individuals, the foramen lies closer to the lower border. The opening of the foramen faces outward, upward, and backward; consequently the foramen is sharp only at its anteroinferior circumference, whereas its posteriorsuperior margin slants in gradually from the outer surface of the mandibular body. All of these details are highly significant clinically (see Chapter 12).

In superior view it can be clearly seen that the alveolar process stemming from the upper border of the body has a sharper curvature than does the bulk of the body itself. Thus the body continues posterolaterally, whereas the alveolar process turns inward toward the sagittal plane. Because of this the posterior end of the alveolar process juts strongly in from the arch of the body. The ramus, continuing along the plane of the mandibular body, is therefore situated well lateral to the plane of the alveolar process in the entire molar region (Fig. 2-44). Thus the anterior border of the ramus continues along the body lateral to the alveolar process as a blunt ridge, the oblique line, running downward and forward to disappear at about the level of the first molar. These features are highly significant for understanding the continuous relations of oral cavity and pharynx as well as for clinical procedures.

On the posterior part of the lower surface of the chin a shallow, oval, roughened depression lies on each side of the midline. These are the digastric fossae for the origins of the anterior bellies of the digastric muscles. Slightly above the lower border on its inner surface the mandibular symphysis is elevated in more or less sharply defined projections, the mental spines, or genial tubercles. These may be fused or distinctly divided into right and left and superior and inferior knobs with small, roughened lateral hollows. The tubercles and adjacent hollows serve as the origins of the genioglossus muscles above and the geniohyoid muscles below.

From the region of the third molar a rough and slightly irregular crest extends diagonally downward and forward on the inner surface of the mandibular body. It is, as a rule, most prominent in its superior and posterior parts. If well developed, it reaches the lower border of the mandible in the region of the chin, passing between digastric fossa and mental spines. From this crest, the mylohyoid line, the mylohyoid muscle takes its origin. Since this muscle forms the floor of the oral cavity, the bone above the line is part of the wall of the oral cavity, whereas the bone below this line forms the lateral wall of the submandibular space and therefore is accessible from the neck. The area below the mylohyoid line is slightly concave and is termed the submandibular fossa because of its relation to the submandibular gland. A shallow depression above the anterior part of the mylohyoid line, the sublingual fossa, is in relation to the sublingual gland.

In the region of the mandibular angle the bone is irregularly rough on the outer as well as on the inner surface. Depressions alternate with more or less pronounced ridges that frequently extend to the border, ending in small knoblike elevations. The irregularities are caused by the two muscles attached to the mandibular angle, the masseter muscle on the outer side and the medial (internal) pterygoid muscle on the inner side.

The upper end of the ramus is divided into the condylar and coronoid processes by the semilunar, sigmoid, or mandibular notch. The posterior, or condylar, process carries the mandibular condyle, or mandibular head, an irregularly cylindroid structure the axis of which extends medially and posteriorly from laterally and anteriorly. The axes of the two condyles form an obtuse angle of 150 to 160 degrees, which is open to the front. The connection of the mandibular head with the mandibular ramus is the slightly constricted mandibular neck. Above the neck the condyle itself is slightly bent anteriorly so that the articulating surface faces upward and forward. The sharp border of the mandibular notch continuing backward and upward meets the lateral pole of the condyle. Medial to this crest and on the anterior surface of the mandibular neck a depression is found to which most of the fibers of the lateral (external) pterygoid muscle are attached; it is the pterygoid fovea.

The coronoid process is a thin, triangular plate either sharply pointed or ending in a backwardly curved hook. Thus its posterior border is concave. Its anterior border is convex above then becomes concave below, the concavity being an important landmark for palpation in block anesthesia (see Chapter 12).

Almost exactly in the center of the inner surface of the mandibular ramus the mandibular canal starts with a wide opening, the mandibular foramen. At its anterior circumference a variable bony process, the mandibular lingula, is found. At its posteroinferior circumference a narrow, sharply demarcated groove, the mylohyoid groove, commences and runs in a straight line downward and forward. It ends below the posterior end of the mylohyoid line and sometimes is closed to form a canal for some part of its length. It houses the mylohyoid nerve.

At the tip of the coronoid process a crest begins that runs straight down, traversing the coronoid process and then continuing on the medial surface of the ramus, becoming increasingly prominent in its downward course. Behind the last molar it bends into an almost horizontal plane and widens to a rough triangular field, the retromolar triangle. The prominent medial and lateral borders of the triangle continue into the buccal and lingual alveolar crests of the last molar. The vertical crest on the medial surface of the ramus serves as the attachment of the deep tendon of the temporal muscle and therefore is best designated as the temporal crest. Between it and the anterior border of the ramus is a depression, the retromolar fossa, which is variable in its width and depth. The retromolar fossa continues downward and forward into a shallow groove between the alveolar process and the oblique line.

Another ridge begins on the inner surface of the mandibular ramus at the inner pole of the mandibular condyle, crosses the mandibular neck in a forward and downward course, and continues to the region above and in front of the mandibular foramen, where it fuses with the elevation of the temporal crest. This ridge is of variable height and, in contrast to the temporal crest, smooth and blunt. Because of its relation to the neck of the mandible and because it is here that this ridge is most prominent, it may be designated as the ridge or crest of the mandibular neck. It is the main buttress of the mandibular ramus (see Fig. 2-68), transmitting the forces of mastication from the base of the alveolar process in a trajectory* to the mandibular head and, from there, to the base of the skull. The trajectory, consisting of strengthened and parallel trabeculae of the spongy bone, bulges toward the inner surface of the mandibular ramus, thus causing the elevation described as the ridge of the mandibular neck. The compact bone itself along this crest is also thickened. Behind and below the ridge the bone is depressed to a shallow groove, the groove of the mandibular neck, which is bounded posteriorly and inferiorly by a more or less prominent, fairly sharp ridge to

---

*Tracts of strengthened trabeculae of the spongy bone, coinciding with the lines of stress or trajectories, are themselves designated as trajectories.

which the posterior fibers of the sphenomandibular ligament are attached. The groove itself leads into the mandibular foramen. However, this groove owes its existence only to the prominences of the bone in front and behind it and does not contain the lower alveolar nerve.

The mandibular canal, which houses the inferior alveolar nerve and blood vessels, begins at the mandibular foramen, curves downward and forward, and turns into a horizontal course below the roots of the molars. In the region of the premolars the mandibular canal splits into two canals of unequal width: the narrower incisive canal continues the course of the mandibular canal toward the midline; the wider branch, the mental canal, turns laterally, superiorly, and posteriorly, to open at the mental foramen.

The alveolar process consists of two compact bony plates, the external and internal alveolar plates. These two plates are joined to each other by the radial interdental and, in the molar region, by the interradicular septa, thus forming the sockets for the teeth much in the same manner as in the upper jaw. The outer alveolar plate is free distally to the level of the second molar. In the region of the second and, especially, the third molar, however, the bony substance of the oblique line is superimposed on the outer alveolar plate because of the divergence of the mandibular body and the alveolar process. This relation between alveolar process and ramus gives the impression that the outer alveolar plate is of a considerable thickness in the distal part of the molar region.

Hyoid bone

The hyoid bone has been called the skeleton of the tongue, but this narrow designation obscures its multiple functions. It is a U-shaped bone (as the name indicates) that consists of an unpaired body (basihyoid) and greater and lesser horns, or cornua, on each side (Fig. 2-45). The hyoid is intercalated between the tongue above and the larynx below and has the distinctive feature of being subcutaneous externally and submucous internally. It is suspended in this position partially by the stylohyoid ligaments, which continue from the tips of the styloid processes of the temporal bones to the lesser horns of the hyoid.

The body of the bone is essentially an anteriorly curved, roughly quadrilateral plate. Its upper border is usually sharp and often has a slight notch in the midline. Its lower border is thicker and concave, and it lies in a plane anterior to the upper border. The anterior surface is overlaid by a prominent, forwardly curved bony ridge, which divides the surface into an upper, nearly horizontal, plane and a lower vertical plane. The ridge is sometimes sharply demarcated and it forms a continuous, downwardly curved line with the lesser cornua, stylohyoid ligaments, and styloid processes. The sling thus formed represents the remains of the second visceral arch. The rest of the hyoid bone, including the long greater cornua, represents the third arch with its body telescoped up inside the arch above. A median vertical crest is often present crossing the body of the bone from top to bottom. This divides the anterior surface into four hollows, which house the numerous muscle attachments. Occasionally the

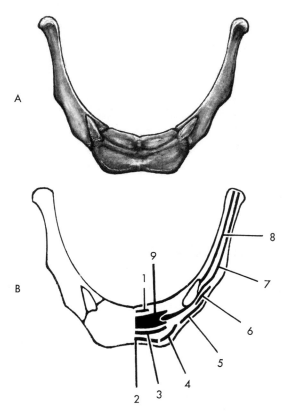

Fig. 2-45. Hyoid bone. **A,** Note greater cornua with tubercles at tips; lesser cornua with connecting ridge dividing body into upper horizontal portion and lower vertical portion. **B,** Relations of muscle attachments: *1,* geniohyoglossus; *2,* sternohyoid; *3,* mylohyoid; *4,* omohyoid; *5,* thyrohyoid; *6,* stylohyoid and digastric sling; *7,* hyoglossus; *8,* middle constrictor of pharynx; *9,* geniohyoid.

upper portion of the crest is raised in a projecting bony knob, which may represent the glossohyal, or lingual, process found embedded in the tongue in many mammals. The posterior surface is strongly scooped out; this hollow houses a bursa. Its smooth surface faces down and back, and it is perforated by numerous tiny vascular foramina.

The greater cornua are long bony bars flattened from above downward. They extend backward from the lateral margins of the body on each side and are linked to the body by cartilage, which is replaced by bone in later life. They terminate in a rounded tubercle and serve as anchorages for muscles, membranes, and ligaments.

The lesser cornua are short bony cones that slant up, back, and out from their bases seated at the upper ends of the junctions between the body and the greater cornua. They are linked to the body by fibrous tissue and sometimes to the greater horns by synovial joints.

The hyoid bone is tied by musculature to the tongue, mandible, and cranium above and to the thyroid cartilage, sternum, and scapula below. It is thus highly mobile and acts as a readily adjustable but stable base for muscular action in chewing, swallowing, and speech (see Chapters 3, 4, and 6).

SUTURES OF THE SKULL

Of all the bones of the skull, only the mandible is movable against the complex of the other bones of the skull. The mandible, therefore, is joined to the skull by a diarthrosis. The other bones of the skull are united by synarthroses to form the cranium, a rigid though resilient complex. The connections of the bones of the cranium are achieved partly by interposition of cartilage, synchondrosis, and partly by interposition of connective tissue, syndesmosis. Most of the syndesmotic junctions between the bones of the skull are specialized and are called sutures.

Synchondroses are found in several locations at the base of the skull of the fetus and the young child. The different parts of the sphenoid and occipital bones are joined to each other by cartilage. All these synchondroses disappear by ossification, partly at the end of the intrauterine period and partly in the first years of extrauterine life, with the exception of the spheno-occipital synchondrosis, which joins the sphenoid to the occipital bone. The cartilaginous plate between these two bones persists up to the sixteenth to twentieth year of life and is an important site of growth of the antero-posterior elongation of the base of the skull. The function of the cartilages at the synchondroses can be compared with that of the cartilaginous epiphyseal plates in tubular (long) bones.

In a suture the two bones are joined to each other by a thin layer of dense connective tissue that is continuous with the periosteum on the two surfaces of the bones. The sutural connective tissue, besides forming a firm connection between bones, is the site of growth for the two adjacent bones. This intricate function of the sutural connective tissue explains its rather complicated structure (see Fig. 2-77). A cross section through a growing suture reveals a differentiation of the sutural connective tissue into three zones. The two outer zones, adjacent to the bones, consist of parallel bundles of fibers arranged at right angles to the bone and continuing into the bone as Sharpey's fibers. An intermediate zone consists of an irregular feltwork of fibers that is rich in cells and in which the straight bundles from either side seem to end. It seems that there is a division of labor in the sutural connective tissue; the regular fibrous layers in the periphery serve as the firm connection of the two bones, whereas the central layer with its feltwork of collagenous and precollagenous fibers and its richness in cells serves as the zone of proliferation.

The sutures are divided into different types according to the shape of the borders of the bones united in the suture. The three most important types are the simple sutures, the serrated sutures, and the squamous sutures. (1) If the borders of the bones are smooth or nearly smooth, the suture is called a simple suture, or harmonia. (2) If the borders of the bones are beset by processes that interdigitate with similar processes of the other bone, it is a serrated suture. (3) A squamous suture is formed by a beveling of the two joining bones so that one bone overlaps the other in a variably wide zone.

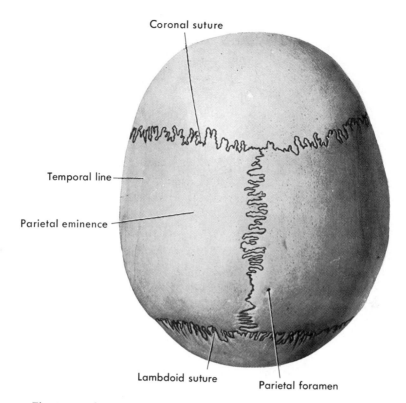

Coronal suture

Temporal line

Parietal eminence

Lambdoid suture

Parietal foramen

Fig. 2-46. Calvaria, external aspect. (Tandler: Lehrbuch der Anatomie.)

The serrations of a serrated suture are always simple near the inner surface of the skull (see Fig. 2-5). A middle layer of the bones has a peg and socket formation, whereas the outer layer is often highly complicated by the formation of secondary and even tertiary processes of the interdigitating spikes (Fig. 2-46). Especially the lambdoid suture and the parts of the coronal suture corresponding to the middle third of the anterior border of the parietal bone are highly complex. The sagittal suture is simple in its most anterior part and in a variably long part between the parietal foramina; otherwise it is highly complex. The complicated interdigitations develop in all probability by reinforcing apposition of bone on the outer surface of the cranium after growth of the cranial cavity has ceased.

That the sutures are sites of growth of the skull explains their disappearance by ossification at the end of the period of growth. Thereafter, the bones of the skull are united by synostosis, and the cranium truly represents *one* bone. The disappearance or ossification or closure of the sutures occurs in a certain order.

At about 30 years of age the closure of the sutures of the cerebral part of the cranium shows in the sagittal suture at a point corresponding to the parietal foramina and part of the coronal suture at the midline. Here, as in most other sutures, the synostosis occurs at the inner surface some years before the suture disappears at the outer surface. At about 40 years of age the sphenofrontal, occipitomastoid, and lambdoid sutures close. In the facial part of the cranium the closure of sutures starts as a rule in the middle thirties at the posterior end of the median palatine suture. Then the sutures between the palatine bone and the pterygoid process, most of the sutures around the nasal bones, and later the transverse palatine and zygomaticotemporal sutures may close.

Some sutures remain "open" even in older age groups; for instance, the squamous sutures, the lateroinferior parts of the lambdoid suture, the middle parts of the parietofrontal (coronal) sutures, and the parietomastoid and sphenotemporal sutures. In the facial skeleton the zygomaticofrontal and nasofrontal sutures frequently persist, as does the most anterior part of the intermaxillary suture. However, the "closure" of the other sutures deprives the "open" sutures of any significance as sites of growth of the cranium.

The connections of the pyramidal part of the temporal bone with the adjacent bones in the cranial base are established by a rather thick, dense connective tissue that often contains some cartilage cells and is then designated as fibrocartilage. These modified sutures are commonly referred to as fissures because of the clefts visible between the bones in a dry skull. The connection between the temporal pyramid and

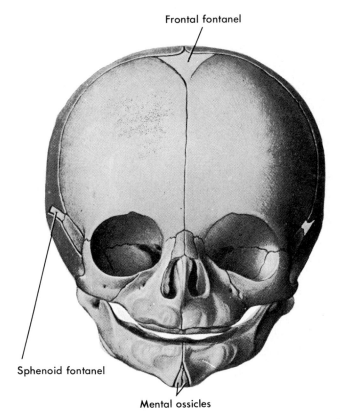

Fig. 2-47. Skull of newborn infant, anterior aspect, showing fontanels. (Sicher and Tandler: Anatomic für Zahnärzte.)

greater wing of the sphenoid bone is the sphenopetrosal fissure, and that between pyramid and occipital bone is the petro-occipital fissure. These two fissures converge at the tip of the pyramid, and here the human skull shows a rather large, irregular defect, foramen lacerum, lacerated foramen. This foramen, however, is closed in the living by a thick plate of fibrous tissue or fibrocartilage.

The bones of the cranial vault start their development in the membranous capsule of the brain from centers of ossification, which are situated at a fairly great distance from each other. At the time of birth the bones that had grown by apposition at their free borders are already aligned for the most part in relatively wide linear sutures (Figs. 2-47 and 2-48). The future corners of these bones, however, are still rounded and therefore the as yet unossified membranous and, at one point, cartilaginous parts of the brain capsule persist between the bones. They are called fontanels. The largest fontanel is found in the midline between the anterior corners of the parietal bones and the posterior corners of the paired frontal bones. It is the diamond-shaped frontal, or anterior, fontanel. A second one is found at the point where the two parietal bones and the occipital bone join. It is triangular and smaller than the frontal fontanel and is called the occipital, or posterior, fontanel. The third fontanel, the sphenoid, or anter-

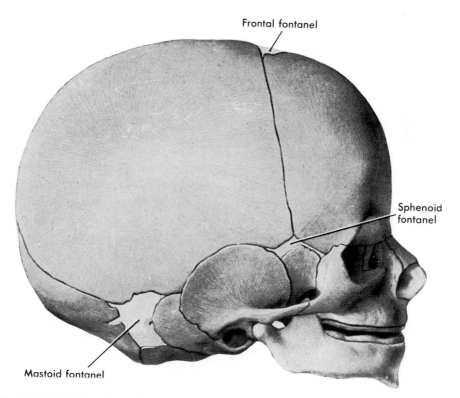

Fig. 2-48. Skull of newborn infant, lateral aspect, showing fontanels. (Sicher and Tandler: Anatomic für Zahnärzte.)

olateral, fontanel, is found at the anterolateral corner of the parietal bone, between it and the frontal, temporal, and sphenoid bones. These three fontanels, of which the first two are unpaired and the third paired, are membranous. The last fontanel is found at the posterolateral corner of the parietal bone between it and the temporal and occipital bones. Here cartilage, derived from the primordial skeleton of the cranium, fills the space between the bones. This is the mastoid, or posterolateral, fontanel, so called because it is situated behind the mastoid part of the temporal bone. The frontal and occipital fontanels can be easily felt in the newborn infant, whereas the sphenoid fontanel is obscured by the covering temporal muscle. The mastoid fontanel cannot easily be palpated because of the more equal consistency of cartilage and bone. The palpation of the frontal and occipital fontanels, which can be differentiated by their shape, plays a great role in obstetrics because it permits the determination of the position of the child's head during delivery. All fontanels close in the first 2 years of postnatal life.

At the site of future sutures supernumerary centers of ossification sometimes develop in the membranous capsule of the brain. They lead to the formation of smaller or larger supernumerary bones, which are termed sutural, or Wormian, bones. In some skulls many of these irregular bones can be observed, joined to each other and to the typical bones of the skull by irregular sutures. The site where these sutural bones are observed most frequently is the point where occipital and parietal bones meet.

CAVITIES OF THE SKULL
Cranial cavity

The floor of the cranial cavity is formed by the cranial base; the roof is formed by the cranial vault or calvaria. The cranial vault is of fairly even thickness, with the exception of the area that is surrounded by the temporal line, the temporal fossa. Especially in the lower parts of the temporal fossa the bone is, as a rule, far thinner than elsewhere. The reduction in the massiveness of the bone is compensated for by the protective layer of the temporal muscle and fascia. The inner surface of the cranial vault (see Fig. 2-5) shows the sulcus for the superior sagittal sinus running along the midline, widening and deepening in anteroposterior direction. Along this groove a variable number of granular foveolae are found. Laterally, narrow furrows for the branches of the middle meningeal artery ascend, branching toward the midline.

In the lower area of the temporal fossa, prominences can be found that are brought about by the bulging of the inferior frontal and superior temporal convolutions of the brain. This is the only area of the skull where the surface structure of the brain may exert an influence on the modeling of the outer surface of the skull. Such prominences are found in 90% of female skulls and in 80% of the heavier skulls of white men. It has been said that musicians show a highly developed upper temporal gyrus and therefore a marked bulge in the corresponding area of the temporal fossa, but this correlation is questionable.

The inner aspect of the cranial base (Fig. 2-49) is divided into the three paired

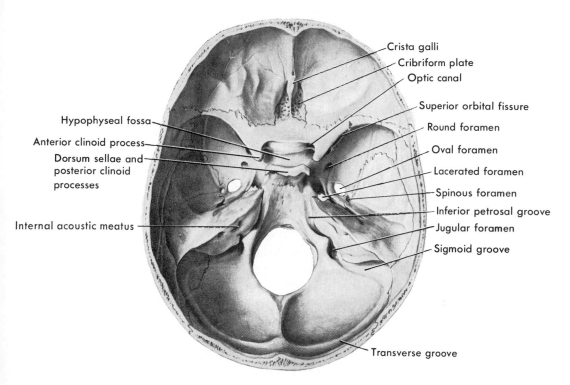

Crista galli
Cribriform plate
Optic canal
Superior orbital fissure
Round foramen
Oval foramen
Lacerated foramen
Spinous foramen
Inferior petrosal groove
Jugular foramen
Sigmoid groove

Hypophyseal fossa
Anterior clinoid process
Dorsum sellae and posterior clinoid processes
Internal acoustic meatus

Transverse groove

Fig. 2-49. Cranial base, superior aspect. (Sicher and Tandler: Anatomie für Zahnärzte.)

cranial fossae. They are arranged in such a way that the floor of the middle fossae is below the level of that of the anterior fossae and above the level of the posterior fossae. The anterior and posterior fossae of the right and left sides continue widely into one another, whereas right and left middle fossae connect only over the narrow sella turcica. The anterior and middle fossae house part of the cerebrum and are, therefore, characterized by the presence of digitated impressions and cerebral juga. This surface modeling is absent in the posterior fossae, which are in contact with the cerebellum.

The anterior fossae are bounded posteriorly by the sharp posterior borders of the lesser wings of the sphenoid bone and by the sphenoid limbus. In continuation of the lesser wing the parietal bone is, in some skulls, elevated into a crest that corresponds to the Sylvian fissure of the brain, the Sylvian crest.

In the midline the crista galli of the ethmoid bone juts into the interior of the cranial cavity. A blind pit, the foramen cecum, in front of the crista galli contains, in the adult, only connective tissue. In the fetus and sometimes in early childhood, the pit opens into the nasal cavity and contains a small vein. In front of the foramen cecum begins the sagittal crest, which soon divides into two lips to accommodate the anterior and narrowest part of the superior sagittal sinus. On the right and left sides of the crista galli the floor of the anterior fossae is considerably depressed by a cleft extending down to the lamina cribrosa of the ethmoid bone. Through the openings in this plate enter the olfactory nerves from the nasal cavity. In the most anterior part of the cribriform plate the anterior ethmoid nerve and the accompanying vessels enter the cranial cavity from the orbit and pass into the nasal cavity through a slit in the anteromedial part of this ethmoid sieve. Behind the depressed area of the cribriform plate the sphenoid plane extends backward to the sphenoid limbus. The lateral area of each anterior cranial fossa is slightly convex and forms the separating wall between the cranial cavity and orbit. In this region cerebral juga and digitated impressions are always prominent.

The middle cranial fossa reaches from the edge of the lesser sphenoid wing anteriorly to the superior crest of the petrosal bone posteriorly. The fossa narrows toward the midline because of the convergence of these two bordering bony crests. In the midline the hypophyseal fossa links the right with the left middle cranial fossa. Under the floor of the hypophyseal fossa lies the sphenoid sinus. Below the lateral parts of the middle cranial fossa lie the temporal surfaces of the craniomandibular articulation and, more medially, the tympanic cavity. In the region of the mandibular fossae the bone is always translucent. Anteriorly the floor of the middle fossa forms the roof of the infratemporal fossae.

The most important communications of the middle cranial fossa with neighboring cavities and spaces of the skull are as follows. The optic canal (optic foramen) perforates the root of the lesser wing immediately behind the sphenoid limbus. It leads anteriorly, laterally, and slightly inferior into the orbit and permits the passage of the optic nerve and ophthalmic artery. Below the posterior free edge of the lesser wing of the sphenoid bone, and between the lesser and greater wings, a second communication between the middle cranial fossa and orbit is established by the superior orbital fissure. The lateral narrow part of this fissure is closed by connective tissue. Through the wide, medial part of the fissure, the three nerves for the muscles of the eyeball, the oculomotor, trochlear, and abducent nerves, and the ophthalmic nerve, the first division of the trigeminal nerve, pass into the orbit. The ophthalmic veins enter the middle cranial fossa through the same opening to reach the cavernous sinus. Behind the medial part of the superior orbital fissure the greater wing of the sphenoid bone is perforated by the round foramen. It is, in reality, a short canal that perforates the bone obliquely, running in an almost horizontal plane, only slightly descending anteriorly. The round foramen emits the maxillary nerve, the second division of the trigeminal nerve, into the pterygopalatine fossa. Behind the round foramen, and slightly lateral to it, the oval foramen leads from the middle cranial into the infratemporal fossa. The oval foramen, situated close to the posteromedial border of the greater sphenoid wing, serves as the passage of the mandibular nerve, which is the third division of the trigeminal nerve. Immediately behind and lateral to the oval foramen, the angular spine of the greater sphenoid wing is perforated by the narrow foramen spinosum, through which the middle meningeal artery enters the cranial cavity.

At the apex of the temporal pyramid the dry skull shows a defect, the foramen lacerum; in the living it is closed by a fibrocartilaginous plate, continuous with the

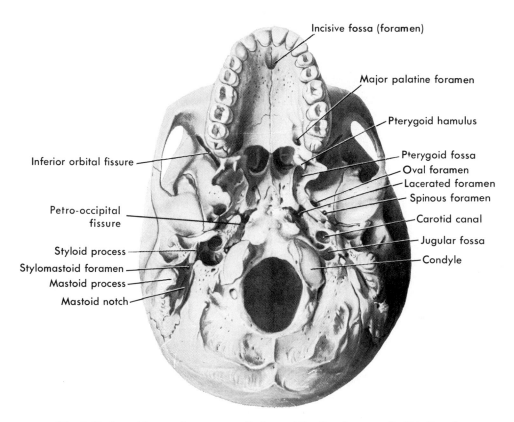

Incisive fossa (foramen)

Major palatine foramen

Pterygoid hamulus

Inferior orbital fissure

Pterygoid fossa

Oval foramen

Lacerated foramen

Spinous foramen

Petro-occipital fissure

Carotid canal

Jugular fossa

Styloid process

Condyle

Stylomastoid foramen

Mastoid process

Mastoid notch

Fig. 2-50. Cranial base, inferior aspect. (Sicher and Tandler: Anatomie für Zahnärzte.)

tissue in the sphenopetrosal and petro-occipital fissures. The internal carotid artery reaches the cranial cavity through the carotid canal, which opens at the tip of the petrosal bone. The artery then continues on the cranial surface of the fibrocartilage of the foramen lacerum. It is, therefore, a fallacy to state that the internal carotid artery passes through the foramen lacerum.

On the anterior surface of the temporal pyramid are the two small openings through which the greater and lesser (superficial) petrosal nerves enter the middle cranial fossa. The former is a branch of the facial nerve; the latter arises in the tympanic cavity. The greater petrosal nerve leaves the cranial cavity by perforating the fibrocartilaginous tissue of the foramen lacerum; the lesser petrosal nerve passes through the tissue of the sphenopetrosal fissure.

The posterior cranial fossa opens in the midline through the foramen occipitale magnum, the great occipital foramen, toward the vertebral canal. The spinal cord connects with the medulla oblongata through this foramen. The vertebral arteries and the spinal accessory nerves enter the cranial cavity through the great foramen on either side of the spinal cord. The hypoglossal canal perforates the lateral wall of the occipital foramen just above the occipital condyles; through this canal runs the hypoglossal nerve. The hypoglossal canal is sometimes subdivided by bony plates into two or three separate openings, which, however, unite in most skulls to a common canal near its lateral end.

Two opposing notches in the fissure between petrosal and occipital bones form the jugular foramen. It is partly or entirely divided into an anteromedial and posterolateral part by the intrajugular processes. The former is smaller and serves as passage for the glossopharyngeal, vagus, and accessory nerves. The latter is larger and emits the internal jugular vein. Because of the asymmetry of the right and left sigmoid sinuses and the right and left internal jugular veins, the right and left venous parts of the jugular foramen are rarely of equal size. In the majority of skulls the right foramen is wider. In a shallow groove along the petro-occipital fissure runs the inferior petrosal sinus, which connects the cavernous sinus with the superior bulb of the internal jugular vein immediately outside the jugular foramen. The inferior petrosal sinus sometimes leaves the posterior cranial fossa through the neural part of the jugular foramen, but as a rule it runs immediately in front of the anteromedial, or neural, part of the jugular foramen through a widened part of the petro-occipital fissure. Some authors describe this passage for the sinus as the most anterior portion of the jugular foramen and divide it, therefore, into three parts. At the posterior circumference of the venous part of the jugular foramen opens the condylar canal, which contains a communication between the sigmoid sinus and deep cervical veins, the condylar emissarium. Another, the mastoid emissarium, connects the middle part of the sigmoid sinus with one of the deep veins on the outside of the skull behind the mastoid process. It perforates the mastoid part of the temporal bone or is contained in the occipitomastoid suture.

The internal acoustic meatus opens on the posterior surface of the pyramid. Here enter the facial and statoacoustic nerves and the internal auditory artery. The facial nerve emerges, after a long course through the petrosal bone, at the stylomastoid foramen. The statoacoustic nerve and the auditory artery end in the inner ear. Laterally and slightly below the internal acoustic meatus lies the slitlike opening for the vestibular aqueduct.

If one applies the term cranial base to the floor of the cranial cavity, only the posterior part of this region can be seen in an inferior view. The facial skeleton is joined to and covers the anterior part of the cranial base.

The central part of the visible cranial base behind the facial skeleton (Fig. 2-50) is occupied by the foramen magnum. Posterior to the foramen magnum extends the nuchal plane, divided by the external occipital crest into a right and left half. The plane reaches posteriorly to the superior nuchal lines, which join in the midline to form the external occipital protuberance. The inferior nuchal line, running parallel to the superior line halfway between the occipital protuberance and the posterior border of the foramen magnum, and one or two sagittal crests on either side, divide the nuchal plane into several fields to which are inserted the posterior muscles of the neck.

The anterolateral margins of the foramen magnum are flanked by the occipital condyles for the articulation with the superior facets of the atlas. In the fossa behind each condyle commences a short canal that empties into the terminal part of the sigmoid sulcus. This canal contains an emissary vein connecting the sinus with one of the deep cervical veins. Another of these emissaries sometimes is found in the midline along the external occipital crest. It opens in the skull into the occipital sinus and connects with occipital extracranial veins.

Above the condyles the lateral opening of the hypoglossal canal is found; in front of the condyles and foramen magnum a rough, approximately rectangular area of bone extends to the site of the spheno-occipital synchondrosis. After the synchondrosis has ossified (between the eighteenth and twentieth year), its former site is seen a bit behind the most posterior extent of the vomer where it joins the body of the sphenoid bone. The bone behind this rim is the inferior surface of the basal part of the occipital bone. In the midline and about halfway between the anterior border of the occipital foramen and the spheno-occipital synchondrosis or its vestiges is a slight elevation, the pharyngeal tubercle, to which the pharyngeal raphe is attached. The rough depressed area on either side of this tubercle is the field of insertion of the longus capitis muscle; the rectus capitis anterior muscle inserts in a second, smaller posterior depression.

The lateral field of the posterior region of the cranial base is formed by the mastoid part of the temporal bone, with the mastoid process projecting inferiorly. A furrow medial to the mastoid process serves as the area of attachment of the posterior belly of the digastric muscle. A sharper and narrower furrow medial to the digastric groove contains the occipital artery.

In front of the mastoid area is the inferior surface of the petrosal part of the temporal bone to which the styloid process and tympanic bone are joined laterally. At the stylomastoid foramen, between the styloid and mastoid processes, opens the facial canal. Anterior and medial to the styloid process extends the sharp tympanic crest. Behind it and medial to the styloid process lies the jugular fossa; anteromedial to this depression is the entrance into the carotid canal. The carotid canal and jugular fossa are separated by a crest and, farther medially, by a triangular depression, the fossula petrosa. In the jugular fossa lies the superior bulb of the internal jugular vein; into the carotid canal enters the internal carotid artery. The fossula petrosa houses the superior ganglion of the glossopharyngeal nerve, which sends a fine branch, the tympanic nerve, into a small canal beginning in this fossa. Posterior and medial to this region the petro-occipital fissure is widened to the jugular foramen through which glossopharyngeal, vagus, and accessory nerves and the internal jugular vein pass. The nerves emerge through the anteromedial part and the vein through the wider posterolateral part of the jugular foramen. In front of the jugular foramen there is, in most skulls, a separate opening for the inferior petrosal sinus.

The external acoustic meatus is found in front of the mastoid process. In front of the tympanic crest extends the mandibular fossa; it is divided by the petrotympanic fissure into posterior and anterior halves. Only the latter is included in the craniomandibular articulation and extends anteriorly onto the articular tubercle. Lateral to the tubercle arises the zygomatic arch. It is formed, in its posterior part, by the temporal bone and, in its anterior part, by the zygomatic bone; it thus forms a link between the neurocranium and splanchnocranium.

In front of the articular eminence extends the roof of the infratemporal fossa formed by the inferior surfaces of the temporal squama and of the greater wing of the sphenoid bone. The infratemporal surface of the greater wing is bounded laterally by the infratemporal crest, a rough line at which the basal surface of the skull sharply bends into its lateral surface. Anteromedially the infratemporal plane reaches to the inferior orbital fissure, the communication of the infratemporal space with the orbit. Posteromedially the boundary is marked by the sphenopetrosal fissure, which widens medially at the apex of the pyramid into the foramen lacerum. This foramen and the sphenopetrosal fissure are closed in the living by the basal fibrocartilage, which is perforated only by the greater and lesser (superficial) petrosal nerves.

The posterior part of the greater wing, inserted between the squama and the pyramid of the temporal bone, juts inferiorly as the angular spine. In front of it is the narrow foramen spinosum for the passage of the middle meningeal artery; the foramen ovale, medial and anterior to the foramen spinosum, leads the mandibular nerve into the infratemporal space.

At the medial corner of the infratemporal plane the pterygoid process projects downward as a buttress of the upper jaw; its inferior end is attached to the maxillary skeleton. The two plates of the pterygoid process are separated posteriorly by the pterygoid fossa. The medial plate ends in the pterygoid hamulus, around which winds the tendon of the tensor palati muscle. The muscle arises, in part, from a small triangular fossa, the scaphoid fossa, right at the base of the pterygoid process, above the pterygoid fossa. The lateral pterygoid plate serves as the origin of lateral and medial pterygoid muscles. The root of the pterygoid process is perforated by the pterygoid canal.

Orbit

The eye socket, or orbit (Figs. 2-3 and 2-51), can be described as a slightly irregular, four-sided pyramid. Its base is the plane of the orbital opening, the axis is directed posteriorly and medially, and the apex is situated at the optic canal. The four sides of the pyramid are not sharply separated from each other, the line angles being slightly rounded.

The entrance to the orbit is bounded by the frontal, zygomatic, and maxillary bones. The frontal bone forms the upper boundary and the upper part of the medial and lateral boundaries. The superior border is blunt in its medial part and sharper in its greater lateral part. Between the medial third and middle third, the supraorbital rim is crossed by the supraorbital notch, which may be closed to a supraorbital foramen. At its lateral end the supraorbital rim extends onto the zygomatic process of the frontal bone and then continues into the anterior edge of the frontal process of the zygomatic bone, which forms the lateral boundary of the orbital entrance. Its inferior border is formed by the zygomatic bone in its lateral half and by the maxillary bone in its medial half. At the lower inner corner, the inferior border continues upward into the lacrimal crest of the frontal process of the maxillary bone.

The circumference of the orbital opening is not situated in one frontal plane. The upper border juts out anteriorly more than any of the other borders; the lateral border, on the other hand, is situated far more posteriorly than the others. The medial border is the least distinct. The peculiar behavior of the ridges bounding the orbital opening explains the fact that the eyeball is not equally protected against injury on all its sides. The best protection is afforded by the supraorbital ridge and the bridge of the nose, which protect the eye superiorly and medially. The protection from below is satisfactory. On the lateral side, however, where the walls recede, the eye is exposed to a high degree. This lack of protection of the outer surface is the price paid by man for the lateral extension of his visual field.

The roof of the orbit is, in its greater anterior part, formed by the orbital plate of the frontal bone. Only a small triangular area, close to the apex of the orbit, is formed by the inferior surface of the lesser wing of the sphenoid bone, which is perforated by the optic canal. The roof of the orbit is slightly concave in its posterior part and strongly concave in its anterior part. The deepest concavity at the anterolateral corner of the roof, the lacrimal fossa, is occupied by the lacrimal gland. At the anteromedial corner of the roof the pulley of the superior oblique muscle of the eyeball is fastened to a small depression or sometimes to a small spine, the trochlear fovea or trochlear spine.

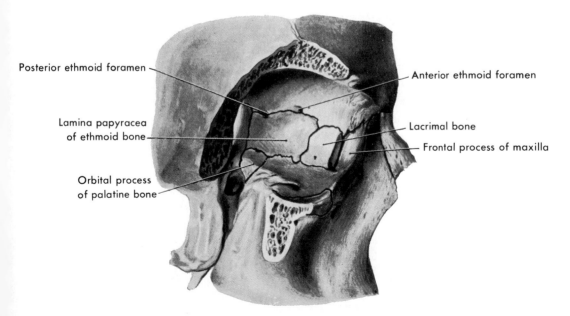

Fig. 2-51. Medial wall of the orbit. (Sicher and Tandler: Anatomie für Zahnärzte.)

The lateral wall of the orbit is almost flat. Two bones participate in its formation, the orbital surface of the greater wing of the sphenoid bone and, in front of it, the orbital surface of the frontal process of the zygomatic bone. The most posterior part of the lateral wall is separated from the roof by the superior orbital fissure. Through the wide medial part of the fissure pass the oculomotor, trochlear, and abducent nerves, the ophthalmic nerve, and the ophthalmic veins. The lateral wall of the orbit is separated from the floor by the inferior orbital fissure, which extends over half to two thirds of the length of the orbit, beginning just below the medial end of the superior orbital fissure. The inferior orbital fissure is almost entirely closed by connective tissue containing the smooth orbital muscle of Müller. Through the inferior orbital fissure pass the infraorbital nerve and artery, the zygomatic nerve, and, finally, a vein connecting the inferior ophthalmic vein with the pterygoid venous plexus. Close to the floor of the orbit, the zygomatic nerve enters the small zygomatic foramen to divide within the bone into its zygomaticofacial and zygomaticotemporal branches.

Zygomatic, maxillary, and palatine bones join in forming the floor of the orbit (Fig. 2-51). The palatine bone participates with a small triangular surface of its orbital process at the posterior corner of the floor. From this area the floor slopes gently anteriorly and, sometimes, laterally. Its major part is formed by the orbital surface of the maxilla and, in the region of the anterolateral corner, by the zygomatic bone. A groove starting from the infraorbital fissure runs anteriorly at the floor of the orbit; it houses the infraorbital nerve and vessels. Farther anteriorly the sulcus is roofed by a thin lamella of bone that gradually gains in thickness. Thus the infraorbital sulcus leads into the infraorbital canal, which then opens at the infraorbital foramen.

In order from the front backward, the medial orbital wall is formed by the maxilla, lacrimal bone, ethmoid bone, and sphenoid bone. The maxilla participates with a narrow posterior area of the frontal process behind the anterior lacrimal crest. Then follows the lacrimal bone. The lacrimal groove, between the two lacrimal crests on the frontal process of the maxilla and on the lacrimal bone itself, leads into the nasolacrimal canal. To the posterior border of the lacrimal bone is joined the rectangular lamina papyracea of the ethmoid bone. Between its upper border and the frontal bone are the anterior and posterior ethmoid foramina for the passage of the ethmoid nerves and vessels. The most posterior part of the medial orbital wall is contributed by the lesser wing and by part of the body of the sphenoid bone, just in front of and below the optic canal.

Temporal and infratemporal fossae

The *temporal fossa* (see Fig. 2-2) is a shallow depression on the lateral surface of the skull, bordered by the semicircular inferior temporal line. Its anterior and inferior part is deepest and has the sharpest boundary, formed by the concave temporal surface of the ascending, or frontal, process of the zygomatic bone. The floor of the fossa is formed by the parietal bone, the squama of the temporal bone, the temporal surface of the greater wing of the sphenoid bone, and the small temporal surface of the frontal bone behind its temporal line. The entire temporal fossa serves as the field of origin for the temporal muscle. It reaches downward to the level of the zygomatic arch laterally and to the infratemporal crest of the greater sphenoid wing medially.

The *infratemporal fossa* is an important compartment that lies immediately below the temporal fossa. It is bounded anteriorly by the posterolateral surface of the maxilla medial to its zygomatic process, which includes the maxillary tuberosity. Most of this wall is a thin partition between the fossa and the maxillary sinus. It ends above at the inferior orbital fissure and medially at the pterygomaxillary fissure. The medial boundary of the fossa is the lateral pterygoid plate anteriorly; there is no bony boundary posteriorly. The lateral wall is the ramus of the mandible. The roof of the fossa is the flat, horizontal part of the greater wing of the sphenoid bone and a small triangular portion of the temporal squama. The roof extends from the medial rim of the foramen ovale laterally to the infratemporal crest, which separates it sharply from the temporal fossa above. The roof is perforated by the foramen ovale immediately behind the root of the pterygoid process, by the foramen spinosum at the sphenoidal spine posterolateral to the above, and by the variable foramen of Vesalius, which transmits an emissary vein anteromedial to the foramen ovale (see Chapter 14 for the significance of emissary veins).

The most important structures contained in the infratemporal fossa are the pterygoid muscles, the (internal) maxillary artery, the pterygoid venous plexus, and the ramification of the mandibular nerve. The infratemporal fossa is accessible through the defects of its lateral skeletal wall. A needle can be inserted into the fossa either through the space between the anterior border of the mandibular ramus and maxillary tuber or through the opening between the zygomatic arch and mandibular (semilunar) notch.

The skeletal communications of the infratemporal fossa with other cavities of the skull are as follows: the inferior orbital fissure serves as the passage of the infraorbital nerve and artery and for the zygomatic nerve from the infratemporal space into the orbit. The mandibular nerve enters through the oval foramen; the middle meningeal artery reaches the cranial cavity from the infratemporal fossa through the foramen spinosum. Between the maxillary tuberosity and the anterior border of the pterygoid process the pterygomaxillary fissure connects the infratemporal fossa with the pterygopalatine fossa. The maxillary artery enters the pterygopalatine fossa through this gap to split into its terminal branches. The infraorbital and zygomatic nerves emerge from the fissure to cross the superomedial corner of the infratemporal fossa and enter the orbit through the inferior orbital fissure.

Pterygopalatine fossa

The pterygopalatine fossa (Fig. 2-52) is a narrow funnel-shaped space below the cranial base that is bounded anteriorly by the medial part of the maxillary tuberosity, posteriorly by the anterior or sphenomaxillary surface of the pterygoid process of the sphenoid bone, and medially by the lateral surface of the vertical plate of the palatine bone. Its roof is formed by the root of the greater sphenoid wing. A lateral boundary is

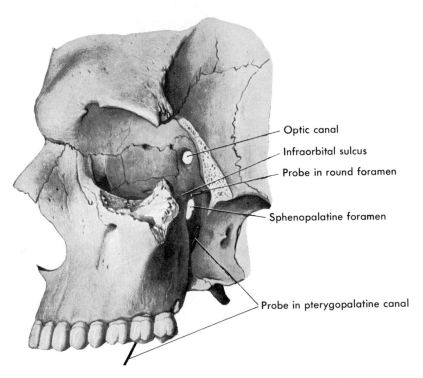

Fig. 2-52. Pterygopalatine fossa. (Sicher: Leitungsanästhesie.)

missing; here the pterygopalatine fossa communicates with the infratemporal fossa through the pterygomaxillary fissure.

The pterygopalatine space is widest in its upper part and narrows downward and continues into the pterygopalatine canal between the medial surface of the maxilla and the lateral surface of the vertical plate of the palatine bone. The canal opens into the oral cavity through the greater and lesser palatine foramina. The pterygopalatine fossa contains the ramification of the maxillary nerve, the terminal branches of the maxillary artery, and the pterygopalatine (sphenopalatine) ganglion.

The maxillary nerve enters the pterygopalatine fossa through the foramen rotundum. Below the opening of this canal and medial to it opens the pterygoid canal, leading the pterygoid or Vidian nerve to the pterygopalatine, or Meckel's ganglion. A pterygoid artery, one of the terminal branches of the internal maxillary artery, can be traced posteriorly into the Vidian canal. The palatine nerves and the descending palatine artery reach the oral cavity through the pterygopalatine canal. Through the sphenopalatine foramen between the orbital and sphenoid processes of the palatine bone and the inferior surface of the body of the sphenoid bone the pterygopalatine (sphenopalatine) nerves and artery pass into the nasal cavity.

Despite its deep location, the pterygopalatine fossa and thus the maxillary nerve are accessible for the injection of anesthetics. The pterygopalatine fossa can be reached by passing a needle through the infratemporal fossa and the pterygomaxillary hiatus. An alternative way into the space leads from the oral cavity through the greater palatine foramen and the pterygopalatine canal.

Nasal cavities

The nasal cavities are interposed between the cranial cavity above and the oral cavity below and between the orbits and maxillary sinuses on the right and left. They communicate with the outside through the anterior nasal or piriform aperture. The posterior nasal openings, the choanae, open into the pharyngeal space. The nasal cavities are separated by the nasal septum (see Fig. 2-55). The bony septum consists of the vertical plate of the ethmoid bone and of the vomer. The vertical or perpendicular ethmoid plate is continuous above with the cribriform plate. Its anterosuperior border is joined to the inner surface of the nasal bones, its posterior border to the crest of the sphenoid bone. Its posteroinferior border is in contact with the vomer; its anteroinferior border is free in the dry skull, but in the living it joins the septal cartilage. The alae of the vomer are in contact with the inferior surface of the sphenoid bone on either side of the sphenoid rostrum. The anterior border of the vomer descends anteriorly; its superoposterior half meets the perpendicular plate of the ethmoid bone; its inferoanterior half, forming an angle with the anteroinferior border of the perpendicular ethmoid plate, is connected to the cartilage of the nasal septum. The inferior border of the vomer rests on the nasal crest of the palatine and maxillary bones. The free posterior border of the vomer is smooth and slightly concave and marks the boundary between the right and the left choana.

The floor of the nasal cavity (see Fig. 2-60) is smooth and concave in transverse direction. Its greater anterior part is formed by the palatine process of the maxilla; its smaller posterior part is formed by the horizontal plate of the palatine bone. About 12 to 15 mm. from the anterior nasal spine, the nasal floor is perforated by the incisive, or nasopalatine, canal. It commences close to the septum and leads into the oral cavity where right and left canals open in a common opening, the anterior palatine, or incisive, fossa. From the nasal opening of this canal, remnants of the incisive suture can sometimes be traced laterally and anteriorly. The slightly elevated area in front of this sutural remnant is formed by the homologue of the premaxilla.

The roof of the nasal cavity is, at its highest middle part, formed by the cribriform plate of the ethmoid bone. Anteriorly the nasal part of the frontal bone and the concave inner surface of the nasal bones and posteriorly the body of the sphenoid bone form the sloping parts of the roof.

The lateral wall of the nasal cavity (Fig. 2-53) is occupied by the nasal conchae. The plates of the conchae are attached to the lateral nasal wall and project into the nasal cavity. The plates are vertical and slightly curved; their medial surface, directed toward the septum, is convex; their lateral surface is concave. The inferior concha is an independent bone; the middle and superior conchae and a variable supreme concha are parts of the ethmoid bone. The middle and superior conchae and superior and supreme concha are separated from each other only incompletely by fissures that start

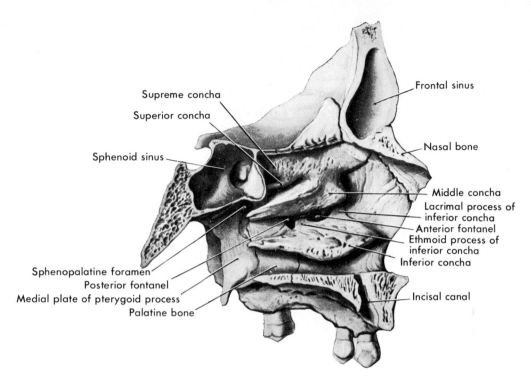

Fig. 2-53. Nasal cavity, left lateral wall. (Sicher and Tandler: Anatomie für Zahnärzte.)

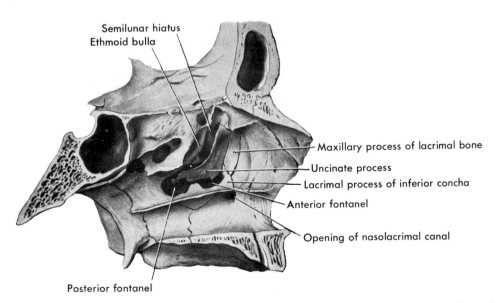

Fig. 2-54. Nasal cavity, left lateral wall after removal of lower and middle nasal concha. (Sicher and Tandler: Anatomie für Zahnärzte.)

at the posterior border of the conchal plate of the ethmoid bone. These fissures ascend anteriorly and end at some distance behind the anterior end of the plate. The space between the conchae and the nasal septum is the common nasal passage or meatus; the fissures between the lateral surface of each concha and the lateral wall of the nasal cavity are called the lower, middle, upper, and, if present, supreme nasal meatuses or passages. The nasal cavity extends upward and backward into the narrow space between the anterolateral surface of the sphenoid body and the ethmoid bone. This space is the sphenoethmoid recess, into which the sphenoid sinus opens.

Without removing the free parts of the conchae, only small parts of the lateral nasal wall are visible. The lowermost part of the lateral wall can be seen below the free end of the inferior concha and above the nasal floor. In front of the middle concha a variably large portion of the lateral nasal walls is formed by the frontal process of the maxilla. The space between the frontal process of the maxilla and septum, in front of the anterior end of the middle concha, is called the atrium of the middle nasal meatus.

Removing the free parts of the conchae (Fig. 2-54) exposes the region that, in the isolated maxilla, contains the hiatus of the maxillary sinus. This large irregular opening is, in the complete skull, narrowed considerably by thin processes of neighboring bones. The lower corner is closed by the maxillary process of the inferior concha, and the posterior corner is closed by the maxillary process of the vertical plate of the palatine bone. The remaining gap is divided into two openings by an oblique bridge formed by two processes crossing the opening, the ethmoid process of the inferior concha and the uncinate process of the ethmoid bone. In the living the two remaining openings are almost entirely closed by the fused mucous membranes of the nasal cavity and the maxillary sinus; they are termed anterior and posterior nasal fontanels. In the anterosuperior part of the posterior fontanel, and thus above the posterior end of the uncinate process, is the permanent communication of the nasal cavity with the maxillary sinus. It is situated at the inferoposterior end of the semilunar hiatus, a curved narrow sulcus between the uncinate process and the ethmoid bulla. Accessory openings of the maxillary sinus may be present and are located in the posterior area of the posterior fontanel in the middle meatus. The semilunar hiatus narrows anterosuperiorly to the infundibulum, which leads upward into the frontal sinus. Anterior ethmoid cells open into the hiatus, and middle cells open into the middle meatus above and behind the semilunar hiatus, whereas posterior ethmoid cells communicate with the superior or, if present, supreme nasal meatus.

In front of the uncinate process of the ethmoid bone, the nasal process of the lacrimal bone descends and joins the ascending lacrimal process of the inferior concha. These two processes close the nasolacrimal canal against the nasal cavity. The opening of the canal is found below the line of attachment of the inferior concha, that is, the inferior nasal meatus. By removing the entire labyrinth of the ethmoid bone, the medial surface of the lacrimal bone and the lamina papyracea, which separate nasal cavity and the ethmoid cells from the orbit, can be exposed.

The common anterior opening of the bony nasal cavities is the piriform aperture.

It is heart-shaped with the apex of the heart pointing upward. Its borders are formed by the free borders of the nasal bones and the anterior border of the maxilla. This border curves from the base of the frontal process outward and downward to return in a curve medially. The border terminates on a bony spine that forms half of the anterior nasal spine.

The posterior openings of the nasal cavities are the choanae. Each choana is an oval opening with the long axis extending vertically. The boundaries of each choana are as follows: below, the sharp concave posterior border of the horizontal plate of the palatine bone; medially, the posterior free border of the vomer; laterally, the medial plate of the pterygoid process of the sphenoid bone; above, the inferior surface of the body of the sphenoid bone, covered in part by the wing of the vomer medially and by the vaginal process of the pterygoid process laterally.

It has been pointed out that the skeletal housings for the organ complexes of the head completely surround the upper airway (see Chapter 1). For continuity in concept, it seems best to describe the nasal cavity and associated sinuses as the passageway seen in the living.

The external nose is supported not only by bony but also by cartilaginous skeletal parts. The root of the nose forms the boundary toward the forehead and is more or less deeply saddled. A straight nose, its bridge continuing from the forehead, was once the ideal of Greek sculptors. The bridge of the nose ends in the nasal apex. The lateral surfaces of the nose are separated from the cheeks at the nasal base; the movable area

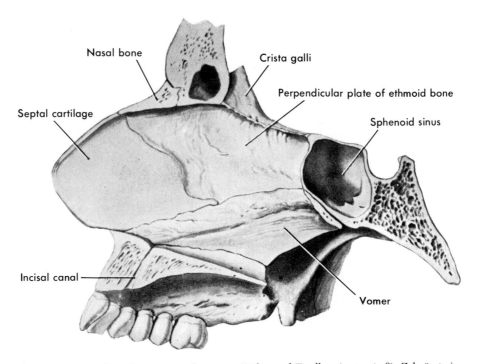

Fig. 2-55. Bony and cartilaginous nasal septum. (Sicher and Tandler: Anatomie für Zahnärzte.)

near the tip of the nose is known as the nasal wing, bounded against the superior parts by a superiorly convex groove. The free margin of the nasal wing borders the nostrils or nares, which are separated by the mobile part of the nasal septum.

One of the cartilages of the nasal skeleton completes the nasal septum; it is the roughly quadrilateral septal cartilage (Fig. 2-55), which fits into the angle between the perpendicular plate of the ethmoid bone and the vomer. The posterior corner of this cartilage extends upward and backward, reaching, in children, far between the perpendicular plate and the vomer but decreasing in size with advancing age. This projection of the septal cartilage is the sphenoid process. The lower border of the septal cartilage is free, and the inner parts of the alar cartilage are attached to it by connective tissue. The anterosuperior border of the septal cartilage, supporting the lower part of the nasal bridge, is often grooved in the midline (Fig. 2-57). From here the cartilage is bent backward on either side as if it were split, and it forms a triangular plate that is the skeleton on the lateral surface of the nose above the nasal wing. The upper border of the lateral cartilage (Figs. 2-56 and 2-57) joins the lower border of the nasal bone and the adjacent anterior border of the frontal process of the maxilla; the lower border is connected with the alar cartilage by the intervention of dense connective tissue.

The wing of the nose and the lowermost part of the nasal septum between the nostrils are supported by the paired major alar cartilages (Figs. 2-56 and 2-57). Each of these cartilages is formed like a C, the opening of which faces backward. The medial crus is narrow; the lateral crus is wide. The medial crus touches and partly extends below the lower border of the septal cartilage. It is movably connected to the septum and forms, together with that of the other side, the skeleton of the mobile part of the nasal septum.

The wide lateral crus of the alar cartilage is the skeleton of the nasal wing. The upper border is connected with the lateral nasal cartilage; the lower border is free but does not reach the border of the wing, which is formed by a double layer of skin only. The posterior border of the lateral crus of the alar cartilage does not reach the bone at the border of the piriform aperture but is connected with it by dense connective tissue, in which are embedded smaller irregular pieces of cartilage, the minor alar cartilages (Fig. 2-56).

At the lower border of the septum and immediately in front of the entrance to the incisal canal, an isolated small irregular cartilage lies underneath the mucous membrane. It is the vomeronasal cartilage, a vestige of the cartilaginous capsule of the rudimentary Jacobson's organ.

Examination of the nasal cavity in the living or on the cadaver shows that the region immediately above the nostrils, the nasal vestibule, is lined by a continuation of the skin. The keratinization of this part of the skin is slightly reduced; hairs (here called vibrissae) and sebaceous glands, however, are present in great numbers. In the adult male the hairs are long and strong. At the upper border of the vestibule, which coincides with the upper border of the nasal wing the alar cartilage bulges slightly into the interior. The bulge is known as limen nasi, the threshold of the nose. Above and

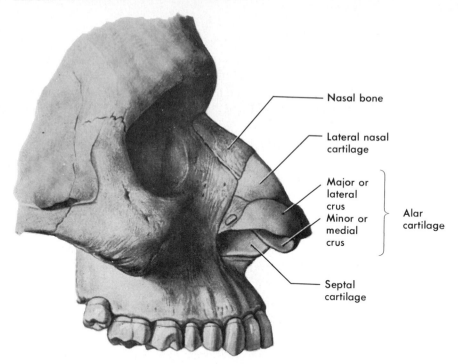

Fig. 2-56. Cartilaginous skeleton of outer nose, lateral view. (Sicher and Tandler: Anatomie für Zahnärzte.)

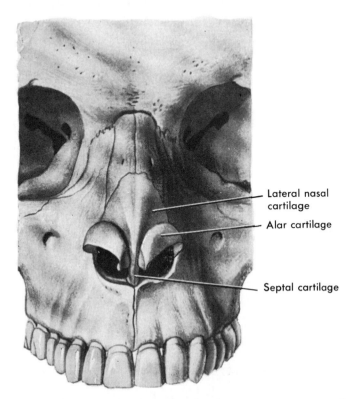

Fig. 2-57. Cartilaginous skeleton of outer nose, anterior view. (Sicher and Tandler: Anatomie für Zahnärzte.)

behind it commences the mucous membrane of the nasal cavity. The transition between the cutaneous and mucous lining is gradual.

The mucous membrane of the nasal cavity can be differentiated into the "convex" and "concave" mucosa. The mucosa at the convexities of the conchae is thick and richly vascularized; the veins, especially, form dense networks that often have been compared with a cavernous erectile body. In addition the "convex" mucosa is connected with the periosteum by a rather thick submucous layer in which numerous glands are embedded. In contrast to the convex mucosa, the mucosa that covers the concave areas of the nasal cavity is thinner and contains few glands and blood vessels; its lamina propria is fused with the periosteum to one layer of connective tissue. The mucous membrane covering the nasal septum is intermediate between the extreme types of convex and concave mucosa.

The glands of the nasal cavity are, for the greatest part, mucous glands; only in a rather small area of the superior concha and the opposite part of the septum, that is, in the olfactory area, are found the olfactory glands of Bowman, which probably elaborate a specific secretion. The mucous glands are especially numerous at the convexity of the conchae and on the agger nasi, a small bulge on the lateral nasal wall in front of the attachment of the middle concha. On the septum opposite the anterior end of the middle concha, aggregated glands cause a small protrusion, the septal tubercle of Zuckerkandl.

The shape of the nasal cavity in the living conforms generally to that of the skeleton, with the three conchae projecting from the lateral wall and the three nasal passages below and lateral to each concha (Fig. 2-58). Sometimes a fourth supreme concha and a corresponding passage are present. The common space between conchae and septum continues behind the conchae as the nasopharyngeal meatus and opens at the choana into the pharynx. In normal breathing most of the air passes through the lower part of the common nasal passage between the conchae and septum and through the lower meatus. Only in forced inspiration does the air penetrate into and pass through the upper regions of the nasal cavity and then come into direct contact with the olfactory area close to the roof.

On the lateral wall the anterior and posterior nasal fontanels of the skeleton are closed in the living by the fusion of the mucous membrane of the nasal cavity with that of the maxillary sinus. Defects of this closing membrane are frequent, generally situated in the region of the posterior fontanel. These defects form the accessory openings of the maxillary sinus. After removing the middle concha, the semilunar hiatus is exposed, situated between the roundly protruding ethmoid bulla above and the sharp border of the uncinate process below. The semilunar hiatus leads upward and forward into the infundibulum and through it into the frontal sinus. The maxillary sinus opens at the posteroinferior end of the semilunar hiatus.

If one removes the inferior concha, one can observe the nasal opening of the nasolacrimal duct. Because of the oblique course of the duct through the mucous membrane, the opening is slitlike and flanked anteriorly and superiorly by a fold of the mucous membrane, often described as Hasner's valve.

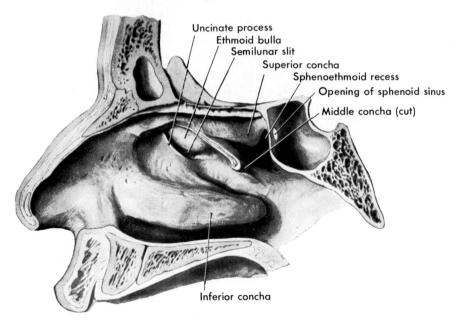

Fig. 2-58. Right lateral nasal wall after removal of middle nasal concha. (Sicher and Tandler: Anatomie für Zahnärzte.)

The posterior end of the nasal cavity is sometimes marked by a shallow and insignificant groove on its lateral wall behind the posterior end of the middle and lower conchae. This groove is the posterior sulcus, which runs obliquely downward and backward.

Paranasal sinuses

The paranasal sinuses are pneumatic (air-filled) cavities that are restricted to the skull in man. They are lined by respiratory mucous membrane continuous with that of the nasal cavity. They can be considered the "spaces between the braces," the braces being the pillars and plates that underlie the basic stress-bearing design of the skeleton of the head (see the section on architectural analysis of the skull in this chapter). They develop and expand as invagination of the nasal mucosa follows the outward growth of the facial bones and the eruption of teeth. This invagination is brought about by resorption of bone on inner surfaces, apposition on outer surfaces, and remodeling to accommodate the biomechanical stresses of adult masticatory function. Thus in the human skull the sinuses are in immediate connection with the nasal cavity as are the cavities of the middle ear in immediate connection with the nasopharynx via the auditory tube.

The sphenoid sinuses, the frontal sinuses, the ethmoid cells, and the maxillary sinuses are listed as paranasal sinuses. The lining of all these cavities is a thin membrane, a fusion of the periosteum and the mucous membrane, sometimes called a mucoperiosteum. The membrane is inelastic, poor in glands and blood vessels, and covered by a ciliated, pseudostratified columnar epithelium, the typical respiratory epithelium. The glands are, as a rule, somewhat more numerous in the neighborhood of the opening, by which the pneumatic sinuses communicate with the nasal cavity.

Sphenoid sinus. The sphenoid sinus (Fig. 2-58) is, as a rule, a slightly irregular, cube-shaped space. It starts its development from the sphenoethmoid recess into which it opens with a round ostium 2 to 3 mm. in diameter. Right and left sphenoid sinuses are separated by a septum that is only rarely situated in the midplane. The deviation of the septum is caused by the asymmetrical enlargement of the two sinuses. If the sphenoid sinus is of average size, it extends posteriorly to the anterior border of the sella turcica. If it is large, it extends posteriorly below the hypophyseal fossa, which then bulges into the sinus as a transverse prominence. Sometimes a posterior extension of the sinus may even hollow out the anterior part of the occipital bone. Laterally the sinus may gradually invade the root of the lesser and greater wings of the sphenoid bone; downward it may extend into the pterygoid process. In such cases of extreme development the sphenoid sinus comes into close relation to the optic canal, the foramen rotundum, and the pterygoid canal; these canals may protrude to a variable degree into the lumen of the sinus. The optic nerve, the ophthalmic nerve (second division of the trigeminal nerve), and the pterygoid nerve may in such cases be involved in infections of the sphenoid sinus.

Frontal sinus. The frontal sinus, which commences its development from the anterosuperior end of the infundibulum, is at first situated in the medial part of the superciliary arch. The prominence of the superciliary arch, however, is not exactly correlated to the size of the sinus. If the frontal sinus enlarges, it extends upward and laterally between inner and outer plates of the frontal bone. In extreme cases the sinus may develop an extension into the anterior parts of the orbital roof. The septum between right and left frontal sinus is, like the sphenoid septum, almost always asymmetrically placed. The walls of the frontal sinus are rarely smooth; sickle-shaped crests of the bone persist, especially at its upper wall. The main cavity, therefore, extends into incompletely separated recesses.

Ethmoid cells. The ethmoid cells are variable in their number, shape, and size. Diagrammatically an anterior, middle, and posterior group can be differentiated. The anterior cells open into the infundibulum and the semilunar hiatus; the middle cells communicate directly with the middle nasal meatus above the bulla; the posterior cells open into the superior, and into the supreme nasal passage, if it is present.

In describing the ethmoid bone, it was mentioned that many of the ethmoid cells are not contained entirely in the ethmoid bone itself. Instead, the walls of some of these cells are completed by the neighboring bones. In other words, the ethmoid cells extend into the bones that join the ethmoid bone. The upper cells thus extend into the frontal bone; posterior cells may extend into the sphenoid bone and the palatine bone; inferior cells may extend into the maxilla; anterior cells are closed by the lacrimal bone.

In abnormal cases ethmoid cells extending into neighboring bones may enlarge to

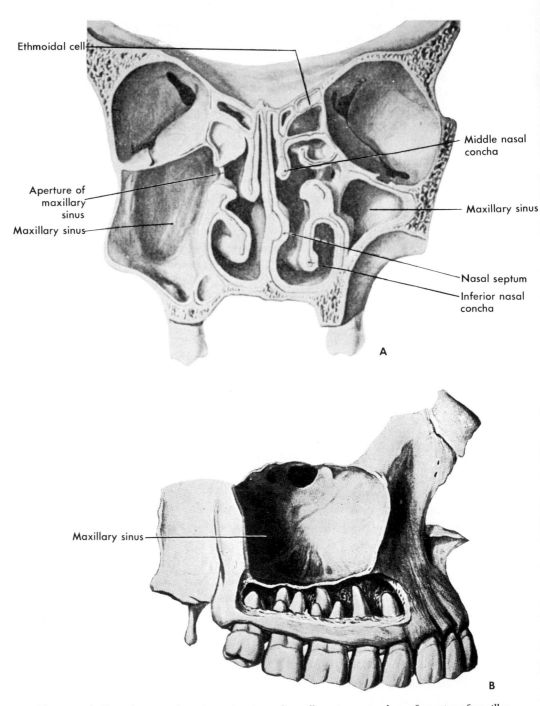

Fig. 2-59. A, Frontal section through nasal cavity and maxillary sinuses in plane of opening of maxillary sinus into nasal cavity. Note conspicuous asymmetry of right and left maxillary sinuses. B, Relations of a large maxillary sinus to maxillary teeth. (Sicher and Tandler.)

become wide cavities. If an anterosuperior cell extends into the frontal bone, it imitates a second frontal sinus. A "doubling" of the sinus can also occur in the maxilla and has been observed, although rarely, in the sphenoid bone. In these cases of double frontal, maxillary, or sphenoid sinus, the typical sinus can always be recognized by the typical location of its communication with the nasal cavity although the size of the sinus in such cases may be greatly reduced. The "second" sinus can always be recognized as an abnormally enlarged ethmoid cell. Cases are known in which the frontal sinus was entirely replaced by an expanded anterior ethmoid cell.

Maxillary sinus. The maxillary sinus, or antrum, is the largest of the paranasal sinuses and normally occupies the entire body of the maxilla. Structurally the sinus is described as a three-sided pyramid (Fig. 2-59), the base of which is the vertical lateral nasal wall and the apex of which extends into the zygomatic process of the maxilla. The three sides of the pyramid face upward, backward, and forward. The upper wall, the roof of the maxillary sinus, is at the same time the floor of the orbit. The posterior wall bulges as the maxillary tuber; the anterior wall is depressed by the canine fossa.

The maxillary sinus opens into the posteroinferior end of the semilunar hiatus. The opening is situated close to the roof of the sinus (Fig. 2-59) and is, therefore, unfavorable for drainage of the sinus. The location of the ostium of the maxillary sinus has little to do with the upright posture of man. Its position can be explained by the fact that at the time when the development of the maxillary sinus commences, the greater inferior part of the body of the maxilla is occupied by the germs of the deciduous teeth so that the pneumatization of the maxilla necessarily starts in its uppermost part immediately below the orbital floor. While the maxilla grows and the teeth move downward, the sinus expands inferiorly, but the site of the first appearance of the sinus persists as the communication with the nasal cavity. An accessory ostium in the middle nasal meatus is slightly more favorably situated for drainage of the sinus, but it is not far below the level of the normal opening.

The medial wall of the maxillary sinus, separating it from the nasal cavity, is generally slightly convex toward the sinus (Fig. 2-60). This wall is not entirely formed by bone but consists of a double layer of mucous membrane in the region of the anterior and posterior fontanels (Figs. 2-53 and 2-54,) in front of and behind the uncinate process. The roof of the sinus is flat and slopes slightly anteriorly and laterally. The posterior wall bulges posteriorly toward the infratemporal fossa. The anterior wall, depressed by the canine fossa on the anterior surface of the maxilla, is convex toward the interior of the sinus. The depth of the canine fossa and the size of the maxillary sinus are in inverse proportion. Sickle-shaped bony crests frequently arise on the floor of the maxillary sinus (Fig. 2-60, *B*) and may extend to a variable height on its lateral wall. The crests partition the lower part of the sinus into several niches. The presence of such "septa" may interfere with the easy removal of a root that has been dislocated into the sinus. If the maxillary sinus is of average size, its floor is at the level of the nasal floor or slightly below it.

The size and shape of the maxillary sinus vary considerably. Expansion of the sinus leads first to a thinning of its walls and later to the development of smaller or larger recesses. The smallest of these extensions is found at the posterosuperior corner, where it may invade the orbital process of the palatine bone.

Expanding laterally, the maxillary sinus may hollow out the entire zygomatic process of the maxilla and may even extend into the zygomatic bone. Where roof and

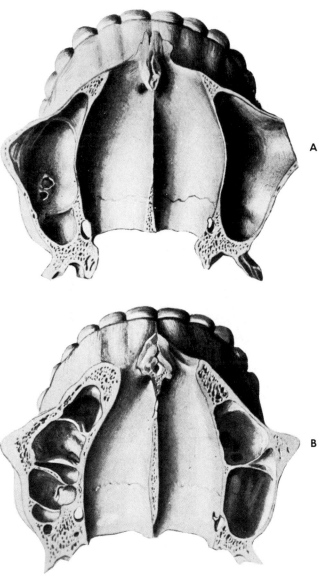

Fig. 2-60. Horizontal sections through facial skeleton above nasal floor. **A,** Apices of left second molar are exposed at floor of sinus. **B,** Sickle-shaped bony partitions of alveolar recess of sinus. Note also the three cross sections through pillars of upper facial skeleton. (Sicher and Tandler: Anatomie für Zahnärzte.)

anterior wall of the sinus meet, the enlargement of the sinus extends into the infraorbital rim. Then the infraorbital canal, which normally slightly protrudes into the sinus, may be more or less isolated from the roof of the sinus (see Fig. 11-9, A). Extension of the sinus medially and anteriorly leads to an increasing prominence of the nasolacrimal duct into the sinus.

An inferior extension of the sinus into the base of the alveolar process is of special practical significance, because it establishes more intimate relations of the sinus with the maxillary teeth. In extreme cases the sinus even extends into the alveolar process between the roots of the teeth so that their sockets protrude into the cavity. The bony floor of the sinus may even become defective above the apices of the roots (Fig. 2-60, A). The periapical tissue of a root is then in direct contact with the lining membrane of the sinus (p. 440). The implications of the intimate relation between sinus and teeth are self-evident.

An extension of the sinus may also remove the inner walls of the narrow canals containing the alveolar nerves in the posterior and anterior walls of the sinus. Then the alveolar nerves are no longer separated from the sinus by bone but are, for some distance, in direct contact with the mucoperiosteal lining of the sinus. Even the wall of the infraorbital canal may become dehiscent so that an involvement of the infraorbital nerve during a sinus infection is possible. The maxillary sinus is sometimes considerably narrowed (Fig. 2-59, A). The most common corollary of a reduction of the size of the maxillary sinus is an abnormal depth of the canine fossa. It seems that in such skulls, the removal of the mechanically nonfunctional bone of the maxillary body progressed faster than normal by resorption from the outer surface in "competition" with the removal of bone by the expanding sinus from within.

In other individuals the lateral wall of the nasal cavity bulges more than normal toward the maxillary sinus so that the width of the nasal cavity increases at the expense of the maxillary sinus. A third reason for smallness of the maxillary sinus is a

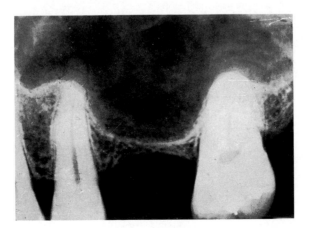

Fig. 2-61. Radiograph of upper jaw; maxillary sinus expanded toward alveolar crest after loss of first molar. (Orban: Oral histology and embryology.)

failure of the formation of the alveolar recess of the sinus. In these cases the floor of the sinus is at a higher level than that of the nasal cavity.

The maxillary sinuses are frequently asymmetrical (Fig. 2-59, A). Cases are known of extreme size of the sinus on one side and severe reduction of the sinus on the other.

After loss of teeth, the maxillary sinus may expand into the part of the alveolar process that, by the loss of a tooth, has lost some of its mechanical function (Fig. 2-61). Recesses of the sinus may then reach far downward between the remaining teeth, and the floor of such an extension of the main cavity of the sinus may be thin. Such extensions of the sinus are explained by the fact that they develop as "replacements" of functionless bone.

Oral cavity

The oral cavity is only incompletely bounded by bones. Its lateral and anterior walls are formed by the inner surface of the alveolar processes, which join at the midline. The lingual surfaces of the teeth complete these walls. Of the inner surface of the mandible, the area above the mylohyoid line also participates in bounding the oral cavity.

In the anterior region the transition between the roof of the bony oral cavity and alveolar process is gradual, whereas the alveolar process and hard palate join at almost right angles in the molar region.

The roof of the oral cavity (Fig. 2-62) is formed by the hard or bony palate, consisting of the palatine processes of the maxillae and the horizontal plates of the palatine bones. These four bony parts are joined together in a cross-shaped suture. Between the bones of the right and left halves of the hard palate extends the median palatine suture, and between maxillae and palatine bones extends the transverse

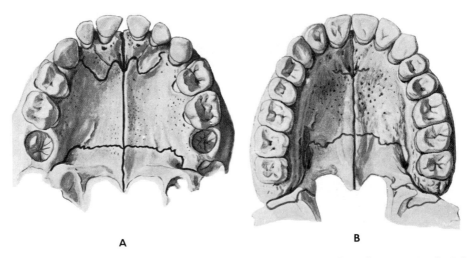

A   B

Fig. 2-62. Palatine sutures. **A,** In 5-year-old child. **B,** In adult. (Sicher and Tandler: Anatomie für Zahnärzte.)

palatine suture. The posterior border of the hard palate is a doubly curved line, concave posteriorly; in the midline projects the posterior nasal spine.

The incisive fossa, or anterior palatine foramen, opens in the midline, behind and between the upper central incisors. It is the common opening of the two incisive canals. It contains the nasopalatine nerves and arteries and the variable vestiges of the epithelial nasopalatine ducts or Stensen's organs. Close to the posterior border of the hard palate and in the furrow between the alveolar process and hard palate opens the pterygopalatine canal. Its opening is the greater palatine foramen through which palatine nerves and the descending palatine artery emerge. The bone behind the greater palatine foramen is often elevated to the sharp palatine crest, which flattens out medially. Behind this crest one or two small side branches of the pterygopalatine canal open through the lesser palatine foramina. They contain branches of the palatine nerves for the soft palate and tonsil. The hard palate is often elevated along the midline to a variably high and variably wide bony prominence, the palatine torus. The remnants of the incisive suture (Fig. 2-62, A) can be followed in young persons from the incisive foramen to the interstice between the lateral incisor and canine, or to the alveolus of the canine itself. The bone in front of the suture corresponds to the palatine process of the premaxilla.

ARCHITECTURAL ANALYSIS OF THE SKULL

General plan

The skull is a stress-bearing construct. Whether an animal punctures, shears, or chews its food, considerable and complicated forces are generated. The common engineering solution to the resistance of force is manifest in the design of "frames and trusses." The basic frame is a triangle, a form in two dimensions. Three members (bars) with joints at their angles resist distortion of the triangle from forces applied in any direction in the same two-dimensional plane. Increase in the number of members weakens the frame; a rectangle so jointed collapses when similar angular force is applied (Fig. 2-65). The basic truss is a tetrahedron (three-sided pyramid), which is simply four triangles (base included), a form in three dimensions. It resists distortion from forces applied in any direction in three planes of space. Increase in number of members weakens the truss; a cube collapses when similar angular force is applied.

The structural strategy of the skull is a biologic compromise that accommodates multiple competing functional demands. Most evident are the protective housings for the brain and each of the functionally oriented special sense organs, the separate corridors for the airway and foodway, and the variety of entrances and exits for arteries, veins, and nerves. In addition, the masticatory system is deeply rooted within this assemblage. Though its force-resisting triangles and tetrahedrons may be somewhat warped to bypass obstructing organs, the trusswork can be readily traced throughout the skull as pillars of reinforced bone (Figs. 2-63 to 2-65).

In frontal view several frames can be clearly outlined (Fig. 2-63). A central triangle dominates the facial skeleton. Its sides are formed by canine buttresses, which begin at the anterior corners of the dentition and run up between nasal and orbital spaces to meet at the glabella, bulging in the midline of the frontal bone. This, in turn, is backed by the vertical temporal squama. The base of the central triangle is formed by the thickened anterior strip across the palate between the canines. A large inverted triangle can be traced on each side of this central frame. Its medial side is the canine buttress in common with the central frame. Its lateral side diverges as the zygomatic process of the maxilla, which is continuous upward through the reinforced middle strip of the zygomatic bone to meet the frontal bone at its zygomatic process. The base of this inverted triangle is the bulky superciliary bar, which forms the upper margin of

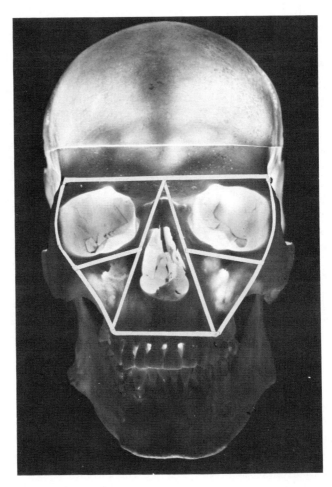

Fig. 2-63. Dissecting with light, frontal view. Light inside skull reveals buttressing. Note triangular arrangement of cranial buttresses, drawn in white outlines.

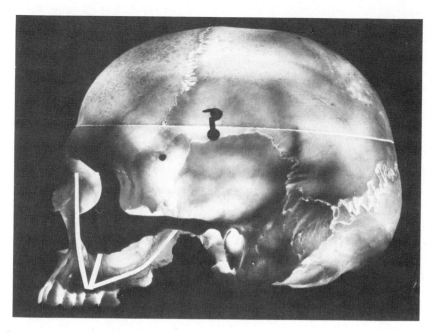

Fig. 2-64. Dissecting with light, lateral view. White outlines indicate pyramidal arrangement: canine buttress, anterior; zygomatic buttress, lateral; pterygoid buttress, posterior. Note zygomatic arch joining facial buttressing with base of skull.

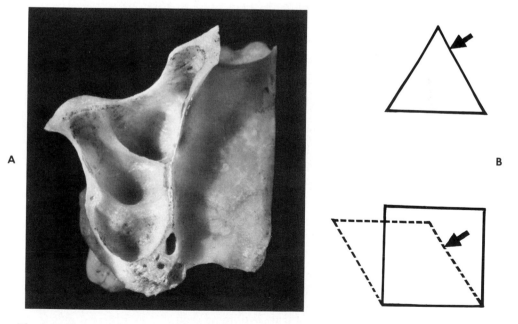

A

B

Fig. 2-65. Frames and trusses. **A,** Horizontal section of left maxilla exposes triangular arrangement with canine buttress above, zygomatic buttress at left, and maxillary tuberosity junction with pterygoid buttress below; flat plane of nasal floor at right. **B,** Triangle with arms riveted at angles; force *(arrow)* cannot distort triangle; square collapses as arms turn on rivets with similar force applied.

the orbit. A shorter triangle can be seen fitted within the greater frame. Its sides are the same below, but its base cuts it short at the thickened lower margin of the orbit (Fig. 2-63). Now it can be seen that this trusswork already meets several of the essential requirements specified previously. It frames nasal, orbital, and sinus spaces while providing an optimal force-resisting framework for masticatory stress.

In the lateral view this functional plan can be followed in depth (Fig. 2-64). Canine and zygomatic buttresses can be seen diverging from the dentition. Posteriorly the bulbous maxillary tuberosity can be seen, strongly braced by the pterygoid process, which takes up the force on the posterior dentition like a flying buttress diverging upward to the cranial base.

The plan of this three-dimensional trusswork is convincingly demonstrated in a horizontal section of the maxilla (Fig. 2-65). A three-sided pyramid (tetrahedron) cut in half yields a triangular plane which, in the maxilla, is reinforced as a bony pillar at each angle; these are the canine buttress, the zygomatic buttress, and the maxillary tuberosity, which butts against the pterygoid buttress. Between these buttresses the bone is thin and forms the walls of the various cavities.

The mandible completes the framework of the skull. It contributes the movable part of a complicated lever system. To meet this function it is designed as a strong central bar, like the shaft of a long bone, running forward in a continuous curve from condyle to condyle. The bar is reinforced at its midline symphysis by the bulging chin, which resists the squeezing action of the lateral pterygoids at the condylar ends of the horseshoe-shaped curve. This central bar supports three processes. Thus two thinner plates are pinched off above and below for the attachment of masticatory muscles. The temporalis inserts on the coronoid process, which is reinforced by the narrow temporal crest; the masseter and the medial pterygoids insert on the mandibular angle, which is a slightly thicker plate since it must resist the pull of two muscles. The alveolar process for the attachment of the dental arch is a continuous process pulled up from the bar with the eruption of teeth.

This basic framework of the mandible is unmistakably demonstrated in the senile jaw (see Chapter 17; Figs. 17-1, 17-3, and 17-4). With the loss of teeth the alveolar process disappears. Since masticatory function is thus severely reduced, the masticatory muscles atrophy from disuse. This is accompanied by extensive resorption of their mandibular insertions. Coronoid and angular plates recede, and little but the central bar of bone remains.

Internal construction

Bone tissue is both resistant and resilient. It is thus well adapted to withstand all the kinds of stress—that is, pressure, tension, and shear—generated by the living, vigorous animal. But bone is also remarkably plastic. It grows and is continuously remodeled during life by the sculpturing activity of deposition and resorption along the bone surfaces. In the direction and control of growth, the bony surfaces are augmented by precisely placed cartilaginous (epiphyseal) plates, such as those near the ends of long bones and between the bones at the base of the skull. Sutures between bones further increase the workable surfaces in the cranium. They join bones by fibrous connective tissue and are therefore tension bearing.

Individual bones provide the mechanical units of the skeleton. They have evolved by the natural selection of adaptive engineering, which has produced both the stabilizing framework of the vertebrate body and the lever systems for its complex movements. Thus most bones are designed with a dense outer casing of compact or cortical bone housing an inner meshwork of trabecular, spongy, or cancellous bone. Exceptions are found where bones are so thin that only a compact plate is possible, as in certain bones of the skull.

Compact bone is rigorously organized. It is composed of bony lamellae (layers) lying parallel on the surface. They overlie deeper tubular constructs of concentric lamellae surrounding longitudinal central canals like alternating plywood layers. These structures, called Haversian systems or osteones, run side by side and are oriented along lines of force transmission. Such a cylinder resists bending in any direction and, since it is hollow in its central axis where pressure and tension from bending are neutralized, it is also provided with a protected channel for its vascularization (Fig. 2-66). Even in areas where distinct osteones cannot be traced because of local remodeling or filling in of interstices between incongruent osteone surfaces, or where bone is too thin, etc., the pattern of bony strips adhere to lines of force transmission called trajectories.

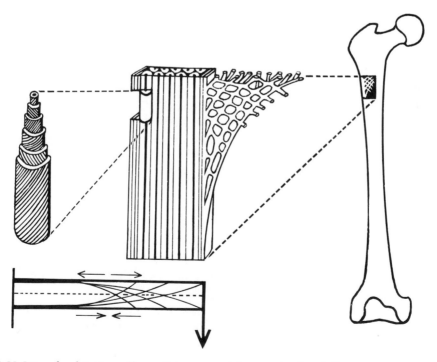

Fig. 2-66. Internal architecture of bone. Note osteone, left; cortical and medullary bone, center; a bone, right; arched force trajectories on loaded beam, below.

Spongy bone projects this stress-bearing organization into the interior of the bone. Here it dissipates the stress transferred to it by the osteones, or carries loads to the osteones from stresses at the joints. Its trabeculae (little beams) spring from the inner cortical layers like the flying buttresses of Gothic cathedrals to span the medullary spaces to opposite sides (Fig. 2-66). These struts and braces are continuous with the osteones, and the pattern of their trajectories traces the dispersion of the stresses.

In the maxilla the rodlike structures converge from local areas of masticatory stress to concentrate in the pillars that form the trusses that characterize the facial skeleton (Fig. 2-63).

In the mandible, where the form is comparable to that of a long bone, the arrangement is dramatically displayed (Fig. 2-67). The trabecular pattern is remarkably similar to that of the femur. The head of the femur is offset from the axis of the bone, and the trabeculae cross in arches springing from the thick cortical shaft of the bone to opposite surfaces of the articular surfaces of the femoral head. In this way the pressure of the body weight is directly supported by trabeculae, and pressure from the gluteal muscles, etc., which pull transversely into the pelvis is similarly supported (Fig. 2-67). The head of the mandible faces upward and forward, offset on the bent mandibular neck. Its trabeculae can be seen to cross in arches springing from cortical bone in exactly the same pattern as that of the femur (Fig. 2-67). A transverse section of the femoral condyles, where the articular surfaces are not offset, shows the trabecular struts running straight to the articular surface, and they are braced by transverse trabecular ties (Fig. 2-67). Similarly, a transverse section of the mandibular condyle is supported by parallel vertical struts and cross ties (Fig. 2-67). Both articular surfaces are obviously pressure bearing and thus are identically structured.

The mandible resists bending forces with its strong, compact layer. The compact shell is filled with cancellous bone, forming and surrounding the sockets of the teeth. The masticatory pressure exerted on the teeth is transmitted as tension on the alveolar bone proper, or cribriform plate, through the bundles of the periodontal ligament. The alveolar bone proper tends to sink into the mandible if the tooth is under pressure; this tendency is counteracted by the spongy bone around the alveolar bone proper. These trabeculae arise on the outer surface of the alveolar bone proper. Some connect the sockets of two adjacent teeth and may be horizontal and regular or irregular. Others are arranged in an approximately cone-shaped field and end mainly on the compact alveolar plates. Because of their specific function, the spongy trabeculae and the compact alveolar plates are designated as supporting bone of the alveolar process.

Some of the spongy trabeculae surrounding the apical part of the sockets unite as a trajectory that runs backward below the sockets and then diagonally upward and backward through the ramus to end in the condyle (Fig. 2-68). In this way the masticatory pressure is finally transmitted to the base of the skull over the craniomandibular articulation. This most important trajectory of the mandible, the dental trajectory, bulges on the inner surface of the ramus as a blunt crest, the crest or ridge of the mandibular neck.

Other trajectories of the mandible are formed in response to the forces exerted by the muscles of mastication. One is found in the region of the mandibular angle; another begins at the tip of the coronoid process and fans out into the mandibular body. Between these trajectories there is a region of the mandible, above and in front of the angle, where the cancellous bone is relatively free of stresses. In this region the trabeculae of the spongy bone are thin and the marrow spaces wide, a fact that can also be verified by studying roentgenograms.

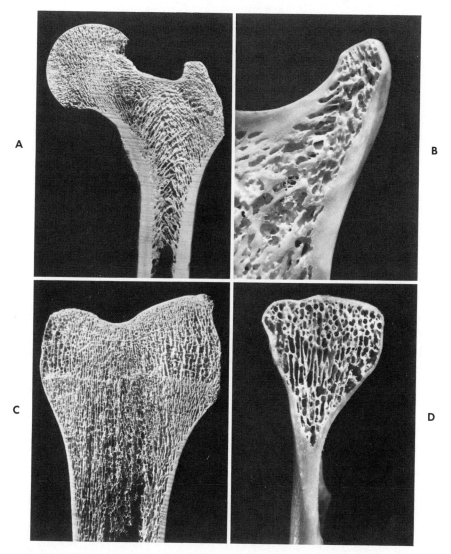

Fig. 2-67. Joint adaptations for pressure bearing. **A,** Frontal section of head of femur. Note gothic archlike crossing of trabecular struts from cortical bone below to articular surface above. **B,** Sagittal section of head of mandible. Note similar archlike crossing of trabeculae from cortical bone below to articular surface above. **C,** Frontal section of femoral condyles. Note vertical trabecular struts to articular surface braced by cross ties. **D,** Frontal section of mandibular condyle. Note similar vertical struts braced by cross ties.

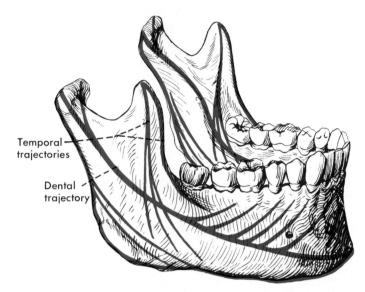

Fig. 2-68. Trajectories of the mandible. (Modified from Sicher and Tandler: Anatomie für Zahnärzte.)

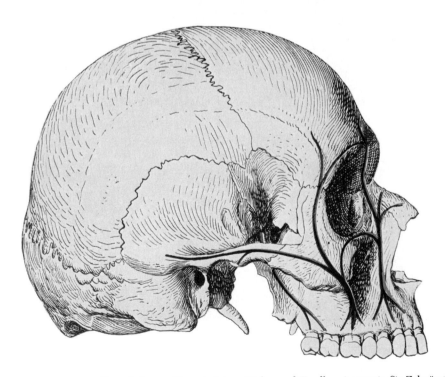

Fig. 2-69. Supporting pillars of the maxillary skeleton. (Sicher and Tandler: Anatomie für Zahnärzte.)

The region of the chin is especially endangered if bending forces act on the mandibular body. Forceful forward thrust of the mandible causes a measurable deformation, namely, a contraction of the mandible by the inward pulling component of the two lateral pterygoid muscles. In response to these forces the region of the chin is strengthened not only by the rather massive compacta of the mental protuberance, but also by trajectories of the spongiosa. These tracts of trabeculae cross each other at right angles, running from the right lower border of the chin upward to the left into the alveolar process and vice versa.

The upper jaw and the skeleton of the upper face form, biologically and mechanically, a unit anchored to the base of the skull. On each side of the skull are three vertical pillars that have already been described. All of them arise in the basal part of the alveolar process, and all of them abut to the base of the cranium (Fig. 2-69).

Seen in basal view, the connection between the posterior end of the horizontal arm of the zygomatic pillar and the upper end of the pterygoid pillar is a thickened reinforcement of the bone in front of the foramen ovale connecting the articular eminence with the root of the pterygoid process (see Fig. 2-50). The hard palate connects the system of pillars of one side to that of the other side and thereby forms a vaulted supporting arch between the bases of the right and left alveolar processes.

SEX DIFFERENCES OF THE SKULL

Sex differences of the skull are referable mainly to the average weakness of the musculature in the female skull. Pronounced in the great apes and perhaps in extinct and primitive races of man, the differences in the development of musculature between male and female skulls are greatly reduced in recent races of man. This is the reason that the diagnosis of sex is dubious or even impossible in a certain small number of modern human skulls.

Reduced to a simple statement it can be said that the female skull is characterized by a weaker development of its superstructures (Figs. 2-70 and 2-71). All bony ridges, crests, and processes are smaller and smoother in the female skull than in the male skull. This is especially true for the temporal line, mastoid process, nuchal lines, external occipital protuberance, and the modeling of the mandibular angle. Also, in the woman the superciliary arches or ridges are developed to a much lesser degree and sometimes are even entirely missing. Roughness and irregularity of the lower border of the zygomatic bone, at the origin of the masseter muscle, are strongly characteristic of the male skull, but smoothness of this region does not by itself allow the diagnosis of the skull as female.

The lack or the weaker development of frontal and occipital superstructures also causes a fairly characteristic difference in the profile of the female and the male cranium. In the male skull (Fig. 2-71) the contour, if followed from the root of the nose upward and backward and then downward to the occipital protuberance, forms a fairly smooth and even curve, which is interrupted only by inconstant depressions behind the coronal suture and above the occipital bone. The contour in the female skull (Fig. 2-70) is more angular. The forehead ascends more steeply than in the male

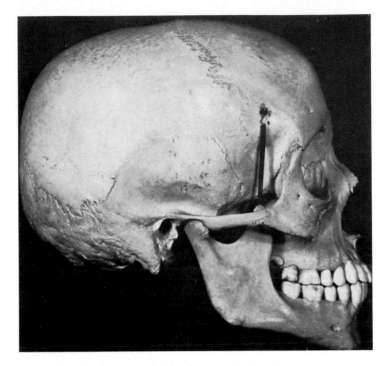

Fig. 2-70. Young adult female skull, lateral aspect.

skull, and the profile line then turns more sharply into the horizontal. In the occipital region a similar more abrupt change of the curve into the vertical direction can be observed. This outline of the female skull, caused by the weakness of cranial super-structures, is, therefore, more closely similar to the outline of the skull of a child (Fig. 2-72) than is that of the male skull, in which the reinforcement of the superstructures continues beyond the time and extent valid for the female skull. It may be worthwhile to stress the fact that these differences are merely superficial and correlated to muscular activity.

The average weight and volume of the female brain are slightly below the figures for the male. This difference is probably correlated with the smaller number of neurons needed to innervate the female's smaller muscle mass, which explains the slightly smaller capacity of the female skull.

ANTHROPOLOGIC REMARKS
Cephalometry and craniometry

Cephalometry, measurements taken on the head of the living person directly or by radiographs, and craniometry, measurements of the skull of a deceased person, have been used more and more frequently in an effort to study the growth of the skull under normal and abnormal conditions and to analyze the disharmonies in the pattern of the skull manifested, for instance, in the different types of malocclusion. A short explanation of the landmarks used for such measurements is therefore of interest to the dentist and especially to the orthodontist.

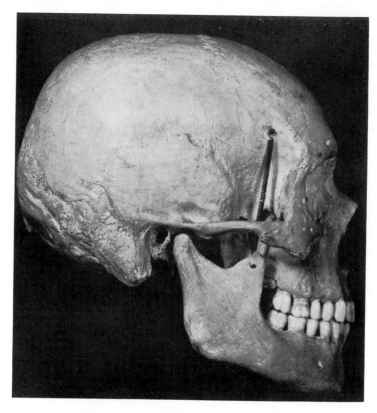

Fig. 2-71. Young adult male skull, lateral aspect.

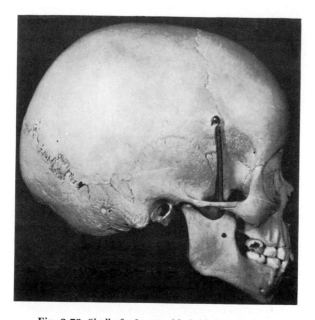

Fig. 2-72. Skull of a 3-year-old child, lateral view.

The head or skull has to be oriented in a fixed position in space if comparable measurements or pictures are to be taken. To achieve this, the skull is brought into the Frankfurt horizontal plane, which passes through the two orbital points and poria. Orbitale is the lowest point at the infraorbital rim; porion is defined as the most lateral point on the roof of the external auditory meatus, vertically over the middle of the meatus. Because of the asymmetries of almost every skull, these four points are rarely in one plane. The rule, therefore, is to plan the Frankfurt horizontal through the two poria and one orbitale. Then the skull is in nearly the same position as in a living person standing upright and looking into the far distance.

On the living the orbitale can be determined with a sufficient amount of accuracy. Instead of the porion, however, the tragion has to be used. This is the most forward point in the supratragal notch. The tragus itself is that roughly triangular part of the outer ear that projects backward and slightly outward at the anterior circumference of the entrance into the ear passage. The tragion lies at an average of 2.5 mm. above and in front of the bony porion. A second landmark, which in the living can be used instead of the porion on the bony skull, is the "cartilaginous porion," the midpoint on the upper border of the entrance into the external auditory meatus (Figs. 2-73 to 2-75).

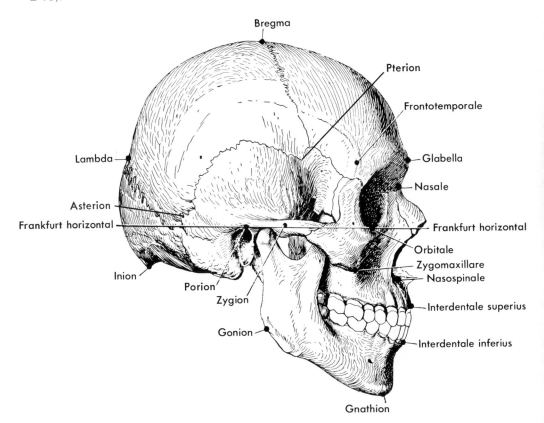

Fig. 2-73. Lateral aspect of skull with Frankfurt horizontal and anthropologic landmarks. (Sicher and Tandler: Anatomie für Zahnärzte.)

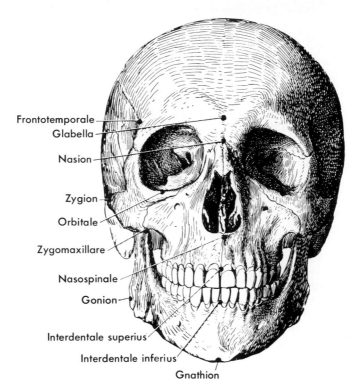

Fig. 2-74. Anterior aspect of skull with anthropologic landmarks. (Sicher and Tandler: Anatomie für Zahnärzte.)

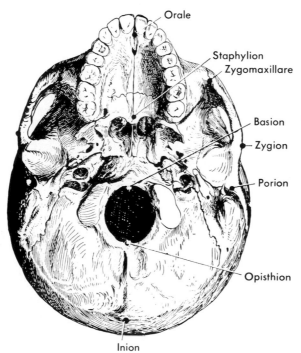

Fig. 2-75. Inferior aspect of cranium with anthropologic landmarks. (Sicher and Tandler: Anatomie für Zahnärzte.)

The following points serve as landmarks on the brain capsule or calvaria:

1. *Glabella* is the most anterior point on the midsagittal plane between the superciliary arches. In the living it is found above the root of the nose and between the median ends of the eyebrows.
2. *Bregma* is the point at which sagittal and coronal sutures meet.
3. *Lambda* is the point at which sagittal and lambdoid sutures meet.
4. *Opisthocranion* is the point in the midline that projects farthest backward. It marks the posterior end of the maximum cranial length measured from the glabella in front. It can be determined in the living.
5. *Inion* is defined as the crossing point of the midline with a tangent to the upper convexities of the superior nuchal lines. It can be determined in the living with some degree of accuracy.
6. *Asterion* is the sutural point at which the parietal, occipital, and temporal bones meet.
7. *Opisthion* is the midline point at the posterior border of the occipital foramen.
8. *Basion* is the midline point at the anterior margin of the occipital foramen. Since this point is not always defined on lateral radiographs of the head, another landmark is used as the posterior end of the cranial base, namely, the Bolton point.
9. *Bolton point* marks the height of the curvature posterior to the condyle between it and the basal surface of the occipital bone.
10. *Porion* is the most lateral point on the roof of the external auditory meatus vertically over the middle of the meatus. Since this point cannot be determined in the living, either the tragion or the cartilaginous porion is used.
11. *Tragion* is the most forward point in the supratragal notch.
12. *Cartilaginous porion* is the midpoint on the upper border of the entrance into the external auditory meatus.
13. *Frontotemporale* is the most anterior point of the temporal line, situated approximately at the root of the zygomatic process of the frontal bone. This point can be determined in the living.
14. *Pterion* is the midpoint of the sphenoparietal suture.

In the facial part of the skull, the following measuring points are of importance:

1. *Nasion* is the midpoint of the nasofrontal suture or, in a simpler definition, the point where internasal and nasofrontal sutures meet. It can be determined approximately in the living where it corresponds to the deepest part of the depression just below the level of the eyebrows.
2. *Nasospinale* is the midpoint on a line that connects the lowest points of the border of the piriform aperture on either side. It is situated at the base of the anterior nasal spine. In the living, the subnasale can be used instead of the nasospinale, which, however, is fairly well defined on radiographs.
3. *Subnasale* is the point where the lower border of the nasal septum meets the root of the upper lip.

4. *Interdentale superius* is the midline point on the tip of the septum between the right and left upper central incisors. In the living, the tip of the inter-dental papilla between these two teeth is used, although this point is about 2 mm. distant from the border of the bone.

5. *Interdentale inferius* is the midline point on the tip of the alveolar septum between the right and left lower central incisors. For measurements on the living, the tip of the interdental papilla in the midline is used.

6. *Prosthion* is that point of the upper alveolar process that projects most ante-riorly in the midline. This point is not to be used in measurements of facial height. It serves as a landmark to measure facial length, that is, anteropos-terior extension of the face.

7. *Orbitale* is the lowest point of the infraorbital margin. It can be determined in the living with a fair degree of accuracy.

8. *Zygomaxillare* is the lowermost point of the zygomaticomaxillary suture. It can be determined in the living, though only approximately, by palpation from the oral vestibule.

9. *Zygion* is the most lateral projection of the zygomatic arch. This point can be determined approximately in the living.

10. *Staphylion* is a midline point of a line connecting the most anterior points of the posterior border of the hard palate on either side. This point is situated at the base of the variable posterior nasal spine.

11. *Orale* is the midpoint of a line connecting the posterior borders of the sockets of the upper central incisors. This point can be located approximately in the living.

12. *Gnathion* is the lowest point of the mandible in the midline. It can be pal-pated in the living. For its determination on lateral head plates, the definition is given as the midpoint between the most anterior and inferior points of the bony chin.

13. *Gonion* is the apex or the point of maximum curvature at the mandibular angle. It can be determined in the living. In a lateral radiograph of the head or in the goniometer, the gonion can be located by bisecting the angle between tangents to the lower and posterior borders of the mandible.

14. *Condylion laterale* and *mediale* are the lateral and medial poles of the man-dibular condyle.

15. Orthodontists use the most posterior points of *incurvations of upper and lower jaws* in the midline and name the maxillary point (a) and the mandibular point (b).

The following linear measurements of the neurocranium may be mentioned:

1. *Maximum cranial length* is the distance from glabella to opisthocranion, the most prominent point of the occipital bone in the midline.

2. *Length of the cranial base* is the distance of nasion from basion; on the radio-graph it is measured between nasion and Bolton point.

3. *Maximum cranial breadth* is measured wherever it is found between the two most prominent points on either side of the cranium.

4. *Minimum frontal breadth* is the distance between the two frontotemporalia.
5. *Basiobregmatic height* is the distance between basion and bregma.

The following linear measurements of the facial skeleton may be mentioned:

1. *Upper facial length* is the distance of prosthion from basion; on a radiographic head plate, from prosthion to Bolton point.
2. *Lower facial length* is the distance of gnathion from basion or Bolton point.
3. *Zygomatic breadth* is the distance between the two zygia.
4. *Midfacial breadth* is the distance between the two zygomaxillaria.
5. *Facial height* is the distance of nasion from gnathion.
6. *Upper facial height* is the distance between nasion and interdentale superius.
7. *Upper alveolar height* is the distance between nasospinale and interdentale superius.
8. *Lower facial height* is the distance between interdentale superius and gnathion.
9. *Maxilloalveolar length* is the distance of prosthion from the midpoint of the tangent to the posterior margin of the sockets of the upper third molars. The latter point is also termed *alveolon*.
10. *Maxilloalveolar breadth* is the maximum distance measured on the outer surface of the upper alveolar processes.
11. *Palate length* is the distance between orale and staphylion.
12. *Palate breadth* is the distance of the inner borders of the sockets of the two upper second molars, endomolaria.
13. *Palate height* is the distance of the maximum arching of the palate from the line connecting the two endomolaria.
14. *Condylar breadth of the mandible* is the distance of right and left condylion laterale.
15. *Angular breadth of the mandible* is the distance between right and left gonia.
16. *Anterior mandibular breadth* is the distance of inner borders of right and left mental foramina.
17. *Mandibular length* is the distance of the most anterior point of the mental protuberance from a vertical plane tangential to the most posterior points of the condyles and at a right angle to a tangent to the lower border of the mandible.
18. *Mental height* is the distance of interdentale inferius to gnathion.
19. *Height of the mandibular ramus* is the distance of gonion to the highest point of the condyle.
20. *Breadth of mandibular ramus* is the smallest breadth of the ramus measured at a right angle to its height.

To describe proportions independent of absolute size, indices are used in anthropology. An index is the ratio of a smaller to a larger linear measurement expressed in terms of a percentage. If, for instance, the relation of cranial breadth to cranial length in the skull of a deceased person is to be evaluated, the *cranial index* is computed according to the following formula:

$$\frac{\text{Maximum cranial breadth} \times 100}{\text{Maximum cranial length}}$$

In measurements in the living, the maximum head length and maximum head breadth are used to compute the *cephalic index*. According to the cephalic and cranial indices the skulls are divided into long, or dolichocephalic, skulls and short, or brachycephalic, skulls; a middle type is called mesocephalic.

Ultradolichocephalic	X-64.9
Hyperdolichocephalic	65.0-69.9
Dolichocephalic	70.0-74.9
Mesocephalic	75.0-79.9
Brachycephalic	80.0-84.9
Hyperbrachycephalic	85.0-89.9
Ultrabrachycephalic	90.0-X

Another index permits classification of skulls according to the height of the cranial vault as seen in profile. The index gives the ratio of a basion-bregma height to maximum cranial length. The formula for computing the index is as follows:

$$\frac{\text{Basion-bregma height} \times 100}{\text{Maximum cranial length}}$$

According to the value of this index, the skulls are classified as chamecephalic or low skulls and hypsicephalic or high skulls, and a middle type is called orthocephalic.

Chamecephalic	X-69.9
Orthocephalic	70.0-74.9
Hypsicephalic	75.0-X

The height of the cranial vault as seen in an anterior view is expressed by the ratio of basion-bregma height to maximum cranial breadth. According to the computed index, the skulls are classified as lowly arched, or tapeinocephalic, skulls and highly arched, or acrocephalic, skulls. A middle class is called metriocephalic.

Tapeinocephalic	X-91.9
Metriocephalic	92.0-97.9
Acrocephalic	98.0-X

The *facial index* characterizing the proportions of the face is computed by the following formula:

$$\frac{\text{Facial height} \times 100}{\text{Zygomatic breadth}}$$

The index shows whether the face is high and narrow, leptoprosopic, or low and wide, euryprosopic. A middle type is the mesoprosopic.

Hypereuryprosopic	X-79.9
Euryprosopic	80.0-84.9
Mesoprosopic	85.0-89.9
Leptoprosopic	90.0-94.9
Hyperleptoprosopic	95.0-X

The *palatine index* is computed according to the following formula:

$$\frac{\text{Palate breadth} \times 100}{\text{Palate length}}$$

This index enables the classification of skulls into those with a narrow palate, leptostaphyline, and those with a wide palate, brachystaphyline.

Leptostaphyline	X-79.9
Mesostaphyline	80.0-84.9
Brachystaphyline	85.0-X

The arching of the palate is characterized by the *palate height index* according to the following formula:

$$\frac{\text{Palate height} \times 100}{\text{Palate breadth}}$$

A low palate is chamestaphyline, a high palate is hypsistaphyline, the intermediate group is orthostaphyline.

Chamestaphyline	X-27.9
Orthostaphyline	28.0-39.9
Hypsistaphyline	40.0-X

There are a great number of other indices useful in the description and classification of skulls that do not need a specific definition. As an example, the ratio of breadth and height of the mandibular ramus or that of mandibular length and breadth may be mentioned. It is also possible to compare the upper or lower facial breadth with the middle facial height to characterize the lateral outline of the face.

Especially in the facial skeleton, angular measurements are revealing because they characterize most concisely the relation of the facial profile to a vertical plane; in other words, they show the degree of prognathism (Fig. 2-76).

The *total profile angle* is the angle between a line connecting nasion and prosthion and the Frankfurt horizontal. According to the size of this angle, the skulls are classified as prognathous if the jaws protrude strongly or orthognathous if the jaws do not protrude or protrude only slightly, and the intermediate type is called mesognathous. The following classes are recognized:

Hyperprognathous	X-69.9°
Prognathous	70.0°-79.9°
Mesognathous	80.0°-84.9°
Orthognathous	85.0°-92.9°
Hyperorthognathous	93.0°-X

Another possibility to characterize the position of the upper face is to measure the angle of the triangle nasion-prosthion-basion at the prosthion. This angle is known as *Rivet's angle*. If this measurement is taken as a basis, the following classification is valid:

Prognathous	X-69.9°
Mesognathous	70.0°-72.9°
Orthognathous	73.0°-X

It is desirable separately to determine the inclination of the nasal and the alveolar part of the upper facial skeleton. To do this, the *nasal profile angle* and the *alveolar profile angle* are measured. The nasal profile angle is the angle formed by the line from nasion to nasospinale with the Frankfurt horizontal. The alveolar profile angle is

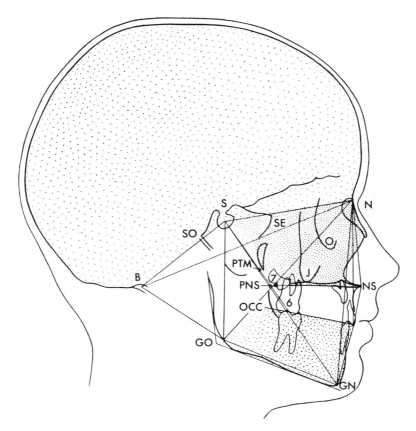

Fig. 2-76. Anthropologic landmarks on craniometric radiograph: *B*, Bolton point; *GN*, gnathion; *GO*, gonion; *J*, area corresponding approximately to zygomaxillare; *N*, nasion; *NS*, nasospinale; *O*, orbitale; *OCC*, occlusal plane; *PNS*, posterior nasal spine; *PTM*, pterygomaxillary (sphenomaxillary) gap; *S*, sella; *SE*, sphenoethmoid junction; *SO*, spheno-occipital junction; *6*, first molar; *7*, second molar. (Courtesy Dr. A. G. Brodie.)

the angle formed by the nasospinale-prosthion line with the Frankfurt horizontal. The classification according to the nasal profile angle is as follows:

Hyperprognathous	X-69.9°
Prognathous	70.0°-79.9°
Mesognathous	80.0°-84.9°
Orthognathous	85.0°-92.9°
Hyperorthognathous	93.0°-X

The classification according to the alveolar profile angle is as follows:

Ultraprognathous	X-59.9°
Hyperprognathous	60.0°-69.9°
Prognathous	70.0°-79.9°
Mesognathous	80.0°-84.9°
Orthognathous	85.0°-92.9°
Hyperorthognathous	93.0°-X

The mandibular profile angle is the angle between a line connecting the interdentale inferius with the anteriorly most prominent chin point and the Frankfurt horizontal. This angle can be measured only if the occlusal position of the mandible can be secured. If this is impossible, for instance, because of a lack or mutilation of the teeth of a skull, an angle is determined between the line interdentale inferius to the anterior chin point and the tangent to the lower border of the mandible; this latter measurement has no great value. Its integration into the facial profile depends on the unknown position of the occlusal plane.

The *condylar angle of the mandible* is the angle between a tangent to the lower and a tangent to the posterior border of the mandible. The term *condylar angle* was selected because this angle indicates the inclination of the condyle, an important growth site of the mandible, to the plane of the mandibular body.

The *basal mandibular angle* is the angle between the two gnathion-gonion lines.

Of interest also is the angle that the axes of the two mandibular condyles include.

GROWTH OF THE SKULL
General features of skeletal growth

Bones of the human skeleton arise, for the most part, in hyaline cartilage, but in certain restricted places they also arise in condensed mesenchyme. Thus a soft tissue "model" is always present first; this is gradually replaced by hard bone tissue. The growth of bone involves three interdependent factors: (1) growth of the model tissue, (2) growth of the bone tissue, and (3) remodeling of bone.

In the long bones of the body the tissue of the model is cartilage, hence the bones are called endochondral, or cartilage, bones. Early growth of the cartilage model before any bone tissue appears and later growth of the derivatives of the model, epiphyseal and articular cartilages, determine the size of the bone, especially its length. But since the cartilage is destroyed as it is being replaced by bone, the growth of the bone tissue itself plays an equally important part in growth. Increase in thickness and the addition of ridges and other projections for the attachment of muscles and ligaments are also the consequences of the growth of bone tissue. The final refined outer contour and internal structure are sculptured out by remodeling. This is a process of selective apposition and resorption of bone, that is, cellular activity at the surface that lays down bone or removes it.

In the flat bones of the skull the tissue of the model is connective tissue (condensed mesenchyme); hence these bones are called intramembranous, or dermal, bone, since they form close beneath the skin. Here the growth of the connective tissue membrane is followed closely by the invading bone, just as it is in the cartilage matrix, and the derivative of the membrane model can be considered the suture.

Growth of the skull is best understood as a phenomenon occuring in two skeletal units that go to make up a functional whole, the cranium and the mandible that works against it. The whole grows as a coordinated composite from many sites in both model tissues, cartilage and membrane. Thus the bones of the base arise in cartilage just as do the limb bones and vertebrae, while the bones of the roof and face arise directly in the connective tissue membrane.

In this view the many bones of the cranium are seen in the same light as the many bony pieces that go to make up any single adult long bone; both fuse to become a more or less single unit with age. Thus in early life the humerus consists of eight distinct bony pieces (the head, shaft, greater and lesser tubercles, capitulum, trochlea, and medial and lateral epicondyles) separated by cartilage plates. These elements grow and fuse to become a single bone, completed as late as the twentieth year. The femur even resembles the mandible in some ways. Although it arises from five centers, its head sits on a bent neck and a bony process for muscle insertions projects from each side of the immediately continuous shaft (see section on architectural analysis of the skull in this chapter).

The change in the size and shape of the newborn skull to the adult form is brought about by several distinctive features of the growth process. Since all bones are embedded in soft tissue blankets, the growth-promoting fields are not in the bone itself but in the tissues contiguous with the bone, that is, the periosteum, endosteum, suture, and synchondrosis. All the surfaces of a bone are active in growth at one time or another, and at various rates at various times. But a bone does not simply get bigger by the symmetrical addition of bone on all its surface contours. There is a differential mode of enlargement that changes the size and shape as well as the position of a bone in relation to other bones, and this changes the whole form of the skull. As a normal consequence bones are moved, "translated," because of the growth of the bone itself, or the growth of adjacent or distant bones. Even parts of a bone are "relocated" by apposition of bone on one side and resorption on the opposite side so that bone tissue that once formed the back of a bone finally comes to lie at its front surface. All of these processes must have clinical relevance, especially in orthodontics, so that teeth are moved, "relocated," with the flow of skull growth and not against it.

The present problem in explaining growth is the lack of knowledge of the exact nature of growth control. Genetic processes ultimately direct growth and form. But the manner by which genetic dictates are channeled down through the continuous change of adjacent growing environments to monitor the specific pattern of formation of a bone remains elusive. Thus, although skeletal development cannot be an independent process insulated from the effects of growth of surrounding organs, all inputs do not bear equal weight in affecting the growth of a bone. Some influences on cranial growth stand out above others. To begin with, it appears that the cartilage growth discs in the skull base can grow to some extent, even though the brain that the base nestles does not, as in cases of anencephaly. This certainly suggests that basal cartilage has at least a modicum of innate genetic potential monitoring its growth. Furthermore, experimental tampering with cartilage growth sites in laboratory animals changes the growth pattern of the whole skull. Long flat skulls can be shortened, rounded and bent, buckling up at the base to simulate a basal angle like that at the sella turcica in the human skull. On the other hand, the dermal bones of the calvaria do not enlarge in the absence of brain expansion. Nor do facial bones enlarge in the absence of the normal growth of the organs they house, including the musculature and particularly the tongue. Here it is revealing to find that no amount of experimental manipulation of sutures can change the general form of the skull.

An enlightening diagram of the growth plan of the skull pictures two features. First, the base is drawn as a forward continuation of the vertebral axis, since it is composed of midline bony blocks separated by cartilage growth plates that are set in continuous series with the perichordal growth plates of the vertebrae. This is entirely reasonable because the notochord around which all vertebrae form extends forward through the cranial base up into the future body of the sphenoid bone in the embryo. Both the microscopic appearance and the mode of growth of these basicranial plates resemble the epiphyseal growth plates of long bones. Second, the axial core is surrounded by an outer casing of membrane bones separated by growing sutures. The casing houses the brain above, and the facial and oral structures below, the base.

Such a working blueprint provides a preliminary explanation for the adaptive value of two different modes of bone formation. The firm cartilage core affords the same central supportive function to the skull as the vertebral column does to the rest of the body. It establishes the stable base from which surrounding structures extend in growth. Its developmental process is comparatively slow and steady, passing through a tight sequence of distinct stages: cartilage grows, cartilage calcifies, bone invades cartilage, cartilage is removed as bone replaces it. In this way the supportive function is never relinquished but actually increases as rigidity grows with the growing demands of increased mass.

Dermal bone, on the other hand, expands rapidly since it arises and grows directly in connective tissue sheets with no intervening stages. Thus though the connective tissue affords little pressure support, it is well adapted for the speedy spread of bone.

The brain case triples in size in the first two years, then growth declines to completion by about the sixth year. At about this time growth of the diminutive face becomes active; the permanent dentition is appearing and growth of the face and jaws accelerates. Thus growing bones above and below the skull base overlap at their slow-growing ends, brain case growth declining as facial growth accelerates.

In some ways the mandible is a unique bone. It develops primarily as a membrane bone, that is, within the connective tissue lateral to the primary skeleton of the first branchial arch, Meckel's cartilage. Although at first the mesenchymal cells of the mandibular arch differentiate into osteoblasts and form bony trabeculae, later other undifferentiated mesenchymal cells differentiate into chondroblasts and form cartilage at the future condylar process of the mandible and to a lesser degree in other areas. When this cartilage has been established it contributes a new model tissue for the growth of the mandible. Its growth is essential in developing the overall size of the lower jaw, and as it grows it is replaced by bone. Growth of bone tissue is necessary not only to replace the growing cartilage, but also to form the angular process of the mandible, the coronoid process, most of the alveolar process, and the reinforcements of the mandible, for instance, in the region of the chin. Modeling resorption at the neck of the mandible, at the anterior border of the coronoid process, and in other areas is equally important.

Thus, though it might seem that the mandible behaves much like any other long or tubular bone, at least after the time the secondary cartilage appears in the condylar area, this is only partially true. This cartilage does not grow in the same manner as does cartilage in other parts of the skeleton, such as articular cartilage, epiphyseal cartilage, and the cartilage in the base of the skull (that is, between the four parts of the occipital bone, between parts of the sphenoid bone, and between the sphenoid and occipital bones). Articular, epiphyseal, and cranial base cartilages enlarge by interstitial, or expansive, growth. This means that cells of the cartilage, chondrocytes, proliferate by mitotic division, form new cartilaginous intercellular substance, and thus spread the cartilage apart. Expansive, or interstitial, growth, therefore, depends on the division of already differentiated cells, the chondrocytes. On the other hand, it is known that cartilage can and does grow by what is aptly called appositional, or additive, growth; for instance, a costal cartilage grows longer by expansion but thicker by apposition. That means that in the deepest layers of the growing perichondrium, undifferentiated mesenchymal cells gradually differentiate into chondroblasts and then into chondrocytes. In other words, interstitial growth of cartilage depends on the proliferation of differentiated cells, chondrocytes; appositional growth of cartilage depends on differentiation of proliferated cells, mesenchymal cells into chondrocytes. Appositional growth of cartilage is, of course, restricted to surfaces covered by a perichondrium. The growing cartilage at the mandibular condyle, developing within the primary undifferentiated mesenchyme of the embryo, is covered throughout life by connective tissue that is but a highly differentiated perichondrium that later takes over as the articulating cushion of the condyle. This fact makes the cartilage in the mandibular condyle unique in the mammalian, thus in the human, skeleton. It is unique because this cartilage grows mainly, possibly entirely, by apposition. The cartilage in the mandibular condyle is added to by differentiation of mesenchymal cells into cartilage cells. There is no, or possibly just occasional, mitotic division of differentiated cartilage cells.

There is a great biologic difference between interstitial and appositional growth of cartilage. In interstitial growth of cartilage, differentiated cells divide and form new cartilaginous intercellular substance; in appositional growth of cartilage, undifferentiated mesenchymal cells differentiate into cartilage cells. It is hardly possible to exaggerate the importance of this difference. Differentiation, among many other things, implies the acquisition or activation of new enzyme systems in a cell. In mitotic division, cells of a certain degree of differentiation divide. These cells, before division, had acquired certain enzyme systems, and their daughter cells possess the same enzyme systems. In appositional growth of cartilage, undifferentiated mesenchymal cells acquire new enzyme systems that change them into cartilage cells. They do not differentiate into fibroblasts; they differentiate along a new line of cell ancestry into chondroblasts and then chondrocytes.

Since by its growth the mandibular cartilage increases the overall length of the mandible and at the same time the height of the mandibular ramus, the mechanism of its growth is highly significant. In chondrodystrophic dwarfs, for instance, the inhibition of body growth is due to a genetic inhibition of the interstitial growth of hyaline cartilage. Appositional growth of cartilage is not impaired at all or is not impaired to the same degree. The skull of dwarfs of this type is characterized by the short cranial base, the growth of which depends largely on the interstitial growth of the cartilage in the basicranial synchondroses. Consequently, the forehead bulges and, because the cartilaginous nasal septum cannot enlarge normally, the nose is deeply saddled. The mandible of such dwarfs, however, develops to a fairly normal size, although its growth, too, depends on cartilaginous growth. The mandible often even protrudes in chondrodystrophic dwarfs because its growth cartilage enlarges by appositional growth. The same relation of upper face and mandible is also clearly seen in partly chondrodystrophic breeds of dogs, for example, bulldogs.

Growth of the cranium, except for its base, occurs at the sutures. Apposition of bone is active across the entire surface of the suture and so is not limited to its outer portion. At the same time, however, there is selective apposition and resorption on both the outer and the inner surfaces of the cranial bones. In the first years of life resorption is restricted to small areas on the inner surfaces of the vault bones, whereas in other areas of the inner surface apposition takes place. Later the entire inner surface of the cranial cavity shows apposition, which continues for a long time.

The detailed structure of the growing suture has been described as consisting of as many as five distinguishable layers: (1) a layer of proliferating bone-forming cells depositing new bone along the sutural edge of the bone, (2) a layer of fibrous tissue running across the suture connecting the outer and inner fibrous periosteum of the bone, (3) a middle layer rich in proliferating connective tissue cells and small blood vessels, (4) again a fibrous periosteal layer for the adjoining bone, and (5) the layer of

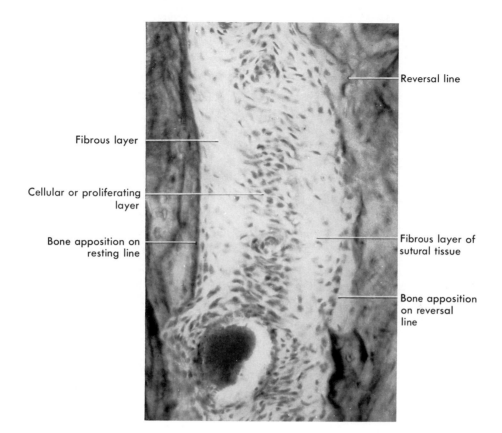

Reversal line

Fibrous layer

Cellular or proliferating layer

Bone apposition on resting line

Fibrous layer of sutural tissue

Bone apposition on reversal line

Fig. 2-77. Part of premaxillomaxillary suture of Rhesus monkey. (Courtesy Dr. A. G. Brodie; Weinmann and Sicher: Bone and bones.)

proliferating bone-forming cells against the sutural edge of the adjoining bone (Fig. 2-77). Thus the suture has an active growth site for each bone, while the middle layer contributes to the interstitial growth of the sutural junction itself, and hence to the expansion of the cranium.

The complexity of the skull, in a phylogenetic, ontogenetic, and functional sense, is especially apparent if one tries to understand its growth. This is why it has taken so long to acquire a fairly clear picture of the intricate changes in the different parts of the skull during its development and growth. The single fact that the bony capsule of the brain is inseparably linked with the masticatory facial skeleton, so that these two parts of the skull are integrated into one anatomic and biologic unit, accounts for many complications. These complications arise because the growth of the capsule of the brain is entirely dependent on that of the brain itself, whereas the growth of the masticatory skeleton is, to a great extent, dependent on muscular influences, dentition, and the growth of the tongue. Not only do the two parts of the skull follow different paths of development, but also the timing of their growth rates is entirely divergent. The brain, has, at the age of 12 years, almost completed its growth by reaching about 90% of its ultimate weight and volume. At this age, however, the dentition and therefore the jaws are only beginning their final phase of growth, which will end 8 or 10 years later.

Thus the skull shows an overall pattern of remarkable plasticity in its growth. This is an adaptation that meets all the spatial and mechanical requirements of the contained components mentioned previously in the context of the basic adjustment of the skull to the upright body axis. Although the growth of any particular part of the skull is integrated with the growth of the whole, it is most convenient to discuss skull growth under the following headings:

1. Growth of the brain capsule in a strict sense; that is, the growth of the inner plate of the bones of the cranium.
2. Growth of the cranial superstructures. The outer plates of the cranial bones serving mechanical functions show striking divergences from the growth of the inner lamina in many areas. These divergences are much more marked in the primitive and extinct races of mankind than in modern man.
3. Growth of the facial skeleton. It follows, in many ways, independent curves in space and time. An additional complication is produced by differences in the mechanism of growth of the upper facial skeleton and that of the mandible.
4. Growth of the facial skeleton and tooth eruption; that is, the interplay between skeletal growth and eruption and movements of teeth.
5. Growth of the pneumatic, or air-containing, cavities of the skull. These have to be discussed separately because they may expand at an age when other processes of growth have long ceased.

Growth of the brain capsule

It has been mentioned before that the brain advances in its growth much more rapidly than the facial skeleton and that by the age of 12 years the brain has reached 90% of its final volume. The rate of the growth of the brain and its capsule decreases considerably as early as the third or fourth year of life.

If radiographs of the same child are taken at regular intervals, it can be shown that the growth of the brain capsule is fairly concentric (Fig. 2-78). The cranial base is taken as the fixed point, and the superposition of the pictures is done by superposing the sella turcica. Much has been said about the impossibility of finding a truly fixed point of reference during the growth of the skull, but the difficulties in this respect have been magnified, since we are mostly concerned with changes of the different parts of the skull relative to each other. It is possible to study these changes by selecting the most convenient basis for comparison. Although the cranial base grows with the growing skull, it furnishes the most convenient "reference point" for growth studies. It is, furthermore, entirely reasonable to take the sella, and thus the hypophyseal region, as a starting point for comparative studies because this region of the brain and of the axial skeleton seems to be truly a crucial point in the development of the vertebrates.

The mechanisms of the enlargement of the cranial base on one hand and the cranial vault on the other have already been described. It is principally the growth of cartilage that lengthens and widens the diameters of the base; in the cranial vault, it is growth of connective tissue. The cartilaginous growth occurs mainly in the sphenoethmoid, spheno-occipital, and intraoccipital synchondroses. The intersphenoid synchondroses disappear soon after birth, and the intraoccipital synchondroses disappear in the fourth and sixth year. The cartilaginous plate between the occipital and sphenoid bones, which is not entirely replaced by bone until about the eighteenth year of life (16 to 20 years), is the most important of the growth cartilages.

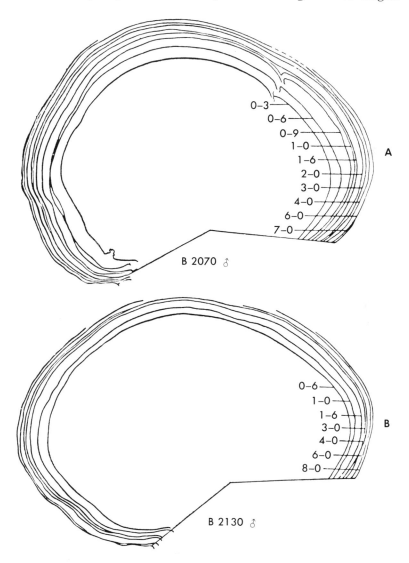

Fig. 2-78. Concentric growth of cranial vault. Superposed outlines of skull from craniometric radiographs of same individual at different ages. **A,** From 3 months to 7 years of age. **B,** From 6 months to 8 years of age. (After Brodie; Weinmann and Sicher: Bone and bones.)

The cranial vault expands, as was described before, by sutural growth. It has to be realized that the ossification of the proliferating sutural connective tissue, or the replacement of the proliferating cartilage by bone, is but a secondary phase in the growth of the skull. Apposition of bone should properly be considered as growth of the single bony parts of the skull. The role of the connective tissue is the more important because only through this role can one understand the selective influence of different diseases and hereditary factors on the growth of either the cranial base or the cranial vault.

Especially in the first years of life, when the rate of growth of the skull is greatest, the changes in the curvature of the bones forming the convexity of the skull are significant. It is clear that these bones have to flatten while they expand to fit the increasing radius of curvature of the growing brain. Expansion occurs by sutural growth only. Flattening is accomplished by resorption at the inner surface in the areas close to the sutural borders and apposition of bone on the inner surface in the central areas. Resorption on the cerebral surface has been denied by some investigators. But though resorption does take place, it seems to be active only in the first years of postnatal life. Later, when the rate of growth of the brain decreases rapidly and therefore when the change in curvature is only slight, the change is brought about solely by differential apposition. Then, apposition on the cerebral surface in the central areas of the bones and increased apposition on the external surfaces in the marginal areas suffice to bring about the slight changes leading to the definitive flattening of the bones.

The concomitant thickening of the bones of the cranial vault occurs by apposition on both surfaces of the bones, except during the early period when restricted resorption is active in the border areas of the single bones. It is especially noteworthy that on the inner surface of the skull, on the bones of the cranial vault as well as on those forming the cranial base, apposition of bone predominates. This is the best indication that the enlargement of the cranial cavity occurs mainly by sutural growth.

The continual apposition of bone on the inner surfaces of the cranial capsule is said to progress even after cranial growth has ceased, slightly reducing the cranial cavity. It is claimed that this is due to a "shrinkage" of the brain during its maturation. It is known that the specific gravity of the brain increases after it has reached its ultimate volume, and this could be associated with a slight decrease of the volume. It is, however, also possible that sutural growth continues after brain and cranial cavity have reached their final volume. Sutural growth then would allow for the strengthening of the cranial walls by internal apposition without reducing the cranial capacity.

After infancy, since apposition occurs on the entire surface of the cranium, the gradual deepening of the vascular grooves and the development of the digitated impressions are due not to a hollowing out of the grooves but to a heightening of their borders.

It is clear that growth of the brain capsule is dependent on the growth of the brain. The expanding brain causes an increase of the intracranial pressure. However, it would be erroneous to view this in a strictly mechanical sense, the growing brain "spreading" the cranial bones apart. The slight daily increase of intracranial pressure, acting against living and, therefore, reactive tissues merely acts as stimulus for the growth of interosseous tissues, cartilage or connective tissue. By their growth—that is, by the growth of the brain capsule—the pressure is shortly eliminated and never, under normal conditions, can it build up to a degree that would endanger the growing brain.

Growth of the cranial superstructures

The increase in thickness of the cranial bones is not uniform. In many regions a progressive divergence develops between the inner plate, the brain capsule in a stricter sense, and the outer plate, which is largely under mechanical influences. These divergences are found, for instance, in the nuchal region where the nuchal crests and especially the external occipital protuberance develop under the influence of the posterior musculature of the neck. Such divergence between the two plates of the cranial bones is most pronounced in two regions, the supraorbital and the otic and mastoid areas.

At birth the outer and inner plates of the frontal bone are parallel (Fig. 2-79), a superciliary arch does not exist, and a frontal sinus is absent. Later, the outer plate in the supraorbital region grows faster than the inner plate by apposition of bone on the outer surface. The outer plate *seems* gradually to bend away from the inner plate,

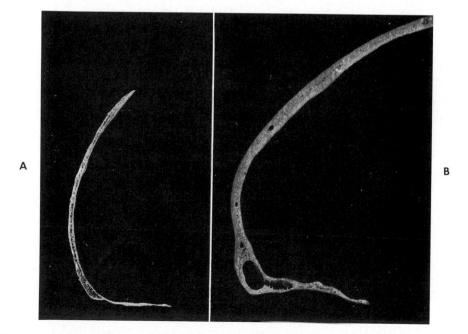

Fig. 2-79. Sagittal sections through frontal bone at approximate level of trochlear fovea. **A,** Newborn infant. **B,** Young adult. (Weinmann and Sicher: Bone and bones.)

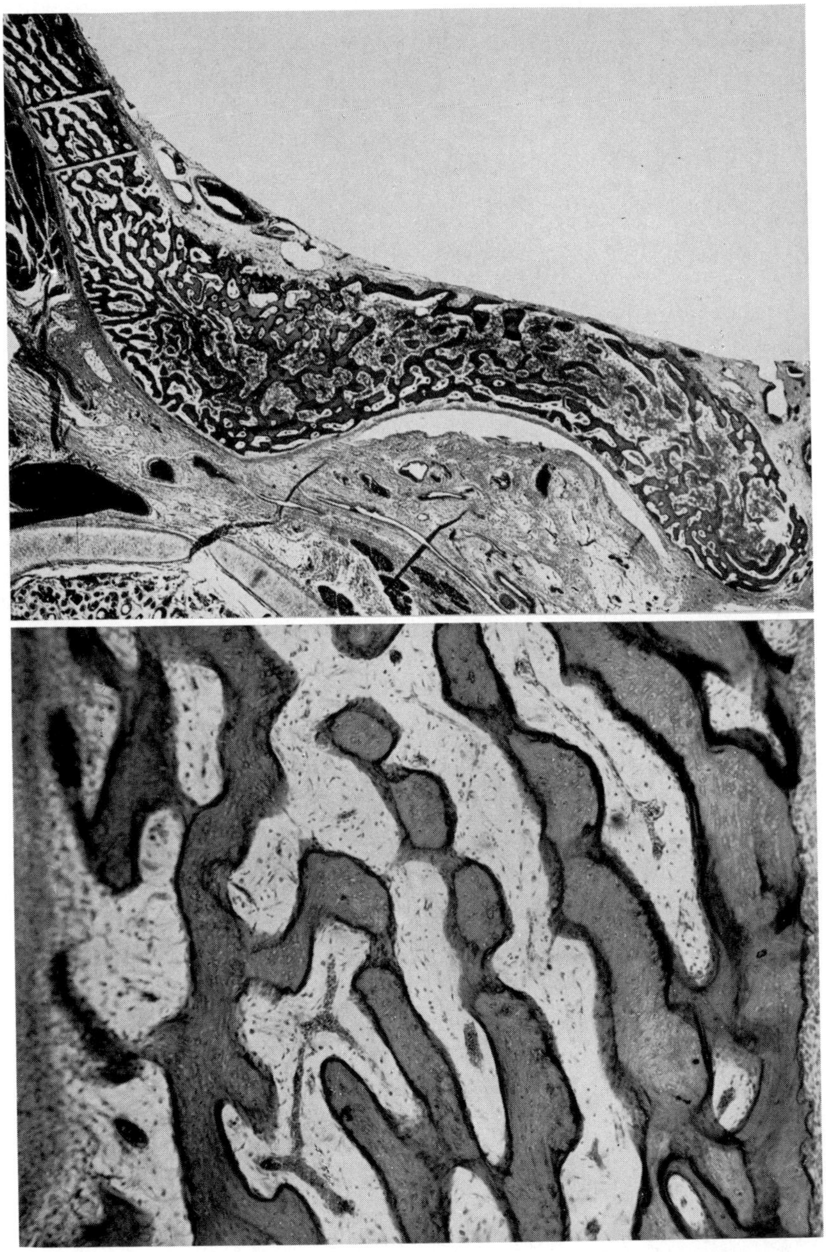

Fig. 2-80. Frontal section through temporal squama of newborn infant. **A,** General view. Note signs of resorption on cerebral surface and signs of apposition on periosteal surface of bone. **B,** High magnification of area between the two lines in **A.** Note apposition on periosteal surface at left and resorption on cerebral surface at right. (Weinmann and Sicher: Bone and bones.)

forming a blunt ridge above the upper border of the orbital entrance. At first, spongy bone and later the frontal sinus occupy the space between the internal and external plates of the frontal bone. It is highly probable that the accentuation of the outer plate in this region occurs as a response to the growing masticatory forces, which are transmitted to the most anterior part of the cranial base by the frontal processes of the maxilla and the zygomatic bone. The changes, confined to the outer plate of the frontal bone, are the reason for the difference in the external shape of the forehead in the child and the adult; it is high and bulging in the infant and more sloping or receding in the adult. The described changes do not advance as far in the female skull as in the male skull, which accounts for the "infantile" shape of the female skull.

The changes in the otic and mastoid region (Figs. 2-80 to 2-82) are even more striking. In the newborn infant the lack of any superstructure in this part of the skull is shown by the following facts:

1. A mastoid process has not yet started to develop.
2. The stylomastoid foramen is found on the lateral surface of the skull, unprotected because of the lack of the mastoid process. This explains injuries to the facial nerve, for instance, during forceps delivery.
3. The articular surface faces laterally and downward, instead of being horizontal as in the adult. An articular eminence is not yet present.
4. The bony part of the external auditory meatus is absent, because the tympanic bone is represented by a bony ring only.

The changes in the mastoid region start soon after birth and are well advanced by

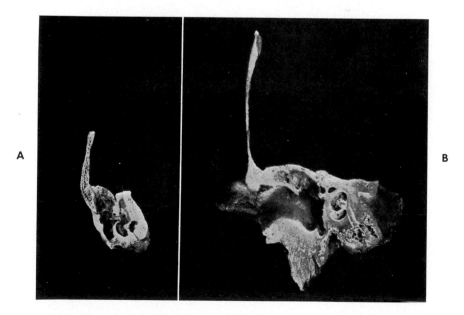

A   B

Fig. 2-81. Frontal sections of temporal bone through center of the external acoustic passage. **A**, Newborn infant. **B**, Adult. (Weinmann and Sicher: Bone and bones.)

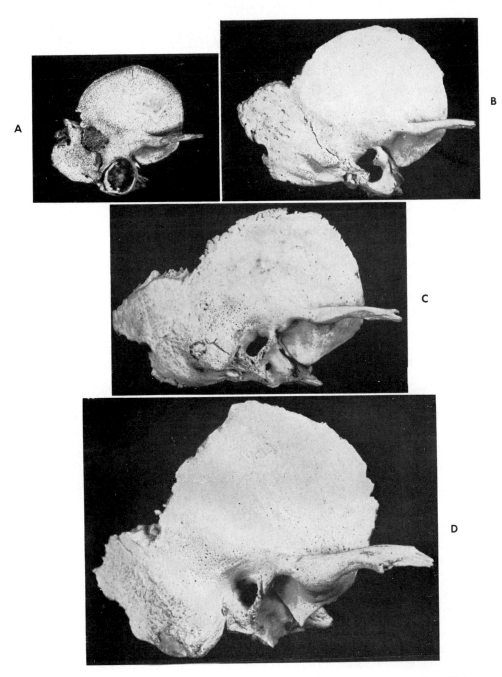

Fig. 2-82. Four stages in development of temporal bone. **A,** Newborn infant. **B,** 1 year of age. **C,** 4 years of age. **D,** Adult. (Weinmann and Sicher: Bone and bones.)

the second year of life. Accentuated apposition of bone laterally above the tympanic membrane, extending anteriorly to the root of the zygomatic process and posteriorly onto the mastoid surface, gradually "folds" the outer and inner plates of the temporal bone. At the same time resorption on the cerebral surface of the temporal squama widens the cranial cavity in this region (Fig. 2-80). By this remodeling the originally oblique outer plate in this region is divided into an upper, almost vertical, part and a lower horizontal part (Fig. 2-81). In the most anterior region this leads to a change in the position of the articular surface for the mandible, which gradually shifts into a horizontal plane, and at the same time the articular eminence develops. It is clear that this change coincides with the beginning of masticatory function.

In the tympanic region the same "folding" of the outer bony plate of the temporal squama leads to the development of the roof of the bony part of the external auditory meatus, the floor of which develops simultaneously by the outward growth of the tympanic bone (Fig. 2-82). This bone, at first a C-shaped ring, grows into a curved plate, still C-shaped in cross section, which forms the floor and anterior and posterior walls of the bony auditory passage. Its roof is the squama of the temporal bone. In the course of this change of the tympanic ring to the tympanic bone, a defect persists for a few years in the floor of the bony acoustic meatus (Fig. 2-82, C). This defect, which normally closes in the third or fourth year of life, may remain open and should not be confused with a traumatic defect. Remnants of it persist in almost 20% of adult skulls.

In the mastoid region the "folding" of the outer plate of the temporal bone is coincident with the outgrowth of the cone-shaped mastoid process on the lateral side of the stylomastoid foramen. The foramen moves simultaneously to the base of the skull, and the facial nerve is then safely protected from injury. The development of the mastoid process is correlated with the acquisition of the upright posture and gait and provides the necessary area of attachment for the sternocleidomastoid muscle, one function of which is to aid in balancing the head.

Growth of the facial skeleton

The growth curve of the facial skeleton is widely different from that of the neurocranium. At birth, the cranium overshadows the face because of the advanced development of the brain and the lack of function of the masticatory apparatus. The brain and, with it, its capsule triple in volume in the first 2 years of life and then slow down in their growth until, after the seventh year of life, the annual increment is almost negligible. After the first years of life the facial skeleton not only grows faster than the brain case, but it also retains a considerable rate of growth to the eighteenth year and probably ceases its growth much later. These differences are easily visualized in comparing the head of an infant with that of an adult. The bulging forehead of the former and the sloping forehead of the latter and the insignificance of the maxillary and mandibular skeleton in the infant, and their more or less prominent position in the adult are the external expressions of the different tempo of growth of the two main parts of the skull.

The facial skeleton increases during the growth period in all three dimensions of space: height, width, and depth or length. The detailed mechanism by which the coordination and simultaneity of the enlargement of the face in the three planes are achieved is one of the fascinating chapters of biology. Before going into details, however, one point has to be stressed, namely, a certain regularity of this process of growth or the maintenance of the original pattern of the facial skeleton and its relations to the skull. It has been shown, for instance, by the study of radiographs of the same child at different ages, that the plane of the palate, the occlusal plane, and the plane of the lower mandibular border maintain a fairly constant angular relation to the base of the skull. In other words, during the growth of the facial skeleton, these structures and planes shift roughly parallel to themselves.

During the growth of the skeleton of the upper face, the central problem is the shift and enlargement of the maxillary complex, that is, maxillae and palatine bones. In part, the enlargement of the maxillary skeleton in an anteroposterior diameter is simultaneous with the growth of the base of the skull in the same dimension. This growth, however, is achieved only to a small degree in that part of the base that is anterior to the spheno-occipital synchondrosis. Since the latter is situated behind the area of attachment of the facial to the cranial skeleton, growth in this location will affect the relations of the facial skeleton to the neurocranium more than it will affect the absolute growth of the face.

In the early development of facial bones of the maxillary region, the cartilaginous nasal capsule, a part of the chondrocranium, plays an important role as a growing template for these bones. Later, only the cartilaginous nasal septum remains of the nasal capsule. As in the cranial complex, cartilaginous growth and connective tissue (sutural) growth are correlated. So growth of the nasal septum and sutural growth are correlated, with the nasal cartilage apparently playing the leading role.

Most important sites of growth for the maxillary complex are three sutures on either side: the frontomaxillary suture between the frontal process of the maxilla and the frontal bone; the zygomaticomaxillary suture between the maxilla and the zygomatic bone and, secondarily, the zygomaticotemporal suture in the zygomatic arch; and the complex at the maxillary tuberosity, involving the pterygopalatine suture between the pterygoid process of the sphenoid bone and the pyramidal process of the palatine bone (Fig. 2-83). It is significant that these sutures are parallel to each other and directed from above and anteriorly to downward and posteriorly. Growth in these sutures will accommodate the shifting of the maxillary complex downward and anteriorly. While this "shift" occurs, apposition of bone on the entire posterior surface of the maxilla, the maxillary tuberosity, increases the anteroposterior dimensions of the maxillary body.

Growth in the described sutures and the nasal septum increases height and length or depth, that is, the vertical and anteroposterior dimensions, of the nasal part of the maxillae and palatine bones only. The subnasal part increases in height by apposition of bone on the free borders of the alveolar process simultaneously with the eruption of the teeth (Fig. 2-84). In an average skull, sutural growth contributes more to the

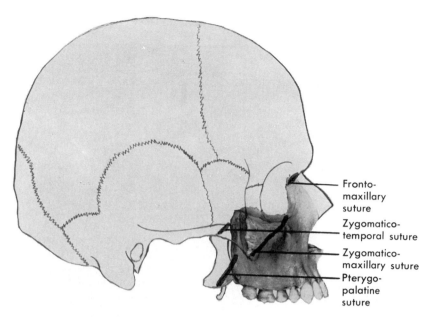

Fronto-
maxillary
suture

Zygomatico-
temporal suture

Zygomatico-
maxillary suture

Pterygo-
palatine
suture

Fig. 2-83. Sutural sites of maxillary growth (red). Photograph of maxilla of 16-year-old boy placed into diagrammatic outline of a skull. (Weinmann and Sicher: Bone and bones.)

increase in length, growth on the alveolar border more to the increase in height. In other words, sutural growth contributes more to the forward shift, and growth at the alveolar border contributes more to the downward shift of the upper jaw.

At the same time regulatory bone apposition and modeling resorption take place. Sutural growth alone evidently does not suffice to achieve the normal height of the nasal cavity; at the same time the orbits, which are relatively large at birth, would gain too much in height by growth at the sutures between frontal bone and zygomatic and maxillary bones. As correcting processes, apposition of bone on the orbital floor and resorption on the nasal floor can be observed (Figs. 2-85 to 2-87). The latter, in turn, is compensated for by apposition on the oral surface of the palate. Thus the palate "shifts" downward by the additive effect of sutural and septal growth and of continued rebuilding. The apposition of bone at the orbital floor is also proof of the reality of sutural growth.

The downward and forward growth of the subnasal part of the maxillary body is accompanied by intensive apposition of bone at the free borders of the alveolar process. While the alveolar process grows in height at its free borders and the teeth continue to erupt, the basal part of the alveolar process becomes part of the maxillary body. The apposition at the alveolar crests not only contributes to the increase in height of the upper facial skeleton, but it also allows for proper adjustment of the alveolar process and the dental arch, especially during the eruption of the permanent dentition. During this time of change in the proportionate size of the members of the two dentitions, such an adjustment is especially necessary. At the same time, the

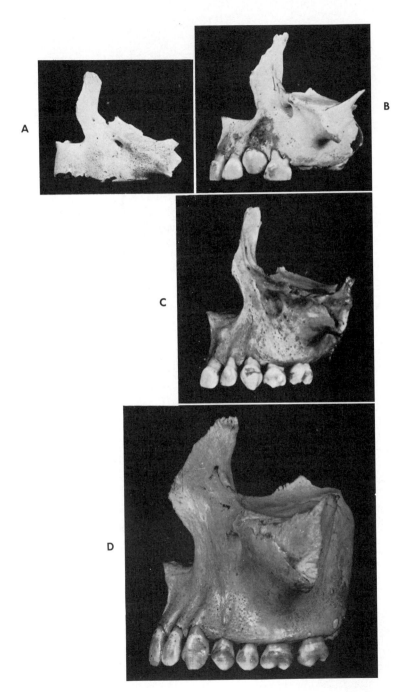

Fig. 2-84. Four stages in the development of maxilla. **A,** Newborn infant. **B,** 18 months of age. **C,** 4 years of age. **D,** 16 years of age.

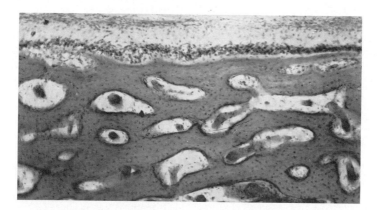

Fig. 2-85. Section through orbital floor of a 9-month-old child. Note layer of osteoblasts and seam of osteoid tissue, denoting rapid appositional growth. (Weinmann and Sicher: Bone and bones.)

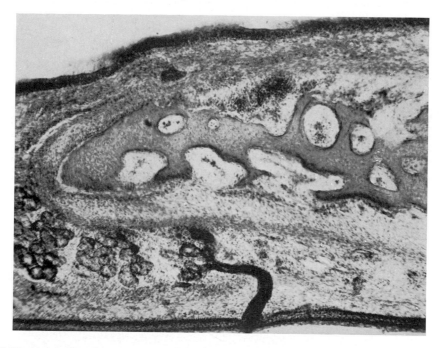

Fig. 2-86. Section through posterior end of hard palate of a human fetus of the seventh month. Note resorption of bone on nasal surfaces and apposition of bone on oral surfaces of trabeculae and apposition of bone at posterior margin. (Weinmann and Sicher: Bone and bones.)

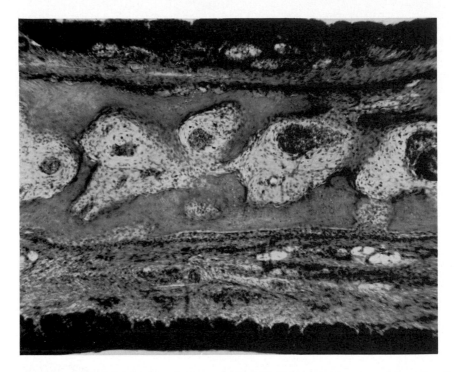

Fig. 2-87. Section through hard palate of a 9-month-old child. Note resorption on nasal (upper) surfaces and apposition on oral (lower) surfaces of the two bony plates that form hard palate. (Weinmann and Sicher: Bone and bones.)

growth of the alveolar process accounts for the transition from the flat curve of the infantile to the more highly arched curve of the adult palate. The downward shift of the hard palate, by resorption on its nasal and apposition on its oral surface, tends to obscure the downward growth of the alveolar process. The palate maintains a relation to the alveolar process that allows the most efficient buttressing of the dental arches by the pterygoid processes that, in turn, are correlated in their downward growth to the downward shift of the palate.

If the described phenomena explain the vertical and anteroposterior growth of the maxillary complex, the increase in transverse diameter, especially of the nasal part, has still to be accounted for. It is relatively slight in the anterior parts of the maxillary skeleton, which are, so to speak, shifted bodily and undergo only moderate adjusting changes by local apposition and resorption, for example, on the surfaces of the growing alveolar processes. The widening of the maxillary skeleton in its posterior parts, coincident with its growth in anteroposterior diameter, that is, the posterior divergence of the bony parts anchoring the dental arches, presents a problem because of the junction of the maxillary complex to the pterygoid processes of the sphenoid bone. Although the median palatine suture provides a site of adjusting the increasing transverse diameter, the pterygoid processes are but a part of the unpaired sphenoid bone. The adjustment of maxillary and interpterygoid width during growth is achieved by the downward divergence of the pterygoid processes. The growth of the pterygoid processes in postnatal life occurs by apposition at the free borders and surfaces and by corresponding modeling resorption. Because of the downward divergence of these processes, their increase in length by apposition at their lower ends will necessarily increase the distance of their inferior ends from one another. It is interesting that the distance of the upper ends of these processes from each other, a distance that equals twice the width of the upper border of the nasal choanae, increases only slightly after birth, an increase that can easily be accounted for by resorptive processes in this region.

It is evident that growth in the median palatine suture is simultaneous with and correlated to the widening of the downward-shifting and anteroposteriorly elongating maxillary complex. It is, furthermore, apparent that adjusting growth occurs in all the other sutures of the facial skeleton, as, for instance, between ethmoid, zygomatic, lacrimal, and nasal bones and those in contact with them.

The widening of the nasal cavities, especially of their lower part, lags for some time behind that of the dental arches. In children the bilateral width of the posterior part of the maxillae is relatively much greater than the distance between the lower ends of the pterygoid processes. This incongruence of lower nasal width and width of the developing alveolar processes is expressed in a lateral shift of the developing molars and thus a lateral bulging of the growing maxillary tuberosity. With the downgrowth of the maxillae, the downward shift of the hard palate, the lengthening of the divergent pterygoid processes, and the widening of the nasal cavity, the posterior end of the alveolar process is brought more and more in line with the lower end of the pterygoid process. Since this alignment is proportionate to the vertical growth of the upper face, the posterior end of the alveolar process and the pterygoid process coincide more in individuals with a high face (leptoprosopic type) than in those with a low face (euryprosopic type).

The problem of a human premaxilla has been resurrected again. The question of whether or not man has a premaxilla really involves two distinct questions. (1) Does man, in fetal or postnatal life, have an *independent* premaxilla? (2) Does man possess the *homologue* of the premaxillary bone of other mammals? The first question has to be answered in the negative. As a matter of fact, we know today that either the maxillary ossification center fuses with that of the maxilla per se almost immediately after its appearance or that—and this may be an individual variation—there is only one ossification center for both bony elements. The significance of this fact is the elimination in man of a site of growth in the upper face, namely the premaxillomaxillary suture.

However, man does possess the homologue of a premaxilla, the bone that carries the upper incisor teeth. Apart from other obvious homologies, the presence of a premaxilla, or the derivation of the human maxilla from the fusion of a premaxillary and a maxillary element, is still manifest in the development of separate premaxillary and maxillary palatine shelves that fuse to the maxillary palatine process. The line of fusion, the incisive fissure, is still plainly visible in the skulls of young persons.

Growth of the mandible

The growth of the upper facial skeleton is obviously closely correlated with that of the mandible. Mandibular growth can even be considered the leading factor of facial growth. The mechanism of mandibular growth, however, is entirely different from that of the maxillary part of the face. In the maxilla, the growth is largely sutural. In the mandible, however, a major growth site is at the surface of the cartilage in the mandibular condyle. The fact that proliferation of connective tissue and interstitial growth of the septal cartilage are the chief factors of growth in the upper facial skeleton but that appositional growth of cartilage is the chief factor of growth of the mandible explains a certain independence of the growth of these two parts of the facial skeleton and their different reactions to pathologic influences.

At birth, the mandible still consists of two halves separated in the midline by the symphyseal cartilage and connective tissue in which the mental bones develop. In postnatal life this suturelike junction does not seem to play any significant role as a site of growth. Although the mandible develops as a membrane bone lateral to, and at some distance from, Meckel's cartilage, secondary centers of hyaline cartilage differ-

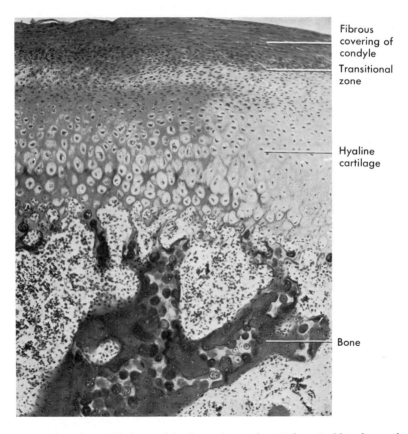

Fibrous
covering of
condyle

Transitional
zone

Hyaline
cartilage

Bone

Fig. 2-88. Section through mandibular condyle of a newborn infant. (Orban: Oral histology and embryology.)

entiate in the growing mandible to take an important part in its growth. The second-ary cartilages at the tip of the coronoid process and at the mandibular angle disappear long before birth, but the cartilage in the condyle persists as the most important growth site of the mandible. The secondary appearance of the condylar cartilage is evidently an adaptation to growth of the mandible at a site of pressure, namely, at the articular end; throughout the body secondary cartilages appear at sites subjected to pressure and intermittent motion.

Since the condylar cartilage of the mandible is covered by a thick layer of con-nective tissue, dense in the superficial and loose in the deep layers (Fig. 2-88), the cartilage cannot be compared with an articular cartilage of tubular bones or to an epiphyseal plate, even though growth of the mandible does occur in the condyle by growth of the cartilage and its gradual replacement by bone just as in the cartilages of tubular bones. The covering of connective tissue enables the cartilage to increase in thickness almost entirely by appositional growth, whereas the cartilages of long bones, both articular and epiphyseal, and the cartilages at the cranial base thicken by interstitial growth only. The hyaline cartilage in the head of the mandible, therefore, holds a unique position and differs widely from that of other cartilaginous growth centers in its reaction to certain pathologic conditions.

Growth of the condylar cartilage contributes to the increase in height of the man-dibular ramus, to the increase of the overall length of the mandible, and to the increase of intercondylar distance. The longitudinal growth can be measured either by taking the distance between condyle and chin point (gnathion) or by measuring the distance from the gnathion to a point where a perpendicular tangent to the posterior surface of the condyle meets the gnathion-gonion line (Fig. 2-89, A). Condylar growth has this combined effect on height and length of the mandible because the condyle is linked to the body of the mandible by the obliquely ascending ramus.

The overall length of the mandible increases by condylar growth, but not the length of the mandibular body; nor does the condylar growth contribute to the nec-essary increase of the anteroposterior width of the ramus itself. Here, appositional growth of bone on the entire posterior border of the ramus is the mechanism for adjusting the width of the ramus and the length of the body to the growing height of the ramus (Fig. 2-90, B). Appositional growth at the tip and the upper borders of the coronoid process keeps pace with the heightening of the ramus. At the same time, resorption along the anterior border of the coronoid process and the ramus corrects the anteroposterior dimension of the ramus and increases the alveolar space distally. This is an excellent example of "relocation" of a segment of bone, since bone tissue that once formed the upper, posterior border of the ramus now rests in the posterior body of the jaw (Fig. 2-90).

The height of the mandibular body, measured from the lower border of the man-dible to the free border of the alveolar process, increases almost exclusively by appo-sition of bone at the free borders of the alveolar process, which grows into the space opened by the growth of the mandibular ramus in height. Growth at the condyle results in a downward and forward shift of the entire mandible so that upper and lower teeth and alveolar processes tend to become ever more distant from each other. The alveolar processes maintain normal distance by growth at their free borders, and the teeth maintain contact by continued vertical eruption. During the growth in height of the alveolar process and the concomitant eruption of the teeth, more and more of the alveolar process, vacated by the moving teeth, is incorporated into the mandibular body. This process is also responsible for the increasing distance between the mandibular canal and the apices of premolars and first and second permanent molars.

The projecting chin is as unique to man as is upright posture. In the adjustment of skull balance on the erect vertebral column the jaws have been severely retruded, leaving the lower border of the mandible everted to allow space for the vital structures behind, such as the tongue, pharynx, and airway. The anterior end of the lower

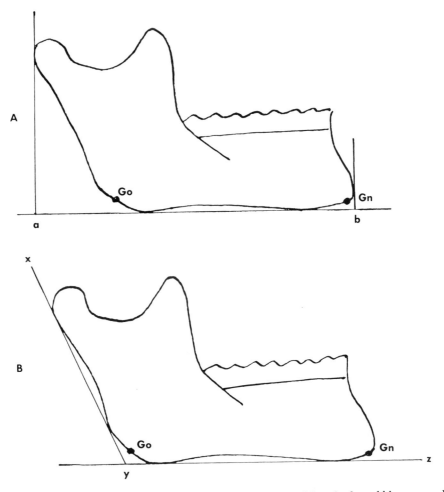

Fig. 2-89. Diagrams of mandible: *Gn*, gnathion; *Go*, gonion; *ab*, overall length of mandible; *xyz*, condylar angle. (Weinmann and Sicher: Bone and bones.)

border is subjected to bending from the squeezing action of the masticatory muscles, which are all close to the back end of the mandible. The bending is braced lingually by the "simian shelf" of bone in horizontally postured animals like the baboon. But because lingual space is crowded in man, bony reinforcement is added labially as the mental protuberance, or chin. The remodeling growth process sculpturing the chin is beautifully demonstrated in the marked resorption of bone across the alveolar area above and bony apposition at the chin below. At the same time, depending on how far the whole jaw is carried forward with condylar growth, a variable amount of space is provided for some lingual apposition.

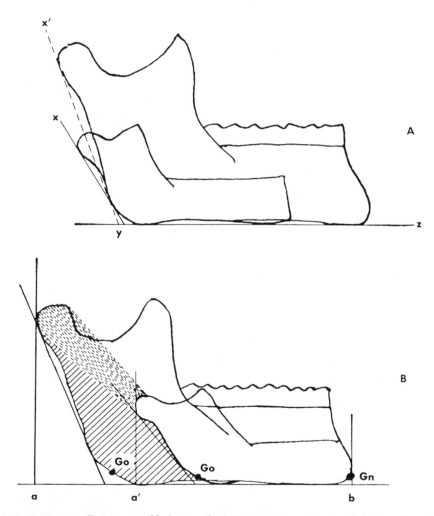

Fig. 2-90. Diagrams to illustrate mandibular growth. **A,** Superposition at gonion of outlines of an infantile and an adult mandible. Decrease of condylar angle xyz to $x'yz$. Outline of gonial angle remains unchanged. **B,** Superposition at gnathion of outlines of an infantile and an adult mandible. Stippled area, increment of ramus by cartilaginous growth; hatched area, increment of ramus by appositional growth of bone. (Weinmann and Sicher: Bone and bones.)

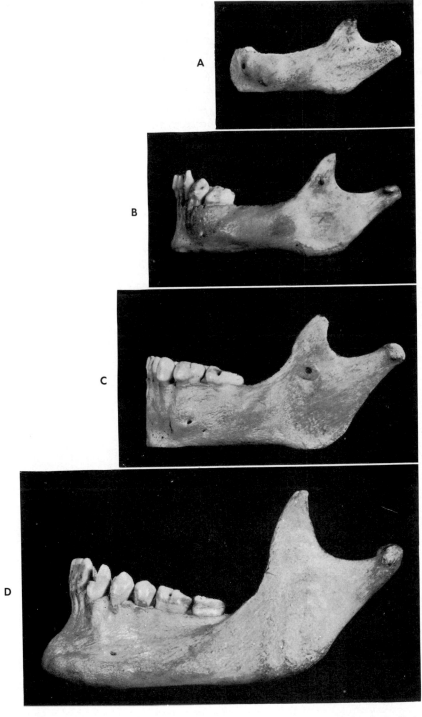

Fig. 2-91. Four stages in development of mandible. **A,** Newborn infant, **B,** 18 months of age. **C,** 4 years of age. **D,** 16 years of age.

Apposition of bone at the lower mandibular border and in the region of the chin serves not so much for the enlargement as for the modeling and strengthening of the lower jaw. Changes in the shape of the alveolar process, especially during the replacement of the deciduous by the permanent teeth, occur during the vertical growth of the alveolar process. It is, therefore, incorrect to visualize this adaptation as a direct horizontal change of the deciduous maxillary or mandibular arch. Instead, this permanent arch is an entirely new formation adjusted to the permanent dentition during its vertical growth (Fig. 2-91).

Serial radiographs have shown that the contour of the mandibular angle does not appreciably change for some time (Fig. 2-92). This observation seems to contradict the often repeated assertion that the mandibular angle decreases during the period of growth. In reality, there is merely a difference in the definition of the term "mandibular angle" and the method of measuring it. Anthropologically the mandibular angle is measured by placing the mandible on a table to which a hinged leaf is fastened (Fig. 2-90, *B*). This leaf is placed in such a position that it touches the posterior border of the mandibular ramus at two points, one near the condyle and the other near the mandibular angle. The inclination of the movable leaf to the table is then measured as mandibular angle. This angle does change despite the fact that the contour of the angular region is fairly stable. The confusion can be easily eliminated by calling the contour of the angular region the "gonial" angle, whereas the anthropologic angle is called the "condylar" angle. Only the condylar angle is an angle in the geometric

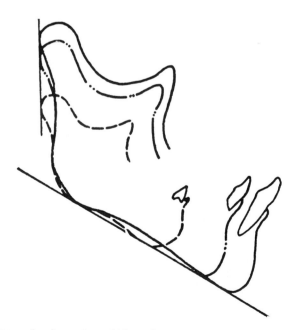

Fig. 2-92. Superposition of outlines of mandible in three stages of growth. Note stability of contour of gonial angle and change in inclination of condylar process to lower border of mandible. (After Brodie; Weinmann and Sicher: Bone and bones.)

sense. It is significant for the constancy of the pattern during growth that the gonial angle does remain fairly constant, but it is equally significant that the condylar angle decreases during the period of growth (Figs. 2-90, *A*, and 2-91).

The changes of the condylar angle are caused by a change in the direction of growth of the condylar cartilage. In the first years of life the plane of growth is inclined more than in later years. In other words, at first the increase of mandibular length exceeds the increase in mandibular height. During this period the condylar angle is wide. After the length of the dental arch has almost been established, the face continues to grow in height. It is the change in the direction of condylar growth that causes the gradual decrease of the condylar angle with increase in height now predominating over increase in length.

Since the two halves of the mandible diverge posteriorly, the growth of the mandible in its anteroposterior diameter is necessarily associated with an increase in transverse diameter, or intercondylar distance.

The growth of the mandible at the condylar cartilage is indispensable for the normal vertical growth of the upper face. Growth at the condyle moves the mandibular body forward and downward and thus opens the space below the cranial base into which mandibular and maxillary alveolar processes grow and teeth erupt. Therefore disorders of mandibular growth lead secondarily to changes in the upper face. In the majority of individuals these changes involve only the subnasal part of the maxilla.

After loss of all teeth, especially if no denture is worn, the condylar angle widens again. This change is often referred to as a senile change. It is, however, not the age of the individual but the loss of function that plays the decisive role; in other words, the change is to be defined as disuse atrophy. The loss of bone where masseter and medial pterygoid muscles attach at the lower and posterior border of the gonial area leads not only to a widening of the condylar angle, but also to a radical change of the bony outline and thus to a change of the gonial angle.

Facial growth and tooth eruption

The correlation between teeth and jaws has often been interpreted in the sense that the presence of teeth in their proper number and relation is necessary for the normal growth of the jaws. This assumption is erroneous. In many animals it can be observed that the development of the teeth and that of the jaws are highly independent. This same independence in the human being can be demonstrated in cases of anodontia where, despite a total lack of teeth, the jaws develop to a fairly normal size. It is, however, true that development and growth of the alveolar processes are dependent on the development and eruption of the teeth. Not only does no alveolar process, in the strict sense of the word, develop if a tooth or teeth are absent, but the alveolar process also disappears if teeth are lost.

Although the dependence of bone growth on the development of teeth is slight, the reverse relation, that is, the dependence of tooth development, and especially tooth eruption, on growth of bone and bones, is considerable. The influence of the growth of the facial skeleton on the eruption of teeth is threefold. The growth of maxilla and mandible, in an anteroposterior direction, provides the necessary space for the successive eruption of the posterior teeth. Growth in height of the maxilla and mandible, accompanied by the vertical growth of the mandibular ramus, is necessary for the free vertical eruption of the teeth. Finally, growth of bone tissue in the maxilla and mandible is one of the "forces" of eruption.

The correlation between anteroposterior growth of the jaws and eruption of the teeth can best be observed in studying the position and movement of the permanent molars during their eruption. In a child 3 years of age, for instance, the jaws are just long enough to accommodate the deciduous teeth. The first permanent molars, at this time already far advanced in their development, are found in the maxillary tuberosity and in the root of the mandibular ramus. The occlusal surface of the upper molar faces backward and downward, and that of the lower faces forward and upward. During the succeeding years these teeth undergo movements that place their crowns in the right plane; that is, their occlusal surfaces become parallel to those of the deciduous teeth. These rotary movements are possible only if the upper and lower jaws lengthen to such an extent that sufficient space is created behind the last deciduous teeth to receive the first permanent molars. The same process repeats itself after the sixth year of life, when the second molars undergo the last phases of crown development and go through the same rotary movements as did the first molars. The same correlated changes occur for the third time before the eruption of the third molars.

During this last phase of molar eruption, disturbances in the correlation between the growth of the jaws and the eruption of the third molars occur rather frequently. The primary reason for this seems to be that the third molars in modern man are rudimentary and consequently vary greatly in shape and size. Not infrequently one or more of the four third molars are missing. Another consequence is the often delayed development and eruption of the third molars and the great variability in the time of their eruption.

The loss of the third molar, and thus the reduction of the dentition, is but one phase in the reduction of the masticatory apparatus in the evolution of man. The second phase is the reduction of the facial skeleton, most strikingly expressed in the gradual loss of facial protrusion. The reduction in length of the jaws and the reduction of the dentition are not fully correlated. This leads to frequent disharmonies between length of the jaws in an anteroposterior direction and length of the dental arch. It seems that the shortening of the jaws is, in modern man, already further advanced and more firmly fixed than the shortening of the dentition. The reduction of space for the third molars is enhanced in many individuals by the fact that the third molars erupt at a time when the general growth of the individual and that of the jaws is already nearing its end.

The frequent impaction or total embedding of the third molars is thus easily understood. It remains only to be explained why the lower third molar is so much more frequently affected by this discordance between bone growth and tooth development than the upper third molar. The preeruptive position of these two teeth gives a clue to their different behavior. The upper third molar, developing in the maxillary tuberosity, faces downward and backward. If sutural growth of the maxilla at its posterior end is inadequate, the rotation of the third molar into its proper position will be inhibited. If this tooth continues its eruptive movement in the direction of its long axis, it will not encounter any obstacle and will erupt, though in a more or less abnormal axial position.

The lower third molar faces upward and forward during its development. If sufficient space is not provided for its preeruptive rotation, and if it starts to erupt in the direction of its abnormally inclined long axis, its crown moves toward the root or crown of the second molar and its movement is, sooner or later, arrested.

The space for the vertical growth of alveolar processes and for the vertical eruption of the teeth is created and increased by the growth in height of the mandibular ramus. In this way the body of the mandible is moved away from the cranial base, and both maxillary and mandibular alveolar processes grow toward each other. The different rate of growth of the mandibular condyle is responsible for the different rate of vertical eruption under varying conditions. Thus an inhibition of this growth, as in mandibular retrusion, causes an undereruption of the molars and premolars. In mandibular protrusion, in which the mandibular ramus is too high, we find the premolars and molars overerupted.

The influence of growth of *bone tissue*, in contrast to growth of the facial *bones*, on the eruption of teeth is discussed in Chapter 5 (p. 278).

Growth of the pneumatic cavities of the skull

Development and growth of the air-filled cavities of the skull can be understood only if their functional significance is clarified. These spaces develop as evaginations of the nasal cavity or as expansions of the cavity of the middle ear into the adjacent bones. They are lined by an extension of the mucous membrane of the cavity with which they communicate.

The pneumatic spaces can be likened, in a mechanical way, to the large marrow spaces in the tubular bones. The marrow space replaces the central part of the shaft of a long bone, where bony substance would not contribute materially to a greater mechanical efficiency of the bone. A solid bone would carry only a slightly greater load, but it would be heavier and would need stronger muscles for its movement, and thus the level of functional adaptation would be lowered. Mechanical requirements of the same type are at work in certain regions of the skull. Wherever the spongy core of a bone of the skull is not under mechanical forces, the bone tissue is removed. Marrow is not deposited in its place, however; rather, the bone is made hollow by a diverticulum of the adjacent air-conducting passages. This explains the peculiarities in the development and growth of the air spaces of the skull and eliminates many erroneous interpretations. It is, for instance, contrary to the sequence of events to contend that a bone failed to grow to its normal size because the air space contained in it did not fully expand. In reality, just the reverse is true. The growth of the bone was inhibited primarily, and therefore the air space, hollowing it out, remained smaller than normal. It is also a confusion of cause and effect to claim that bones enlarge because the contained air space or sinus expanded. Overgrowth of the bone is primary, and the expansion of the sinus is secondary.

From this point of view it can also be understood that air sinuses enlarge at an age when the normal growth of the individual has ceased. The enlargement of certain sinuses in old age is explained by the fact that at this time the mechanical stresses in the skull diminish, especially if teeth are lost and the masticatory apparatus is weakened. It can also be understood that even in young individuals certain sinuses enlarge, sometimes in a rather irregular manner, if parts of the bone that they occupy lose their mechanical function.

The air spaces that have to be considered in this discussion are the following: frontal sinus, maxillary sinus, and sphenoid sinus, all evaginations of the nasal cavity, and the cells of the mastoid process, originating in the cavity of the middle ear and indirectly communicating with the respiratory tract via the tympanic tube.

The frontal sinus develops at the time when the supraorbital ridge arises as a buttress for the masticatory forces. In the first year of life the outer and inner plates of the frontal bone are closely applied to each other, whereas later, starting in the second year of life, the outer plate is bent away from the inner plate, and a potential space is created between the two compact layers of the bone (see Fig. 2-79). Into this space extends a diverticulum of the most anterior cell of the ethmoid labyrinth, thereby giving rise to the frontal sinus. The enlargement of the sinus proceeds simultaneously with the differentiation of the supraorbital region and is directed upward, medially, and laterally. If the prominence of the superciliary ridges is correlated to the strength of the masticatory stresses, it seems contradictory that the reinforcement of this region is in part counteracted by the hollowing out of the bone. One has to visualize the apposition of bone in the supraorbital region not only as a reinforcement, but also as a forward shift of the supraorbital buttress. Since this shift is effected by continuous apposition of bone at the outer surface, much of this new bone is of only temporary value. After the sinus has developed, the result is a sufficiently strong bar of bone in the correct forward position.

The two frontal sinuses are almost always asymmetrical and are separated from each other by a thin, irregularly bent septum. In later years, when reduction or loss of function of the masticatory apparatus permits a further thinning of the compact plates of the frontal bone, the sinus expands more and more and may hollow out the orbital roof to a variable extent. This senile enlargement of the sinus furnishes additional evidence that mechanical causes determine the origin and growth of the air spaces. A thinning of the bones of the skull is a general feature of old age. Flat and wide depressions on the outer surface of the parietal bones, for instance, can often be observed in the skulls of deceased elderly persons and are sometimes even visible in the living. Here the decrease in substance is effected by resorption at the outer surface of the bone. In areas where air spaces are contained in the bone, the bony plates are thinned out from within.

The sphenoid sinus of the adult is, in reality, the fusion of a posterosuperior recess of the nasal cavity with a cavity occupying the body of the sphenoid bone. In the newborn infant the body of the sphenoid bone proper consists of uniformly arranged spongy bone. A "sphenoid sinus" is restricted to a small cavity in front of the sphenoid body. It is surrounded by a thin concave bony plate, the sphenoid concha, which later fuses with the anterior surface of the sphenoid bone. In the second year of postnatal life, the hollowing out of the body of the sphenoid bone commences and thereby the sphenoid sinus in the strict sense is developed. The enlargement of the sinus proceeds in many persons far into old age. In middle age the sphenoid sinuses occupy the central part of the sphenoid body, separated from each other by a thin, rarely symmetrical septum. They reach posteriorly to the level of the hypophyseal fossa, which causes a bulge into the cavity of the sinus at its superoposterior wall. Later, the sinus may expand considerably in all directions. It may invade the occipital bone, the roots of the lesser sphenoid wings, and the pterygoid processes. If the expansion hollows out the root of the lesser wing, the sinus may gradually envelop the optic canal, with the exception of a thin plate of bone connecting the bony wall of the optic canal with the cerebral surface of the lesser wing. A similar relation can develop between an inferior or pterygoid recess of the sphenoid sinus and the pterygoid canal. It is evident that these close relations of the sinus and the nerves contained in the optic and pterygoid canals are of clinical importance.

The maxillary sinus develops as an evagination from the middle nasal meatus in the last months of fetal life. At birth the sinus is still an insignificant cavity smaller than a pea (Fig. 2-93). Its growth is largely dependent on the eruption of the deciduous, and later the permanent, teeth. The germs of the deciduous teeth and, later, although to a lesser degree, those of the permanent teeth occupy the maxillary body. Only after eruption of these teeth can the maxillary sinus expand into the space formerly occupied by the developing teeth. At puberty the maxillary sinus reaches its average size. At this time the sinus is bounded by thin bony walls toward the orbit, toward the canine fossa, and in the region of the maxillary tuberosity. It reaches downward into the root of the alveolar process.

In most individuals the maxillary sinus continues to expand throughout life. The most frequent expansion penetrates deeper into the alveolar process, thus establishing a more and more intimate relation to the apices of the roots of the second premolars and the three molars. In later age the sinus expands mainly in two directions. The zygomatic process of the maxilla is sometimes hollowed completely and, after closure of the zygomaticomaxillary suture, the sinus may even invade the body of the zygomatic bone. Another expansion of the sinus, the infraorbital recess, is directed anterosuperiorly. If it develops, the infraorbital canal is increasingly carved out from the roof of the maxillary sinus. The canal may then protrude into the sinus, separated from its space by only a thin plate of bone, and defects of even this separating bony plate may develop. Sometimes the maxillary sinus extends into the root of the palatine process to form a palatine recess, and sometimes it extends into the posterior, superior, and medial corner of the maxilla and even into the orbital process of the palatine bone. In most individuals the gradual expansion of the maxillary sinus and

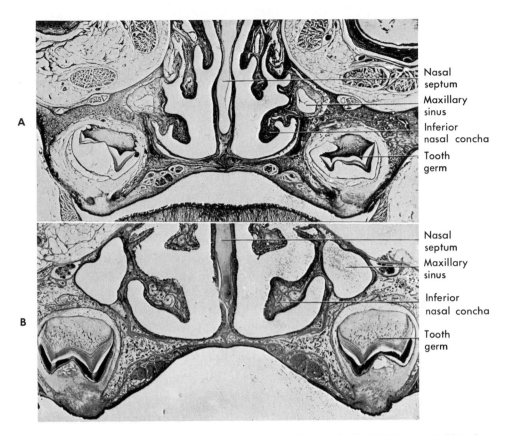

Nasal septum

Maxillary sinus

Inferior nasal concha

Tooth germ

Nasal septum

Maxillary sinus

Inferior nasal concha

Tooth germ

Fig. 2-93. Frontal sections through head. **A,** Newborn infant. **B,** 9-month-old child. (Orban: Oral histology and embryology.)

the thinning of its anterolateral and posterolateral walls open from within the narrow canals of the superior alveolar nerves, so that the nerves themselves are for some distance in immediate contact with the lining membrane of the sinus. This is why an acute inflammation of the sinus is frequently accompanied by pain in groups of maxillary teeth.

The pneumatic cells of the mastoid process develop simultaneously with the mastoid process itself. At birth the mastoid process is absent, and of the pneumatic cavities only the mastoid antrum, a posterosuperior recess of the middle ear cavity, is established. This is the point from which in the second year of life the gradual pneumatization of the mastoid process commences. As yet, the fact that the mastoid process is not hollowed out by one single air cavity but by a system of communicating cells cannot be explained. The size and number of these cells are variable, and occasionally their development is entirely suppressed. The mastoid process in such instances is filled with a variably dense spongiosa.

Variations and anomalies of the neurocranium

Measurements of the skull and head have been used not only for descriptive purposes, but also as a means to differentiate the races of man. It has to be stressed that no one measurement or proportion exists that could be said to be characteristic of a particular human race. The differentiation of racial groups is possible only because a certain combination of a number of somatic characteristics is found more often in one population than in any other. Racial concepts and descriptions are therefore of a statistical nature, and the single individual may or may not conform to the concept of his race.

In the neurocranium great value has been placed and is still being placed on the cephalic or the cranial index. Whether an individual has a long or a short skull and head has seemed to be of great importance. Though dolichocephaly and brachycephaly are characteristic of some races, if they are combined with other physical characteristics, they have no influence at all on the development of the brain. In this connection three examples may be quoted showing that (1) growth of the skull is dependent on the growth of the brain, (2) the attainment of the inherited brain size is, as a rule, not impaired by anomalies of the growth pattern of the skull, and (3) it seems impossible to prevent the brain from growing by artificial disfiguration of the growing head and skull.

In microcephalic individuals, growth of the brain and its capsule is arrested. The idea that the arrest of bone growth, for instance, by premature closure of the sutures, may have prevented the normal growth of the brain has been proved erroneous. As a matter of fact, in at least some of the microcephalic skulls the sutures remain open far beyond the time of their normal fusion. Microcephaly should properly be called "microencephaly," that is, smallness of the brain.

Premature closure of one or several sutures of the cranium has frequently been observed. Not much is known about the time of this abnormal occurrence. However, if the tempo of cerebral growth is considered, one can assume that a premature ossification of a suture that distorts the proportions of the skull and head must occur in the early years of life, probably some time before the sixth year. If one of the sutures of the calvaria closes before the normal size of the brain and its capsule is attained, an important site of growth is eliminated. It is interesting to observe how the loss of a site of growth is compensated for by what could be called an "emergency pattern of growth." Though the change of the pattern permits the attainment of a normal volume of the brain, the shape and proportions of the brain, skull, and head are considerably altered.

A characteristic picture develops, for instance, in consequence of premature ossification of the interparietal, or sagittal, suture. Though nothing definite is known, premature closure of this suture probably occurs in the second year of life by an abnormal posterior continuation of the normal closure of the interfrontal, or metopic, suture. A skull with fused parietals cannot expand sufficiently in the transverse diameter and, to compensate for this loss, it grows long and often shows a characteristic constriction in the postfrontal area. Such skulls are termed "scaphocephalic" because of the resemblance of the calvaria to a boat.

Oxycephaly, or acrocephaly, develops by a premature synostosis of the coronal suture. The interruption of longitudinal growth leads to an overaccentuated growth in height. The synonymous term "turricephaly," from the Latin word for tower, is descriptive of this anomaly of cranial growth.

Many peoples have, at one time or another in the history of mankind, changed the shape of the head of their offspring by artificial means. This habit, known in many regions of the globe, served in all probability to achieve a mystic ideal of head configuration and was sometimes the prerogative of the ruling class. Bandages or wooden appliances of some kind gave the desired result if the treatment started early enough. In other instances, the infant was traditionally held in a fixed position, for instance, bound to a board on his back. The forces of gravity then led to typical changes of the configuration of the head. Nothing is known to indicate that any one of these procedures had any influence on the size and the normal function of the brain, though the shape of the head was sometimes grotesquely changed.

The influence of relatively light forces acting over a long period of time has even led to the belief that dolichocephaly and brachycephaly are not inherited patterns but are mechanically caused. Some evidence has been introduced that tends to substantiate the claim that the habitual position of the infant on his side elongates the head, positioning of the infant on his back shortens the head. However, it seems that these mechanical influences, if they are active, will serve only to accentuate or slightly obscure a genetic pattern of the skull.

Another observation seems to be based on better evidence and is of even greater significance. It has been shown that environment in the widest sense of the word has a definite influence on the cephalic index. The offspring of immigrants into the United States show a tendency toward mesocephaly. The offspring of long-headed Sicilians, for instance, already show in the second generation a tendency to mesocephaly, that is, a shortening of their heads. The descendants of extremely short or round-headed East European Jews, on the other hand, show a tendency to elongation of the head that is also a tendency toward mesocephaly. However, these observations are still controversial.

In attempts to estimate the development of the brain from the proportions of the skull and the head, one more fact has to be considered: in a strict sense, only the inner plates of the cranial bones form the brain capsule, whereas the outer plates develop as cranial superstructures under the influence of mechanical forces impressed on them by the musculature. An analysis of the variations in configuration and inclination of the forehead shows the danger of such reasoning. The opinion often is voiced that a high forehead is a sign of great mental capacity, whereas a low or sloping forehead indicates an underdevelopment of the brain. However, the angle of inclination of the forehead is dependent on two factors, the size of the frontal lobes of the brain and, indirectly, on the development of the masticatory apparatus. In an individual with heavy jaws and strong masticatory muscles, especially if this is combined with a "bimaxillary protrusion" or total facial prognathism, the outer plate of the frontal bone in the supraorbital region grows to a strongly prominent and bulging superciliary arch, serving as a buttress for the masticatory pressure. The accentuation of this frontal superstructure changes the high forehead of a young individual gradually into a more receding forehead.

Variations and anomalies of the facial skeleton

The variations of the facial skeleton can be classified into two main categories. The first category deals with the differences in proportion of facial height and breadth, the second category with the variations of the facial profile angles.

The extreme types of high and narrow and low and broad faces are to some degree correlated with the general body build. There is less correlation between the facial proportions and the cranial index. The correlation between the proportions of the face and those of the body as a whole is explainable by the leading role that the mandible plays in the development of the facial proportions. Height of the mandibular ramus determines not only the variations of the mandible itself, but also those of the upper facial skeleton. While the mandibular ramus gains in height, the body of the mandible grows away from the cranial base and the maxillary body, and into the widening space grow both mandibular and maxillary alveolar processes. The growth of the mandibular ramus in height occurs by growth of the condylar cartilage. The more accentuated cartilaginous growth is, the higher will be the mandibular ramus and thus the entire face. Accentuated cartilaginous growth in the bones of trunk and limbs is responsible for the development of high stature and, in extreme cases, for the establishment of the linear body type.

That the correlation between face and body is not complete is caused by the interference of two factors. Though the growth of the mandible in height and length depends mainly on the growth of the condylar cartilage, this cartilage is not at all comparable to the epiphyseal cartilages of other bones. The latter grow in longitudinal direction only by interstitial growth, whereas the mandibular cartilage grows mainly by apposition. In addition, the final proportions of the face depend to a high degree on the inherited facial breadth. The euryprosopic type has not only a lower, but also an absolutely broader face than the leptoprosopic individual.

The variations in the profile of the human face are caused not only by the variations in the absolute size of facial angles, but also by the independent variations of different parts of the face. Prognathism can be a total facial prognathism or, in the terms of the orthodontic literature, a bimaxillary protrusion. This type of facial development was characteristic for all extinct races of mankind. Its degree is also one of the more important racial characteristics of modern man.

Upper facial prognasthism, or maxillary prognathism, involves the maxillae to a higher degree than the lower part of the face. If only the nasal part of the maxilla protrudes and the alveolar process approaches a more vertical position, the prognathism is diagnosed as nasal, or middle facial, prognathism. In contrast to this type, the alveolar, or subnasal, prognathism shows an isolated obliquity and protrusion of the alveolar process of the upper jaw. Also in the mandible a total and an alveolar mandibular prognathism can be distinguished. In total mandibular prognathism the entire mental plate is obliquely inclined, but in alveolar prognathism only the alveolar process is so inclined.

The reduction of the prognathism leads gradually to orthognathism. The differentiation is arbitrary according to the angular measurements enumerated before (see section on anthropological remarks in this chapter).

One of the most important facts in understanding facial anomalies is that the size of facial angles can vary widely without a break in facial harmony or the harmonious relation between upper and lower face, expressed in the proper occlusal relations of the upper and lower teeth. A total facial prognathism, for instance, may violate our concept of facial esthetics and as such may be an indication for orthodontic interference; however, total facial prognathism cannot be considered an anomaly.

On the other hand, the proportions of upper and lower face can be dissociated either in favor of maxillary or mandibular development. But underdevelopment of the mandible, for instance, or its overgrowth, is independent of facial configuration as expressed in the angulations of the upper face. In other words, a mandibular underdevelopment or overgrowth may occur in individuals with an orthognathous or prognathous face. The disharmonies of the face can best be classified according to Angle's terminology. If the mandible is relatively too short, the lower teeth occlude distally to their upper antagonists. This is a malocclusion of Class II. If the mandible is relatively too long and the chin protrudes too far, the lower teeth are in mesioclusion. This is a malocclusion of Class III.

It is difficult to decide whether in a Class II malocclusion case the disharmony is caused by an arrest in growth of the mandible or whether the mandible appears to be too small because of a primary overdevelopment of the maxilla, or whether, as has been claimed, the disharmony is caused by a displacement of the craniomandibular articulation. The same questions, of course, have to be asked in cases of Class III.

That probably the majority of facial disharmonies develop as a consequence of disturbance of mandibular growth seems indicated by the following facts. The growth of the mandible shows throughout the intrauterine and early postnatal development a characteristic curve that is different from, and to some degree independent of, that of maxillary growth. Young embryos show a typical micrognathism that later, at the time of palatine closure, reverses itself into a temporary mandibular protrusion. Still later, the growth of the mandible again lags behind that of the maxilla, and a fetus in the second half of pregnancy is, as a rule, characterized by a receding chin. Usually before birth, but sometimes only in the first months after birth, the mandible gains in its growth so that the normal proportions of upper and lower jaws are established.

The assumption that most occlusal anomalies are caused by deviations of mandibular growth is supported by two additional facts. (1) Most individuals show facial harmony despite the almost endless cranial variations. This is not only true for variations of facial angles, but also for variations of the cranial base angle between the lines nasion-sella and sella-basion and for anteroposterior relations of the articular eminence and the craniomandibular articulation. (2) It must be remembered that in the mode of growth the mandible is unique because its growth cartilage enlarges by appositional rather than by interstitial growth, that is, by differentiation of proliferated cells rather than by proliferation of differentiated cells.

If the primary cause of facial disharmonies were a disturbance of maxillary growth or a variation in the position of the craniomandibular articulation on the cranial base, some findings frequently associated with Class II and Class III malocclusion could hardly be explained. They are, however, readily understood as a consequence of primary underdevelopment or overgrowth of the mandible. Such observations are, for instance, the general shortness of the face and the undereruption of premolars and molars in distoclusion and the opposite findings in mesioclusion of the mandible. In other words, many individuals with a Class II malocclusion are euryprosopic; most individuals with a Class III malocclusion are leptoprosopic.

That the isolated mandible of most individuals with either one of these common facial disharmonies appears to be normal, and that it falls inside the range of variation of shape and measurements, cannot be used as an argument against the primary significance of the mandible in the causation of these anomalies. It is just as true that the isolated cranium of such individuals would only rarely permit a diagnosis of a facial disharmony if the position of the teeth were disregarded.

There is another aspect to skeletal disproportions or disharmonies. In the mandible and in that complex of bones that constitutes the upper face, there are two most important sites of growth: in the mandible it is the cartilage in the condyle whose appositional growth determines the overall dimensions of the mandible; in the maxilla it is the nasal septum and sutures that join maxilla to frontal bone, to zygomatic bone, to palatine bone, and to sphenoid bone. This complex of sutures plays the same role for the overall dimensions of the maxillary bones as the cartilage in the condyle of the mandible plays for the overall size of the mandible. But apart from any other sites of bone apposition or growth of bone tissue, there are in the maxilla as well as in the mandible sites of bone apposition that are of great importance, namely, the free edges of the alveolar process. The total height of the maxilla or mandible is dependent not only on growth of the sutures or the condylar cartilages, but also on the growth of the alveolar processes that is simultaneous with the eruption of the teeth. These two sites of growth, sutures and condyles on one hand and alveolar processes on the other, are widely separated. Though under normal conditions there is a complete correlation between these sites of growth, this correlation sometimes may be broken. The growth of the mandibular condyle, removing, as it were, the mandibular body from the base of the skull, creates a space between maxilla and mandible into which the alveolar processes of both of these bones grow and into which upper and lower teeth erupt. However, there are many cases in which, for some unknown reason, the alveolar processes, crudely speaking, seem not to be able to take advantage of the space that is provided for their growth and thus do not grow to their full height. This development is characterized by an abnormal increase of the free-way space, or interocclusal clearance: the mandibular ramus grows to a normal height; therefore, the elevators of the mandible, masseter, medial pterygoid, and temporal muscles grow to their normal length, and thus the rest position of the mandibular body is normal. But since mandibular and maxillary alveolar processes have not grown to their full height, too wide a space remains between upper and lower teeth. This disproportion can be diagnosed from far away if one observes the profile at rest and in occlusion, because in occlusion the lips are pursed and the face has a similarity to the face of an edentulous person.

The variations in formation of the palate also play an important role in the orthodontic literature; especially the combination of mouth breathing with high palate and a collapsed, V-shaped upper dental arch is fairly frequent. The pathogenesis of this malformation of the skeleton seems to start with a deficiency of the modeling resorption at the nasal floor. The next consequence is a failure of the normal downward shift of the hard palate by resorption on its superior surface and apposition on its inferior surface. The vertical growth of the alveolar processes at their free borders, however, continues in correlation to the growth of the mandible. There is no balance between the length of the buttressing pterygoid processes and the height of the alveolar process, and the break of this correlation may be responsible for the "collapse" of the growing upper arch. Whether the lack of expansion of the nasal cavity is primary or whether it is the consequence of an impairment of nasal breathing by adenoids, the hypertrophy of the pharyngeal tonsil, is still questionable.

Though the growth of the mandible is to a high degree dependent on the growth of the condylar cartilage, mandibular growth does not entirely cease if the condylar cartilages have been destroyed. In such cases, for instance, after traumatic ankylosis of the craniomandibular joints in early life, the mandible and face attain a characteristic shape. Though the mandible grows, it never gains normal size, the chin recedes considerably, and the face in profile has a birdlike appearance; hence the German term "Vogelgesicht." The mandibular ramus remains relatively short, whereas the height of the mandibular body increases much more. The disproportion in the vertical dimensions of ramus and body causes a deep notching of the lower border of the mandible in front of the mandibular angle. We deal in such cases with an emergency growth pattern of the mandible, which, in essence, is comparable to the growth pattern that was discussed for the cranium after premature closure of a suture. The growth of the cranium, although distorted, continues under the leading influence of cerebral growth. The distorted growth of the mandible in an ankylosis of the jaw occurs mainly under the influence of the growth and function of the tongue and pharynx. The pattern of growth is entirely changed, the body of the mandible gaining in length and height by apposition of bone at the outer surfaces (especially on the lower border) and modeling resorption on the inner surfaces. Accentuation of bone apposition on the lower border of the mandibular body in front of the attachment of the masseter muscle and lack of proportionate apposition at the lower border in the region of the angle may account for the notching of the lower border of the mandible.

CHAPTER 3

The musculature

GENERAL FEATURES
Contractile structures

Muscles are structures specially adapted to produce movement. They have evolved by elaboration of the basic protoplasmic aptitude for contraction. All muscle cells are elongated along their lines of contraction, and three major categories of these fibers are recognized. Cardiac muscle is confined to the heart and so plays no part in the special system of concern here. Visceral (smooth) muscle and skeletal (striated) muscle, on the other hand, move special segments of the digestive tract.

Smooth, involuntary muscle supports the viscera. Its fibers are simpler cells than those of the other muscle types and are comparatively short, averaging about 0.2 mm. in length by 5 μ wide. Each cell has a single centrally located nucleus. The surrounding cytoplasm is filled with fine longitudinal myofibrils, but there is none of the repetitious, symmetrical cross striping that characterizes skeletal muscle. Smooth muscle is innervated by the autonomic or peripheral nervous system. Its fibers contract slowly and can maintain the contracted state for long periods of time without fatigue. Hence the primary function of smooth muscle is to hold organs in place while producing localized movement, as in propelling food along the gut tube.

Striated, or voluntary, muscle moves the skeletal system (with a few exceptions). Each muscle is a highly organized system (Fig. 3-1). Its fibers are complex cells that are enormously elongated, reaching lengths of 30 cm. and widths of 60 μ. Each cell is multinucleated, with its nuclei flattened against the cell walls. These cells are also packed with longitudinal myofibrils, but the fibrils are crossed by repetitious bands continuous across the entire cell. The different transverse striations are identified by differences in staining and optical properties. The details of this complicated organization are not essential here; however, it is important to understand that the unit of contraction is the *sarcomere*. This is a small segment of the cylindrical myofibril (on the order of a 2.8 μ resting length) between two of the special transverse striations called Z *bands* (Zwischenscheibe, between discs). The sarcomere is divided in two equal parts by a central cross stripe called the *H band* (Hensen's line). Fine myosin myofilaments extend outward from the H band to interdigitate with overlapping extremely fine actin myofilaments projecting inward from the Z bands. For present purposes the process of contraction can be summarized as a chemically induced slid-

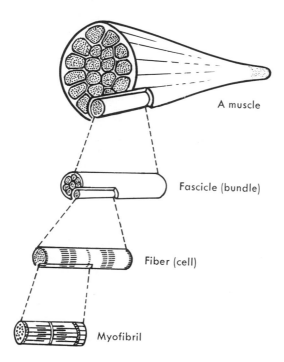

A muscle

Fascicle (bundle)

Fiber (cell)

Myofibril

Fig. 3-1. Organization of a striated muscle.

ing together with increasing overlapping of the filaments. This action pulls the Z bands toward each other (Fig. 3-2). Since sarcomeres run in a continuous series along the whole muscle fiber, contraction of a total muscle is considerable. Skeletal muscle is innervated by the central nervous system. Its fibers contract and relax swiftly. Hence its primary function is to perform extensive, speedy, and skillful movements while it holds the skeletal system in proper postures.

Two main types of skeletal muscles have been defined on the basis of morphology, physiology, and specific histochemical reactions. But even here, the rates of contraction differ:

Type I—small, slow-firing, relatively fatigue-resistant fibers

Type II—large, fast-firing, fatigable fibers.

Attempts at further classification are unclear, but the distribution of the distinct fiber types in specific muscles seems correlated to the muscle's functions. This may be especially important in the oral apparatus since the ratios of the fiber types apparently shift toward Type I in edentulous jaws.

Architecture of skeletal muscles

There are two indispensable parts to a muscle, the contractile (pulling) machinery and the harnessing system. Thus each muscle cell is saddled by a wrapping of loose areolar tissue (endomysium). The cells are gathered in bundles (fascicles) by a thickening continuation of this connective tissue wrapping (perimysium). Finally the wrap-

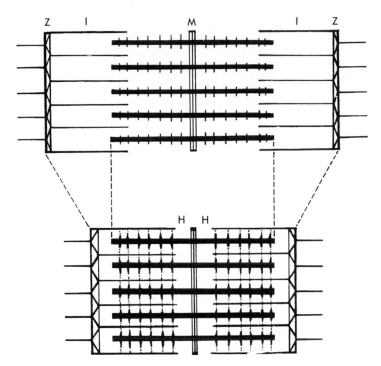

Fig. 3-2. Model of sarcomere, the unit of contraction. Resting state above, contracted state below. Heavy longitudinal lines, myosin filaments; fine longitudinal lines, actin filaments. Areas or "bands" crossing the sarcomere are: Z band, ends of the sarcomere; I band, area containing only actin filaments; H band, area containing no actin filaments; M band, interconnections between myosin filaments. Projections from myofilaments attract actin toward center of sarcomere.

pings are extended peripherally with increasing collagen fiber content to form a firm sheath for the whole muscle (epimysium). The essential features of this system are that: (1) it is continuous with the terminal anchorages of the muscle, (2) it allows fibers and fascicles to slip and slide with minimal interference, (3) it packages the whole muscle to its special contour, and (4) it attaches the muscle to the elements to be moved.

In summary, the gross muscle one dissects is made up of long muscle bundles, or fasciculi, composed of elongated muscle cells or fibers. Each fiber, in turn, is packed with longitudinal myofibrils. Each myofibril is made up of a chain of tiny cylindrical sarcomere segments that activate the contraction. A skeletal muscle is thus a structure of diminishing cordlike elements bound together and oriented along a line of motion (Fig. 3-1).

Attachments of muscles vary according to situation and function. "Fleshy" attachments have muscle cells ending close to the periosteum; tendon attachments are tough, flexible, cablelike concentrations of the collagen fibers of the harness; aponeuroses and septa are flattened extensions of this concentration.

Forms of striated muscles also vary according to situation and function. They may

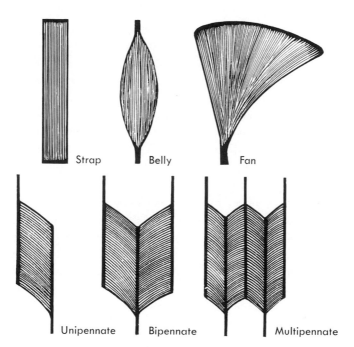

Fig. 3-3. Functional architecture of a muscle. Differences in design depend on: (1) surface on bone available for muscle attachement, (2) speed of contraction, (3) range of movement, and (4) force of contraction.

be straplike (flat), fusiform (bellied), fanlike (triangular), or pennate (featherlike) (Fig. 3-3). Strap muscles have fascicles parallel from end to end (sternohyoid, sartorius of leg). Fusiform muscles have nearly parallel fascicles that converge on a tendon at one or both ends (digastrics, biceps of arm). Fanlike muscles are relatively flat with a wide attachment converging on an apical attachment (temporalis, in lateral view, adductor magnus of leg). Pennate muscles have fascicles oriented obliquely to the line of pull. They attach to tendons, which resemble the shaft, or quill, of a feather. These muscles are termed unipennate when they run obliquely from a linear attachment to one side of a tendon, bipennate when they converge from opposite attachments to both sides of a tendon (temporalis in coronal section, interossei of the hand), and multipennate when fascicles angle in on numerous, alternate, tendinous plates (masseter in coronal section, deltoid of shoulder).

There is also a circular arrangement of striated muscle called a sphincter, which may not have direct attachment to the skeleton. Here the fibers run in a ring around a central opening. Contraction closes the opening as in the pulling of a purse string (orbicularis oris, external anal sphincter).

Actions of muscles

Muscles move parts only by pulling them. Hence the musculoskeletal apparatus is designed in opposing systems. Agonists act together to pull in a given direction;

antagonists pull in the opposite direction to bring parts back to the original position. A muscle is organized in functional units. The unit consists of a number of muscle fibers all innervated by the same motoneuron. These *motor units* vary in size. Muscles controlling fine, swift, subtle movements and adjustments are made up of the smallest number of muscle fibers per motoneuron (muscles of ear ossicles, larynx, and pharynx have less than 10 fibers per motoneuron). Muscles involved in grosser performance have the largest number of muscle fibers per motoneuron (said to reach 2000). Jaw muscles seem to range between these extremes (about 600 to 900). Movements are made by activating an increasing number of motor units while, at the same time, reducing the action of the antagonists.

The tension, or force, developed by a muscle changes with its length. Since muscle length depends on the contractile unit, the sarcomere, tension will fall if the unit is so stretched that myofilaments barely overlap or so shortened that overlapping buckles up the filaments. Optimum tension occurs at complete undistorted overlap (Fig. 3-2). However, an additional contribution to tension may be made by the harnessing system, which resists extensive stretch. Optimum length of the whole muscle seems to be within the range of normal functional movements in the body. This is obviously highly significant in jaw muscles since here muscle length depends on "normal" space relations between upper and lower jaws.

JAW MUSCLES

All muscles that are attached to the mandible have an influence on its movements and positions. These muscles belong to two groups: the supramandibular muscles, or elevators of the mandible, and the inframandibular muscles, or depressors of the mandible. Of the latter, only the stylo-hyoid muscle does not directly influence the mandible, but indirectly it has, in conjunction with the infrahyoid muscles, an important influence on mandibular movements by stabilizing the hyoid bone during its functional excursions, just as the cervical muscles stabilize the cranium. It is from either cranium or hyoid bone that the mandibular muscles act on the mandible itself.

Supramandibular muscles

Knowledge of the *action* of individual masticatory muscles is necessary to an understanding of their contribution to *function* during the movements of the mandible. These muscles, in conjunction with the suprahyoid musculature, work in groups (as do other muscles in the body) and not as individual units. An analysis of their function is possible only after the description of the craniomandibular articulation (see Chapter 4).

Traditionally four powerful muscles—the masseter, the temporalis, the medial (internal) pterygoid, and the lateral (external) pterygoid—are called the "muscles of mastication" (which is misleading, since lowering the jaw requires additional musculature). Two of these, the masseter and medial pterygoid, are associated as a sling, and for the most part they pull in an upward and forward direction. The most massive

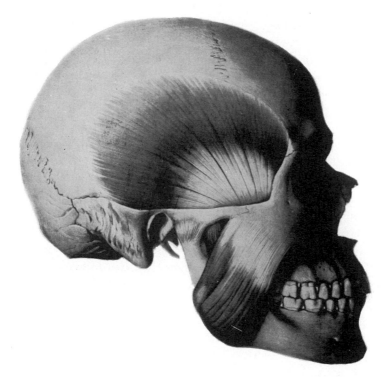

Fig. 3-4. Masseter and temporal muscles. (Sicher and Tandler: Anatomie für Zahnärzte.)

portion of the temporalis lies anteriorly, and it pulls upward in a practically vertical direction. The pull of the lateral pterygoid is forward in a practically horizontal direction (see details in Chapter 4). The resultant of the vertical component of the temporalis and the horizontal component of the lateral pterygoid is upward and forward, which is in coordination with the masseter-pterygoid sling.

Masseter muscle. The masseter muscle (Fig. 3-4), the most superficial of the masticatory muscles, stretches as a rectangular plate from the zygomatic arch to the outer surface of the mandibular ramus. The muscle can be divided, though incompletely, into a superficial and a deep portion. The superficial portion arises from the lower border of the zygomatic bone with strong tendinous fibers. If the masseter is well developed, the most anterior fibers may arise from the outer corner of the zygomatic process of the maxilla, and the area of origin of the muscle may extend back as a narrow strip on the outer surface of the zygomatic bone. Posteriorly the origin of the superficial portion ends with the zygomatic bone and never passes the zygomatico-temporal suture. The fibers have a general direction downward and backward to insert in the angular region of the mandible. The attachment occupies the lower third or fourth of the posterior border of the ramus, the lower border anteriorly to the level of the second molar, and the outer surface of the ramus in its lower half. The field of insertion shows ridges to which the tendons insert and grooves between the ridges to which the fleshy fibers insert.

The superficial muscle plate is covered on its outer surface by a strong tendinous layer that extends from the zygomatic bone over a third or half of the muscle. The tendon ends with a downwardly convex border or in a zigzag line. If the overlying tissues are not too thick, the border of the tendon can be seen when the muscle is tensed because of the contrast of the flat tendon to the strongly bulging muscle fibers below the tendon. In its depth, the superficial portion is formed by alternate tendinous plates and fleshy bundles so that the intimate structure of the muscle is rather intricate, presenting a herringbone pattern in coronal section (multipennate). Usually three tendons of origin alternate with two tendons of insertion. The effect of the alternation of muscle fibers and layers of tendon is to shorten the average length of the contractile elements and, at the same time, to enlarge the number of muscle fibers and the functional cross section of the muscle. The functional cross section of a muscle may be defined as the total of the cross sections of its muscle fibers and is correlated with the power of the muscle. The absolute shortening of the muscle, on the other hand, is proportionate to the length of its fibers. Muscles composed of long parallel muscle fibers, arranged in the long axis of the muscle, will therefore primarily act as fast movers. Muscles composed of fibers arranged at an angle to the long axis of the muscle will consist of relatively more and shorter fibers and will, therefore, primarily be muscles of great power. The specific structure of the masseter muscle suggests that it belongs to the second category.

The deep portion of the masseter can be separated from the superficial portion only in the posterior part of the muscle. Anteriorly the two layers fuse. By separating the two layers, a variably deep pouch is opened, which is filled by a small amount of loose connective tissue. The fibers of the deep portion arise from the entire length of the zygomatic arch back to the anterior end of the articular eminence. The fibers take their origin from the inner surface of the zygomatic arch and, at its most posterior part, also from its lower border. Immediately in front of the mandibular joint, the deep portion is not covered by the superficial portion and can be seen as a triangular muscle field, the fibers of which run almost vertically downward and thus are at an angle to the fibers of the superficial muscle plate, which are directed downward and backward. The field of insertion of the deep portion is above that of the superficial part and reaches to the base of the coronoid process. The craniomandibular articulation and the mandibular neck are never covered by the muscle.

The masseteric nerve reaches and enters the muscle from its deep surface after passing through the semilunar notch of the mandible behind the tendon of the temporal muscle. The nerve supplies the deep portion, perforates it, dividing it into an anterior and a posterior part, and then enters the superficial portion. The masseteric artery, a branch of the (internal) maxillary artery, and the masseteric veins follow the course of the nerve.

The deep part of the masseter muscle is inseparably fused with the most superficial fibers of the temporal muscle. Some authors distinguish this complex of muscle fibers, namely, the deep layer of the masseter and the most superficial fibers of the temporal muscle, as a separate muscle unit, terming it the zygomaticomandibular

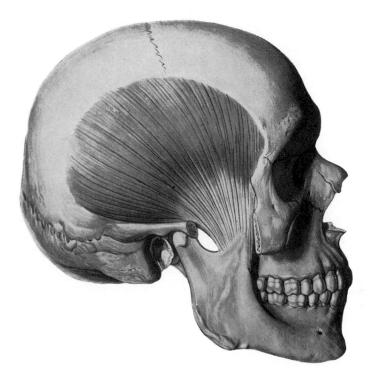

Fig. 3-5. Temporal muscle after removal of zygomatic arch. (Sicher and Tandler: Anatomie für Zahnärzte.)

muscle. In many animals the distinction of this muscle is easier than in man. It is described as a muscle originating from the lower border and medial surface of the zygomatic arch and inserting on the basal part of the coronoid process and the adjacent parts of the mandibular ramus.

If the masseter muscle is strong, the area of its insertion is slightly widened. At its anterior border a bundle of fibers arising from the superficial tendinous plate extends its insertion anteriorly along the lower border of the mandible so that the anterior border of the muscle is not straight but anteriorly concave (not shown in Fig. 3-4). Posterior fibers may end behind the posterior border of the mandibular ramus, joining fibers of the medial pterygoid muscle in a tendinous raphe.

The action of the muscle is that of a powerful elevator of the lower jaw closing the jaws and exerting pressure on the teeth, especially in the molar region. The superficial portion exerts pressure at a right angle to the posteriorly ascending occlusal plane of the molars, the curve of Spee. The fibers of the deep portion are directed downward and forward if the mandible is in protruded position. The deep portion therefore has a retracting component that is important during the closing movement, a combination of elevation and retrusion.

Temporal muscle. The fan-shaped temporal muscle (Fig. 3-5) has its origin from a wide field on the lateral surface of the skull that is surrounded by the inferior temporal line. This field, the temporal fossa, comprises a narrow strip of the parietal bone, the greater part of the temporal squama, the temporal surface of the frontal bone, and the temporal surface of the greater wing of the sphenoid bone. Some fibers may arise from the most posterior part of the temporal surface on the frontal process of the zygomatic bone. On the sphenoid bone the field of origin reaches downward to, and including, the infratemporal crest. In addition, many muscle fibers originate from an aponeurosis fused to the inner surface of the temporal fascia, especially in its upper part.

The bundles of the temporal muscle converge toward the opening between the zygomatic arch and the lateral surface of the skull, in the center of which the apex of the coronoid process is situated. The anterior fibers, which form the bulk of the muscle, are vertical; the fibers in the middle part of the muscle are increasingly oblique. The most posterior fibers run horizontally forward to bend sharply downward in front of the articular eminence to reach the mandible (see Fig. 4-14).

The temporal muscle inserts on the coronoid process of the mandible and on a flat tendinous plate that is an extension of the coronoid process upward into the depth of the muscle. This plate springs from the edge of the process, extending from the deepest point in the mandibular (semilunar) notch forward to the apex of the process. Fibers arising from the temporal surface of the skull insert on the medial surface of the plate; fibers arising from the temporal fascia insert on the plate's lateral surface. This presents a bipennate arrangement in a coronal section of the muscle. Thus the fibers of the temporalis are actually much shorter than most illustrations indicate, but they are longer than those of the masseter or medial pterygoid. In addition, two bulky, tendinous extensions of the muscle reach far down the ramus anteriorly and medially toward the posterior end of the alveolar process (Fig. 3-6). These two tendons are separated from each other by a downwardly widening cleft. The outer or superficial tendon is attached to the anterior border of the coronoid process and mandibular ramus. The inner or deep tendon is inserted to the temporal crest of the mandible. The deep tendon is, as a rule, stronger and longer than the superficial one. It juts medially and reaches downward into the region of the lower wisdom tooth. The retromolar fossa of the mandible between the superficial and deep tendon is free from the insertion of the temporal muscle (Figs. 3-6 and 3-9). All these relations are clinically important (see Chapter 12).

It has already been mentioned that the most superficial and, at the same time, shortest fibers of the temporal muscle, in part arising from the inner surface of the zygomatic arch, and the deepest fibers of the masseter muscle are fused; together they form the zygomaticomandibular muscle.

The innervation of the temporal muscle is provided by the temporal nerves of the mandibular nerve. The posterior two of the three temporal nerves commonly present arise as separate filaments from the mandibular nerve immediately after it emerges through the oval foramen. The anterior temporal nerve is, at its beginning, united with the buccal nerve; the common trunk runs close to the base of the skull from the foramen ovale anteriorly and laterally. It is held in place by a fibrous ligament that may ossify, and it then bounds the temporobuccal foramen, foramen crotaphiticobuc-

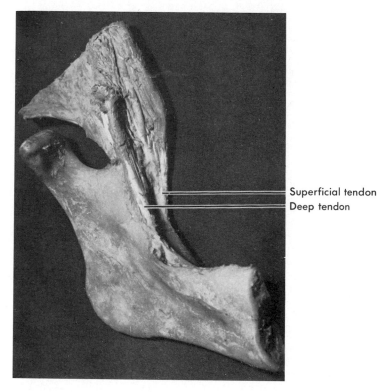

Superficial tendon
Deep tendon

Fig. 3-6. The two tendons of the temporal muscle, medial view.

cinatorium (see Fig. 2-14). As a rule, the anterior temporal nerve separates from the buccal nerve after it has passed between the two heads of the lateral pterygoid muscle.

The blood supply of the temporal muscle is furnished by the middle and deep temporal arteries. The middle temporal artery is a branch of the superficial temporal artery. The deep temporal arteries are branches of the (internal) maxillary artery.

The temporal muscle, built more for movement than for power, is mainly an elevator of the mandible. Its middle fibers have a retracting component because of their oblique direction downward and forward. Its most posterior fibers are bent around the root of the zygomatic process, and only their direction below this pulley is significant. (See Chapter 4.)

The temporal fascia is set in a frame formed by the inferior temporal line and the upper border of the zygomatic arch. Its upper part is thin and aponeurotic, and its fibers, fused to the periosteum, extend toward the superior temporal line without reaching it. Farther down, the temporal fascia thickens considerably and finally splits into two layers; the superficial layer continues into the periosteum on the outer surface, the deep layer into that of the inner surface of the zygomatic arch. The two layers are joined by irregular bands of connective tissue, and the communicating spaces between the layers are filled with fat. The outer layer is, by far, the stronger

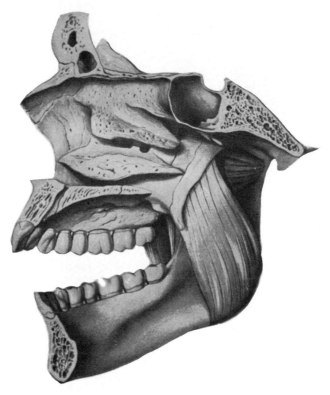

Fig. 3-7. Medial pterygoid muscle, medial view. (Sicher and Tandler: Anatomic für Zahnärzte.)

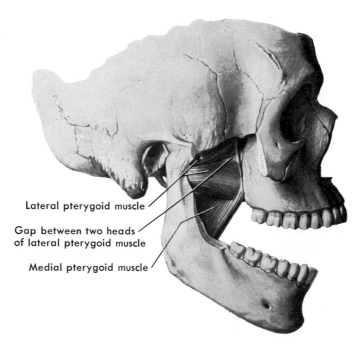

Lateral pterygoid muscle

Gap between two heads
of lateral pterygoid muscle

Medial pterygoid muscle

Fig. 3-8. Lateral and medial (external and internal) pterygoid muscles, lateral aspect, after removal of zygomatic arch and coronoid process. (Sicher and Tandler: Anatomie für Zahnärzte.)

and gives, to the palpating finger, almost the impression of bone. The temporal fascia is not directly comparable to other muscle fasciae since it is also the suspensory sling for the zygomatic arch.

Medial pterygoid muscle. The medial (internal) pterygoid muscle (Figs. 3-7 and 3-8), situated on the medial side of the mandibular ramus, is anatomically and functionally a counterpart of the masseter muscle. It is a rectangular, powerful muscle, although it is not as strong as the masseter. Its main origin is in the pterygoid fossa. The fibers at its inner surface arise by strong tendons; others arise directly from the medial surface of the lateral pterygoid plate. The tendon that covers the medial surface of the muscle at its origin is just as wide as the tensor palati muscle, with which it is in contact. Anterior fibers arise by strong tendons from the outer and inferior surfaces of the pyramidal process of the palatine bone and even from the adjacent parts of the maxillary tuberosity (Fig. 3-8). These features are important in surgical repositioning of the maxilla.

The fibers of the medial pterygoid muscle run downward, backward, and outward and are inserted to the medial surface of the mandibular angle. The field of insertion is approximately triangular. It is bounded by the lower half of the posterior border of the mandibular ramus and by two lines that start at the mandibular foramen. One line runs horizontally back to the posterior border of the ramus; the other runs downward and forward to the lower border of the mandible just in front of the mandibular angle. It has been mentioned that fibers of the medial pterygoid muscle may meet fibers of the masseter in a tendinous inscription behind and below the mandibular angle.

The internal structure of the medial pterygoid muscle is also complicated by the alternation of sagitally oriented fleshy and tendinous parts so that many muscle fibers, arising from one tendon and ending on another, are arranged at an angle to the general direction of the muscle. Usually three tendons of origin alternating with three of insertion can be identified. This arrangement, which makes the muscle appear as if its fibers were braided, tends to increase the power of the muscle (the muscle being multipennate).

The nerve supplying the medial pterygoid muscle reaches it at its posterior border or slightly in front of it. The medial pterygoid nerve leaves the mandibular nerve immediately below the foramen ovale, and is closely connected with the otic ganglion (see Fig. 9-16). The artery supplying the muscle is a branch of the maxillary artery.

The muscle is a synergist of the masseter muscle, especially of its superficial part, and, therefore, an elevator of the mandible. Despite the oblique direction of its fibers, this muscle is not able to shift the mandible to one side in synergism with the lateral pterygoid because its main pull is directed upward.

Lateral pterygoid muscle. The lateral pterygoid muscle (Figs. 3-8 and 3-9) arises from two heads. The larger inferior head originates from the outer surface of the lateral pterygoid plate, and the smaller superior head originates from the infratemporal surface of the greater sphenoid wing medial to the infratemporal crest. The fibers of the upper head at first run downward, then backward and outward in close relation to the cranial base. When they reach the anterior limit of the joint, the fibers

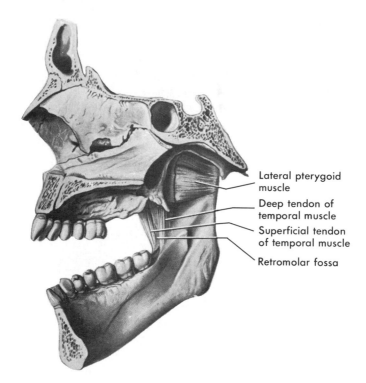

Fig. 3-9. Lateral pterygoid muscle and tendons of temporal muscle, medial view. (Sicher and Tandler: Anatomie für Zahnärzte.)

bend horizontally back to the neck of the mandible. The fibers of the lower head converge upward and outward, the upper fibers running more horizontally, the lower fibers more and more steeply ascending. The two heads, separated anteriorly by a variably wide gap, fuse in front of the craniomandibular joint and there can be separated only artificially.

Only part of the upper head, namely, its uppermost and most medial fibers, is attached to the anteromedial surface of the articular capsule and thus indirectly to the anterior border of the articular disc. The majority of the fibers, that is, the greater part of the superior head and the entire inferior head, are inserted to a roughened fovea on the anterior surface of the mandibular neck. It should be noted that only protracting muscle fibers are attached to capsule and disc; retracting fiber bundles (of masseter and temporal muscles) are attached only to the mandible itself.

The nerve to the lateral pterygoid muscle branches off the masseteric or the buccal nerve. The blood supply is a branch of the maxillary artery.

The muscle pulls the head of the mandible and the articular disc forward, downward, and inward along the posterior slope of the articular eminence (Chapter 4).

Inframandibular muscles

The inframandibular muscles are arranged between the skull and mandible and the hyoid bone. Their function is either to elevate the hyoid bone and, with it, the larynx or to depress the mandible. Whether one or the other movement is effected

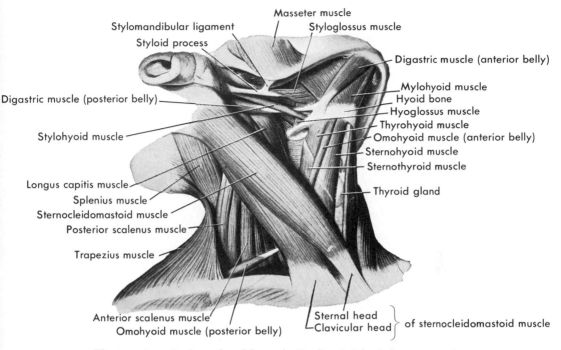

Fig. 3-10. Superficial muscles of the neck. (Tandler: Lehrbuch der Anatomie.)

depends on the state of contraction of other muscles. If the mandible is fixed in its position by the action of the masseter, temporal, and medial pterygoid muscles, the inframandibulars will elevate the hyoid bone and the larynx. If, on the other hand, the infrahyoid muscles—sternohyoid, omohyoid, sternothryoid, and thyrohyoid— and the stylohyoid muscles are contracted, the hyoid bone is stabilized, and the inframandibular muscles that extend to the mandible will depress and retract the lower jaw. (See Chapter 4.) The inframandibular muscles are the digastric, the genio-hyoid, the mylohyoid, and the stylohyoid.

Digastric muscle. As indicated by its name, the digastric muscle (Fig. 3-10) con-sists of two fleshy parts, a posterior and an anterior belly, which are connected by a strong round tendon. The posterior belly arises from the mastoid notch medial to the mastoid process; the intermediate tendon is fixed by a fascial pulley to the hyoid bone, and the anterior belly finds its attachment in the digastric fossa of the mandible at its lower border close to the midline. The two bellies of the muscle form an obtuse angle that is maintained by the pulley of fascia, which partially fixes the tendon in its relation to the hyoid bone but allows the tendon to slide in the fascial sling.

The posterior belly is much longer than the anterior belly, almost circular in cross section, and only slightly flattened in lateromedial direction. Gradually tapering ante-riorly, the posterior belly continues into the round intermediate tendon.

The anterior belly, arising from the intermediate tendon, is much shorter than the posterior belly. It consists, in most individuals, of a thicker lateral and a thinner medial part. Its insertion into the digastric fossa of the mandible is partly fleshy and partly tendinous. The transverse diameter of the anterior belly varies considerably. If this part of the muscle is broad, right and left muscles touch or almost touch each other at their insertion. If the anterior belly of the digastric muscle is narrow, there is a distance between right and left muscles, and the submental region is not triangular but irregularly quadrilateral.

The intermediate tendon is not directly attached to the hyoid bone but is fastened to it by strengthened fibers of the cervical fascia, which form a loop around the tendon, sometimes separated from it by a synovial bursa. The tendon, therefore, can slide in this loop within limits. The fibers of this pulley are attached to the greater horn and the lateral part of the body of the hyoid bone. The length of the fascial loop varies considerably; thus, the distance of the tendon from the hyoid bone and the angle between the posterior and anterior bellies of the digastric muscle also vary. The longer the loop and, therefore, the greater the distance between hyoid bone and tendon, the more obtuse is the angle between the two bellies of the muscle.

The digastric muscle has a double innervation. The posterior belly is supplied by a branch of the facial nerve entering the muscle close to its posterior end. The anterior belly is supplied by a branch of the mylohyoid nerve of the mandibular nerve.

Variations of the digastric muscle are frequent. They are, however, almost entirely confined to its anterior belly. The most frequent aberration from the typical shape consists of oblique connections between the two anterior bellies, sometimes symmetrical, more often asymmetrical. The accessory muscle bundles may occupy the entire space between right and left anterior digastric bellies.

Geniohyoid muscle. The geniohyoid muscle (see Fig. 5-8) arises above the anterior end of the mylohyoid line from the inner surface of the mandible, close to the midline and lateral to and including the interior mental spines, by a short and strong tendon. The muscle, in contact with that of the other side, proceeds straight posteriorly and slightly downward and is attached to the upper half of the hyoid body (see Fig. 2-45). Posteriorly the muscle gradually widens and assumes a triangular shape in cross section.

The muscle is supplied by branches of the first and second cervical nerves, which reach it via the hypoglossal nerve. The geniohyoid muscle pulls the hyoid bone upward and forward or it exerts a downward and backward pull on the mandible, depending on the fixation of either the mandible or the hyoid bone by other muscles.

Mylohyoid muscle. The mylohyoid muscle (Figs. 3-10 to 3-14) forms, anatomically and functionally, the floor of the oral cavity; hence the old term for it was oral diaphragm. The right and left muscles are united in the midline between mandible and hyoid bone by a tendinous strip, the mylohyoid raphe.

The muscle arises from the mylohyoid line on the inner surface of the mandible. Its most posterior fibers take their origin from the region of the alveolus of the lower third molar. The origin of the anterior fibers descends toward the lower border of the mandible. The posterior fibers of the coarsely bundled muscle run steeply downward, medially, and slightly forward, and are attached to the body of the hyoid bone; the majority of the fibers, however, join those of the contralateral muscle in the mylohyoid raphe. The muscle plate is considerably thicker in its posterior part. Slit-like defects in the anterior part of the muscle are not rare. The free, sharply defined posterior border of the muscle, reaching from the third molar socket to the body of the hyoid bone, is an important topographic and surgical landmark. Because of the origin high up on the inner surface of the mandible, the muscle plate of the mylohyoid and the inner surface of the mandible bound a niche, the mylohyoid, or submandibular, niche. It is deepest posteriorly and more shallow anteriorly.

The mylohyoid muscle is supplied by branches of the mylohyoid nerve of the mandibular nerve. The innervating branches enter the muscle from its inferolateral surface. The submental artery, a branch of the facial artery, sends twigs into the muscle.

Only the posterior bundles of the mylohyoid muscle, running almost vertically from the mandible to the hyoid bone, have a slight influence on these bones. If the mandible is fixed, they lift the hyoid bone; if the hyoid bone is held in place, they help

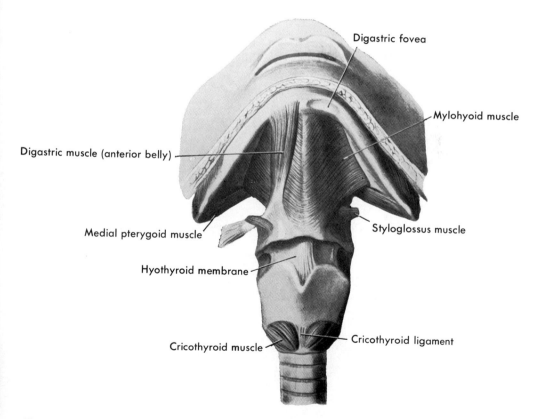

Fig. 3-11. Mylohyoid muscle and anterior belly of digastric muscle, inferior view. (Sicher and Tandler: Anatomie für Zahnärzte.)

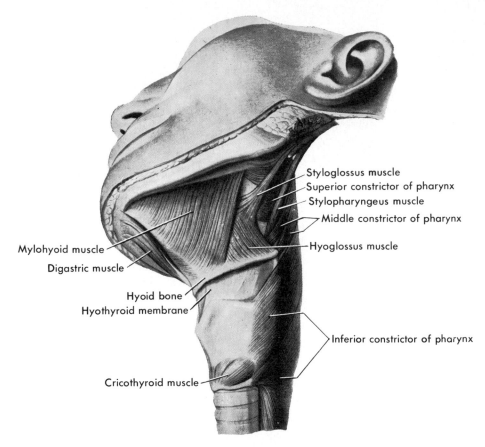

Styloglossus muscle
Superior constrictor of pharynx
Stylopharyngeus muscle
Middle constrictor of pharynx
Hyoglossus muscle

Mylohyoid muscle
Digastric muscle

Hyoid bone
Hyothyroid membrane

Inferior constrictor of pharynx

Cricothyroid muscle

Fig. 3-12. Mylohyoid muscle and muscles of tongue and pharynx, lateral view. (Sicher and Tandler: Anatomie für Zahnärzte.)

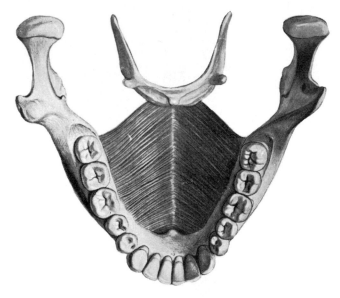

Fig. 3-13. Mylohyoid muscle, superior view. (Sicher and Tandler: Anatomie für Zahnärzte.)

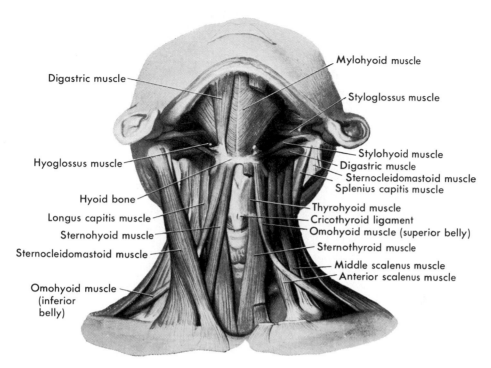

Fig. 3-14. Infrahyoid muscles, anterior view. (Tandler: Lehrbuch der Anatomie.)

in depressing the mandible. The anterior larger but thinner part of the mylohyoid muscle has no action on the lower jaw or the hyoid bone. In contracting, the downward convex plate of this portion, consisting of the right and left fibers joined in the median raphe, flattens its curvature, and thus the floor of the oral cavity is elevated and with it the tongue that rests on it. The mylohyoid muscle is, therefore, primarily an elevator of the tongue.

Stylohyoid muscle. The stylohyoid muscle (Fig. 3-10) arises from the lateral and inferior surface of the styloid process. It is a thin round muscle that converges with the posterior belly of the digastric muscle anteriorly and inferiorly. It lies first superior and medial to the digastric muscle and then close to its upper border. Where the stylohyoid muscle reaches the intermediate tendon of the digastric muscle, it splits in most individuals into two slips that enclose the tendon of the digastric muscle and insert onto the greater horn of the hyoid bone where it joins the body (see Figs. 4-21 and 6-4). The nerve supply of the stylohyoid muscle is derived from the facial nerve. The branch supplying the stylohyoid muscle enters the muscle near its anteroinferior end. The function of the stylohyoid muscle is the elevation and retraction of the hyoid bone or its stabilization in cooperation with other hyoid muscles.

Infrahyoid muscles

The infrahyoid muscles extend between the hyoid bone above and the sternum, clavicle, and scapula below. The two superficial muscles, sternohyoid and omohyoid, directly connect the hyoid bone with the sternum and the scapula, respectively; the deep layer connects the sternum to the thyroid cartilage. Thus, the deep layer is divided into two muscles, the sternothyroid and the thyrohyoid.

The function of the infrahyoid muscles is twofold; they may either depress the hyoid bone and, with it, the larynx, or they may, together with the stylohyoid, hold the hyoid bone in its position relative to the trunk. The hyoid bone then is made the stable point from which the suprahyoids, with the exception of the stylohyoid muscle, can act on the mandible. Although the larynx generally moves with the hyoid bone, the attachment of the deep layer of the infrahyoids to the thyroid cartilage allows for some independent movement between the larynx and hyoid bone. The infrahyoid muscles are supplied by the first, second, and third cervical nerves. These fibers reach the sternohyoid, sternothyroid, and omohyoid muscles via the cervical ansa (hypoglossal loop). The nerve to the thyrohyoid muscle leaves the hypoglossal nerve as a separate branch.

Sternohyoid muscle. The sternohyoid muscle (Fig. 3-14) is, as are all infrahyoid muscles, a flat band. It arises from a line extending from the lateral part of the inner surface of the sternum close to its upper border over the sternoclavicular capsule to the sternal end of the clavicle. The line of origin is about an inch long. The right and left muscles, separated rather widely at the origin, converge in their upward course but remain separated from each other by a variably wide strip of fascia, sometimes referred to as the white line of the neck, linea alba colli (see Fig. 15-2). In its upper part, the sternohyoid muscle becomes narrower and slightly thicker and is, finally, attached to the inferior border of the hyoid bone, close to the midline. The muscle is in most cases partly divided by a narrow tendinous inscription, nearer to its sterno-clavicular attachment. This inscription is sometimes seen only at the deep surface of the muscle.

Omohyoid muscle. The long, narrow, two-bellied omohyoid muscle (Figs. 3-10 and 3-14) originates at the upper border of the scapula, medial to the suprascapular notch. The inferior or posterior belly runs obliquely upward and forward, crossing the posterior triangle of the neck. Deep to the sternocleidomastoid muscle the flat posterior belly ends in a more rounded, short tendon which, in turn, continues into the superior or anterior belly. This part of the muscle forms, with the posterior belly, an obtuse angle that opens posteriorly and superiorly. The superior belly is more steeply directed upward and forward until the muscle reaches the inferior border of the hyoid bone. There it is attached just lateral to the attachment of the sternohyoid muscle. The intermediate tendon is fixed to the clavicle by a rather firm layer of the deep cervical fascia, the omoclavicular fascia, which covers the internal jugular vein. The vein is firmly attached to the fascia, so that the omohyoid muscle can widen the lumen of the vein.

Sternothyroid muscle. The origin of the sternothyroid muscle (Fig. 3-14) is found on the posterior surface of the manubrium sterni at the level of the first rib. The line of its origin begins at the midline of the sternum and extends over the entire length of the cartilage of the first rib. Sometimes the origins of the right and left muscles even cross the midline so that their most caudal parts overlap. The muscle is wider than the superficial sternohyoid muscle and reaches, slightly deviating laterally, the thyroid cartilage, where its fibers end at the oblique line. The sternothyroid muscle is, like the sternohyoid, divided into two parts by an oblique tendinous inscription fairly close to its lower end.

Thyrohyoid muscle. The thyrohyoid muscle (Fig. 3-14) originates from the oblique line of the thyroid cartilage and is inserted to the lateral part of the body and to the medical part of the greater horn of the hyoid bone. The muscle is an irregularly rectangular plate; its medial part is covered by the sternohyoid and omohyoid muscles.

FACIAL MUSCULATURE

A group of muscles in the head have in common their superficial arrangement and especially their attachment to, or their influence on, the skin. To this group belongs also the platysma muscle, which extends from the face over the entire length of the neck to the chest. These superficial muscles can be divided into several groups. The first is made up of the platysma muscle alone; a second group has sphincter-like arrangements around the mouth, nostrils, and eyes; a third is concerned with the movements of the outer ear; the fourth and last group belongs to the scalp. Almost all of these muscles have an influence on facial expression and are, therefore, collectively called the muscles of facial expression. Beyond this, however, they perform major functions such as closing of the eyelids, closing and opening of the lips, auxiliary functions during intake of food and its mastication, and in speaking. All these muscles are supplied by the facial nerve.

The superficial muscles of the head are distinguished by their great variability. The muscles are variable not only as to their strength, but also as to their shape. In some persons many of these muscles consist only of a few pale muscle bundles, whereas in others they form solid, though thin, muscle plates or bands of a dark red color. In many cases it is difficult to separate one muscle from the other either because two neighboring muscles fuse to become one muscular unit or because they exchange fiber bundles. An added difficulty is that the terminal parts of some of these muscles are interlaced, for instance, lateral to the corners of the mouth. The dissection of these muscles is, for all these reasons, a rather difficult undertaking. The difficulties are increased by the peculiar way of insertion of these muscles into the skin and of some bundles into the mucous membrane. They insert, as a rule, by isolated, thin, and sometimes elastic tendons that are continuations of the individual muscle bundles. These tendons are frequently separated from one another by lobules of fat and can be traced only with great care. Where the tendons are attached to the skin in lines or in a small concentrated area the skin is either folded or pulled inward to form a small fovea, which is seen as a dimple. The creasing of the skin along certain lines, repeated over and over again, leads finally to the formation of permanent folds. The two most important of these are the nasolabial and labiomental folds. The folds become deeper and sharper with advancing age because of the loss of elastic tissue in the skin (see Fig. 5-1).

Inconstant folds are caused by habitual wrinkling of the skin in certain areas for

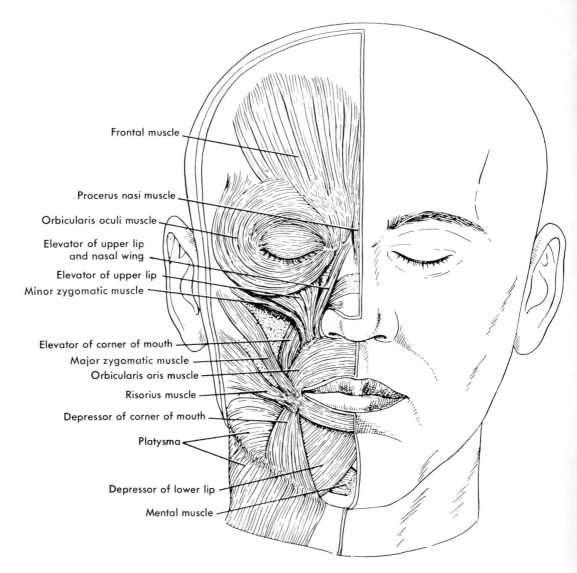

Frontal muscle

Procerus nasi muscle

Orbicularis oculi muscle

Elevator of upper lip
and nasal wing

Elevator of upper lip

Minor zygomatic muscle

Elevator of corner of mouth

Major zygomatic muscle

Orbicularis oris muscle

Risorius muscle

Depressor of corner of mouth

Platysma

Depressor of lower lip

Mental muscle

Fig. 3-15. Muscles of facial expression, superficial layer. (Modified and redrawn from Sicher and Tandler: Anatomie für Zahnärzte.)

instance, the horizontal folds on the forehead and the vertical folds between the brows. They, too, become permanent when, by long-repeated action or by advancing age, the elastic fibers of the skin degenerate. The same origin can be established for the fine small divergent folds radiating from the outer corners of the eye, crow's feet, which are characteristic for elderly persons as well as for those who are used to squinting in bright sunlight.

Platysma muscle. The platysma is a flat and wide muscle plate that covers most of the lateral and anterior regions of the neck. Its posterior border reaches from the acromion to the angle of the jaw, its anterior border from the region of the sterno-clavicular joint to the chin. At the lower end the bundles of the muscles cross the clavicle and cover a variably wide part of the infraclavicular region, where they end with thin tendons in the skin. At its upper border (Fig. 3-15) many of the platysma fibers find attachment on the lower border of the mandible; the rest continue into the face. The bony attachment (Fig. 3-18) reaches from the mental tubercle to a point approximately between the first and second molars. Bundles of the anterior part of the muscle that fail to attach themselves to the mandible may continue into the depressor anguli oris (triangular muscle) and intermingle with its fibers. As a rule, only the fibers that reach the face posterior to this bony attachment continue upward and anteriorly. At the level of the lower lip these fibers bend forward and cross each other in a rather intricate manner. The most anterior and posterior bundles of this part continue into the lower lip, and the middle fibers sometimes reach the upper lip after interlacing with fibers of the buccinator muscle lateral to the corner of the mouth.

The platysma muscle is supplied by the descending, or cervical, branch of the facial nerve, which forms, with a branch of the transversus colli nerve, the superficial cervical loop, or facial ansa. In contracting, the platysma muscle raises the skin of the neck into several parallel folds that are directed from above and in front down and backward. In addition, the muscle has some influence on facial expression by pulling the corner of the mouth down and sideward. It is more than doubtful whether the platysma, because of its mandibular attachment, can be considered an auxiliary depressor of the lower jaw. The mandibular attachment is, in all probability, the fixed point of the muscle bundles. It is more likely that the platysma facilitates venous flow in the neck by keeping skin and fascia fairly taut between mandible and clavicle. It has to be remembered that venous flow in the neck is mainly by suction during the inspiratory phase of thoracic movements.

Variations of the platysma are frequent. Smaller or larger defects of the muscle are often seen; in some cases the muscles of the right and left sides may overlap in the submental region, the fibers of the right muscles being, in the majority of cases, superficial.

Musculus transversus menti. The transverse muscle of the chin is present in about one half of individuals. It consists of an unpaired muscle band reaching from one mental tubercle to the other. The muscle is 8 to 10 mm. wide. The fibers, crossing the midline immediately below the bony chin, often continue into bundles of the depressor anguli oris (triangularis). The muscle may aid the two depressor muscles of the corner of the mouth when they act symmetrically.

Muscles of the mouth and nose

Of the muscles of the mouth and nose, the oral muscles are, by far, the more important in man. They can be subdivided into two groups: one group closes the lips and consists of the various parts of the orbicularis oris muscle; the second group opens the lips and consists of radially arranged muscles. The radial muscles can be divided into superficial and deep muscles of the upper and lower lips. The superficial muscles of the upper lip are zygomaticus minor, levator labii superioris, and levator labii superioris alaeque nasi (all three formerly called quadratus labii superioris) and the zygomaticus major muscle; in the deep layer of the upper lip lies the levator anguli oris (canine) muscle. The superficial muscle of the lower lip is the depressor anguli oris (triangular) muscle. The deep muscles are the depressor labii inferioris (quadratus labii inferioris) and the mental muscle. Two muscles extend to the corner of the mouth. The superficial of the two is the variable risorious muscle; the deep one is the buccinator muscle, the muscle of the cheek.

The bundles of the oral muscles insert partly into the skin and partly into the mucous membrane of the lips and their immediate vicinity. One area has to be considered as a rather concentrated attachment of many fibers of converging muscles. This insertion field is situated immediately lateral to and slightly above the corner of the mouth and can be felt through the mucous membrane as a somewhat circumscribed firm body; it is known as the muscular or tendinous node of the cheek. It continues downward as a tendinous strip of varying length.

The often repeated claim that most bundles of one muscle continue into the neighboring muscles is generally erroneous; it rests on the lack of delicate dissections. Such an arrangement is restricted to specific areas.

Elevators of the upper lip (musculus quadratus labii superioris, or square muscle of the upper lip). This muscle (Figs. 3-15 and 3-16) arises in a long line from the frontal process of the maxilla laterally to the zygomatic bone. According to its origin it was formerly divided into three heads, but now it is divided into three muscles: the first, the levator of the upper lip and nasal wing (the angular head), arises from the frontal process of the maxilla; the second, the levator of the upper lip (the infraorbital head), is attached to the maxillary body in a line paralleling the infraorbital margin and slightly below it, extending laterally to the zygomatic process of the maxilla; the third, the minor zygomatic muscle (the zygomatic head), originates from the most prominent part of the zygomatic bone. In the majority of persons these three muscles are separated from each other, the space between the levator of upper lip and minor zygomatic muscles (infraorbital and zygomatic heads) being wider than that between the levator of upper lip and levator of upper lip and nasal wing (infraorbital and angular heads). Farther down, the three muscles may fuse to form a solid muscular plate; often, however, they can be separated all the way to their insertion.

The levator labii superioris alaeque nasi, elevator of upper lip and nasal wing (angular head), is a narrow band of muscle fibers arising from the frontal process of the maxilla at the level of the medial palpebral ligament. From here the bundles run steeply downward to insert, in great part, into the skin of the wing of the nose. Some fibers surround the lateral circumference of the nostril and may even reach its posterior border. Such muscle bundles interlace with those of the nasal muscle. The muscle bundles that do not terminate in the skin of the nose can be followed into the upper lip, where they end in the neighborhood of the philtrum, interwoven with fibers of the orbicularis oris muscle.

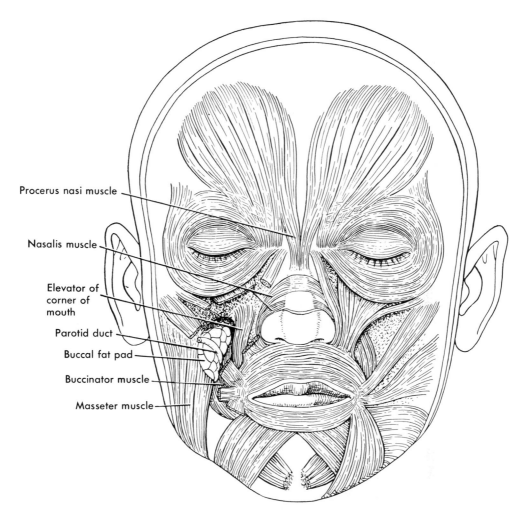

Fig. 3-16. Muscles of facial expression: superficial layer on left side of face; deep layer on right side (Modified and redrawn from Sicher and Tandler: Anatomie für Zahnärzte.)

The levator labii superioris, elevator of upper lip (infraorbital head), consists of fibers that converge downward. They pass under the nasolabial sulcus and then curve into the skin to insert in an area below the sulcus and parallel to it, reaching almost to the vermilion zone of the lip. Many of the fibers interlace with those of the orbicularis oris muscle.

The zygomaticus minor (zygomatic head), as a rule the weakest of the three muscles, is also the most variable. If it is well developed, it arises from the height of the zygomatic bone in front of the origin of the major zygomatic muscle and courses obliquely downward and medially. Its fibers overlap to a variable degree those of the elevator of the upper lip (infraorbital head) and end in the skin of the upper lip at a variable distance from the midline, lateral to and partly below the wing of the nose. One of the most frequent variations of the zygomatic head is the replacement of some or all of its fibers by aberrant fibers of the orbicularis oculi muscle. A minor zygomatic muscle is missing in about 20% of the persons examined.

The action of the three muscles, formerly called heads of the square muscle of the upper lip, is to raise the lip and the corner of the mouth and the wing of the nose and so to widen the nostril. By their action the skin is folded in a line parallel to and above the area of their insertion into the skin. The fold is the nasolabial fold.

Musculus zygomaticus major (zygomatic muscle). This muscle (Figs. 3-15 and 3-16) is one of the most constant and best-developed muscles of the middle face. Even in individuals in whom most of the muscles of facial expression consist of weak and pale muscle bundles, the zygomatic major muscle is characterized by its darker red color. The muscle arises from the temporal process of the zygomatic bone, that is, on the lateral surface of the face, at some distance behind the origin of the minor zygomatic muscle (Fig. 3-18). From its origin, the flat band of the major zygomatic muscle runs downward and forward to the corner of the mouth, where it is frequently divided by the levator anguli oris (canine muscle) into a superficial and a deep part. The more superficial fibers end in a line extending the insertion of the upper square muscle laterally, that is, below and parallel to the nasolabial sulcus, to the level of the corner of the mouth. Many of the deep fibers end in the mucous membrane of the upper lip; some bundles, however, may pass through the tendinous node and reach the mucous membrane of the lower lip to intermingle with fibers of the orbicularis oris.

The greater zygomatic muscle pulls the corner of the mouth upward and laterally.

Musculus risorius (risorius muscle). This muscle, the "smiling" or "grinning" muscle (Figs. 3-15 and 3-16), arises from the fascia of the masseter muscle behind its anterior border. The bundles of the risorius muscle converge toward the corner of the mouth so that the muscle gains in thickness. As a whole, the muscle is triangular, and its general direction is horizontal. Lateral to the corner of the mouth most of its fibers pass into and through the tendinous node, partly interlacing with fibers of the adjacent muscles. The majority of the tendons end in the skin and mucous membrane of the upper lip and in the mucous membrane just lateral to the corner of the mouth. Some bundles enter and end in the lower lip.

The risorius muscle is highly variable, often reduced to a few bundles widely separated from each other, or is even lacking. Sometimes the muscle is strengthened, or even replaced, by bundles of the platysma muscle, which turn into a horizontal course at the level of the corner of the mouth. The risorius pulls the corner of the mouth laterally, hence its name, "grinning" muscle.

Musculus levator anguli oris (canine muscle). This muscle, the elevator of the corner of the mouth (Figs. 3-15 and 3-16), represents the deep layer of the muscles of the upper lip and is, as a rule, well developed. It arises on the anterior surface of the maxillary body from the canine fossa below the infraorbital foramen (Fig. 3-18). The muscle band narrows slightly in its course downward and laterally. Above and lateral to the corner of the mouth, the fibers enter the tendinous node after crossing and often dividing the greater zygomatic muscle. In the node the fibers of the levator anguli oris interlace with fibers of the neighboring muscles, and most fibers end in the skin and the mucous membrane of the lower lip.

The canine muscle elevates the corner of the mouth and pulls it slightly medially.

Musculus depressor anguli oris (triangular muscle of the lower lip). This muscle, the depressor of the corner of the mouth (Figs. 3-15 and 3-16), originates from the outer surface and above the lower border of the mandible at, and just above, the line to which fibers of the platysma muscle are attached (Fig. 3-18). This line reaches from the mental tubercle to a plane below the first molar. At their origin the muscle bundles interdigitate, often regularly, with those of the platysma. The muscle forms a triangular plate with its posterior border, ascending vertically to the corner of the mouth, and its anterior border can be followed obliquely upward and backward. The convergence of the bundle causes the muscle to become thicker at its upper end close to the tendinous node. Through the node the bundles of the muscle continue as fine tendons, mostly into the upper lip, where they end in the skin of its lateral half. Some tendons continue into fibers of the elevator of the corner of the mouth (canine muscle), and some end in the skin of the corner of the mouth itself.

The depressor anguli oris pulls the corner of the mouth downward and inward.

Musculus depressor labii inferioris (square muscle of the lower lip). This wide, flat muscle, the depressor of the lower lip (Figs. 3-15 and 3-16), originates from the uppermost level of the rough line that serves as the attachment of the platysma and triangular muscles (Fig. 3-18). From here the fiber bundles run, parallel to each other, upward and medially into the lower lip. The lateroinferior part of the muscle is entirely covered by the depressor anguli oris muscle; its superomedial part is visible medial to, and above, the medial border of the depressor anguli oris. The most medial fibers of the depressor of the lower lip may pass the midline, crossing the corresponding muscle fibers of the other side. The insertion of the greater part of this muscle occurs in tiers to the skin of the lower lip, above the mentolabial fold. Some of the fibers end in the skin of the chin. Deep fibers find their insertion in the mucous membrane of the lower lip.

This muscle pulls the lower lip down and slightly laterally.

Musculus mentalis (mental muscle or chin muscle). This muscle (Figs. 3-16 and 3-17) arises from an oval area in the depth of the mental fossa. Its lower margin is usually raised to form a slight bony ridge (Fig. 3-18). From their origin the fibers of each mental muscle project in their course toward the skin; at the same time they converge and interlace with those of the contralateral muscle to end, after crossing the midline, in the skin of the chin. Only the most lateral fibers end in the skin of the same side. The superior fibers of the muscle course downward in anteriorly concave arches looping under the lower border of the orbicularis oris muscle to reach the skin (Fig. 3-17). The inferior fibers gradually assume a course increasingly inclined anteriorly and downward, the most inferior fibers even passing the lower border of the mandible to end in the skin on the inferior surface of the chin.

The muscle elevates the skin of the chin and lifts and rolls the lower lip outward.

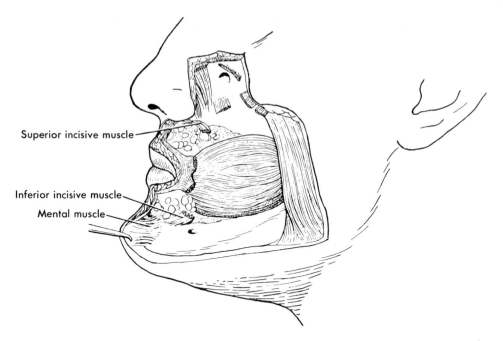

Fig. 3-17. Incisive muscles and mental muscle in their relation to vestibular fornix. (Redrawn from Sicher and Tandler: Anatomie für Zahnärzte.)

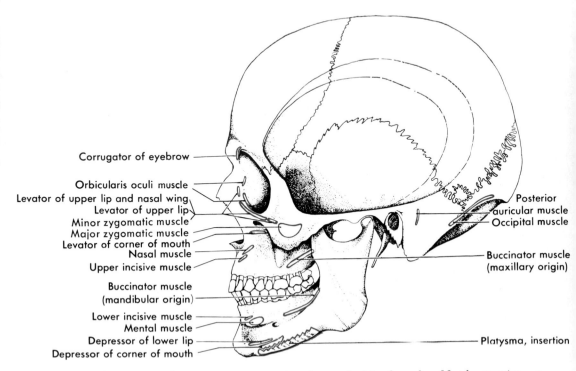

Fig. 3-18. Semidiagrammatic representation of areas of origin of muscles of facial expression.

Since its origin extends to a level higher than that of the fornix of the vestibule, the mental muscle, in contracting, renders the lower vestibule shallow. Its reflex contraction may, therefore, interfere greatly with dental work on the labial surface of the lower front teeth.

Musculus buccinatorius (buccinator muscle or cheek muscle). This muscle (Fig. 3-17) forms the mobile and adaptive substance of the cheek. It is a wide, rather thin muscle plate that arises from a horseshoe-shaped line. The line can be followed along the base of the alveolar process from the level of the first upper molar distally to the suture between the maxilla and palatine bone (Fig. 3-18). From here, the line of origin reaches the lower surface of the pyramidal process of the palatine bone and continues on a short ligament, spanning from the lower surface of the pyramidal process of the palatine bone to the tip of the pterygoid hamulus. This ligament or tendinous arch forms, with the concavity of the hamulus, an opening for the tendon of the tensor palati muscle. A ligament extends from the pterygoid hamulus, downward and outward, to end on the mandible at the lower end of the temporal crest behind the third molar tooth. It is called the pterygomandibular raphe and can be compared with a tendinous inscription from which fibers of the buccinator muscle and part of the upper constrictor of the pharynx take origin. On the mandible (Fig. 3-18) the line of attachment of the buccinator muscle crosses the lower end of the retromolar fossa laterally and then follows the oblique line downward and forward. At the base of the alveolar process, it turns horizontally forward to a level corresponding to the mesial end of the first molar.

The muscle bundles arising from this horseshoe-shaped line run in a generally forward direction but are not arranged parallel to each other. The bundles arising from the upper jaw have a tendency to descend in their forward course, whereas those arising from the lower jaw ascend slightly toward the corner of the mouth. Thus the bundles partly overlap each other in the anterior part of the muscle, which, therefore, is thicker than its posterior part. Close to the corner of the mouth, the fibers end in a rather intricate manner. Most of them insert into the mucous membrane of the cheek in and around the tendinous node and the tendinous line. Other fibers, however, interlace with those of the neighboring muscles and terminate in the skin of the upper and lower lips near the commissure.

Opposite the upper second molar the buccinator muscle is perforated by the parotid duct. In many other places the muscle bundles are forced apart by smaller or larger buccal glands, the bodies of which lie in part or entirely on the outer surface of the muscle. The motor nerve supply of the buccinator muscle is derived from the facial nerve. The sensory buccal nerve of the mandibular nerve divides into its branches on the lateral surface of the muscle. The single branches perforate the buccinator muscle and end in the mucous membrane of the cheek.

The buccinator muscle pulls the corner of the mouth laterally and posteriorly. Its main function, however, is to keep the cheek taut during all the phases of opening and closing of the mouth. Relaxing during the opening of the jaws, the muscle gradually contracts during the closing phase and thus maintains the necessary tension of the cheek so that the cheek is prevented from folding in and being bitten by the teeth. Paralysis of the buccinator muscle by a lesion of the facial nerve leads, invariably, to repeated and severe lacerations of the mucous membrane of the cheek during mastication.

Musculus orbicularis oris (oral sphincter). This muscle (Figs. 3-15 and 3-16) occupies the entire width of the lips. It has no direct attachment to the skeleton. Its fibers can be divided into an upper and a lower group that cross each other at acute angles lateral to the corner of the mouth. In addition, the majority of upper and lower fibers are confined to one side only, interlacing at the midline with the fibers of the other side. Thus, the muscle is a unit only functionally, not anatomically.

The bundles of the orbicularis oris muscle that correspond to the red zone of the lips are finer and more densely arranged than are those in the periphery. In many individuals the former are paler than the latter. The fibers in the upper lip find their medial end in an area corresponding to the philtrum of the upper lip, in a densely woven connective tissue strip that begins at the lower end of the nasal septum. Here the fibers of the muscle cross the midline and, in part, may reach the nasal septum itself. Some authors have called these fibers the depressor of the nasal septum. The deepest fibers of the muscle, which can be easily exposed by removing the mucous membrane of the lip, cross from right to left without interruption. Such continuous fibers are found in the upper as well as the lower lip.

In the midline the fibers of the lower lip show an arrangement similar to that in the upper lip. In addition they interlace with fibers of the depressor of the lower lip in an intricate pattern.

Laterally the fibers of both lips cross each other at acute angles, and the majority of the fibers end in the tendinous strip and node. Other fibers, however, after crossing fibers of the adjacent muscles, continue by intercalated tendons into fibers of the radial muscles, for instance, the major zygomatic, risorius, and depressor anguli oris muscles.

The orbicularis oris muscle closes the lips. It is, moreover, able to narrow the lips and press them against the teeth, or to protrude the lips, or to purse them. The varying functions of the muscle are made possible, in part, by the independence of its several portions and, in part, by the combination of its action with that of the other muscles of the lips.

Musculi incisivi (incisive muscles). These muscles (Fig. 3-17) of the upper and lower lips arise from the alveolar process and course laterally, closely following the peripheral bundles of the orbicular oris muscles to end in the tendinous node. Because of their close relation to the orbicularis oris muscle, they are sometimes referred to as its accessory skeletal heads.

The upper incisive muscle arises from the alveolar eminence of the canine, close to the alveolar crest (Fig. 3-18). It curves over the fornix of the upper vestibule to reach the orbicularis oris muscle. The lower incisive muscle originates at the height of the canine alveolus (Fig. 3-18) just above the origin of the mental muscle. The field of its origin is also relatively close to the alveolar border, as is that of the mentalis muscle. Its course simulates that of the upper incisive muscle.

The action of these weak muscles is not well circumscribed. However, in contracting, they press on the fornix vestibuli and make the vestibulum oris shallow in the
respective areas. Thus, like the mental muscle, they can make it difficult for the
dentist to work on the labial surfaces of upper or lower front teeth.

Musculus nasalis (nasal muscle). This muscle (Fig. 3-16) originates from the alveolar eminences of the lateral incisor and canine of the upper jaw at the base of the
alveolar process (Fig. 3-18). From here, the fibers diverge upward and medially
toward the wing of the nose. The muscle can be divided into two parts: the alar part,
musculus dilator naris, ends in the wing of the nose; the transverse part, musculus
compressor naris, passes over the lower part of the bridge of the nose to join the nasal
muscle of the other side.

The alar, or inferior, part of the nasal muscle ends at the lateral and posterior
circumference of the nostril; its most medial fibers reach the posterior end of the
mobile septum of the nose; the lateral fibers end in the skin of the nasal wing.

The transverse upper part of the nasal muscle continues upward and medially
toward the bridge of the nose into a thin and wide aponeurosis that is continuous with
that of the other side. Thus the transverse parts of the nasal muscles form a slinglike
band across the cartilaginous part of the nasal bridge.

Muscles of the eyelids and eyebrows

Four muscles can be grouped under the heading of muscles of the eyelids and
eyebrows. The orbicularis oculi muscle functions as the closer of the eyelids; the other
three, depressor supercilii, corrugator supercilii, and procerus muscle, move the
brow.

Musculus orbicularis oculi (sphincter of the eyelids). This muscle (Figs. 3-15 and
3-16) surrounds the opening of the lids in wide sweeping arches. It can be divided into
two main parts, the palpebral and the orbital portions. The first is situated in the lids;
the second extends far beyond the lids into the forehead, temporal region, and
cheek.

The origin of the muscle fibers is concentrated in the region of the inner canthus,
where they arise from the frontal process of the maxilla and the lacrimal bone. Other
fibers come from the wall of the lacrimal sac and from the medial palpebral ligament.
One bundle, the lacrimal part (Horner's muscle), arises from the posterior lacrimal
crest of the lacrimal bone behind the lacrimal sac. The bundles of the palpebral part
end in the skin in the region of the lateral corner of the eye, sometimes in an irregular
raphe that extends for a variable distance from the outer canthus laterally. The lateral
fibers of the orbital part diverge and continue into neighboring muscles or end separately in the skin.

Musculus depressor supercilii. This muscle, the depressor of the brow, is often
described as the most medial bundle of the orbital part of the orbicularis oculi muscle.
These fibers, arising from the lacrimal crest of the maxillary frontal process, run
almost vertically upward and end in the skin of the head of the eyebrow, which they
pull downward.

Musculus procerus nasi (slender muscle of the nose). This muscle (Fig. 3-16) arises from the nasal bone close to the midline and runs straight upward. The narrow muscle soon widens by divergence of its fibers. The bundles end in the skin of the head of the brow and of the forehead in the glabellar region between the eyebrows.

The muscle depresses the medial wider part, the head of the eyebrow.

Musculus corrugator supercilii. This muscle, the wrinkler of the eyebrow, is a horizontal muscle that arises from the frontal bone at the medial end of the superciliary arch (Fig. 3-18). The bundles of the muscle course laterally, some laterally and upward, ending in the outer part, the tail, of the eyebrow and the skin of the forehead immediately above it. Many of its fibers interlace with those of the frontal muscle.

The muscle pulls the eyebrow medially and is responsible for the vertical folds between the brows at the root of the nose.

Muscles of the outer ear

The muscles that are able to move the outer ear are vestigial in man and are therefore highly variable. The variations consist not only of aberrations of the typical muscles, but also in the appearance of accessory muscles, many of which have been described in the literature. A short description of the three typical muscles, the auricularis anterior, superior, and posterior, will suffice.

Musculus auricularis anterior. This muscle, the protractor of the outer ear, arises from the aponeurotic tendon of the scalp in the temporal region. Its fibers run horizontally backward and are inserted to the cartilage of the outer ear at its anterior border and medial surface above the entrance to the auditory passage. This muscle is, as a rule, small and weak.

Musculus auricularis superior. This muscle, the elevator of the outer ear, is normally the largest of this group. It arises above the ear in a broad line from the aponeurotic tendon of the scalp and sends its converging muscle bundles to the medial surface of the auricular cartilage.

Musculus auricularis posterior. This muscle, the retractor of the outer ear, is a small but strong muscle. It has its origin from the lateral part of the superior nuchal line and the base of the mastoid process and is directed horizontally forward (Fig. 3-18). Its termination is on the medial surface of the cartilaginous outer ear.

Only a few people can contract these outer ear muscles voluntarily, most frequently the posterior auricular muscle, which pulls the auricle backward. The muscles are, however, often involuntarily contracted if other muscles of facial expression are in action.

Muscles of the scalp

Four muscles, the paired frontal and occipital muscles, and their common tendon cover the vault of the skull like a cap. Together they form the epicranius muscle; their common tendon is known as galea aponeurotica, the tendinous skull cap.

Musculus frontalis (frontal belly). This muscle (Figs. 3-15 and 3-16) arises from the anterior border of the galea aponeurotica and ends in the skin of the eyebrow and of the root of the nose. Many of its fibers interlace and are connected with those of adjacent muscles; its most medial fibers may have connections with the procerus nasi muscle and the elevator of upper lip and nasal wing. The two frontal muscles are usually almost in contact at the midline or may even fuse.

Musculus occipitalis (occipital belly). This muscle arises at the supreme nuchal line from the base of the mastoid process to a point close to the midline (Fig. 3-18). Its fibers form an irregularly quadrilateral plate and continue upward into the fibers of the aponeurotic cap.

The galea aponeurotica, the common tendon of the fronto-occipital muscles, consists mostly of sagittal fibers. Transverse fibers are found in a greater number only in the lateral part of the galea, where the anterior and superior auricular muscles, arising from it, exert a transverse pull. Laterally, the galea has no sharp boundary but thins out gradually and is, above the zygomatic arch, fused to the superficial fascia. The galea aponeurotica is loosely fixed to the underlying periosteum and, farther laterally, to the upper part of the temporal fascia. The skin, however, is tightly fixed to the galea and moves with it. Blood or pus may accumulate in great volume underneath the galea, but such fluids remain confined to small areas in the dense subcutaneous tissue between galea and skin.

Occipital and frontal muscles, acting together, lift the eyebrow and fold the skin of the forehead in horizontal creases. The action is such that the occipital muscles tighten and hold the epicranial aponeurosis, transforming it into a fixed basis from which the frontal muscles act on the skin. Fully contracted, the fronto-occipital muscles also gain some influence on the upper eyelids, which they lift in an exaggerated fashion.

CHAPTER 4

The craniomandibular articulation

STRUCTURAL DESIGN

Jaw movement is analyzed as an action between two rigid components jointed together in a particular way, the movable mandible against the stabilized cranium. Since the adult human mandible is a single bone with the same type of joint at each end, the term *craniomandibular joint* is distinctly preferable to the customary designation "temporomandibular" joint. This latter label reinforces the unconscious habit of thinking of only one side in most jaw joint discussions, a habit early acquired in beginning anatomy courses where joint dissections are carried out on sagitally sectioned heads. In the living, the articulation of one side cannot possibly move without movement of, and a restricting effect from and on, the opposite side. Nevertheless, in principle the mandible works like a Class III lever with its joint as the fulcrum (see Chapter 5 and Fig. 5-16).

The jaw articulation is distinguished from most other synovial joints of the body by the coincidence of certain characteristic features. In the first place its articular surfaces are covered not by hyaline cartilage as elsewhere (clavicular articulations excepted), but by a dense, avascular, fibrous tissue that may contain a variable number of cartilage cells. It is thereby designated fibrocartilage. In addition, the two jointed components carry teeth whose shape, position, and occlusion introduce a unique influence on specific positions and movements within the joint. The joint is further distinguished by the marked differences in the shapes of the two articulating components. Finally, a fibrocartilaginous disc is interposed between upper and lower articular surfaces; this disc compensates for the incongruities in opposing parts and allows sliding, pivoting, and rotating movements between the bony components. Thus, in terms of joint mechanics, the craniomandibular articulation is a peculiar, bilateral, roving fulcrum around which moments of force turn in a complex jaw-lever system.

The articular surface of the mandible is seated on its ovoid condylar process (Fig. 4-1, *A*). The lateral pole of the condyle is roughened and often bluntly pointed, and it projects only moderately from the plane of the ramus. The medial pole is usually rounded, and it extends strongly inward from the plane of the ramus. It is braced from below in this extension by the prominent ridge of the mandibular neck (see Figs. 2-41 and 2-42). In lateral view the condyle appears tilted forward on the mandibular neck with its articular surface on its anterosuperior aspect. The articular surface thus faces the posterior slope of the articular eminence when the jaw is held with the teeth in complete occlusion against the skull (Figs. 4-3, A and 4-4). The articular surface continues medially down and around the rounded medial pole of the condyle. This medial articular surface faces the entoglenoid process of the temporal bone when the jaw is held in the occluded position (Fig. 4-3, B). The condyle is about 15 to 20 mm. from side to side and about 8 to 10 mm. from front to back. Its long axis lies at a right

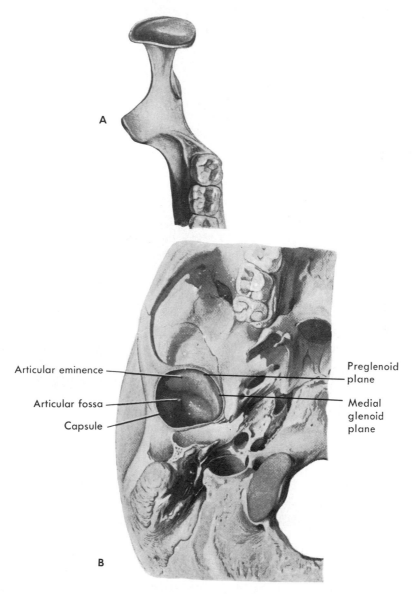

A

Articular eminence

Articular fossa

Capsule

Preglenoid plane

Medial glenoid plane

B

Fig. 4-1. A, Articulating surface of mandible with line of attachment of capsule. B, Articulating surface of temporal bone with line of attachment of capsule. (Sicher and Tandler: Anatomie für Zahnärtze.)

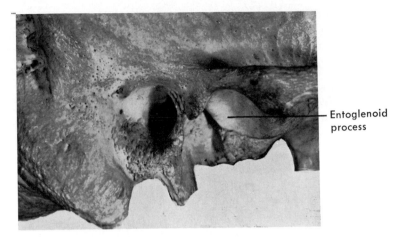

— Entoglenoid
process

Fig. 4-2. Note well-developed postglenoid process and entoglenoid process walling the fossa.

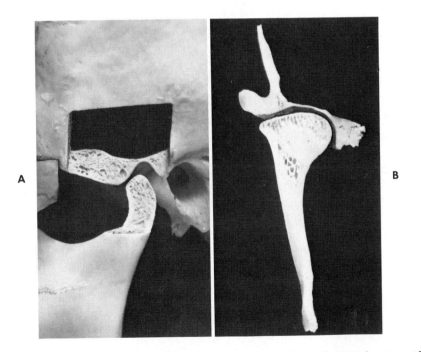

Fig. 4-3. Sections through the bones of the left craniomandibular articulation. **A,** Sagittal section with teeth in full occlusion. Note (1) forwardly bent condyle facing posterior slope of articular eminence, (2) closest match of opposing articular surfaces (close packed position), and (3) bulkiness of articular eminence versus thinness of bone in depth of fossa. **B,** Transverse section with teeth in full occlusion. Note (1) increased curvature around projecting medial pole of condyle facing entoglenoid process at right and (2) thinness of bone between articular fossa and area of temporal lobe of the brain.

angle with the plane of the ramus. It therefore does not lie in the frontal plane of the skull since the two sides of the jaw spread widely posteriorly (see Fig. 2-44). Thus if the long axes of the two condyles are extended medially, they meet approximately at basion on the anterior limit of the foramen magnum. This forms an angle, open toward the front, varying from 145 to 160 degrees. The condyle is usually strongly convex anteroposteriorly and mildly convex mediolaterally, the convexity increasing around the medial pole. The mediolateral convexity is often irregular, with medial and lateral slopes divided by a more or less prominent anteroposterior ridge. Variations from the general form are frequent, but the bony variations seen on dried skulls are not good reflections of the articular surface in life, where irregularities in the bone are filled in with fibrocartilage to produce a smooth, even covering.

The articular surface, or *facies articularis*, of the temporal bone is more complicated. It is situated on the inferior aspect of the temporal squama, anterior to the tympanic element of the temporal complex (Fig. 4-1, *B*). This is a continuous surface consisting of three regions: (1) the posterior slope to the height of convexity of the *articular eminence*, just anterior to the mandibular (glenoid) fossa; (2) the flattening preglenoid plane continuing anteriorly from the height of the eminence; and (3) the *entoglenoid process* continuous with the narrow *medial glenoid plane* on its inferior edge (Figs. 4-1, *B*, 4-2, and 4-3, *B*).

The anatomic terminology used in discussions of the joint has often been most confusing. Elaboration of the above terms will demonstrate their usefulness for clarity and accuracy in description. To begin with, an unequivocal distinction must be made between the labels *articular tubercle* and *articular eminence*. The articular tubercle is *nonarticulating!* It is a small, rough, bony knob raised on the outer end of the anterior root of the zygomatic process of the temporal bone (see Fig. 2-21). It projects below the level of the articular surface (see Fig. 4-9) and, as such tubercles do elsewhere, it serves as the attachment of collateral ligaments of the joint. The articular eminence, on the other hand, is the entire transverse bony bar that forms the anterior root of the zygoma (see section on the temporal bone, Chapter 2). This is the articular surface most heavily traveled by condyle and disc as they ride forward and backward in normal jaw function. The *preglenoid plane** is the slightly hollowed, almost horizontal articular surface continuing anteriorly from the height of the eminence. The medial glenoid plane has been identified previously (Fig. 4-1, *B*).

The boundary between the squama and the tympanic bone is formed laterally by the tympanosquamosal suture. Medially the inferior edge or process of the tympanic roof, the tegmen tympani, protrudes between the tympanic bone and temporal squama to divide the simple fissure into an anterior petrosquamosal and a posterior petrotympanic fissure (see Fig. 2-21). The posterior part of the fossa is elevated to form a ridge, the posterior articular ridge or lip. This ridge increases in height laterally to form the thickened, cone-shaped prominence called the postglenoid process immediately anterior to the external acoustic meatus (Fig. 4-2).

---

*This term, as first introduced by Weidenreich in describing *Homo erectus pekinensis*, included the entire bony roof of the infratemporal fossa.

The lateral border of the fossa is usually raised to form a narrow crest joining the articular tubercle in front with the postglenoid process behind. Medially the articular fossa narrows considerably and is bounded by a bony wall, the entoglenoid pocess, that leans against the angular spine of the sphenoid bone. The medial articular wall is sometimes elevated to a triangular process then called the temporal spine (Fig. 2-82, D). The roof of the fossa, separating it from the middle cranial fossa, is always thin (Figs. 4-3 and 4-4) and, even in heavy skulls, translucent. This is clear evidence that the articular fossa, although containing the posterior rim of the disc and the condyle, is not a stress-bearing functional part of the craniomandibular articulation; this function in the articulation is always between the condyle and disc, on one hand, and the articular eminence and its extended planes, on the other.

The articular eminence is strongly convex in an anteroposterior direction and somewhat concave in a transverse direction. The degree of its convexity is highly variable, with the radius of the curvature varying from 5 to 15 mm. Medial and lateral borders of the articular eminence are sometimes accentuated by fine bony ridges. The anterior boundary of the articular eminence is, as a rule, indistinct. The entire articulating surface of the temporal bone is covered by a layer of fibrous tissue that is thickest at the posterior slope and the summit of the articular eminence (Fig. 4-4). That the fibrous tissue is hardly thicker than a periosteum where it lines the roof of the articular fossa is added evidence that the fossa does not function as a stress-bearing part of the craniomandibular articulation.

The articular disc (Fig. 4-4) is an oval fibrous plate of great firmness. Its central part is always considerably thinner than its periphery; the posterior border is especially thick. The disc varies in thickness, and its variations seem to be correlated to the prominence of the articular eminence: the more prominent the articular eminence, the thicker the disc. Posteriorly the disc continues into a thick layer of loose and vascularized connective tissue that reaches to and fuses with the posterior wall of the articular capsule, the retrodiscal pad (Fig. 4-4).

The fibrous layers covering both mandibular and temporal surfaces are avascular. Blood vessels are also absent in the firm central area of the articular disc. The lack of blood vessels demonstrates clearly that there is considerable pressure in this joint as, indeed, there is in all joints. Avascular connective tissue is adapted to resist pressure, although it is not as highly specialized as cartilage. The differentiation of islands of cartilage in the fibrous layers and, more rarely, in the disc occurs as a rule in older age groups and may be regarded as a response of the tissue to pressure and friction. The lack of blood vessels and, therefore, of blood circulation does not, however, mean that there is no lymph or tissue fluid circulation in these tissues. In this respect they may be compared with the cornea of the eye. Pressure that is sustained too long in one or that is too heavy, will interfere with the circulation of the tissue fluid and will lead to degenerative changes in these avascular tissues.

The fibrous capsule of the mandibular joint is rather thin (Fig. 4-5). Mainly the lateral surface of the fibrous capsule is strengthened by a distinct ligament, the temporomandibular ligament.

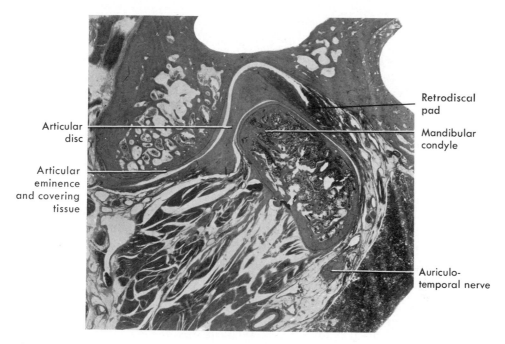

Retrodiscal
pad

Articular
disc

Mandibular
condyle

Articular
eminence
and covering
tissue

Auriculo-
temporal nerve

Fig. 4-4. Sagittal section through craniomandibular articulation of a 28-year-old man. (Courtesy S. W. Chase.)

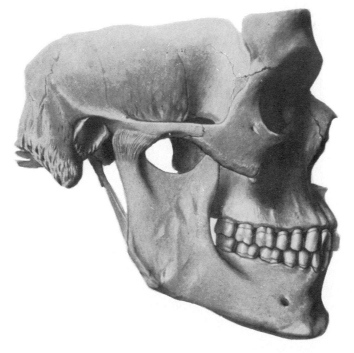

Fig. 4-5. Right craniomandibular articulation. (Sicher and Tandler: Anatomie für Zahnärzte.)

The temporomandibular ligament* has been specialized into two separate layers, a wide, lateral or superficial layer and a medial or deep band (Fig. 4-9). The lateral fan-shaped portion arises broadly from the outer surface of the articular tubercle at the root of the zygomatic arch. There is often a slightly raised ridge of attachment in this area. The ligamentous fascicles converge to run obliquely downward and backward and insert at the back of the mandibular neck behind and below the lateral condylar pole. Medial to this portion a narrow band of the ligament arises on the crest of the articular tubercle. It is continuous anteromedially with the anterior attachment of the disc on the temporal squama. Its fibers run horizontally back as a flat strap to attach with the disc on the lateral pole of the mandibular condyle and to the back of the disc (Figs. 4-10 and 4-11). There is no comparable reinforcement on the medial side of the condyle, but a medial horizontal band is present at a lower level. Evidently this is because right and left craniomandibular articulations function as *one* joint (see discussion of postures and movements of the mandible). The ligament is thus part of a system of "check reins" limiting joint movements. The oblique band is the radius of the arc of the eminence; it keeps the condyle close. The horizontal band prevents backward displacement.

The fibrous capsule is attached to the border of the temporal articulating surface and to the neck of the mandible (Fig. 4-1). Of interest is the fact that the capsular attachment is not just to the edge of postglenoid lip and process, but to their entire anterior surfaces. This makes it clear that there is never contact between condyle and postglenoid process. All claims that the postglenoid process serves as a fulcrum in lateral movements of the mandible are entirely without foundation.

Repeated claims of "the condyle bracing itself on the postglenoid process" evidently arose from attempts to study mandibular movements on the dry skull. There is only one way of fitting the mandible to the cranium, and that is by bringing mandibular and maxillary teeth into occlusion. Then the teeth and only the teeth hold the mandible, and there is no bony contact at the sites of the joints. Any attempt to move the mandible disturbs the holding contact of the occluding teeth. Then the mandible slips upward and backward, and the condyle or condyles fit snugly into the articular fossa and "brace" themselves against the postglenoid process or processes. It should, therefore, be understood that studies of mandibular movements on the dry skull are futile and must necessarily lead to grave mistakes.

The relations of the capsule to the disc and of the disc to the condyle are as interesting as they are significant. Anteriorly disc and capsule are fused and can be separated only artificially and arbitrarily. This fusion allows the attachment of some fiber bundles of the lateral (external) pterygoid muscle to the disc. Posteriorly disc and capsule are connected by a pad of loose, vascularized, and innervated connective tissue. This loose connection gives the disc the necessary freedom of anterior movement. Laterally and medially the disc and capsule are independently attached to the

---

*The precise term for the ligament is temporomandibular since it extends from the temporal bone to the mandible, which makes the distinction from other mandibular ligaments. The term for the joint itself is craniomandibular, as noted previously.

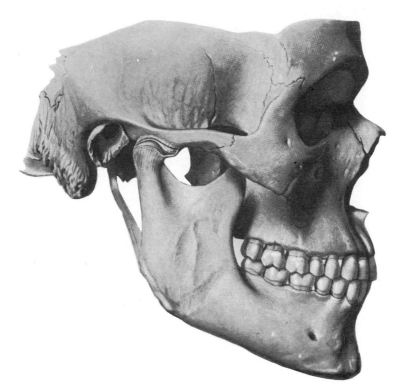

Fig. 4-6. Right craniomandibular articulation after opening into joint cavities. (Sicher and Tandler: Anatomie für Zahnärzte.)

lateral and medial poles of the condyle. This direct and firm attachment of the disc to the poles of the condyle assures the simultaneity of movements of mandible and discs. The discs follow the movements of the mandible passively as long as the muscles function harmoniously (Figs. 4-6 and 4-7). However, the attachment of the disc to the two poles of the condyle is not rigid enough to prevent small shifting movements of the condyles against the disc in a horizontal plane during the hinge or rotatory movement of the mandible in the lower compartments.

The synovial capsule of the craniomandibular joint lines the fibrous capsule and covers the loose connective tissue between it and the posterior border of the disc. At the mandibular neck (Fig. 4-4), as is the rule for convex articular bodies, the synovial capsule inserts at some distance from the articulating surface itself and reflects on, and covers, the bone to the borderline of the articulating facet. Thus part of the mandibular neck is covered by the synovial capsule and, therefore, is intracapsular, a fact that is important in prognosis and treatment of fractures of the condylar process. The area included in the articulation is more extensive on the posterior surface of the neck than on its anterior surface. The synovial capsule forms small folds and villi, especially in the region of the retrodiscal pad.

Two ligaments are described as accessory ligaments of the craniomandibular artic-

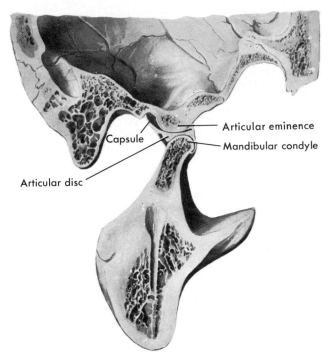

Articular eminence

Capsule

Mandibular condyle

Articular disc

Fig. 4-7. Frozen section through left craniomandibular articulation, mouth opened maximally. (Sicher and Tandler: Anatomie für Zahnärzte.)

ulation, namely, the sphenomandibular and the stylomandibular ligaments (Fig. 4-8). Neither one has any influence on the movements of the mandible. The sphenomandibular ligament, a remnant of Meckel's cartilage, arises from the angular spine of the sphenoid bone and is directed downward and outward. It spreads fanlike toward the mandible, to which it is inserted at the mandibular lingula, at the lower border of the mandibular foramen, and at the lower border of the groove of the mandibular neck. In most persons it is a thin layer of connective tissue with indistinct anterior and posterior borders. However, it has an influence on the spread of the injected fluid in block anesthesia of the lower and alveolar nerve. The stylomandibular ligament is a reinforced part of a fascial lamella that extends from the styloid process and stylohyoid ligament to the region of the mandibular angle. Part of its fibers are attached to the mandible itself, but the majority continue into the fascia on the medial surface of the medial pterygoid muscle. The upper border of the stylomandibular ligament is often sharp and thickened. The ligament is relaxed when the mouth is closed and is tense only in extreme protrusion of the mandible. At the end of the opening movement, the stylomandibular ligament is in its most relaxed state. This ligament is an important landmark for the exposure of the external carotid artery in the retromandibular fossa.

Blood and nerve supply. As in all other joints, the surrounding vessels and nerves contribute to service the capsule of the craniomandibular articulation. Branches from

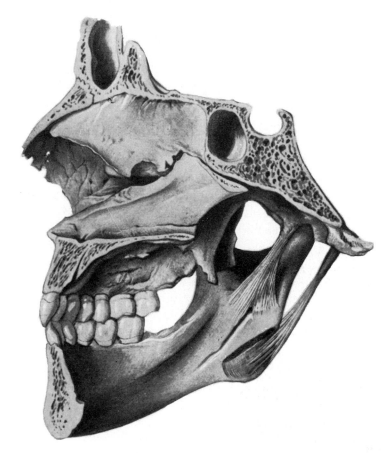

Fig. 4-8. Sphenomandibular and stylomandibular "ligaments." (Sicher and Tandler: Anatomie für Zahnärzte.)

the superficial temporal and maxillary arteries supply the capsule posteriorly, whereas twigs from the masseteric artery enter anteriorly. An unusually rich plexus of veins is found at the posterior part of the capsule, which serves to equalize pressure in the tissues by filling and emptying as the condyle rocks rhythmically forward and backward in chewing. The majority of sensory nerves to the capsule arise from the auriculotemporal nerve. Anteriorly, however, branches are regularly contributed by the mixed masseteric nerve and sometimes by the posterior deep temporal nerve.

POSTURES AND MOVEMENTS OF THE MANDIBLE

A primary tenet of mechanics (Newton's third law) holds that all orderly movement must spring from a stable base that resists displacement with a force equal and opposite to the force of the movement. Such bases are supplied by the joints of the body. They act as fulcra around which moments of force can turn. A crucial feature in the functioning of the human jaw arises from the fact that the craniomandibular connection is *one* operating unit composed of right and left joint complexes. Then, since the mandible is a single bone, the joints of each side are coordinated so that each contributes to every movement. Although it is easily accepted, this fact is often lost sight of when studying jaw movements because the joints are far apart and on opposite sides of the head. The mechanism can be distinctly demonstrated in the knee joint, where the condyles, meeting anteriorly, are barely an inch apart posteriorly. Just as in the jaw, both femoral condyles rotate around a common transverse axis in flexion and extension. Furthermore, in full extension, the femur rotates around a vertical axis in which the lateral condyle rides forward on a sliding articular cartilage, just as in the jaw in a lateral excursion.

Close examination of synovial joints has shown that no articular surfaces are perfectly flat and that the surface curvatures vary from point to point. Furthermore, no opposing surfaces are completely congruous; the entire surfaces never fit together perfectly. In joint movements the small areas of contact are constantly shifting so that pressure is not concentrated in one spot for long. However, as one surface travels over its counterpart, the fit varies. In certain positions of the bones, broad areas of the two articulating surfaces are exactly matched. This is called the "close-packed" position, and at this time the joint transmits pressure most effectively (see Fig. 4-3, A).

Synovial joints have been officially classified into as many as seven types, according to the contours of their articular surfaces. Extensive studies in articular mechanics have narrowed this down to two fundamental forms, ovoid and sellate. The ovoid form is egg shaped; its curvature changes along the longitudinal plane whether it is convex or concave. The sellate form is saddle shaped; its curvature is convex in one plane and concave at a right angle to this plane. The articular surface of the mandibular condyle is thus an ovoid form; it is strongly convex anteroposteriorly and, although slightly convex mediolaterally, the curvature increases notably around its medial pole. The articular surface of the temporal bone is sellate; it is strongly convex anteroposteriorly and also concave mediolaterally. But most significantly the broadest area of contact (close-packed position) is found on the posterior slope of the articular eminence and the anterior slope of the condyle, where pressure is transmitted through the thinnest part of the disc when the teeth are in fullest occlusion (Figs. 4-3, A, and 4-4).

Since the craniomandibular joint is a bilateral articulation, both sides sustain pressure, but the load varies from side to side with changes in jaw position during mastication. Recent research suggests that the articulation *contralateral* to the chewing side may bear the greater pressure when biting hard.

The articulation of each side of the jaw is a composite that encloses two joints within its single capsule, an upper joint between articular eminence and disc and a lower joint between disc and mandibular condyle. In essence, then, it can be said that the functional jaw articulation is a double-double joint. The joint of each side is fitted with a temporomandibular ligament on its lateral surface. The ligament is made up of two distinct elements as noted previously. The outer element is the strong oblique band arising from a roughened surface on the lateral side of the articular tubercle and inserting on the neck of the mandible below the lateral condylar pole (Figs. 4-9 and 4-10). The inner element is an almost horizontal band arising on the tubercle medial

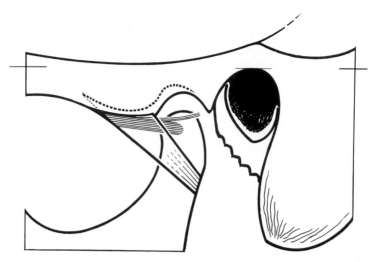

Fig. 4-9. Diagram of adaptive construction of temporomandibular ligament. Condyle is pulled out of position and disc is omitted for clarity. Outline of articular eminence (surface) is represented by heavy interrupted line. Outer, oblique band runs from articular tubercle to condylar neck. Inner, horizontal band (*hatched*) runs from anterolateral attachment of disc to lateral condylar pole and back of disc.

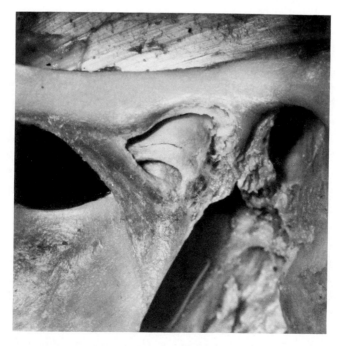

Fig. 4-10. Lateral view of temporomandibular ligament complex. Outer oblique band runs from tubercle down and back of neck of condyle. Disc and faint outline of the inner horizontal band can be seen.

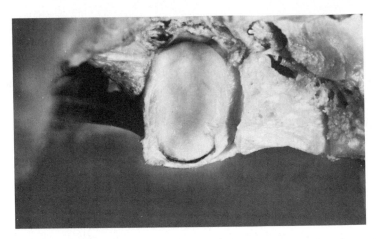

Fig. 4-11. View of joint from above. The joint has been turned down from lateral view so that its outer (lateral) surface is at bottom of picture. Entire roof of joint and zygomatic arch have been removed. Note (1) anterior attachment of horizontal band at left in position of the removed tubercle and (2) posterior attachment of the band into back of disc. A similar band on the medial side is at a lower level.

to, and fused with, the oblique band from which it separates to insert on the lateral condylar pole. A strong part of its upper segment continues backward and then curves medially to insert into the posterolateral aspect of the disc (Fig. 4-11). A smooth glistening surface is grooved on the lateral surface of the disc where this upper band rides. The band may sometimes be partially fused with the disc. This arrangement has a strong restraining function in retrusion that seems to be part of the adaptation of the jaw to the crowding of the retromandibular space in the overall adjustment of the skull to upright posture. It prevents posterior displacement of the condyle into the delicate neurovascular mass at the back of the joint between jaw and ear canal. A thickening of the capsule on the medial side of the joint is rather weak and may have little limiting effect on joint mobility, but a horizontal band similar to that on the lateral side of the joint is present. It arises from the anteromedial corner of the disc attachment above the insertion of the lateral pterygoid. It also inserts by curving around the back of the disc. In addition, the insertion of the lateral pterygoid muscle into the anteromedial corner of the capsule and disc may act as an adjustable "ligament," limiting posterior movement.

Postures

Before functional movements and specific muscular contributions to their performance can be evaluated, certain consistent physiologic postures, or positions and relations, of the jaw must be clearly defined. The term *posture* is preferable, since it emphasizes the disposition of the parts of the body with reference to each other, which is precisely the feature to be analyzed. The most commonly discussed of these postures are usually labeled *rest position* and *hinge position*, along with *centric* and other *occlusal positions*. Unfortunately the terminology of some of these positions is confusing and controversial in the current literature. Here only the simplest and least equivocal terms will be used.

Resting posture (rest position). The resting posture of the mandible is the position the lower jaw assumes when the mandibular musculature is at "rest," provided that the individual stands or sits at ease in the upright posture and holds the head so that the gaze is toward the horizon. This proviso is essential because it specifies that the entire head and neck also be in normal rest position. If the head is flexed forward, the bunched-up soft structures between chin and chest tend to shove the mandible forward from its rest position. If the head is extended backward, the opposite displacement occurs. Then such structures as skin, fascia, and facial muscles (for example, platysma) are stretched and pull the mandible down and back from the rest position. Therefore it must be clearly understood that the term "resting posture" does not imply a fixed or static position. The position varies continuously depending on numerous factors, including momentary bodily postures, immediately preceding activities, fatigue, and perhaps even the time of day. That any such position is *precisely* reproducible with any degree of confidence is wholly an illusion.

In this resting posture the teeth are clearly not in contact. The space between upper and lower teeth is called the *free-way space*, or interocclusal clearance. This normally measures from 2 to 5 mm. between incisors. In this position the lips touch lightly. Thus it is also clear that rest position is entirely independent of the number, form, position, or even the presence or absence of teeth. Instead, rest position is entirely dependent on the resting tonus of the mandibular musculature and gravity. No muscle is ever *totally* atonal (except perhaps under the influence of certain drugs, deep anesthesia, or unconsciousness). The residual tension of a muscle "at rest" is termed resting tonus, but this too must be defined with care.

Resting tonus is due both to the innate turgor and elasticity of muscular and fibrous tissue and to the discontinuous contractions of muscle bundles in response to an alert nervous system. But in addition, in antigravity muscles such as those of the jaw, intermittent reflex contraction of a number of muscle fibers is always present. Thus as some fibers become fatigued, others take up the tension so that a given percentage of the fibers maintains the normal resting posture of the jaw. The great significance of this phenomenon is that it establishes a mechanism that maintains, *at all times*, firm contact between articulating joint surfaces and thus ensures the integrity of the articulation. This mechanism becomes especially critical in all highly movable joints where the stability of the articulation cannot be greatly dependent on other features of joint structure (for example, the shoulder joint). Thus, in normal rest position of the jaw, the anterosuperior articular surfaces of the mandibular condyles are pulled toward the posterior slopes of the articular eminences of the temporal bone. As has been shown, these surfaces are protected by thickened, pressure-bearing, avascular, articular coverings. The thinnest parts of the articular discs intervene between these surfaces, and all are held in these relations by the conditions of resting tonus specified above.

This is simply one instance of the general physiologic principle in which the proper relations of all body parts are maintained by muscle tone. Though considerably lower during sleep, tonus is even then not entirely lost. Obviously, as muscle tonus is constant under constant conditions, so are the rest positions of the mandible. In aberrant conditions, such as disease, exhaustion, or nervous tension, these relationships may change. Certainly it is well understood that "constancy" in a living organism means simply that the *range* of variation is small but constant. Variability in nature is the means of biologic adaptation, the loss of which is incompatible with life itself.

Clinically, the range of the resting posture is of great significance because it specifies the crucial limits to any "bite-raising" prosthetic procedures. If the bite is "opened" (raised) as far as the rest position (meaning that the teeth touch in this position), the mandibular musculature is severely stressed. Constant contact of the teeth, however light, causes the neural end organs in the periodontium to signal this contact to the motor nucleus of the fifth nerve in the brainstem. This disrupts the normal, long-established neural firing pattern. The disrupted pattern then deprives the muscle fibers of their normal resting sequences. Trauma to teeth, supporting structures, and joint structures, as well as muscle spasm and pain, are the obvious consequences.

Hinge posture. The so-called hinge position of the jaw joint is one that can be located with some accuracy. It is the posture in which the condyles rest at the most retruded limit, against the thick back rims of the discs below the front of the fossa when the cusps of the teeth are just cleared of contact. It is from this position that a practically "pure" hinge raising and lowering of the jaw can be made. The simple hinge swinging of the mandible describes a small arc and is accomplished only when the mandible is forcefully retruded. The posteriormost retrusion that the condyle can reach is determined by the length of the tensed inner horizontal band of the craniomandibular ligament. Since the length of this band is constant, the clinical registration of this position can be repeated accurately. The hinge movement rotates around a common horizontal axis, which runs approximately through the centers of both condyles. Because of the appreciable asymmetries between both sides of the skull it is highly unlikely that the axis will ever run exactly through a juncture of horizontal and frontal planes. The location of this position is said to be useful in some clinical procedures. One feature of this is obviously significant; it specifies that the normal rest position of the condyle *must* be some short distance anterior to the hinge position.

Centric occlusal posture. Occlusal postures signify some sort of contact between upper and lower teeth. Centric occlusion denotes a concept of normal mandibular posture in which the dentition is occluded with all teeth fully interdigitated at the same time that all other kinetic components of the oral apparatus are in "harmonious balance." The condyles are slightly backwardly rotated and are at or slightly retruded from the level of their position at rest. Ideally, this is the position that the jaw should reach if it is snapped shut from the open position when the head and neck are in the upright posture. This is most likely to be achieved in healthy young adults with a full complement of teeth and what is classically considered a normal occlusion. It has been shown that in the overwhelming majority of cases, the mandible can be retruded from this position some 0.5 to 1 mm. if the teeth are barely freed. As has been noted above, it is obvious that the normal centric occlusal posture must be slightly forward of the position that the masticatory musculature can actually achieve. Thus the ability to move the mandible slightly backward from the centric occlusal relation is at least one distinct sign of a well-balanced oral apparatus. Although in the past it has been assumed that centric occlusion is identical with the hinge position, this is contradicted by the fundamental facts established above. The hinge position is an extreme position, and it is entirely contrary to well-known principles of biologic constructs that any normal joint be habitually postured in such a strained position. The potential for extreme movements seems unmistakably to be an adaptation installed as a margin of safety by which the integrity of a living structure can be preserved in situations of emergency.

Protrusive occlusal relation. In protrusive, or incisal, occlusion the incisal edges of the four lower incisors contact the incisal edges of the upper centrals and sometimes the laterals. Normally all the other teeth are not in occlusion. The condyles are slightly forwardly rotated and moved downward and forward to a level at or near the peak of the articular eminence.

Lateral occlusal relation. In lateral occlusion the upper and lower posteriors of the ipsilateral side contact along the line of the crests of the buccal and lingual cusps. In unworn teeth the cusps bulge in curves so that contacts are at spots where opposing contours meet. In worn teeth the contours are flattened, and contact lines may be almost continuous. In the natural dentition the teeth of the contralateral side are not in occlusion.

Movements

As with the anatomic terminology, discussions of movements within the jaw joint have lent obscurity to the fundamental features of the activity. Opening and closing of the jaw are most commonly attributed to rotation in the lower compartment of the joint (between condyle and disc) and translation in the upper compartment (between disc and articular eminence). Controverting this view, it has been suggested that *only* rotation occurs in both compartments. This proposition states that the mandible rotates around a transverse axis in the condyle, during which the condyle rotates around a similar axis in the articular eminence.

Physicists point out that the most general type of motion a body can undergo is a combination of translation and rotation. Translation is defined as a motion in which all points of a rigid body move in the same direction with the same velocity, at any given instant, relative to some point outside the body. Rotation is a motion in which some points of a rigid body move in one direction while other points move in the opposite direction, at any given instant.

Now it can be readily seen that a partially lowered mandible *can* translate, that is, move forward or backward over the articular eminence with all points of the jaw moving in the same direction at the same rate, at any given instant. Thus in simple

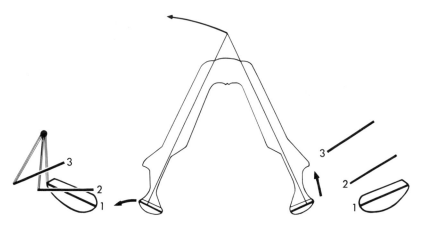

Fig. 4-12. Left lateral movement of jaw. Enlarged condyles at each side exaggerate movements; movement on left, the "chewing" side, is magnified about 4 times that on right. Heavy lines through condyles denote their long axes. On left, horizontal band of craniomandibular ligament (striped) runs from its origin on the tubercle (black spot) to lateral condylar pole. *Left side: 1,* Beginning position; *2,* orbiting around vertical axis (somewhere behind condyle) tenses ligament, which then halts movement; *3,* any further lateral movement must swing from ligament's origin on tubercle. *Right side:* Condyle, orbiting around common axis behind left condyle, moves forward and medially. Heavy arrow opposite lateral pole of left condyle indicates *transverse, bodily shift* of jaw.

lowering and raising of the mandible, the definitive statement must be that the condyle rotates relative to the disc while the disc is rotating relative to the articular eminence with concurrent translation of the mandible relative to the temporal articular facies. It is simply a problem of relative motion, and mandibular movements are completely consistent with the general observations in the physics of motion.

Opening and closing movements are symmetrical; that is, both sides of the craniomandibular articulation are making the same movements. Protrusive and retrusive movements may also be symmetrical. In this case disc and condyles of both sides slide downward and forward and backward and upward, respectively, with condyles and discs always, as in all joints of the body, in firm contact with their opposing articular surfaces. Movements may also be executed asymmetrically, which then produces a lateral movement, a swinging of the jaw to one side. In this case one disc, accompanied by its condyle, slides downward, forward, and medially on to the preglenoid and medial glenoid planes. The disc and condyle on the side to which the jaw is moving (left condyle for left lateral movement) do not travel far from their starting positions on the posterior slope of the eminence. Here the condyle orbits very slightly downward then outward in a small arc around a *vertical* axis somewhere behind the condyle. This imparts a transverse component to the excursion and thus produces a direct lateral shift of the entire mandible to the chewing side (Fig. 4-12). This has been called the Bennett movement, or Bennett shift, and although it may be slight (probably never more than 1.5 mm.) it has been considered significant in certain cases of restorative and prosthetic dentistry.

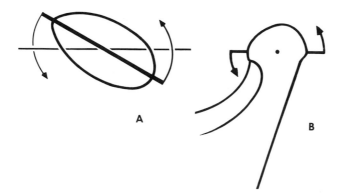

Fig. 4-13. Long axis of condyle relative to frontal plane. **A,** Left condyle from above; transverse line represents axis of opening rotation. **B,** Left condyle in lateral view. Black dot represents axis of opening rotation. Lateral pole lies in front of axis; medial pole lies back of axis. In opening rotation, lateral pole swings down and back while medial pole swings up and forward as indicated by arrows.

The *lower joints* of both sides work together as a common hinge joint. The two discs are the sockets, or "hooks," of the hinges, and each condyle forms the bar in the eye of the hinge on which the jaw swings open and closed. Because of the notable obliquity of the condyles to the frontal plane—the condylar axes converge posteriorly—the hinge movement of the mandible must be accompanied by adjusting movements between condyles and discs. The hinge movement occurs around a horizontal axis that runs approximately through the centers of the two condyles. Thus, during opening, the lateral pole of each condyle, situated *in front of the hinge axis*, must move slightly downward and backward. Concomitantly, the medial poles, situated *behind the hinge axis*, must move slightly upward and forward (Fig. 4-13).

This information is highly significant clinically in radiographic interpretation. Ignorance of these anatomic facts has resulted in the belief that condyle and eminence do lose contact (separate) during normal jaw movements, since a dense lateral pole is seen radiographically to move away from the eminence. But, as pointed out previously, areas of articular contact are constantly shifting during movement in all joints of the body; thus contact is shifting toward the medial pole in simple opening (Fig. 4-13). This prevents concentration of pressure at any point for any length of time. The broad areas of the close-packed position are adapted to withstand the peak of functional pressure (Fig. 4-3, A).

Whether the excursions of lateral and medial condylar poles are equal depends on the precise point through which the hinge axis passes between these poles. Because of appreciable facial and mandibular asymmetries, it is highly improbable that the hinge axis will ever run exactly through a juncture of horizontal and frontal planes.

Under normal conditions, sliding in the upper joints and rotating in the lower joints are probably always combined, but the magnitude of one or the other at a given time varies considerably. Both mandibular joints, always working together as a functional unit, can be classified as a hinge joint with a sliding socket. This definition clarifies the proper role or functional significance of the articular discs; they comprise the movable sockets of the hinge joint between the condyles and discs. The combination of *two* joints on each side of the jaw gives a certain freedom of movement to the mandible in all planes of space. But the fact that the articulating components always work in close contact obviously imposes some limitation of movement because of the two-sided articulation. Furthermore, the magnitude of these movements is not great, since they are effectively limited by all the various fibers of the temporomandibular ligaments of each side in the opened positions, to which is added the contact of the tooth planes in terminal closing positions.

One point cannot be overstressed. Strong contact between articulating bodies is found in all movable joints because muscles are always arranged to pull across joints. This means that condyles, discs, and eminences are in close contact at rest, in all movements, and in all positions. It means further that the moving discs and condyles must follow exactly the surface of the articular eminence. Thus all the movements of the condyles with their discs are entirely dependent on the configuration of the temporal articular facies. But curiously, many movements of the body of the mandible seem relatively independent of the shape of the eminence! This apparent paradox is easily dispelled. Movements of the mandible entail movements in both compartments. Of these only the translatory component is completely dependent on the shape of the eminence, but the addition of vertical and horizontal rotatory components introduces additional degrees of freedom within the frame of this dependency.

There are two outstanding features marking articulations classified as "freely movable joints." First, the articular bony contours of these joints are not predominant in guiding the movements, nor do the capsular ligaments determine the direction of movements. Instead, the musculature dominates in guiding and determining the movements. Second, such joints have the characteristic property of circumduction. The circumductory pathway defines the broadest limits of mobility as the moving part proceeds in a continuous sequence from one extreme position to the next. This is clearly seen in a ball-and-socket joint such as the head of the humerus rolling in the glenoid cavity of the scapula in the shoulder joint. When the rigid arm is swung forward windmill fashion alongside the body (considering the scapula theoretically stable), the limb moves smoothly from flexion through abduction, extension, adduction, and back to flexion. This tour of movement is traveling along the marginal limits of the limb's mobility, and so the movement is limited, though not guided, by the ligaments. Both craniomandibular articulations, operating as a unit, approximate a freely movable joint more complicated than that of the shoulder. In the mandibular complex, the periodontal ligaments are also a limiting factor. Therefore circumduction of the mandible is limited by the ligaments of its teeth as well as those of its joints.

Although it is indispensable for the dextrous performance of intricate acts, great freedom of movement imposes the serious problem of maintaining continuously the firm, normal relations of articulating parts. Ligaments limit the *extent* of movement. The temporomandibular ligaments have been shown to be made up of two distinct parts (Figs. 4-9 to 4-11). The outer oblique band acts as the constant radius of an arc traveled when the condyle slides down and around the articular eminence. Thus it is geared to keep the condyle and disc against the eminence. On extreme opening the condyle moves forward on the flattening articular plane, which increases the radius of the articular arc. This pulls the ligament taut and brings the movement to a halt. On closing, the condyle rotates backward as it glides back and up along the curve of the articular eminence until it reaches the fully closed position on the posterior slope of the eminence. At this point the horizontal band of the craniomandibular ligament begins to come into play (Fig. 4-11). Although the jaw can be forcibly moved farther back, tension of this band soon brings the movement to a halt. But in addition to these limiting ligaments, a most interesting special arrangement of the musculature hugging the joint reveals a mechanism for maintaining the joint integrity common to all highly movable articulations.

The posteriormost segment of the temporalis muscle displays a distinct bundle whose inferior fibers run horizontally straight forward to the anterior edge of the root of the zygoma. Here the undersurface of the fibers is protected by a tendinous layer as the muscle bends sharply downward in an almost vertical direction to attach to the edge of the lowest point in the mandibular notch (Fig. 4-14). In the position of rest,

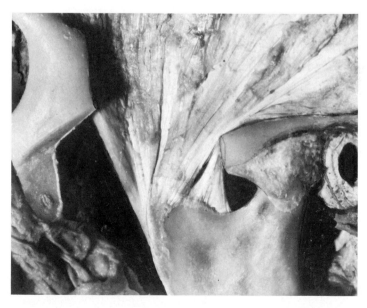

Fig. 4-14. Zygomatic arch has been removed to show special posterior segment of temporalis muscles, left side. Muscle fibers can be seen running horizontally forward above the external auditory meatus. At anterior lip of root of zygoma, muscle inserts into tendon, which turns sharply, in an angle of less than 90 degrees, to run down and slightly back to upper rim of mandibular notch. In this position, contraction of specialized segment can only pull condyle upward and forward to firm contact against back of eminence. Note three distinct divisions of temporalis muscle.

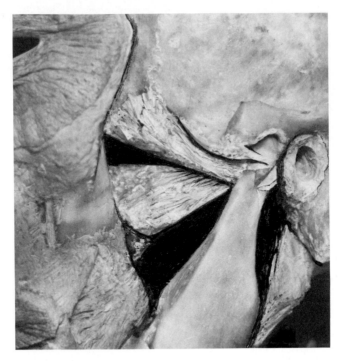

Fig. 4-15. Zygomatic arch and coronoid process have been removed to expose upper head of lateral pterygoid muscle. The muscle runs down and back to lip of root of zygoma, where it turns back to run horizontally to neck of mandible in rest position. As jaw moves forward, vertical direction of the muscle will increase. Hence it can only pull condyle up to firm contact against crest of eminence and preglenoid plane.

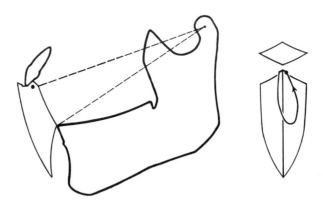

Fig. 4-16. Range of jaw movement. Sagittal view on the left indicates hinge movement (radius from center of condyle to limits of arc indicated in broken lines), wide opening, protrusion, and return to retrusive limit. Black dot under upper incisor marks the rest position. Outlines at right indicate extent of movement in horizontal plane (above) and frontal plane (below). Elliptical path of lateral movement in chewing on left side is indicated. Here, the black dot indicates cusp contact of posteriors, and path deviates along cusp inclines to centric occlusion.

contraction of these fibers can only pull the jaw upward. This seats the condyle firmly against the disc on the posterior slope of the articular eminence. When the jaw opens, the condyle moves downward and forward, and the angle of the posterior temporal fibers unbends or swings toward a more oblique position paralleling more closely the slope of the articular eminence. In this position the fibers can pull the jaw up and back, since the seating function has been diminished. But at this time another highly special and distinct muscular arrangement comes into play.

The lateral pterygoid muscle is divided into two anatomically separate segments. The upper head is of greatest interest here. It arises on the horizontal infratemporal surface of the greater wing of the sphenoid, which is at a level well above the joint. Its fibers run down and back to the anterior limit of the joint capsule, then swing horizontally back to the neck of the mandible (Fig. 4-15). Some of the upper fibers attach to the anteromedial corner of the disc through the capsule. In the position of rest, contraction of these fibers can only pull the jaw (and disc) forward. Then this also seats the condyle firmly against the disc on the posterior slope of the eminence. When the jaw opens and the condyle moves forward, the direction of the fibers of the upper head of the lateral pterygoid becomes more and more vertical. In this position the fibers pull the condyle more strongly up against the articular eminence and preglenoid plane, and the seating function becomes increased.

From the above it can be clearly seen that the special arrangements of both the posterior temporalis and the upper head of the lateral pterygoid muscles may be said to act as adjustable "ligaments" that ensure stability of the joint fulcrum at any instantaneous point of translation and rotation. This is remarkably similar to the function of the short muscles of the highly movable shoulder joint. These hold the head of the humerus firmly in the glenoid cavity of the scapula at all times during circumduction of the arm.

Range of movement. With these biomechanical qualifications of the joints established, the extreme limits of jaw movement (the so-called border movements) can now be considered. These movements are traced from a point at the incisal edge of the lower centrals, since this location is most easily visualized radiographically (Figs. 4-16 to 4-20).

Beginning with the condyles retruded to the extreme hinge position, the mandible can perform a theoretically pure hinge rotation about a fixed axis passing through the approximate centers of both condyles (Fig. 4-17). In opening, the interdental point swings down in an even arc of about 20 to 25 mm. in length. Further opening requires a downward and forward excursion of condyles and discs along the articular eminences, with continued rotation of the condyles within the lower joint compartments. This activity within the joint abruptly changes the course of the incisal point. It then proceeds in an arc of greater curvature directed more anteriorly, in which the lower termination marks the limit of greatest jaw opening (Figs. 4-16 and 4-18).

From this point closing proceeds directly upward and forward with the mandible strained forward in maximal protrusion during its entire path of movement. The interdental point now describes an arc of the least curvature in the sequence. Its upper termination is brought about by contact of the posterior teeth, since the lower anteriors reach forward beyond the upper anteriors with the jaw in its most protruded position (Figs. 4-16 and 4-19). In making this movement, the condyles rotate backward in the lower compartments, and both condyles and discs move slightly posteriorly. From this point the circuit of extreme movement is completed by retrusion to the original point of departure at the most retruded hinge position of the jaw. The path is necessarily uneven because of the shifting contacts of the teeth. Proceeding from the most protruded contact position, where the lower incisors are anterior to the

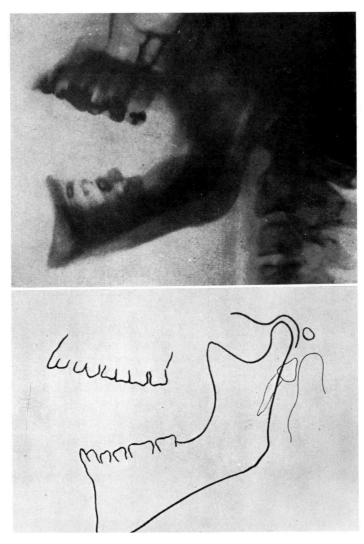

Fig. 4-17. Radiograph and outline drawing of a normal craniomandibular joint, mouth opened as far as possible in forced hinge movement. (Sicher and Tandler: Anatomie für Zahnärzte.)

uppers, the path of the incisal point dips to the edge-to-edge contact of the incisors, rises to the position of complete occlusal interdigitation (Figs. 4-16 and 4-20), then dips again as cusps are cleared to reach back to the terminal hinge position (Fig. 4-16).

Movements in the transverse, or horizontal, plane can be similarly traced. Again beginning with the mandible in its most retruded (terminal hinge) position, the jaw is rotated to one side as far as it will go with teeth just touching. In doing so it turns

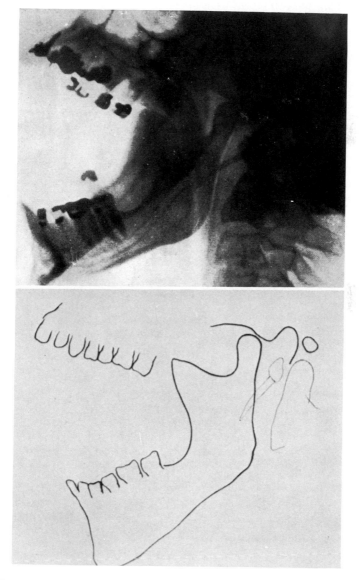

Fig. 4-18. Radiograph and outline drawing of craniomandibular joint, mouth opened maximally. (Sicher and Tandler: Anatomie für Zahnärzte.)

around a vertical axis somewhere behind the condyle on the side of the movement. If this is the left condyle it moves little, orbiting laterally in a small arc with a short radius of curvature. The condyle of the contralateral side, however, orbits in a long, flat arc, since its radius of curvature is much longer. Thus the right condyle slides downward, forward, and inward to the anterior limit of the articular plane. This movement of the jaw carries the incisal point laterally and forward in a mild curve to the right. From this position the jaw is swung toward the midline in full protrusion. Thus the right condyle now slides downward, forward, and inward to the interior limit of its articular plane. This movement carries the incisal point forward and medially in a mild curve to the same point of greatest protrusion visualized in the sagittal view. The reverse action is now carried out by moving the jaw to the extreme of the left lateral excursion; the left lateral condyle thus moves up and back toward the most

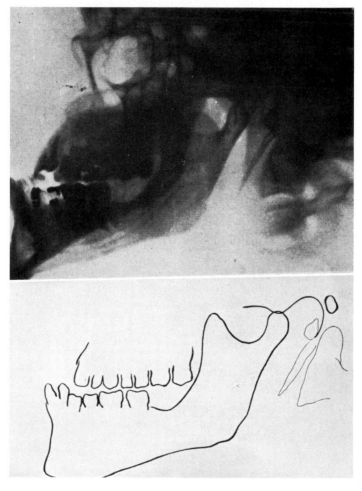

Fig. 4-19. Radiograph and outline drawing of a normal craniomandibular joint, mandible in maximal protrusion. (Sicher and Tandler: Anatomie für Zahnärzte.)

retruded position. Finally, the right condyle follows till the mandible is returned to the original point of departure in the most retruded hinge position. It can be seen that the outline traced by the incisal point in this total excursion is diamond-shaped, and it defines the marginal movements of the jaw in the horizontal (or occlusal) plane. When these lateral movements are made with the jaw at increasing levels of opening, the diamonds become smaller and smaller until they disappear at the point of maximal opening identical with that visualized in sagittal view (Fig. 4-16).

Functional movements. All normal functional movements of the mandible are made well within the boundaries of this envelope of marginal movements up to the point where the teeth come into occlusion (Fig. 4-16). Functional opening and closing

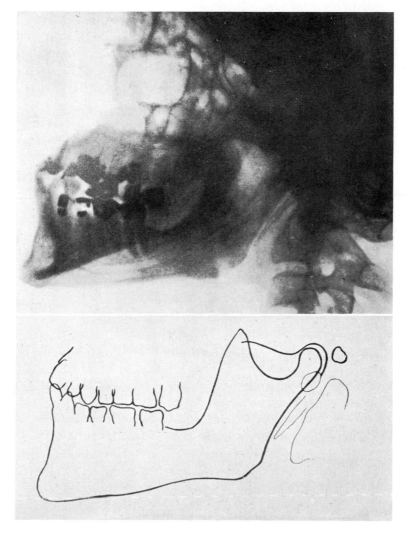

Fig. 4-20. Radiograph and outline drawing of a normal craniomandibular joint in centric occlusal posture. (Sicher and Tandler: Anatomie für Zahnärzte.)

patterns of the mandible merit special attention. Each half of this automatic cycle is a combination of hinge and sliding movements. The detail of this particular way of opening and closing the jaws may be specific to man because even anthropoid apes can apparently open the mandible widely with only a hinge movement. But since in these apes the tympanic bone is high, on a level with the jaw articulation, and since a mastoid process—highly variable, incipient, or even absent—is also at or near this level, *no part of the skull lies behind the mandible*. Hence it is possible for such jaws to swing deeply down and back in a simple hinge movement. In man, however, adaptation to the permanent upright posture and locomotion has resulted in far-reaching changes of the entire skull. A horizontal animal has its face in front of, and its neck behind, the brain case. The vertical human, however, has had his face rotated downward and backward under the brain case, and the neck attachment at the occiput, following the repositioning of the body, has rotated downward and forward under the brain case to achieve the proper balance of the skull in the upright position (Fig. 4-21). This has resulted in the buckling up of the cranial base at the sella turcica to form the familiar slant of the clivus. Consequently the whole skull base at the foramen magnum and occipital condyles is now well below the level of the craniomandibular articulations, bringing the tympanic bone and greatly elongated mastoid process far down and close behind the ramus of the jaw. This greatly narrowed space between jaw and mastoid process is crammed with numerous structures: parotid gland, facial and temporal arteries and veins, auriculotemporal and facial nerves, etc. A wide opening of the jaws in a pure, back-swinging, hinge rotation is now impossible. Thus the strong special bands of the craniomandibular ligament, adapted to these spatial relations, stop a pure hinge movement long before the jaw reaches maximal opening. To compensate for this restriction in hinge movement, the lateral pterygoids have been recruited to contribute an almost immediate effect in the opening movement. They now pull the entire mandible symmetrically downward and forward along the articular eminences, away from the back of the skull, so that the jaw can still open widely by way of the lower compartments of its joints.

Role of the musculature. The *mandibular muscles* determine all the complicated postures and movements of the jaw. Their behavior can be greatly clarified by restating certain fundamentals crucial to purposive muscular activity. In the first place, there are three distinct roles that a muscle can play when activated: it can contract isotonically and shorten to act as a *mover* of a part; it can contract (tense) isotonically yet lengthen to act as a *balancer* for a moving part; and it can contract isometrically, hence neither shorten nor lengthen, to act as a *stabilizer* of a movable part. In the second place, surprisingly large groups of distant muscles must act in the seemingly simplest functional movements. Group action often centers on what engineers term a *force-couple*, in which two muscles or muscle groups, pulling in opposite directions, turn moment arms around some common center. This concept greatly simplifies the analysis of muscle behavior in highly complicated movements.

Six paired muscles, among the many lesser muscles that attach to the jaw, predominate in moving the mandible. The masseter, medial pterygoid, and temporalis

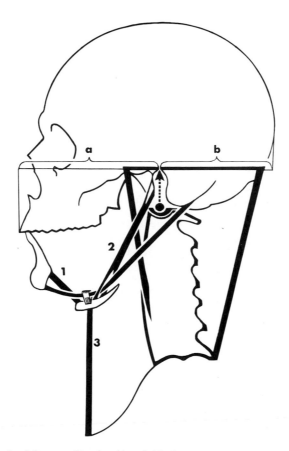

Fig. 4-21. Balance and stabilization of head and hyoid. Black spot at center represents turning axis at occipital condyles projected by arrow to Frankfurt horizontal. Turning moment of skull is appreciably greater anteriorly, *a*, than posteriorly, *b*. To compensate, moment arm of postvertebral musculature is far greater than that of prevertebral musculature *(heavy horizontal line)*. Geniohyoid musculature anteriorly, *1*, and stylohyoid musculature posteriorly, *2*, counterbalance strap musculature from sternum below, *3*. Digastric is entirely free to slide through sling (p. 156) and tunnel (p. 159) on stabilized hyoid base.

muscles elevate the mandible; two of these, the deep portion of the masseter and the posterior portion of the temporalis, also have retrusive capabilities. The lateral pterygoids protrude the mandible. The geniohyoid and especially the digastric muscles depress and retract the mandible. All twelve muscles are active in all mandibular movements—some as movers, some as balancers, some as stabilizers—shifting their roles in accord with the progress of the movement. In close coordination with the above actions, muscles of the neck steady the cranium and hyoid bone to establish stable bases from which opening and closing muscles can pull (Fig. 4-21). Since precise movements of the tongue are an integral part of masticatory activity, the hyoid bone is seen to move in rhythm with the jaw in chewing. It shifts continuously with firm stability to differing positions of mechanical advantage both for jaw opening and bolus manipulation (see Chapters 2, 3, and 6).

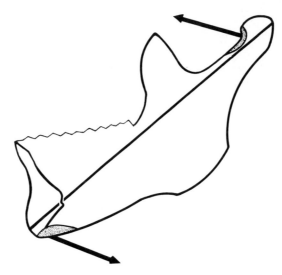

Fig. 4-22. Force-couple in opening movement. Stippled areas represent surface attachments of lateral pterygoid above and digastric below. Arrows indicate vertical turning action of muscles on jaw.

In the opening movement of the jaw the condyles rotate against the discs around a transverse axis as they slide downward and forward along the posterior slope and summit of the articular eminence. The movement is effected by an initial activity of the lateral pterygoids, which first fix the condyles firmly against the posterior slope of the eminence. Immediately this is followed by contraction of the digastric muscles, and the sustained activity of both muscle pairs, acting as a force-couple, turns the mandible around a roving horizontal axis passing through the rami of the mandible (Fig. 4-22). This motion affects all the other muscles anchored to the mandible, but it has also a receding influence on muscles more and more peripheral to the central action. Thus the elevators of the jaw must lengthen to act as mild balancers and so ensure smoothness of performance. At the same instant, muscles of the cranium and hyoid bone must act as holders to establish stable bases from which the force-couple can operate (Fig. 4-21).

In contrast to the opening movement, a forward thrust of the mandible is made by pulling the condyles and discs downward and forward along the articular eminences without the rotation of the condyles around the transverse axis. As before, the lateral pterygoids are active because they are the only protrusors of the jaw, but all the other mandibular muscles must now behave differently. The elevators hold in exactly the necessary adjustment with the balancing depressor-retractors as they lengthen to allow the mandible to slide forward just free of the interlocking dentition (Fig. 4-19). But, again, the more distant muscles of the cranium and hyoid bone must adjust to hold their bony bases stable (Fig. 4-21).

In the lateral movement one condyle and disc slide downward, medially, and forward along the articular eminence while the other rotates laterally around a ver-

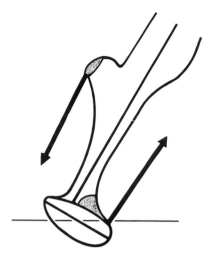

Fig. 4-23. Force-couple stabilizers in lateral movement. Stippled areas represent attachment of horizontal fibers of temporalis above and lateral pterygoid below. Arrows indicate horizontal turning action of muscles on jaw.

tical axis. If one views the mandible from above, it will be seen that the medial pole of the condyle juts far medially from the plane of the jaw while the coronoid process leans laterally. This creates effective moment arms for a coupling action of certain precisely poised muscles. The lateral pterygoid muscle, inserted on the inwardly thrust medial pole of the condyle, pulls inward and forward in the horizontal plane. The oblique fibers of the temporalis muscle, inserted at the posterior tip of the coronoid process, pull outward and backward. These muscles, operating as a force-couple, contribute to the torque of the rotating condyle necessary to effect chewing on this side. But perhaps equally important, they let out slack with a strong lengthening tension to provide maximum stability of the condyle, precariously poised on the back slope of the articular eminence in the closing stroke, during heavy chewing on the same side (Fig. 4-23). If the chin is moved to the left, the holding posterior part of the temporalis muscle forces the left condyle toward its marginal or extreme position under the restricting influence of the temporomandibular ligament, aiding in the Bennett shift. At the same time the right pterygoid muscle pulls the right condyle and disc forward, downward, and medially as the whole jaw is swung, as well as shifted bodily, to the left (see Fig. 4-12). It will be seen that the right pterygoid muscle has also entered the force-couple system. In the closing stroke the force-couple changes in direction and components. The posterior fibers of the right temporalis move the mandible back toward the right while the posterior fibers of the left temporalis hold. At the same time both pterygoids lengthen as balancers, the right one having by far the greatest excursion. The right digastric contracts to aid in this movement. It must be remembered that the cranial and hyoid bone holders are also active participants in this behavior.

In contrast to the usual functional lateral movement, the chin can also be swung to either side from the protruded position. *Both* lateral pterygoids are then contracted to establish the starting position so that all the other mandibular muscles must now behave in a different pattern than before. To swing the chin to the left, the posterior fibers of the left temporalis and the deep portion of the masseter muscles now act as movers, with the left digastric aiding to some extent. The left lateral pterygoid muscle now lengthens to act as a strong balancer. The left condyle is thus moved back to meet the checking of the left craniomandibular ligament. The right lateral pterygoid acts as a holder in a force-couple with the retracting muscles on the left side. Again, all the other mandibular muscles must make minor adjustments as the neck and hyoid muscles act as holders to fix the working bases for jaw movement.

Neural control complex. This condensed discussion of functional jaw movements has shown, in general, *what* the muscles do, but some indication of *how* they come to do it seems crucial at this point. If one opens the jaw widely and then snaps it shut, the muscles move the mandible swiftly and unerringly into the centric occlusal posture. In a mouth with a normal (or average) dentition, there is no initial contact of cusps on inclined planes, no shifting or gliding along these surfaces, no "premature" contact on them, but an instantaneously accurate interdigitation in the medial occlusal position. This is perhaps an extreme example of the nicety of coordination in all normal bodily movements. A common neurologic test of such coordination is made by instructing a patient to touch the tip of his nose with the tip of a forefinger when he is blindfolded. The normal patient does this with no difficulty but with some slight range of error, perhaps as much as 2 mm. off center. Proprioceptive inputs from end organs in the shoulder, elbow, wrist, and finger joints as well as all the muscles of the arm and pectoral girdle must supply all the information that corrects continuously the aim of the forefinger toward the nose tip target. Thus the nervous system is the ultimate governor of all meaningful muscle action, and, although really the realm of neurology, a selective synopsis of its structural organization is essential to clarify the total behavior of jaw musculature.

Four well-established nuclei and several less well-defined subnuclei of the trigeminal nerve are clumped along the length of the brain stem, which includes the entire mesencephalon (midbrain) back into the cervical spinal cord. (1) The *main sensory nucleus* in the pons receives information concerning touch and two-point discrimination from facial and oral surfaces. Its *subnucleus supratrigeminalis* is said to distinguish signals of pressure on teeth, palate, and gingivae and to have an inhibitory effect on motor neurons to jaw muscles. Its *subnucleus paratrigeminalis* moderates motor reflexes initiated by neurons from teeth and jaw points. (2) The descending nucleus, or *spinal sensory nucleus*, receives information concerning pain and temperature from oral and skin surfaces and teeth. The inputs to the nucleus are disposed in an orderly sequence; fibers of the ophthalmic division of the fifth nerve synapse are on cells in the most inferior and ventral part of the upper cervical cord; the maxillary division is directed to cells of the lower part of the medulla; the mandibular division sends fibers to cells found dorsally in the nucleus in the upper part of the medulla.

The cell bodies of these synapsing fibers are situated in the *semilunar ganglion*. They are thus outside the central nervous system as are all other cell bodies of incoming fibers in the cord, which are in the spinal ganglia. But (3) the *mesencephalic nucleus* of the trigeminal nerve is unique in the nervous system. Unlike all the other fibers with cell bodies in ganglia, its cells are in the midbrain, strewn along its entire length. Its incoming fibers carry proprioceptive information from jaw muscles, tendons, periodontal ligaments, and jaw joints. Its terminal fibers synapse directly on the cells of (4) the *motor nucleus* of the fifth nerve. Fibers from cells of the other trigeminal nuclei also synapse on the motoneurons of the fifth nerve, as do inputs from the cerebral cortex, the cerebellum, the reticular formation, and the other cranial nuclei. Hence the motoneuron operates the jaw musculature on the basis of a wide spectrum of incoming information.

The simplest circuit in the spinal cord can be described as a model on which the complex hierarchy of higher circuitry is based. A motoneuron to a muscle (the final common path identified by Sherrington) can be fired by two routes. What is believed to be the usual channel in ordinary voluntary behavior is called the *gamma route*. A moderately sized gamma motor cell in the anterior horn of the cord sends a fiber to the muscle to inervate a highly specialized end organ called a *neuromuscular spindle*. The spindle is composed of some six to eight striated muscle fibers wrapped in a capsule whose ends attach to the connective tissue of the somatic muscle. The middle, or equatorial, part of the spindle is highly modified. The segments of the muscle fibers that cross this area are noncontractile, and the region is heavily nucleated. The capsule is expanded here to accommodate these nuclei; hence the region is called the *nuclear bag*. Moderately sized gamma nerve fibers innervate the contractile ends of the muscular spindle fibers, and large, fast-firing, proprioceptor fibers spiraling around the equatorial, noncontractile portions run up to their cell bodies in the ganglia of the cord. From here their fibers continue to synapse, finally, on the large motor cell in the anterior horn of the spinal cord (Fig. 4-24).

In the peculiar fifth nerve these proprioceptor cells make up the mesencephalic nucleus within the brain stem. The so-called axons of these unipolar cells also synapse on the large, fast-firing cells of the motor nucleus of the fifth nerve, which finally fire the somatic muscle. These last fibers are the ones that form the final common path (Fig. 4-24). It has been demonstrated that the cells of the final common path can be fired more directly from above, without traveling through the spindle. This sequence is called the *alpha route*. As it is a shorter and more direct route, it is faster and believed to operate in "emergency" situations. The advantage of the longer route in routine, coordinated movements is that the spindle remains coupled to the activity. It is thus constantly available for the stretch reflex in all the lengthening and shortening positions of the somatic muscle.

What seems to be the important point of this complex circuitry in the oral apparatus is that every motor cell operates under the influences of excitatory and inhibitory neural inputs from all of the other jaw muscles, their tendons, the jaw joint, the gingivae and oral mucosa, and the periodontal ligaments and their stored memory

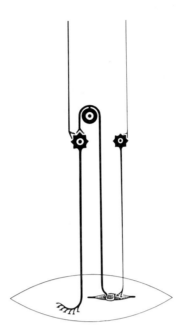

Fig. 4-24. Terminal pathways that activate a muscle. Thick alpha fiber is on left; thin gamma fiber is on right. Thick proprioceptor between connects them by way of muscle spindle. Somatic muscle in fine outline is usually stimulated by gamma route. (From DuBrul, E. L.: Perspect. Biol. Med. **10**:524, 1967.)

circuits. Other cranial nuclei—especially those of the seventh nerve, which operates the facial muscles, and the twelfth nerve, which controls the tongue—are also coupled to the motor nucleus of the fifth nerve. It is because of these interconnections that jaws, teeth, cheeks, and tongue work smoothly to perform feeding functions without the trauma of lip or tongue biting or other disruptions that signify abnormality in the system.

Despite the amassing of all these impressive neuroanatomic details, the exact nature of the mechanism governing the smooth rhythmicity of masticatory movements is still not clear. Traditionally the chewing cycle was attributed to the alternate action of two simple brain stem reflexes: (1) the initial jaw-opening reflex triggered by touch-pressure inputs on lips, teeth, gums, etc., followed immediately by (2) the jaw-closing reflex activated by the opening stretch of the jaw elevators (common stretch reflex). In this view simply putting food to the mouth initiates a self-perpetuating rhythm of open-close. This therefore implies that rhythm coordination is actually governed by structures based *outside* the central nervous system, that is, by the touch-pressure end-organs in oral tissues and by the stretch-tension end-organs in the musculature. But recently the accumulation of extensive experimental evidence emphasizes the probability of a pattern generator *within* the central nervous system associated with the "reticular formation" of the brain stem. Electrical stimulation along this tract evokes activity in the trigeminal and hypoglossal nerves, accompanied by rhythmical masticatory movements. Furthermore, it has been shown that this poorly defined, multisynapsed formation can be activated by appropriate inputs either from higher centers or from the oral cavity.

The patterns of neural firing that instigate the jaw movements are constantly being reinforced by function. They then become firmly implanted as memory circuits. Information relevant to the centric occlusal posture is intermittently signaled into the brain stem at each occlusal contact during the innumerable swallowing sequences and other random contacts throughout the day. These signals are channeled from the periodontal ligaments to act as memory in that all succeeding movements are governed by what has gone on before. Furthermore, as teeth normally wear and drift throughout the life of the dentition, information locating the centric occlusal posture is continually corrected, processed, and rerecorded in the brain at each contact. This feature defines the real problem in the edentulous patient because the precise, corrective feedback from the periodontium has been removed from the system. The patient must then rely solely on the remaining inputs from joints and muscles to position his jaw. But further complicating the picture, a new set of signals is substituted. It brings in information about *pressure* on the mucoperiosteum of the toothless alveolar ridges, whether the pressure be caused by food or by a denture on the bare gums. This introduces an attendant range of error similar to that in the blindfold neurologic test cited above.

The *masticatory movements* of the mandible can now be reviewed with deeper insight. Although the activity may be initiated consciously, the movements are essentially automatic rhythms governed by the complex neural circuitry sketched out above. As in all locomotor sequences, the pattern varies from individual to individual but maintains a remarkable stability within an individual. Again it must be made clear that there is a *range*—an adaptive margin of safety—in every individual pattern. Thus stability means stability of range within which the specific pattern can vary in adjustment to local circumstances. Movements of mastication, just as movements of walking, etc., depend on the proportions and relations of the parts. Structure and function are so inextricably related that different somatotypes (fat, thin, tall, short, etc.), are distinctly characterized by different manners of walking. The point, then, is that different craniofacial proportions, including different dental relations, will establish different masticatory movements even though these may be so minute that they are not readily recognized.

Movements are described beginning from the centric occlusal posture with all teeth in even contact. In this position the elevators of the jaw are under active contraction, whereas in the rest position these muscles are said to be in tonic contraction. There are two major movement sequences of the mandible in which some teeth come into contact: a *cutting* movement, such as that used by incisors and canines to bite off a piece of food, and a *grinding* movement, such as that used by molars and premolars to comminute a piece of food.

Cutting begins with a preparatory opening movement, the extent of which depends on the dimensions of the food. This comprises a forward rotation of the condyles against the discs in the vertical plane and a slight sliding of the discs against the articular eminences in adjustment to the eccentric position of the condyles. This movement unlocks all teeth from occlusion. The sliding or translation now continues as the dominant movement in thrusting the jaw forward to bring the lower incisors forward to the level of the uppers. The jaw is now raised to effect an edge-to-edge incisor contact. This reverses the vertical rotation of the condyles against the discs, which continues, along with a backward translation of the discs against the eminences, as the lower incisal edges glide up and back along the lingual of the uppers. Frequently the contact of the anterior teeth is limited to the incisal edges of the maxillary centrals and the mandibular centrals and laterals. The varying degrees and proportions of vertical rotation and translation of the condyles depend on the degree of vertical overbite and horizontal overjet of upper and lower teeth. Mechanically, the cutting is the result of a shearing force produced between approaching opposed blades formed by the continuous incisal edges of upper and lower incisors.

Grinding must also begin with an opening movement to unlock the occlusion of the overbite of the incisors and canines of the upper jaw and the interdigitated cusps of molars and premolars. The extent of opening depends, as before, on the degree of overbite, height of cusps, and amount of occlusal wear of the teeth. In chewing on the left side, the jaw is rotated horizontally to the left, around a laterally shifting vertical axis behind the left condyle. As described in detail previously, the jaw not only rotates but also shifts bodily to the left in the slight Bennett movement. The right condyle slides downward, forward, and medially as a translatory movement is made between the articular disc and articular eminence. The jaw is next raised to bring the left buccal and lingual rows of cusps into contact. The final act of this automatic movement brings the dentition back with precision into the centric occlusal posture (see Fig. 4-16). The condyles then reverse their movements. The left condyle rotates medially around a medially shifting vertical axis, and the right condyle slides backward, laterally, and upward in the translatory movement between disc and eminence as the jaw shifts bodily to the right. As before, the varying extents and proportions of rotation, vertical and horizontal, and translation depend on the relationships and degrees of wear of the teeth. If the food bolus is small, the translation of the right condyle is minimal.

Normally, contact of the upper and lower teeth can occur only on the chewing side. The teeth on the opposite side will be out of contact. In other words, the occlusion of the natural dentition during grinding is *not* "balanced." Only in the case of extreme wear in which the cusp contours have disappeared to leave the occlusal surfaces flat can a state of balanced occlusion be possible. The human dentition does not differ in this respect from that of the vast majority of other mammals in which the premolarmolar rows function strictly unilaterally.

In *summary*, both masticatory movement complexes—cutting and grinding—can be analyzed in three phases. The first, the opening, or preparatory, phase is a free movement of the jaw. The second phase begins with the beginning closing action and ends at the approach of contact. The third phase is a truly articulatory movement. It occurs with the contact of teeth. The first phase requires little force. Considerable force may be applied during the second and third phases as these phases fuse to produce the masticatory stroke. Furthermore, in actual chewing true contact of teeth probably occurs rarely before many masticatory strokes have been made, depending on the resistance of the food (see Fig. 4-16).

Nicety of muscle integration is of extreme importance during the masticatory stroke because the movement is most often made with great force, but the teeth, not yet in contact, cannot aid in stabilizing the position of the mandible. The powerful holding force of the lateral pterygoids in force-couple combination with the posterior part of the temporalis is essential to prevent displacement of the jaw as its condyles and discs slide backward, precariously balanced on the posterior slope of the articular eminence.

CHAPTER 5

The viscera

ORAL CAVITY

The oral cavity is the space bounded by the lips and cheeks anteriorly and later-ally, by the palate above, and by the muscular floor of the oral cavity below. It communicates with the outside through the opening between the lips, the oral fis-sure, and with the pharynx through the fauces. It is subdivided by the alveolar pro-cesses and the teeth into the oral vestibule and the oral cavity proper. The oral vestibule is the space between the lips and cheeks in the periphery and the teeth and alveolar processes centrally. The oral cavity proper, inside the arches of the teeth, contains the tongue, which is movably attached to the floor.

When the lower jaw is in rest position, the vestibule and oral cavity proper are in communication between the upper and lower teeth. In the occlusal position the communication between these two parts of the oral cavity is restricted to minute clefts between the adjacent teeth in each jaw and to a variable but normally narrow opening behind the last teeth on either side. This statement is valid only in a mouth with a normal full dentition when the teeth are in close contact.

Lips—labia

The upper and lower lips, or labium superius and labium inferius, are composed of muscles and glands, covered by skin on the outside and by mucous membrane on the inside. The glands of the lips, the labial glands, are situated immediately under-neath the mucous membrane.

The upper lip borders onto the nose and is separated from the cheek by a variably deep groove, the nasolabial groove, which on either side starts at the wing of the nose and runs downward and laterally to pass at some distance from the corner of the mouth (Fig. 5-1). In young persons the lower lip has no boundary toward the cheek. Usually with advancing age a furrow develops, which begins at or close to the corner of the mouth, medial to the lower end of the nasolabial sulcus. This furrow runs in a posteriorly convex arch toward the lower border of the mandible, which it rarely reaches. It is known as the labiomarginal sulcus.

The lower lip is separated from the chin proper by a more or less sharp and deep groove that is convex superiorly, the labiomental groove (Fig. 5-1). Its depth depends on the fullness of the lower lip, on the prominence of the bony and soft chin, and on the age of the individual. The labiomental sulcus deepens and sharpens with advancing age, as do all the grooves in the face. The upper and lower lips are connected to each other at the corner of the mouth. The thin connecting fold, the labial commissure, is well visible when the mouth is opened and is a rather vulnerable area.

The skin of the lips ends in a sharp sometimes slightly elevated line, to be replaced by the transitional zone between the skin and mucous membrane, the red or vermilion zone of the lips, a feature characteristic of man only. The epithelium in this zone is thin and not keratinized; the papillae of the connective tissue are numerous, densely arranged, and slender and reach far into the epithelium so that their tips are covered only by a thin layer of the epithelium. The cells of the epithelium, moreover, contain eleidin in the middle and superficial layers, which enhances their translucency. The wide and rich capillaries of the papillae are seen through the thin epithelium, hence the red color of this area.

In the upper lip the red zone protrudes in the midline in a variably sharply limited zone, the tubercle of the upper lip (Fig. 5-1). From here, a shallow depression, the philtrum, can be followed to the nose. In the midline of the lower lip there is a slight indentation corresponding to the tubercle of the upper lip. From here the red zone at first widens and then again narrows toward the corner of the mouth.

The skin of the lip has all the characteristics of the common integument; that is, it contains sweat glands, hairs, and sebaceous glands. The red zone of the lip does not contain hairs or sweat glands. However, in about half of the individuals examined, smaller or larger isolated sebaceous glands can be found.

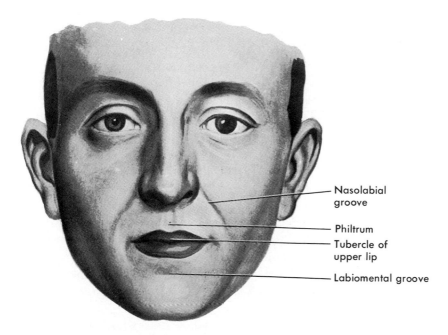

Nasolabial groove

Philtrum

Tubercle of upper lip

Labiomental groove

Fig. 5-1. Semidiagrammatic drawing of adult face. (Sicher and Tandler: Anatomie für Zahnärzte.)

The mucous membrane of the lips is covered by a nonkeratinized stratified squamous epithelium and contains numerous mixed labial glands of variable size, of which the largest can be felt through the thin mucous membrane. They sometimes form an almost continuous layer in the upper as well as the lower lip (see Fig. 5-12).

The skin on the outside and the mucous membrane on the inside are tightly fixed to the connective tissue covering the muscular substance of the lip, the orbicularis oris muscle. Thus neither skin nor mucous membrane can be lifted away from the muscle but follow its movements without much folding.

The thickness of the skin of the face, especially that of the dermis (corium), its connective tissue layer, shows distinct sex differences because of the presence of a mustache and beard in the male. The sexual dimorphism is important to the prosthodontist from an esthetic point of view because the thicker and firmer skin of the male restricts the mobility of the lips, especially that of the upper lip. This is why, as a rule, men show much less of their upper teeth when speaking and laughing than do women, in whom even the gingiva of the upper jaw is often exposed by extreme movements of the lips. The general rule is, however, obscured in a certain percentage of individuals by variations in the length of the lips, length of the teeth, and the relation of the lips and teeth in rest position. The sex difference in thickness and pliability of the facial skin leads to another characteristic behavior of the soft chin in women. If the lower lip is depressed, the region of the chin itself does not move in the male. In most women, however, the hairless and thin skin below the labiomental groove moves visibly downward, and the otherwise smooth contour below the chin is broken by a transverse, often sharp groove. This "postmental" groove also sharpens with age.

Normally upper and lower lips are lightly closed when the mandible is in rest position. The line of contact is slightly above the incisal edge of the upper incisors. The corners of the mouth, in the majority of persons, are found in the region between the upper canine and the first premolar. The variations in the absolute and relative height of the lips are extensive. In most individuals the height of the upper lip is about a third of the distance between the nose and chin. It can, however, be reduced to a fourth and even less of this distance.

Cheeks—buccae

The cheek, the lateral boundary of the oral vestibule, is formed in its mobile part by the buccinator muscle, covered on the inside by mucous membrane, on the outside by skin. In its posterior part the masseter muscle and the parotid gland are interposed between the mucous membrane and buccinator muscle on one side and the skin on the other. Viewed from the outside, the cheek seems to be much larger than when viewed from the vestibule because the zygomatic region above, the mandibular region below, and the parotideomasseteric region behind the vestibule are regarded as parts of the cheek.

As seen from the oral cavity, the cheek is bounded, above and below, by the reflection of its mucous membrane onto the alveolar process. This reflection is the fornix of the vestibule.* The posterior boundary of the cheek is marked by a fold that joins the posterior end of the upper to that of the lower alveolar process. This fold is elevated by the pterygomandibular raphe, a tendinous strip that is attached to the pterygoid hamulus above and to the retromolar triangle below (see Fig. 6-4).

The mucous membrane of the cheek is fixed to the inner fascia of the buccinator muscle by tight strands of connective tissue. The attachment of the mucous membrane to the muscle prevents the formation of folds in the mucous membrane when the buccinator muscle contracts during the closing of the jaws. Instead, the mucous membrane follows closely the movements of the buccinator muscle and shows densely arranged, fine wrinkles if the mouth is closed. In the submucous tissue between the highly elastic lamina propria of the mucous membrane and the fascia of the buccinator muscle, there are numerous mucous and mixed glands (see Fig. 5-13), which frequently reach into the spaces between the muscle bundles and sometimes even protrude to the outer surface of the thin muscle plate. In most persons the buccal glands in the molar region are numerous and may be packed to a rather solid glandular body.

Opposite the second upper molar the parotid duct opens into the oral vestibule. The opening is frequently marked by a variably high elevation of the mucous membrane, the parotid papilla.

In a narrow zone of the buccal mucosa, just lateral to and behind the corner of the mouth, isolated sebaceous glands may be present. They are homologous to the sebaceous glands in the red zone of the lips and occupy mainly the zone of the cheek that developed by a fusion of the upper and lower lips of the embryo. In older individuals these glands are frequently enlarged and visible through the mucous membrane as yellowish bodies. They are then referred to as Fordyce's spots.

The cheek contains a peculiar body of fat tissue, the buccal fat pad of Bichat (see Fig. 5-11). It is a rounded biconvex structure limited by a thin but distinctive capsule. Its anterior part protrudes in front of the anterior border of the masseter. From here it extends between the masseter and buccinator muscles to continue posteriorly and superiorly into the body of fat that occupies the spaces between the masticatory muscles (see Chapter 14). Because of its great volume in the newborn and in infants, it was believed to aid the suckling movement and has been called, accordingly, suckling pad. This function of the fatty body is at least questionable; it can be interpreted as a specific and cushioning fill-in, occupying the wide spaces between the masticatory muscles and the buccinator muscle. It is interesting that even in cases of progressive emaciation this fat persists for a considerably longer time than does the subcutaneous fat, a fact that strengthens the belief in a mechanical function of the masticatory fat pad.

---

*The term mucobuccal fold, used in dental literature, is nondescriptive and should be abolished.

Oral vestibule

The walls of the oral vestibule are best divided into zones according to the behavior of the mucous membrane and its fixation to the deeper structures. The lining of the lips and cheeks is characterized by the tight attachment of the mucous membrane to the epimysium of labial and buccal muscles. From the root of the upper and lower lips and from the upper and lower boundary of the cheek the mucous membrane is reflected onto the upper and lower alveolar processes. The area of reflection, a horseshoe-shaped furrow, is the fornix vestibuli. This region is characterized by the loose

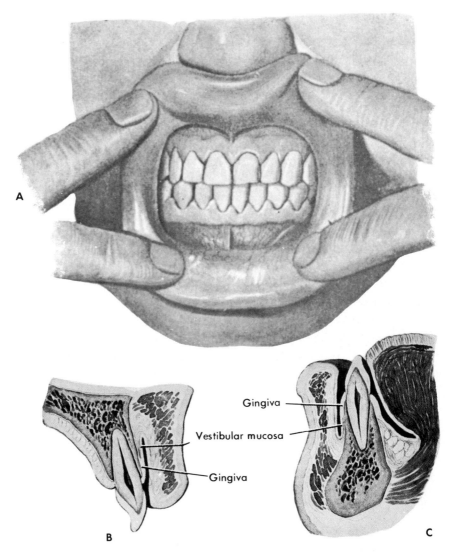

Fig. 5-2. A, Vestibule of adult showing gingiva and alveolar mucosa. **B,** Section through upper incisor and neighboring structures. **C,** Section through lower incisor and neighboring structures. (Sicher and Tandler: Anatomie für Zahnärzte.)

texture of the submucous tissue, which attaches the mucous membrane movably to muscles and bone. The mobility of the lips and cheeks causes this loose attachment, which permits the lips or cheeks to be pulled away from the bone or to be moved upward and downward to a considerable distance. Since the mobility of the cheek decreases gradually in the molar region, the amount of loose connective tissue in the upper as well as in the lower fornix diminishes posteriorly.

The mucous membrane covering the alveolar process to the necks of the teeth may be divided into two sharply distinct areas (Fig. 5-2, A). The peripheral zone adjacent to the fornix is the alveolar mucosa of the vestibule; the area adjacent to the free border is the gingiva, or gum. These two zones are separated from each other by a sharp scalloped line that parallels the free margin of the gingiva, the mucogingival junction. The alveolar mucosa is characterized by its more delicate texture, its mobility, and its dark red color. The gingiva is firm, immovably attached to the bone and the teeth, and is, under normal conditions, of a pale pink color. In addition, the mucous membrane of the vestibule is thinner than the gingiva so that the latter bulges slightly above the surface of the mucosa (Fig. 5-2 B and C). The difference in color of the two regions is caused by the larger number of blood vessels in the alveolar mucosa and by the fact that the epithelium of the gingiva, though not as thick as that of the alveolar mucosa, is, in the great majority of persons, keratinized or parakeratinized. The alveolar mucosa is smooth, although normal gingiva is stippled. Small round prominences are separated by irregular sulci. The appearance is somewhat similar to that of an orange peel.

The tentlike papillae of the gingiva, which fill the interdental spaces, provide, at the same time, the transition between vestibular and oral mucous membrane. The two areas of the mucous membrane are also continuous behind the last teeth. On the vestibular and oral sides the papilla is high, filling the embrasures of the dental arch. Between these areas the edge of the papilla is concave, or col-shaped. *

In the upper jaw the gingiva covers the alveolar tubercle, the rounded bony prominence that forms the posterior end of the upper alveolar process. Here, behind the last molar, the gingiva often is elevated to form the retromolar papilla (Fig. 5-3, A). Toward the mucous covering of the root of the soft palate the retromolar papilla is sharply bounded by the retroalveolar notch, a variably deep groove corresponding to the junction of maxilla and palatine bone at the lower end of the pterygoid process.

In the lower jaw the small retromolar papilla (Fig. 5-3, B), consisting of typical gingival tissue, is situated at the foot of the mandibular ramus and is attached to the most inferior part of the anterior border of the ramus. Immediately behind and above the retromolar papilla the mucosa at the root of the cheek contains an aggregation of buccal glands, the retromolar glands. The prominence caused by the glands is covered by loosely attached mucosa and is thus clearly separable from the firm retromolar papilla. The papilla and the retromolar glandular prominence are often referred to

---

*Col, a pass between two mountain peaks.

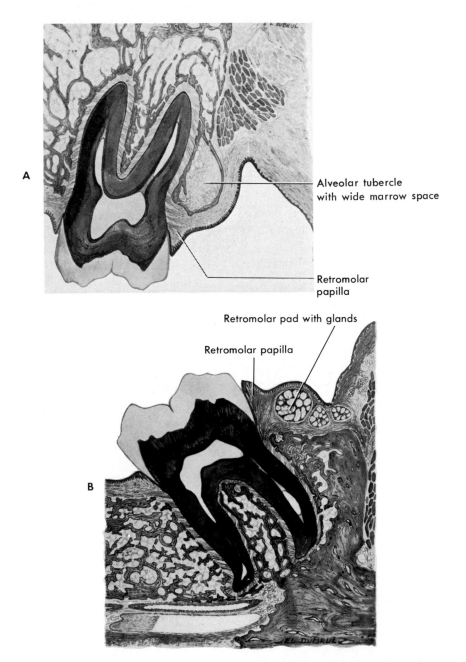

Fig. 5-3. Composite drawing of several mesiodistal sections. **A,** Through upper molars and retromolar papilla. **B,** Through lower molars and retromolar papilla.

as the retromolar pad. The term should be reserved for the glandular part only.

Sagittal folds in the midline connect the alveolar processes with the upper and lower lips (Fig. 5-2, A). The sickle-shaped folds are the upper and lower labial frena or frenula. Of the two, the upper frenum is stronger; the lower may even be reduced to a vestige. Normally the upper frenum does not reach into the area of the gingiva but is restricted to the alveolar mucosa of the vestibule. However, a low attachment of the frenum of the upper lip on the alveolar wall of the vestibule is not infrequent. In cases of a congenital space between the two upper central incisors, median diastema or trema, the insertion of the strongly developed frenum reaches even across the free border of the gingiva between the two separated teeth and connects with the palatine, or incisive, papilla. This is a persistence of the tectolabial frenum, an early developmental stage, when a fold reaches from the roof of the oral cavity to the tubercle of the upper lip.

Sickle-shaped folds of variable height may traverse the fornix of the vestibule as lateral frena in the region of the canines or premolars. The lower lateral frenum is, as a rule, better developed.

All these folds contain a variable amount of loose connective tissue between two layers of the mucous membrane. Muscle bundles are never found in these folds, and larger vessels are likewise absent.

Oral cavity proper

The oral cavity proper is bounded peripherally by the alveolar processes and the teeth. Its roof is formed by the palate, which separates it from the nasal cavity. The floor is muscular and is, in its greater central part, occupied by the attachment of the tongue. Only a semicircular strip of the floor surrounding the root of the tongue on both sides and in front, the sublingual groove, remains accessible. The posterior wall of the oral cavity is formed by the vertical part of the soft palate, which continues on either side into the palatine pillars. Between the free borders of the palate, the pillars, and the base of the tongue, the oral cavity communicates with the pharynx through the narrow isthmus faucium, or oropharyngeal isthmus.

The palate (Fig. 5-4, A) is the roof of the oral cavity continuing posteriorly into its incomplete posterior wall, laterally and anteriorly arching to the alveolar process, and thus continuing into the side walls and the upper part of the anterior wall of the oral cavity. The palate is divided into the hard palate, containing a bony skeleton, and the movable soft palate, or palatine velum. The skeleton of the hard palate consists of the palatine processes of the maxillae and the horizontal plates of the palatine bones.

Orally the hard palate is covered by a rather thick layer of soft tissues. The structure of the mucous membrane and submucosa permit the subdivision of this wide semioval area into different zones. The peripheral zone is a counterpart of the vestibular gingiva, that is, a firm, resistant, smooth band of tissue connected by the interdental and retromolar papillae with the vestibular gingiva. In this area, as in the vestibular gingiva, there is no differentiation between the lamina propria of the mucosa, submucosa, and periosteum; rather, there is a uniform, dense feltwork of collag-

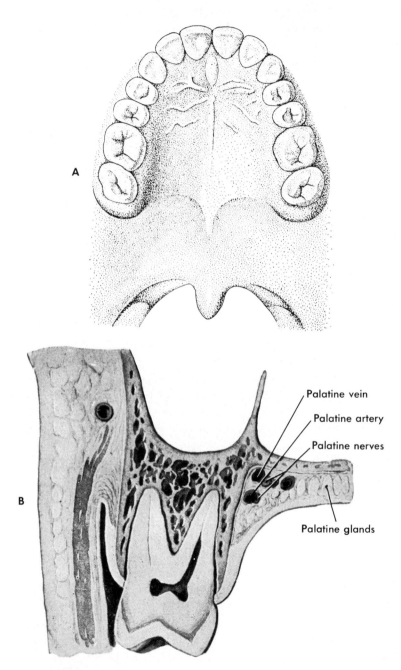

Fig. 5-4. A, Hard and soft palates. **B,** Frontal (buccolingual) section through upper right second molar and neighboring structures. (Sicher and Tandler: Anatomie für Zahnärzte.)

enous connective fibers that extends between bone and the cervical region of the teeth on one side and the keratinized epithelium on the other. A narrow zone along the midline of the palate shows, histologically, a similar appearance. In this zone an oval or pear-shaped smooth prominence, the incisive (or palatine) papilla, can be seen immediately behind the upper central incisors, covering the oral opening of the nasopalatine canals, the incisive fossa. From the papilla a narrow, rather sharp but low ridge, the palatine raphe, extends posteriorly over the entire length of the hard palate.

Irregular, sometimes branching, ridges, radiating from the incisive papilla and the anteriormost parts of the palatine raphe, cross the hard palate in its anterior part and reach laterally to a variable extent (Fig. 5-4, A). These ridges, containing a core of dense and firm connective tissue, are termed transverse palatine folds, or palatine rugae. They are, in man, a vestige of the far higher and regular folds that play an important auxiliary role in the process of mastication in many animals.

In the paired areas between the palatine raphe and palatine gingiva, the palatine mucosa is also fixed immovably to the periosteum of the hard palate. However, in these zones a submucosa is well differentiated. The attachment of the rather thick lamina propria of the mucosa to the periosteum is achieved by strong, tight strands and bands of inelastic connective tissue. The irregular intercommunicating compartments between these fibrous bands are filled by fat or mucous glands. Fat lobules are packed into the spaces in the anterior zone of the hard palate, whereas the glands occupy the spaces in the posterior region (see Fig. 5-14). The boundary between the fatty and glandular zones of the hard palate is, as a rule, a forward convex line connecting the mesial halves of the two first molars. Fat and glands provide a resilient cushion for wide areas of the palatine mucosa.

In the living the horizontal roof of the oral cavity continues in a smooth curve into the anterior and lateral walls. On the skeleton, however, the horizontal roof is, in the molar region, sharply bent into the vertical alveolar process of the upper jaw. This sharp angle changes anteriorly gradually to a gentle slope in the region of the canines and incisors. The incongruity between the skeleton and the surface of the mucosa is caused by the interposition of a rather voluminous mass of loose connective tissue between the periosteum and submucosa proper in the molar region (Fig. 5-4, B), which diminishes gradually anteriorly. This loose connective tissue contains the anterior branches of the palatine nerves and the descending palatine vessels, which enter the space between bone and mucous membrane through the major palatine foramen. The loose connective tissue, which appears triangular or wedge-shaped on a frontal section, is of clinical significance because it is the only zone in the larger posterior part of the hard palate into which a greater amount of an anesthetic solution can be injected than elsewhere without exerting injurious pressure.

The soft palate is a thick fold of mucous membrane containing an intricately arranged musculature of its own. The mucous membrane on its oral surface contains numerous large and densely packed mucous glands. The epithelium of the mucosa on this surface, although it is a stratified squamous epithelium, is not keratinized and is by far thinner than that of the hard palate. This difference in texture of the epithelium, as well as that of the mucous membrane, explains the characteristic difference in color between the hard and soft palate. The thick, densely woven mucosa of the hard palate and the thick keratinized epithelium give to this zone of the oral mucosa a pale pink color, often with a bluish gray hue. The thin and more loosely textured mucosa of the soft palate and its thinner and not keratinized epithelium create a certain translucency. The rich and densely arranged blood vessels and the massive densely packed glands cause the soft palate to appear darker red with a yellowish tint. The boundary between the two differently colored areas is, on either side, a curved line (Fig. 5-4, A) that turns its convexity anteriorly, duplicating, but slightly anterior to, the posterior boundary of the skeleton of the hard palate.

Close to the midline and immediately behind the boundary between the hard and soft palate, a small but sharply demarcated depression or pit can be found in the majority of persons. This small fovea, which is often present only on one side, is the palatine foveola of Stieda; into it empty the ducts of some of the palatine glands. In the lateral area of the root of the soft palate, a short distance medial and posterior to the posterior end of the upper alveolar process, a small prominence can be distinctly felt or even seen. This prominence is elevated by the hamulus of the pterygoid process. The pterygomandibular raphe reaches from the pterygoid hamulus to the posterior end of the lower alveolar process, the retromolar triangle. This tendinous band, interposed between buccinator and pharyngeal muscles, elevates a fold of the mucous membrane that is especially prominent if the mouth is widely opened. This fold, the pterygomandibular fold (Fig. 5-5), stretches from the region of the hamulus to the

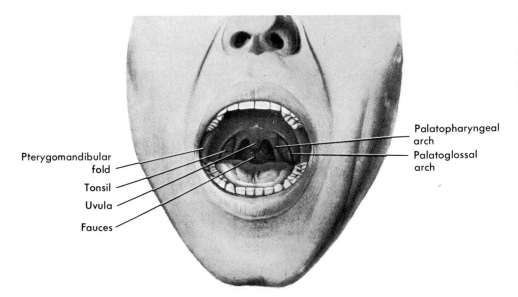

Fig. 5-5. Soft palate, palatine pillars, and tonsils. (Sicher and Tandler: Anatomie für Zahnärzte.)

retromolar pad in an oblique course from above downward and outward. It marks the posterior boundary of the cheek.

The free border of the soft palate is doubly concave and extends in the midline to the palatine uvula (Fig. 5-5). Along the free border the oral mucous membrane continues into the nasal mucosa; the typical oral epithelium, a stratified squamous epithelium, continues for a short distance on the nasal surface, to be then replaced by the characteristic nasal, or respiratory, epithelium, a pseudostratified, ciliated, columnar epithelium.

The simple free border of the soft palate splits laterally on either side into two folds (Fig. 5-5). One, in the plane of the soft palate itself, slants back along the lateral pharyngeal wall finally to flatten out and join its counterpart on the posterior wall. It is the posterior palatine pillar (palatopharyngeal arch or fold). The anterior fold, the anterior palatine pillar (palatoglossal arch or fold), continues downward and anteriorly and, at the same time, laterally, to end on the lateral part of the base of the tongue. Between the two pillars, on the lateral wall of the isthmus faucium, a narrow but high triangular fossa, the tonsillar niche, faces medially and slightly anteriorly. It contains the palatine tonsil. Above this oval body, with its irregular and often deeply cut surface, lies a small triangular part of the tonsillar niche, the supratonsillar recess. Below the tonsil a backward extension of the palatoglossal arch, the triangular fold, forms the inferior boundary of the tonsillar bed.

The maxillary part of the lateral wall of the oral cavity proper is continuous with the oral roof. In the mandibular region the mucous membrane on the lingual surface of the alveolar process is differentiated into the lingual mandibular gingiva and the

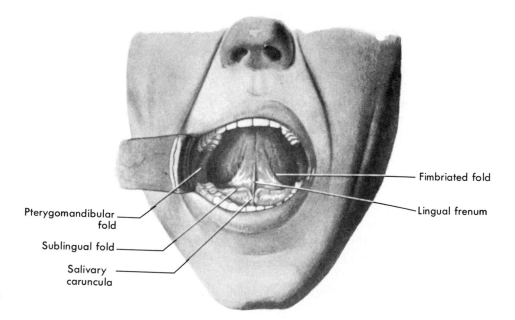

Pterygomandibular fold

Sublingual fold

Salivary caruncula

Fimbriated fold

Lingual frenum

Fig. 5-6. Sublingual region. (Sicher and Tandler: Anatomie für Zahnärtze.)

lingual, or oral, alveolar mucosa. The structure of the gingiva is the same as in other areas; that is, it is a fusion of mucosa, submucosa, and periosteum, covered by a keratinized or parakeratinized stratified squamous epithelium. The inferior boundary of the immovably fixed and firm gingiva is sharp and similar to that found on the vestibular surfaces of the upper and lower jaws. Along this scalloped line the lingual gingiva ends abruptly, to be replaced by a thin mucous membrane that is movably attached to the periosteum by a loosely textured submucous layer (Fig. 5-2, C). The submucosa gains rapidly in volume toward the floor of the mouth, where the lingual alveolar mucosa continues into the mucosa of the sublingual sulcus. The presence of this loose alveolar connective tissue permits the great mobility of the tongue.

The floor of the mouth is visible and accessible only in a horseshoe-shaped area, the sublingual sulcus, surrounding the attachment of the tongue laterally and anteriorly. This groove is traversed in the midline by a thin, sickle-shaped fold reaching upward to the underside of the tongue, the lingual frenum or frenulum (Fig. 5-6). The anterior attachment of this fold reaches only rarely to the mandibular alveolar process. The sublingual area on either side of the lingual frenum is elevated to a plump and irregular prominence, the salivary (or sublingual) eminence, containing the sublingual glands. Along its crest a rather delicate fold can be seen, the sublingual fold, which contains the submandibular, or Wharton's, duct. This fold ends medially close to the lingual frenum in a small papilla, the sublingual (or salivary) caruncula, at which the joined submandibular and major sublingual ducts open.

THE TONGUE

The tongue (Fig. 5-7) is a muscular organ, with its base and the central part of its body attached to the floor of the mouth. Its inferior surface is, therefore, free and accessible only in a peripheral horseshoe-shaped area. This area and the back of the tongue are covered by mucous membrane. The tongue develops from two primordia, the anterior arising from the first branchial arch and the posterior from the second and third branchial arches. This double origin can be recognized in the adult by the differences of surface relief on one hand and by the sensory innervation of the tongue on the other.

The body and tip, or anterior two thirds of the tongue, face upward; the surface of the base of the tongue, or the posterior third, faces backward. The base and body are separated by a shallow V-shaped groove, the terminal sulcus, the angle of the V pointing backward. This furrow not only marks the boundary between two functionally entirely different surface areas, but also corresponds fairly well with that between the trigeminal (anterior two thirds) and glossopharyngeal (posterior third) zones of innervation. In the midline, a variably deep blind pit, the foramen cecum, marks the point from which the development of the thyroid gland started.

The inferior surface of the tongue directed toward and, at rest, in contact with the floor of the mouth is covered by a simple, undifferentiated mucous membrane, which is tightly adherent to the lingual musculature. The lamina propria and the nonkeratinized epithelium are rather thin because of their protected location. In the midline,

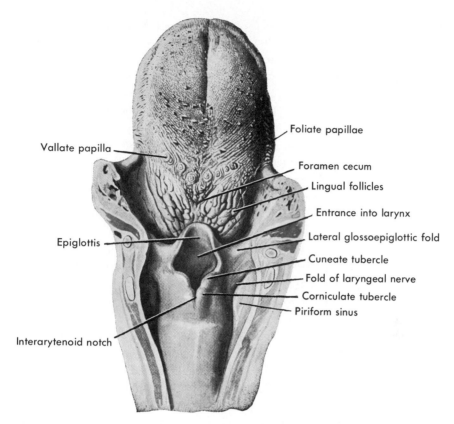

Vallate papilla

Foliate papillae

Foramen cecum

Lingual follicles

Entrance into larynx

Epiglottis

Lateral glossoepiglottic fold

Cuneate tubercle

Fold of laryngeal nerve

Corniculate tubercle

Piriform sinus

Interarytenoid notch

Fig. 5-7. Tongue (flattened out) and entrance into larynx. (Sicher and Tandler: Anatomie für Zahnärzte.)

the frenum linguae arises as a sickle-shaped fold connecting the underside of the tongue with the floor of the mouth (Fig. 5-6). Near the anterior end of the frenum an irregularly scalloped fold can be followed on either side laterally and posteriorly on the inferior surface of the tongue. The folds are termed fimbriated folds. Larger veins can almost always be seen through the thin translucent mucous membrane. They are tortuous so that they can adapt to the stretching movements of the tongue.

The dorsal surface of the tongue can be divided into an anterior horizontal and a posterior vertical part. The first is in contact with the palate; the second faces the pharynx. The first is designated as the palatine surface, the latter as the pharyngeal surface of the tongue.

The palatine surface of the tongue (Fig. 5-7) is situated in front of the terminal sulcus and carries the lingual papillae. Four types of these papillae can be distinguished, one of which, however, is vestigial in man. Immediately in front of the terminal sulcus are the circumvallate, or vallate, papillae, arranged in a V-shaped line, with the largest papilla near or in the midline and decreasing in size laterally and anteriorly. They are mushroom-shaped prominences surrounded by a deeply cut circular trough or furrow; the central prominence is only slightly elevated above the surface of the tongue. The walls of the trough contain numerous taste buds. Into the deepest parts of the furrow empty the serous (von Ebner's) glands. Their function is to rinse the trough and thus to eliminate the soluble parts of food after they have acted on the taste buds.

The entire dorsal surface of the tongue in front of the vallate papillae has a more or less uniform, velvety appearance and is of grayish pink color. The texture and color are caused by the presence of densely arranged hairlike papillae, filiform papillae. These consist of a conical core of connective tissue beset with secondary papillae and covered by a rather thick keratinized epithelium.

The fungiform papillae are singly and irregularly distributed between the filiform papillae. They are small, mushroomlike elevations, not as high as the filiform papillae and characterized by a more deeply red color because of the thinness of the covering epithelium. On their slope are found taste buds in a variable number.

The posterior part of the lateral border of the tongue contains the foliate papillae. These are sharp, low, parallel folds, but are in man usually irregular and insignificant. They are also the site of numerous taste buds.

The pharyngeal surface of the tongue (Fig. 5-7), posterior to the terminal sulcus, is studded with oval or rounded low prominences, separated from each other by irregular, shallow furrows. These prominences are caused by the accumulation of lymphatic tissue and are termed lingual follicles. The sum total of the follicles is designated as lingual tonsil. A narrow pit, the lingual crypt, can be seen in the center of most of the follicles. Into its bottom open the ducts of small mixed glands, the posterior lingual glands, which sometimes reach deeply into the substance of the tongue. The root of the tongue is connected with the palate by the palatoglossal arch and with the epiglottis by the median glossoepiglottic fold. On either side of this sickle-shaped fold are variably deep depressions, the epiglottic valleculae. They are bounded laterally by the lateral glossoepiglottic folds.

Muscles of the tongue

The muscles of the tongue are composed of two groups, extrinsic and intrinsic. Extrinsic muscles arise from the bony skeleton; intrinsic muscles, as the term implies, are confined to the tongue itself. There are four paired extrinsic muscles, genioglossi, styloglossi, palatoglossi, and hyoglossi.

Genioglossus muscle. This is the strongest muscle (Figs. 5-8 and 5-9, A). It arises from the genial tubercle or spine of its side on the posterior surface of the mandibular symphysis. The muscles of both sides form a thick median plate separated by a strong median fibrous septum. The anterior fibers run vertically straight up from their origin at the level of the junction between the free tongue tip and the middle third of the tongue. The posterior fibers run horizontally straight back to the posterior third of the tongue, and the intermediate fibers fan out evenly between vertical and horizontal margins. This makes the muscle triangular in form from the lateral view (see Fig. 6-16). All fibers insert close to the free surface of the tongue along its whole length,

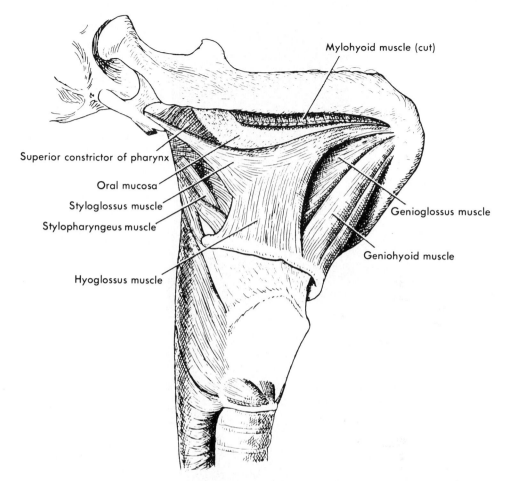

Mylohyoid muscle (cut)

Superior constrictor of pharynx

Oral mucosa

Styloglossus muscle

Stylopharyngeus muscle

Hyoglossus muscle

Genioglossus muscle

Geniohyoid muscle

Fig. 5-8. Extrinsic muscles of tongue and geniohyoid muscle. (Modified and redrawn from Sicher and Tandler: Anatomie für Zahnärzte.)

with the most inferior bundles attaching to the body of the hyoid bone. It is innervated by the hypoglossal nerve.

Styloglossus muscle. This muscle arises from the anterior surface of the styloid process often extending to the stylomandibular ligament. The muscle courses downward, anteriorly and medially. It penetrates the tongue at the angle of junction between the middle and posterior thirds. There it separates into three segments. The first segment turns directly medial and crosses the tongue with transverse intrinsic bundles to become continuous with the muscle of the opposite side. The second segment runs along the side. The third segment spreads downward to interlace with the vertical fibers of the hyoglossus muscle. The styloglossus muscle is a retractor and elevator of the tongue, especially of its angle. Its nerve supply, as in all purely lingual muscles, is the hypoglossal nerve.

Palatoglossus muscle. This muscle arises from the lower surface of the palatine

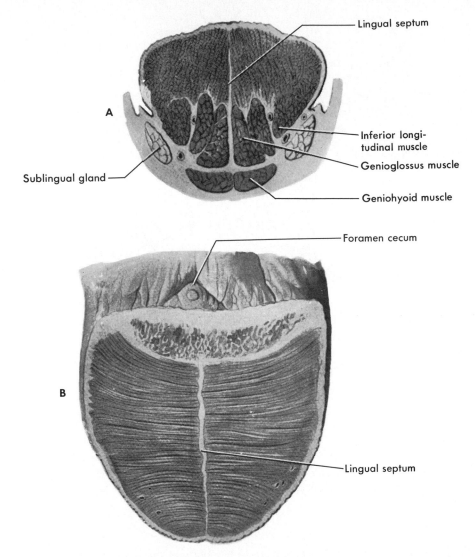

Lingual septum

Inferior longi-
tudinal muscle

Genioglossus muscle

Geniohyoid muscle

Sublingual gland

A

Foramen cecum

B

Lingual septum

Fig. 5-9. A, Cross section through tongue. **B,** Horizontal section through body of tongue: lingual septum and transverse muscle of tongue. (Sicher and Tandler: Anatomie für Zahnärzte.)

aponeurosis (see Fig. 6-17). It runs downward in the curve of the palatoglossal arch to the tongue at its bend. The fibers continue transversely through the tongue, interlacing with transverse intrinsic fibers to meet the muscle of the opposite side. Since the origins of the fibers of both sides may meet in the midline of the palatine aponeurosis and are continuous within the tongue, the muscle acts as a sphincter separating oral and pharyngeal cavities in swallowing as well as in speech. It is supplied by the vagus nerve among others in the pharyngeal plexus.

Hyoglossus muscle. This muscle arises from the upper border of the greater horn of the hyoid bone and from the lateral part of its body and lesser horns (see Figs. 2-45 and 3-12). The muscle is a thin plate with its fibers running upward and slightly forward into the tongue, where they interlace with the third segment of the stylo-glossus muscle. Bundles of the hyoglossus that arise from the lesser horns are referred to as the chondroglossus muscle. The hyoglossus is sometimes perforated by the lingual artery, which may run forward a short distance on the outer surface before it plunges to the inner surface. The artery is most often situated entirely on the inner surface of the hyoglossus muscle, which is a depressor of the tongue. Its nerve supply is the hypoglossal nerve.

Intrinsic muscles of the tongue. These muscles are composed of longitudinal, vertical, and transverse bundles (Fig. 5-9). Longitudinal fibers are found in upper and lower divisions; the superior and inferior longitudinal muscles of the tongue, situated above and below the long second segment of the styloglossus, run to the tongue tip. Transverse fibers arise from the lingual septum for the most part. The lingual septum is a sickle-shaped, flat plate of dense connective tissue embedded in the midline of the tongue. It reaches neither the dorsal surface nor the tip of the tongue. From this origin, the transverse bundles run laterally, intricately interwoven with bundles of other intrinsic muscles. Vertical fibers extend between the upper and lower surfaces of the tongue mainly near its lateral borders, but fibers are also interspersed through the tongue. Action of the intrinsic muscles changes the contour of the tongue mass and contributes to the great versatility of its postures and movements. The nerve supply is the hypoglossal nerve. (For details of functional activity of the tongue see Chapter 6).

GLANDS

In describing the different parts of the oral cavity, many of its glands have been mentioned. Some of these glands are small isolated or more densely packed bodies; others form rather large organs. The smaller glands are situated, for the most part, in the submucous layer and open with numerous narrow ducts on the surface of the mucous membrane. The large glands are farther removed from the inner lining of the oral cavity into which they open with strong, wide ducts. The secretion of all these glands produces the saliva, a fluid which has partly physical and partly chemical functions. Physically, it moistens and lubricates the food; chemically, its enzymes initiate the first phase of digestion and seem to have some antibacterial action related to dental caries.

According to their secretion, the glands may be divided into serous (albuminous) glands, mucous glands, and mixed glands. Anatomically, major and minor salivary glands are distinguished. To the former group belong parotid, submandibular, and sublingual glands; the latter group is subdivided according to their site. They comprise the labial, buccal, palatine, lingual, and incisive glands.

Parotid gland. The bulk of the parotid gland (Figs. 5-10 and 5-11) is situated in the retromandibular fossa. It reaches medially to the styloid process and the muscles arising from it, and upward to the external acoustic meatus, which is situated in a

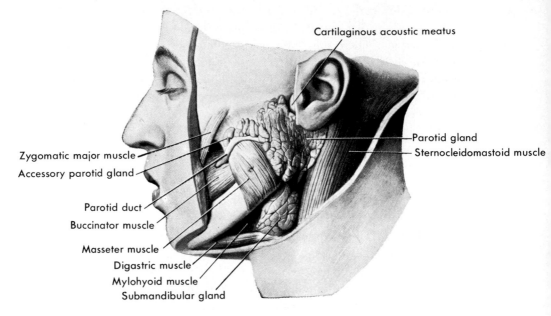

Fig. 5-10. Parotid and submandibular glands. (Sicher and Tandler: Anatomie für Zahnärzte.)

groove of the gland. Surrounding the acoustic meatus on its inferior surface, the gland reaches posteriorly to the mastoid process and the sternocleidomastoid muscle. Anteriorly it is in contact with the posterior border of the medial pterygoid muscle and the mandibular ramus. A part of the gland extends anteriorly on the outer surface of the mandibular ramus and masseter muscle as a thin, triangular layer. The outer surface of the gland is situated superficially, covered only by its capsule, the superficial fascia, and the skin. The upper lobules of the superficial part of the gland cover, in front of the ear, the craniomandibular articulation but never transgress the lower border of the zygomatic arch. The inferior corner of the gland extends below the level of the lower border of the mandible in the space between the mandibular angle and sternocleidomastoid muscle. This inferior extension of the gland is called the cervical lobe. The anterior border of the gland forms a tonguelike lobe, the apex of which is found midway between the lower border of the zygomatic arch and the lower border of the mandible or slightly above this line.

In most persons the parotid gland is divided into a superficial lobe, comprising the bulk of the gland, and a deep lobe. They are connected by a narrow isthmus. Branches of the facial nerve lie between these lobes for a variable, but usually short, distance. The isthmus is found most often in the bifurcation of the facial nerve into an upper temporal and a lower cervical division.

At the apex of the parotid gland on the outer surface of the masseter muscle, the parotid duct (Stensen's duct) emerges from the substance of the gland to course anteriorly until it reaches the anterior border of the masseter muscle at the point

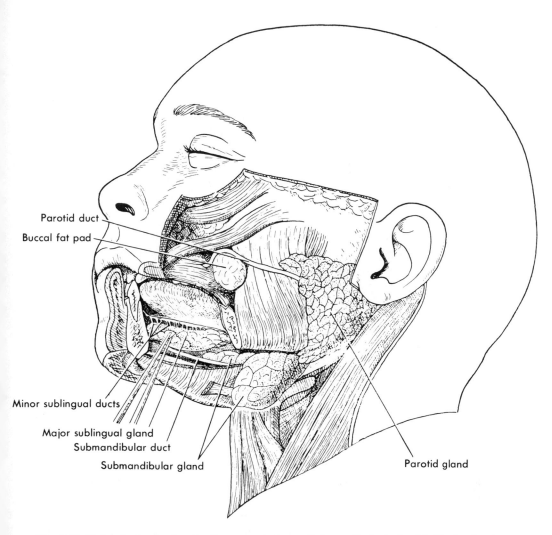

Parotid duct

Buccal fat pad

Minor sublingual ducts

Major sublingual gland

Submandibular duct

Submandibular gland

Parotid gland

Fig. 5-11. Major glands of oral cavity after removal of part of left mandibular body. (Modified and redrawn from Sicher and Tandler: Anatomie für Zahnärzte.)

between its upper and middle thirds. Around the border of the masseter the duct turns sharply medially, often embedded in a furrow of the protruding buccal fat pad (Fig. 5-11). In its medial course, the duct reaches the outer surface of the buccinator muscle, which it then perforates in an oblique direction anteriorly and medially. The parotid duct opens opposite the second upper molar, often at a papilla of the buccal mucosa, the parotid papilla.

In many persons a smaller or larger accessory lobe of the gland is found anterior to the main gland and above the duct into which it opens (Fig. 5-10).

The parotid gland is covered by a capsule, which is by far stronger on the lateral surface of the gland. The capsule is tight and firmly connected with the strong septa dividing the lobes and lobules of the gland from one another. The capsule is fused at the anterior border of the sternocleidomastoid muscle with its fascia but isolated from the other adjacent structures by thin layers of connective tissue. The capsule has to be considered a derivative of the deep fascia. It continues anteriorly as the fascia of the masseter muscle and inferiorly into the investing layer of the deep cervical fascia.

The external carotid artery, retromandibular (posterior facial) vein, and facial nerve are, for some length of their courses, embedded in the substance of the parotid gland. The external carotid artery is covered by the cervical lobe of the gland; in the retromandibular fossa it is situated at first in a groove on the medial surface of the gland, and eventually it enters the substance of the gland itself. The retromandibular vein traverses, superficial to the artery, the gland almost in its entire length from the region of the mandibular neck to the inferior corner of the cervical lobe.

The facial nerve enters the gland immediately on emerging from the stylomastoid foramen in an anterior, inferior, and lateral direction. In the gland the nerve divides into an upper and lower branch and then into the smaller branches after crossing the external carotid artery and retromandibular vein on their lateral side. The branches of the facial nerve leave the gland on its deep surface between the gland and the masseter muscle to emerge at the superior, anterior, and inferior borders of the gland.

Submandibular gland. The submandibular gland (Figs. 5-10 and 5-11) is a round biconvex body that occupies much of the submandibular, or digastric, triangle. Its upper pole, in most persons, lies on the medial surface of the mandible in the submandibular fovea; its lower pole extends beyond the boundaries of the digastric triangle covering the intermediate tendon of the digastric muscle. The inner surface of the submandibular gland is in contact with the stylohyoid, digastric, and styloglossus muscles posteriorly and with the hyoglossus and the posterior border of the mylohyoid muscle anteriorly. From the upper part of the inner surface of the submandibular gland extends the submandibular duct anteriorly and medially, often accompanied by a tonguelike extension of the main body of the gland. The submandibular duct, or Wharton's duct, turns to the superomedial, or oral, surface of the mylohyoid muscle and then courses along the inner surface of the sublingual gland after crossing the lingual nerve superiorly. Wharton's duct opens at the sublingual caruncula either after uniting with the major sublingual duct or emerging close to its opening. The last few millimeters of the duct are often slightly widened.

The submandibular gland is enclosed in a capsule, which, like that of the parotid gland, is in part a derivative of the investing layer of the deep cervical fascia. In contrast to the parotid capsule, that of the submandibular gland is only loosely attached to the substance of the gland itself because of the loose texture of the interlobar and interlobular connective tissue. The gland, therefore, can easily be shelled out of its niche.

The facial artery is closely applied to the inner surface and the upper border of the submandibular gland, running in a groove of the gland, sometimes even embedded in the glandular body itself. It sends branches into the gland and is thus tightly attached to it.

Sublingual gland. The sublingual gland (Fig. 5-11) is a long, flattened body situated close to the medial surface of the mandible which, in this area, shows a shallow depression, the sublingual fovea. On its superior surface the gland is covered by the thin mucous membrane and causes an elevation, the salivary eminence, on the floor of the oral cavity. The sublingual gland is, in fact, a glandular complex, since there is not one common duct for all its lobules. The greater part of the gland, forming the lateral and inferior portion of its substance, empties through the major sublingual duct, Bartholin's duct, which either unites with the submandibular duct or opens close to the latter at the sublingual caruncula.

The smaller, or minor, sublingual glands may be subdivided into two groups. The glands of one group send their ducts into the adjacent submandibular duct and are, sometimes, fused with the anterior extension of the submandibular gland. The other group of lesser sublingual glands lies at the superior surface of the gland. They release short ducts, five to fifteen in number, which open at the crest of the sublingual eminence on the floor of the oral cavity. These minor ducts are also known as ducts of Rivinus.

Labial glands. The labial glands (Fig. 5-12), small isolated mucous or mixed glands, are situated in the submucosa of the upper and lower lips, sometimes slightly protruding toward the vestibulum. They are more numerous in the areas close to the midline. Sometimes they form an almost continuous layer. Some of the larger glands may reach between the bundles of the orbicularis oris muscle.

Buccal glands. The buccal glands (Fig. 5-13) continue the layer of the labial glands posteriorly. In the anterior part of the cheek they are sparse and rather widely and irregularly spaced. In the posterior parts of the cheek they are more numerous and

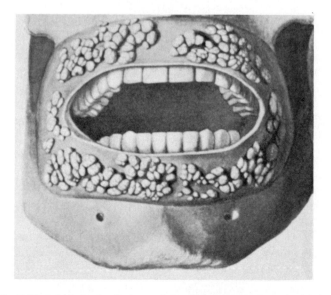

Fig. 5-12. Labial glands. (Sicher and Tandler: Anatomie für Zahnärzte.)

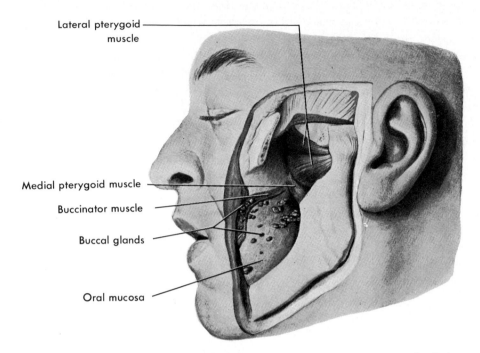

Lateral pterygoid
muscle

Medial pterygoid muscle

Buccinator muscle

Buccal glands

Oral mucosa

Fig. 5-13. Buccal glands dissected from side after removal of part of buccinator muscle. (Sicher and Tandler: Anatomie für Zahnärzte.)

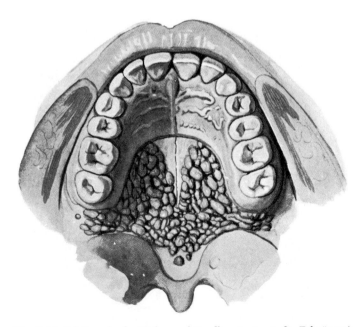

Fig. 5-14. Palatine glands. (Sicher and Tandler: Anatomie für Zahnärzte.)

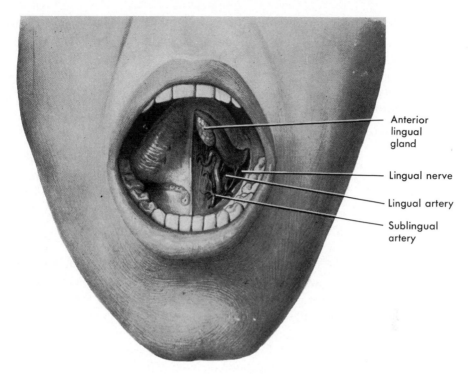

Anterior
lingual
gland

Lingual nerve

Lingual artery

Sublingual
artery

Fig. 5-15. Anterior lingual gland. (Sicher and Tandler: Anatomie für Zahnärzte.)

larger and reach not only between the bundles of the buccinator muscle but, sometimes, even to its outer surface. A group of these glands is situated at the lower
posterior corner of the cheek; these are known as the molar, or retromolar, glands.
The glands of the cheek continue into those of the anterior palatine pillar and, farther,
into the palatine glands.

Palatine glands. The palatine glands (Fig. 5-14) form an almost compact glandular
body situated in the submucous layer of the hard and soft palates. They seldom
extend anteriorly beyond a line that can be drawn from one first molar to the other.
Posteriorly, they increase in size and thickness and reach far into the soft palate. On
the hard palate the bodies of the palatine glands fill the spaces between the connective tissue lamellae connecting the mucous membrane and periosteum, and thus
furnish a cushion for this area of the oral mucosa.

Lingual glands. The lingual glands are found in two locations: in the anterior parts
of the tongue close to its inferior surface and on the base of the tongue near the dorsal
surface. The anterior lingual gland, Nuhn's gland or the gland of Blandin (Fig. 5-15),
is embedded in the substance of the tongue close to the apex and the midline, covered
only by the thin mucous membrane of the inferior surface of the tongue. It is in reality
not a single gland but a compact package of smaller glands that open with several
ducts on the inferior surface of the tongue.

The dorsal group of lingual glands are of two types: first, the von Ebner glands (serous glands), which empty into the bottom of the circular trough of the vallate papillae and, second, the glands at the base of the tongue, which are the mucous posterior lingual glands, the ducts of which open into the lingual crypts.

Incisive glands. The incisive glands are a small group of glands found on the floor of the oral cavity close to the insertion of the lingual frenum behind the lower incisors. Because of this relation these glands were designated incisive glands.

ORAL MUCOUS MEMBRANE

Although the structure of the mucous membrane lining the oral cavity was described in the preceding sections, a summarizing description and a classification of the oral mucosa according to functional and anatomic differences are warranted.

In studying any mucous membrane the following features have to be analyzed: (1) the type of covering epithelium; (2) the structure of the lamina propria, especially as to its density, thickness, and the presence or lack of elastic elements; and (3) the fixation of the mucous membrane to the underlying structures, in other words, the submucous layer. A submucosa as a separate and well-defined layer may be present or absent. Looseness or density of its texture determines whether the mucous membrane is movably or immovably attached to the deeper layers. Presence or absence of adipose tissue or glands also has to be noted.

The oral mucosa may be divided, primarily, into three different types. During mastication some parts of the lining are subjected to strong forces of pressure and friction. These parts, the gingiva and the covering of the hard palate, may be called the *masticatory mucosa*. The second type of oral mucosa is merely the protective lining of a body cavity that communicates with the outside world, without possessing other specific functions. These areas may be called the *lining mucosa*. They comprise the mucosa of the lips and cheeks, the mucosa of the vestibular fornix, the mucosa of the upper and lower alveolar processes peripheral to the gingiva proper, the mucosa of the floor of the mouth that extends to the inner surface of the lower alveolar process, the mucosa of the inferior surface of the tongue, and, finally, the mucous membrane of the soft palate. The third type of mucosa is represented by the covering of the dorsal surface of the tongue and is highly specialized, hence the term *specialized oral mucosa*. In many animals it has a decided masticatory function; in man this function is less significant.

The gingiva and the covering of the hard palate (the latter should not be classed as gums) have in common the thickness and keratinization of the epithelium, the thickness, density, and firmness of the inelastic lamina propria, and, finally, their immovable attachment to the deep structures. In a majority of persons the epithelium of the gingiva is parakeratotic.

As to the structure of the submucosa, these two areas differ markedly. In the gingiva a well-differentiated submucous layer cannot be recognized; instead, the dense and inelastic connective tissue of the lamina propria continues into the depth to fuse with the periosteum of the alveolar process or to attach to the cervical region of the tooth. In contrast to this, the lining of the hard palate has, with the exception of narrow areas, a distinct submucous layer. It is absent only in the peripheral zone, where the tissue is identical with the gingiva, and in a narrow zone along the midline, beginning in front with the palatine, or incisive, papilla and continuing as the palatine raphe over the entire length of the hard palate. Despite the presence of a well-defined submucous layer in the wide lateral fields of the hard palate between the palatine raphe and palatine gingiva, the mucous membrane is immovably and tightly attached to the periosteum of maxillary and palatine bones. This attachment is accomplished by dense bands and trabeculae of connective tissue, which bind the lamina propria of the mucous membrane to the periosteum. The submucous space is thus subdivided into irregular smaller and larger intercommunicating compartments. They are filled with adipose tissue in the anterior part and with glands in the posterior part of the hard palate. Fat and glands in the submucous layer act as a cushion comparable to that which one finds in the subcutaneous tissue of the palm of the hand and the sole of the foot and the corresponding surfaces of fingers and toes.

The presence or absence of a distinct submucous layer permits the subdivision of the masticatory oral mucosa into the simple and the cushioned types. The simple type is represented by the gingiva, the cushioned type by the palatine mucosa.

All of the areas of the lining mucosa are characterized by a relatively thick, non-keratinized epithelium and by the thinness of the lamina propria, but they differ from one another in the structure of the submucosa. Where the lining mucosa covers muscles as on the lips, cheeks, and underside of the tongue, it is immovably fixed to the epimysium or the fascia of the respective muscles. In these areas the mucosa is highly elastic. These two qualities safeguard the smoothness of the mucous lining in any functional phase of the muscle and prevent a folding that would interfere with the function; closing the mouth might, for instance, injure lips or cheeks if such folds protruded between the teeth. The mucosa of the soft palate is a transition between this type of lining mucosa and that which is in the fornix vestibuli and in the sublingual sulcus at the floor of the oral cavity. In the latter zones the submucosa is loose and of considerable volume. Thus the mucous membrane is loosely and movably attached to the deep structures, which allows for a free movement of the lips and cheeks on the one side and of the tongue on the other.

It is thus possible to subdivide the lining mucosa into the two main types of tightly and loosely attached zones. The tightly fixed areas, however, could be subdivided once more according to the absence or presence of a distinct submucous layer. This layer is lacking on the underside of the tongue but is present in the lips, cheeks, and soft palate. In the latter areas the mucous membrane is fixed to the fascia of the muscles or to their epimysium by bands of dense connective tissue between which either fat lobules or glands are situated.

The specialized oral mucosa on the dorsal surface of the tongue, with its papillae and follicles, serving as a sense organ anteriorly and as a lymphatic organ posteriorly, has already been described. It should be added that the mucous membrane on the dorsum of the tongue is tightly attached to the intermuscular and epimysial connective tissue.

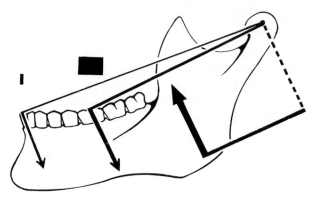

Fig. 5-16. Class III lever action of the mandible. Note: (1) resistance moment arm from condyle to incisor, (2) resistance moment arm from condyle to first molar, (3) effort moment arm from condyle to muscle, and (4) small black block at left = occlusal surface area of incisor, large black block = occlusal surface area of molar. The moment arms are drawn increasingly heavy from front to back, representing increasing forces.

THE TEETH
Functional features of the dentition

The jaw operates essentially as a Class III lever. Its joint is the *fulcrum*, its musculature is the applied force, or *effort force*, and its biting tooth is the *resistance force*. Thus the dentition is but one component of the highly complex oral apparatus. In a Class III lever the effort force lies between fulcrum and resistance force, as the muscles do in the jaw. The torque that tends to turn a lever around its axis of rotation (fulcrum) is called a *moment of force*. This is opposed by a countertorque, the resistance force, which is actually the work that the lever is designed to do. A moment of force is measured as the product of force and the perpendicular distance (moment arm) of the action line of the force from the fulcrum (force × distance). Thus a small effort force with a long moment arm can counterbalance a large resistance force with a short moment arm, and vice versa. Therefore in the jaw lever system, since the effort arm is shorter than the resistance arm, a powerful musculature is present to overcome this mechanical disadvantage (Fig. 5-16).

The dentition as a whole is a working unit made up of individual subunits, the 32 teeth of the intact dental arches. The functional anatomy of the teeth is most interesting in that in some features all teeth are similar while in others they are strikingly different.

Thus to begin with, all the teeth tend to be broadest mesiodistally near their occlusal thirds and broadest buccolingually closer to their cervical thirds. In the first case, the mesiodistal dimension ensures a continuous line of dental contacts, all at the same level, making for the unity of each dental arch (see Figs. 5-81 to 5-86). At the same time the narrowing of the tooth toward its cervical and root regions provides adequate space for the interproximal alveolar supporting tissues lying just below the protecting contact areas (see Figs. 5-79 and 5-80). In the second case, the buccolingual bulging of the tooth near its cervical third provides a sheltering overhang for the protection of the thin margins of the buccal and lingual continuations of the alveolar supporting tissues snugged tightly like gaskets closely below the bulge.

Since teeth are the ultimate tools in the masticatory preparation of food, their individual structural differences clearly reflect the differential functional loading along the length of the jaw lever arm. Since a posterior tooth has a much shorter resistance arm (distance from joint) than does an anterior tooth, we naturally expect a much greater biting pressure on posterior teeth than on anterior teeth because of the increased mechanical advantage. But the posterior teeth also have much larger biting surfaces than do anterior teeth. Pressure is measured by dividing the force applied by the surface over which it is distributed (force/area). Pressure is then actually a measure of the concentration of a force on a surface. *Per unit area,* ten units of force applied to ten units of surface is the same as one unit of force on one unit of surface. Therefore the gradual decrease in occlusal surface from back to front is seen to compensate for a decrease in lever effectiveness with the lengthening of the resistance arm. It tends to equalize biting efficiency along the tooth row (Fig. 5-16). Thus resistance to masticatory pressure is clearly seen in the structural design of teeth as well as in that of the craniomandibular articulation.

General description of the teeth

The human teeth, as well as those of the other mammals, are complicated organs that consist mostly of hard, mineralized tissues. They contain the dental pulp as a core, a tissue rich in nerves and blood vessels. One part of the tooth is exposed in the oral cavity, and the other is contained in a compartment of the jawbone, the socket or alveolus, which corresponds in its shape to that of the individual root. The tooth is fixed in the socket by a highly specialized suspensory ligament.

The bulk of a human tooth is formed by the dentin. That part of the dentinal body which at the height of function is exposed in the oral cavity is covered by the enamel, a derivative of the ectodermal epithelium of the oral cavity. That part of the tooth which is embedded in the socket is covered by the cementum, a tissue almost identical to bone. The suspensory ligament is anchored in the cementum on one side and in the bone of the socket on the other. However, no single fiber reaches from the cementum to the bone.

The part of the tooth covered by enamel is the crown; the part covered by cementum is the root. A slight constriction between the crown and root is the neck of the tooth, or the cervical constriction. At the cervical line enamel and cementum meet; the term cementoenamel junction is preferred by many authors. The dental pulp is contained in a space roughly corresponding to the general shape of the tooth. The space communicates at the tip, or apex, of the root with the surrounding tissues through the apical foramen, continues in the root as the root canal, and widens in the crown to the pulp chamber.

The eruption of teeth is a gradual and continuous process. In young persons not all of the enamel-covered crown is exposed; in old age not only the crown but also parts of the root may have erupted into the oral cavity and may no longer be covered by soft tissues. To simplify description of these relations, new terms have been proposed: anatomic crown and anatomic root refer to the enamel-covered and cementum-covered parts, respectively, of the human tooth. That part of the tooth which at a given moment is exposed to the oral cavity is the functional (clinical) crown; that part which is embedded in, and in organic connection with, the surrounding tissues is the functional (clinical) root. In young persons the functional crown is smaller than the anatomic crown; in older persons the relation is reversed.

Color and size of teeth. The color of the crown is dependent on two factors, the color and the translucency of the enamel. Normal enamel is a light yellowish color and is translucent enough to permit the darker yellow dentin to influence the shade, especially in the areas where the enamel is thin. Thus the cervical parts of the crown are normally darker than the incisal or occlusal parts. When part of the enamel has been worn away and dentin has been exposed, the color of the tooth darkens appreciably because of the imbibition of the dentin with staining materials from food. Lower teeth, especially the anterior teeth, are usually lighter in color than the upper teeth.

Deciduous teeth are more purely white or even bluish white. In the permanent dentition, however, a white or bluish white color of the teeth is often the sign of an imperfect calcification of the enamel, which then partly loses its translucency. Bluish white teeth are considered by some as a sign of a generalized constitutional inferiority and are said to be prevalent in people who are susceptible to tubercular infection.

The size of the human teeth varies individually so much (Fig. 5-17) that only mean values or minimal and maximal measurements can be given. Although the mesiodistal diameter of the crown is, to some extent, correlated to body height, the total length of a tooth, and especially the length of its root, shows no such correlation.

The variations in the length of the root (Fig. 5-17) are of great practical importance. The firmness of a tooth is dependent on the area of the root surface, which in turn varies with the root length. The larger the surface of the cementum, the more bundles of the suspensory ligament find attachment to the root. Exposure in normal or pathologic conditions of an equal part of the root will have less damaging influence if the root is long, but can markedly loosen a tooth with a short root.

Phylogenetic remarks. In structure and development the teeth show their principal similarity to hairs, feathers, and scales. In all of these an ectodermal and a mesodermal blastema combine to form the organ. Primitive teeth show so close a similarity to the placoid scales or dermal teeth of sharks that these appendages of the skin are regarded as the ancestral structures from which the teeth evolved. The oral cavity is lined by a modified continuation of the skin and may, at one time, have been covered by the same placoid scales as the skin itself.

Formation of teeth in many animals, therefore, is not restricted to the borders of the jaws. Futhermore, the teeth develop primarily at the surface of the oral cavity

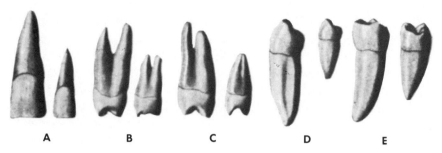

A **B** **C** **D** **E**

Fig. 5-17. Extreme variations in size of various teeth, drawn to natural size. **A,** Upper central incisor. **B,** Upper first premolar. **C,** Upper second premolar. **D,** Lower first premolar. **E,** Lower second premolar. (Sicher and Tandler: Anatomie für Zahnärzte.)

itself and only in later stages of evolution is the epithelial anlage of the tooth invaginated into the deep layers of the oral mucous membrane. Then the tooth develops in the depth and erupts secondarily to the surface from which it originated. As is true of the other organs of the skin, the teeth also were originally temporary structures, destined to be lost after a relatively short period of function and to be replaced whenever and as often as necessary.

Fishes, amphibia, and reptiles show the continuous replacement of teeth, which therefore appear in many generations. This type of replacement is known as polyphyodontism. In mammals (and in the highest extinct reptiles, the Theromorpha) the teeth acquired more permanency, being used now not only to catch or apprehend and hold the food, but also to masticate it. With the acquisition of this function the differentiation of the teeth reaches the highest level and simultaneously the number of generations for replacement is reduced to two, the deciduous and the permanent series. Not even all the teeth are represented in both series. Polyphyodontism has been reduced to diphyodontism.

At the same time there developed a division of labor between different groups of teeth, one group becoming specialized for the apprehension of food, another for its mastication; other teeth differentiated as weapons for attack. Thus the homodont dentition of most reptiles evolved into the heterodont dentition of the mammals, in which the teeth are differentiated into such divergent types as incisors, canines, premolars, and molars.

The acquisition and progressive perfection of masticatory function has also led to a profound change in the attachment of the tooth to the jaw. In fishes and reptiles there is either a simple ligamentous or connective tissue junction of tooth and bone or a solid, ankylotic union between the two. The tooth is almost always fixed to the surface of the jaw. In mammals the tooth develops a root that is enclosed in a bony socket and attached to it by a suspensory ligament. To the two phylogenetically older tissues of the tooth, dentin and enamel, the cementum is now added as a last differentiation, providing for the attachment of the alveolodental ligament.

The higher development and differentiation of the mammalian tooth had to be paid for, to speak in teleologic terms, by the restriction of unlimited replacement to two series of teeth only. Thus the functional life span of teeth became almost identical with the life span of mammals. It is, therefore, interesting to examine some modifications that prolong the functional period of mammalian teeth.

The most perfect adaptation is the continually growing tooth. Here the formation and growth of the tooth continue at its basal end throughout the life of the animal. For instance, the incisors of the rodents (and in some species the premolars and molars also) are worn at their functional end, and the loss is replaced by correlated growth at the basal end and by continual eruption. This mechanism also permits a gradual increase in size of the tooth during the period of growth of the animal. In some species the wear of such "rootless" teeth is insignificant, and the teeth enlarge throughout the animal's life; this occurs in the tusks of elephants.

A transitional type between the short-crowned (brachydont) teeth, for instance, those of carnivores and primates, and the continually growing teeth are the high-crowned (hypsodont) teeth. All stages between brachydont and hypsodont teeth can be observed, especially in herbivorous animals. Browsing animals have lower crowns, whereas grazing animals have higher crowns. In the extremely hypsodont horse the development of the molar roots does not start before the fifth year of life. The life span of these teeth is 20 to 22 years, and their imminent loss coincides with the end of the genetically fixed life span of the animal itself. To assure the fixation of the tooth before the root develops, the enamel of such teeth is covered by cementum. It is interesting that some extinct hominid races did take a step in the direction of hypsodontism. The short-crowned teeth have also been called kynodont teeth (dog teeth), the higher-crowned teeth taurodont teeth (cattle teeth).

A third type of compensation for the short life span of the tooth has been acquired by the elephant and the manatee. It has been called the horizontal replacement of teeth. In these animals only a few of the total number of teeth function at the same time, and when they are worn down more posterior teeth move forward into their place. Here permanent teeth are replaced by permanent teeth.

That man can survive the loss of his teeth is of course due to civilization or self-domestication and the processing of his food. In this respect man and his privileged friend, the dog, behave similarly.

If one looks for a characteristic trend in the evolution of the human dentition as far as it is documented by findings on fossil hominids, one can point to a progressive reduction of the masticatory apparatus. This process seems not to have reached its end even today. The absence of one or more or all of the third molars, wisdom teeth, and the frequent absence of the upper second or lateral incisors can be interpreted as mutations further reducing the human dentition. However, it is questionable whether these mutations foreshadow the establishment of a still more reduced human dentition in the far future.

There is also a definite decrease in the size of the single elements of the dental arches. One example of this latter change is the reversion of the proportions in the molar series. In primitive man the size of the molars increases distally; in modern man the first molar is the largest and the third is the smallest tooth in this series.

Reduction of the dental arches is also correlated, although incompletely, with a reduction of the jaws and, consequently, of certain structures of the head and skull. The shortening of the lower jaw threatened at one period in the evolution of man to encroach on the intramandibular space and thus on the free mobility of the tongue. At this period the reinforcement of the median mandibular region was transposed from the posterior, or internal, surface to the anterior, or external, surface of the mandible. This seems to explain the development of the bony chin, a feature characteristic only of the latest evolutionary types of man.

The shortening of the jaws and the concomitant expansion of the brain and its capsule, both correlated to man's acquisition of upright posture, changed radically the topographic relations between the facial and cerebral parts of the skull. The backward shift of the masticatory skeleton is in turn responsible for the reduction of the super-ciliary ridges, the frontal buttresses of the upper jaw. The reduction of the mastica-tory muscles led to the gradual reduction or even disappearance of bony crests and ridges, which previously served the attachment of this once mighty musculature. In this connection should be mentioned the change of the zygomatic arch, which shifted gradually closer to the lateral surface of the skull.

Terminology.* In the permanent human dentition four types of teeth can be dis-tinguished: the cutting incisors, the pointed canines, the two-pointed premolars, and the many-cusped, or many-pointed molars. Premolars and especially the molars serve for the diminution of food, its grinding and crushing. The cutting incisors bite off morsels of food, and the canines have lost any special function in man and work sometimes with the incisors, sometimes with the premolars.

In the deciduous set of teeth the shape of the incisors and canines conforms in principle with that of their permanent successors. The precursors of the premolars, however, are molariform; that is, they are many-cusped teeth. They are therefore called deciduous molars in the dental literature, which is primarily concerned with the human dentition. Zoologists and comparative anatomists prefer the term decid-uous premolars.

The number of elements of the various groups of teeth in different species of mammals is best given as a dental formula. The formula is written in many different ways. The first letter is used to indicate the tooth category, i for incisors, c for canines, p for premolars and m for molars. If a differentiation is to be made between perma-nent and deciduous teeth, the letter for the permanent teeth is capitalized, whereas the lower case letter is used to indicate the deciduous teeth. It is better to add the subscript d or p, respectively, to the initial letter; for instance, i_d denoting deciduous incisors, p_p permanent premolars.

---

* The terms "cuspid" for canine and "bicuspid" for premolar teeth, which are dental jargon, should be abolished. Human premolars are often *not* bicuspid. The terminology of human dentition should not be different from that used in comparative anatomy. Other changes also seem highly desirable but have met with much resistance.

The formula for the human deciduous dentition is then written:

$$\frac{i_d2,\, c_d1,\, m_d2}{i_d2,\, c_d1,\, m_d2} \qquad OR \qquad i_d\,\frac{2}{2},\, c_d\,\frac{1}{1},\, m_d\,\frac{2}{2}$$

The formula for the human permanent human dentition is written:

$$\frac{i_p2,\, c_p1,\, p_p2,\, m_p3}{i_p2,\, c_p1,\, p_p2,\, m_p3} \qquad OR \qquad i_p\,\frac{2}{2},\, c_p\,\frac{1}{1},\, p_p\,\frac{2}{2},\, m_p\,\frac{3}{3}$$

Dentistry needs an accurate and detailed description of every single tooth, and therefore a special terminology has been developed. Although it is in some ways at variance with the anatomic nomenclature and in other points linguistically not correct, it is used so widely that it could not be changed without much ensuing confusion. The terms refer first of all to the different surfaces of the crowns of the teeth. Of the five free surfaces of any crown, one is the biting, or masticatory, surface. Since it is in contact with the opposing teeth when the jaws are closed, it is called the *occlusal surface*. In the incisors this surface is reduced to a sharp edge, the *occlusal*, or *incisal*, *edge* or *margin*.

On each tooth one surface is turned toward the oval vestibule, the other toward the oral cavity proper. The *vestibular surface* is also called the *labial surface* on incisors and canines and the *buccal surface* on premolars and molars because it is in contact with either lip or cheek. The *oral surface* is generally referred to as the *lingual surface* because it is in contact with the tongue.

The other two free surfaces of each tooth, with the exception of the last molar, are in contact with corresponding surfaces of neighboring teeth. Of these two *approximal surfaces*, or contact surfaces, the one closer to the midline is known as the *mesial surface* and the other as the *distal surface*. The approved international anatomic terminology eliminates these terms. The "mesial" surface in incisors and canines is the *medial*, but in premolars and molars the *anterior* surface. The "distal" surface is, correspondingly, called the *lateral* surface in incisors and canines and the *posterior* surface in premolars and molars. If the term *contact* surfaces could be adopted for "approximal" surfaces, then the criteria of anatomic nomenclature could be satisfied by calling "mesial" surfaces *proximal*, closer to the midline, whereas the term "distal" could be maintained to mean away from the midline. This would make for considerable simplification.

Directions on the crown or root and also the relation of different areas on the crown and root are indicated by the terms *occlusally* and *cervically* on the crown, *cervically* and *apically* on the root.

Special description of permanent teeth*

Upper first (central) incisor (Figs. 5-18 to 5-20). The broad crown of the upper central incisor is shovel-shaped and ends in a sharp incisal edge. When the tooth

---

*The teeth in Figs. 5-18 to 5-46, which are described as typical, belong to the "perfect" dentition of the same young adult male.

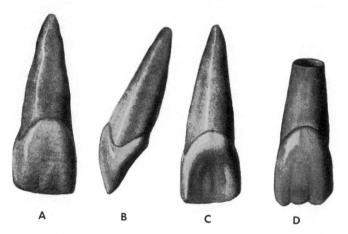

Fig. 5-18. Right upper first incisor. **A,** Labial surface. **B,** Mesial surface. **C,** Lingual surface. **D,** Left upper first incisor of a child with the three incisal cusplets or mamelons. (Sicher and Tandler: Anatomie für Zahnärzte.)

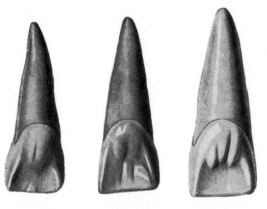

Fig. 5-19. Three variations of dental tubercle of the upper first incisor. (Sicher and Tandler: Anatomie für Zahnärzte.)

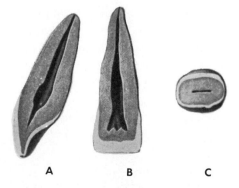

Fig. 5-20. Pulpal spaces of upper first incisor. **A,** Labiolingual section. **B,** Mesiodistal section. **C,** Cross section through crown. (Sicher and Tandler: Anatomie für Zahnärzte.)

erupts, the incisal edge is not straight but is divided into three rounded cusps, or mamelons (Fig. 5-18, *D*), which, however, are soon worn away. From the notches between the three cusplets, two shallow grooves continue over the incisal third or half of the labial surface to disappear at a variable distance from the cervical border.

The labial surface, bordering toward the root in a convex line, widens slowly toward the incisal edge; here the mesial border joins the edge at an almost right angle, whereas the distal corner is markedly rounded. The labial surface is convex in transverse and longitudinal directions. The longitudinal convexity is greatest near the cementoenamel junction and diminishes toward the incisal edge, so that the incisal third often is almost flat. The transverse convexity is generally slight, but as a rule is visibly greater in the mesial half of the labial surface than in the distal half.

In general, the lingual surface is deeply concave. In its cervical third it carries a prominence, the dental tubercle. From here the marginal parts of the lingual surface run as slight ridges toward the incisal edge, forming with the tuberculum a horseshoe-shaped elevation. The shape of the tuberculum itself is highly variable (Fig. 5-19). It may be just the highest area at the junction of the marginal elevations, cingulum, or it may extend tonguelike into the concavity of the lingual surface. It may be simple or divided by furrows into two or more smaller cusplets.

The proximal surfaces of the upper first incisor are roughly triangular, because of the convergence of labial and lingual surfaces toward the incisal edge, and slightly convex; the height of the convexity is close to the incisal edge and forms the contact with the neighboring tooth. The linear angles between the proximal and labial and lingual surfaces are well rounded. The line of the cementoenamel junction on the proximal surfaces is V-shaped, the angle of the V projecting far incisally.

The root of the upper first incisor is roughly cone-shaped and is normally longer than the crown. The root has a labial, a mesiolingual, and a distolingual surface; these, however, often are not well demarcated. The distolingual surface is sometimes grooved. Axes of the crown and root do not coincide. In labial view the axes form an obtuse angle open distally; in proximal view the obtuse angle between the coronary and radicular axes is open lingually.

The root canal (Fig. 5-20) starts at the apical foramen and runs, gradually widening, through the length of the root. It is roughly circular in cross section. In the crown the canal continues into the pulp chamber, which is narrow in labiolingual direction and wide in mesiodistal direction, especially in its most incisal part; it continues toward the incisal edge in three cusplets of the tooth. The horns can be long and may persist even when the chamber itself has been reduced in size by formation of secondary or irregular dentin.

The mean measurements for the upper first incisor are as follows:

Overall length of tooth	24.0 mm.
Length of crown	11.6 mm.
Greatest mesiodistal diameter of crown	8.4 mm.
Cervical mesiodistal diameter	6.7 mm.
Cervical labiolingual diameter	7.3 mm.

Fig. 5-21

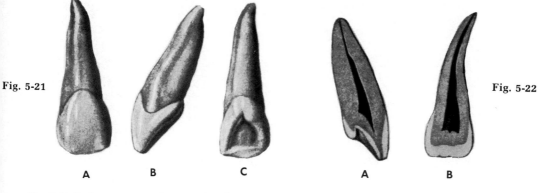

Fig. 5-22

A   B   C   A   B

Fig. 5-21. Right upper second incisor. **A,** Labial surface. **B,** Mesial surface. **C,** Lingual surface. (Sicher and Tandler: Anatomie für Zahnärzte.)

Fig. 5-22. Pulpal spaces of upper second incisor. **A,** Labiolingual section. **B,** Mesiodistal section. (Sicher and Tandler: Anatomie für Zahnärzte.)

Upper second (lateral) incisor (Figs. 5-21 and 5-22). Although it is similar to the first incisor in general outline, the second incisor is not just a small replica of its mesial neighbor. Even if it is fully and typically developed, it has some characteristic features. The crown is more slender and only rarely grooved on its labial surface. The incisal edge is, even before eruption, only indistinctly divided into three mamelons; often there are only two such cusplets, the middle one being rudimentary or missing. The lingual surface is more deeply concave than is that of the first incisor and often has a rather deep pit incisal to the tubercle, which is a feature only rarely seen on the central incisor. The pit is known as the foramen cecum.

The root of the upper second incisor is slender and somewhat compressed in the mesiodistal direction and is often slightly grooved. The angle between the crown and root on the distal side is often more pronounced than on the first incisor. The apical part of the root is frequently bent distally and often distolingually. The bend can be fairly sharp.

The pulp spaces (Fig. 5-22) are, in typical specimens, a reduced image of those of the first incisor, but the widening of the pulp chamber in mesiodistal direction is not as pronounced because of the relatively smaller width of the slender crown.

The wide range of variability of the upper second incisor has to be stressed. The tooth can be reduced to a small cone-shaped crown with a thin, often curved root. Between these peg-shaped incisors and a typical tooth there are many transitional shapes. One fairly frequent variation should be mentioned, in which the crown of the tooth is sharply bent mesially and the tooth looks lacerated or crippled.

The dental tubercle on the lingual surface may reach the size of a well-developed cusp, and then the tooth appears doubled in labiolingual direction. The overdeveloped tubercle is sometimes separated from the rest of the crown by deep and sharp grooves, which may extend for a variable distance along the root. It has been men-

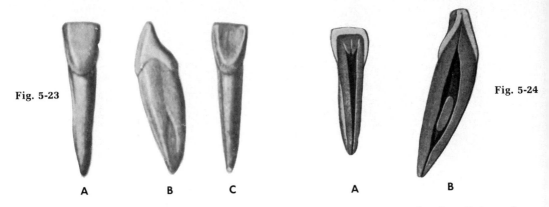

Fig. 5-23. Right lower first incisor. **A,** Labial surface. **B,** Mesial surface. **C,** Lingual surface. (Sicher and Tandler: Anatomie für Zahnärzte.)

Fig. 5-24. Pulpal spaces of lower first incisor. **A,** Mesiodistal section. **B,** Labiolingual section, slightly enlarged. (Sicher and Tandler: Anatomie für Zahnärzte.)

tioned previously that the upper second incisor is fairly often missing on one or both sides.

The mean measurements for the upper second incisor are as follows:

Overall length of tooth	22.5 mm.
Length of crown	9.0-10.2 mm.
Greatest mesiodistal diameter of crown	6.5 mm.
Cervical mesiodistal diameter	5.1 mm.
Cervical labiolingual diameter	6.0 mm.

Lower first (central) incisor (Figs. 5-23 and 5-24). The crown of the lower first incisor is chisel-shaped. The labial surface is slightly convex, its mesial and distal borders meeting the incisal edge at almost right angles. Before the tooth has fully erupted, the incisal edge shows three small and rounded prominences, which soon disappear by attrition. The lingual surface is convex in its cervical part and flatly concave in its greater central and incisal parts. Cervically the convexity forms a low cingulum that continues into ridges at the mesial and distal borders of the lingual surface. The proximal surfaces are triangular with a V-shaped gingival, or cervical, base. Compared with the height of the crown, the proximal surfaces are rather wide at their base. The root of the lower first incisor is markedly flattened in the mesiodistal dimension. Longitudinal grooves are present on the mesial and distal surfaces, the latter usually being deeper.

Corresponding to the shape of the root, the root canal (Fig. 5-24) is a space narrow in mesiodistal direction and extended in labiolingual direction. The relations are reversed in the crown, where the pulp chamber is wider in mesiodistal than in labiolingual direction. The pulp chamber continues occlusally in two or three indistinct and usually short horns. In the widest part of the root the canal is often divided into a labial and a lingual branch by a fusion of its mesial and distal walls. The two branches

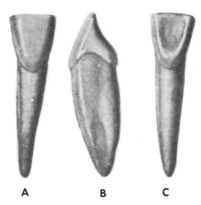

A   B   C

Fig. 5-25. Right lower second incisor. **A,** Labial surface. **B,** Mesial surface. **C,** Lingual surface. (Sicher and Tandler: Anatomie für Zahnärzte.)

may unite again at a variable distance from the root end. Rarely do they open separately at the apex.

The lower first incisor is the smallest tooth of the permanent human dentition. The average measurements for the lower central incisor are as follows:

Overall length of tooth	21.4 mm.
Length of crown	9.4 mm.
Greatest mesiodistal diameter of crown	5.4 mm.
Cervical mesiodistal diameter	3.9 mm.
Cervical labiolingual diameter	5.9 mm.

Lower second (lateral) incisor (Fig. 5-25). The second mandibular incisor, generally shaped like the first, is slightly larger than its mesial neighbor. The most conspicuous difference between these two teeth is the enhanced divergence of the mesial and distal surfaces in the second incisor. The mesial surface is nearly vertical; the distal surface deviates distally toward the incisal edge. Thus the distal corner at the incisal edge is elongated and forms a more acute angle than does the mesial corner.

The average measurements for the lower lateral incisor are as follows:

Overall length of tooth	23.2 mm.
Length of crown	9.9 mm.
Greatest mesiodistal diameter of crown	5.9 mm.
Cervical mesiodistal diameter	4.2 mm.
Cervical labiolingual diameter	6.2 mm.

Upper canine (Figs. 5-26 and 5-27). The upper canine has a pointed cusp instead of an occlusal edge. Mesial and distal edges of the cusp are asymmetrical; the mesial edge is shorter and not as steeply inclined as the longer distal edge. The most prominent points at the proximal surfaces, mediating the contact with the neighboring teeth, are found at the corners between the mesial and distal arms of the modified incisal edge and the proximal surfaces in a stricter sense. The asymmetry of the cusp causes the contact points to be at different levels, the mesial being farther occlusal than the distal. The latter is more prominent than the former. The labial surface is, on the whole, convex, the middle region often heightened to a longitudinal ridge that ends at the tip of the cusp. The middle ridge is often accompanied mesially and distally by shallow grooves so that the labial surface appears to be divided into three parts, or lobes.

Although the lingual surface is generally concave, it is often divided into two shallow grooves by a rather prominent ridge connecting the lingual tuberculum with the cusp. A strong development of the middle ridge can considerably reduce these grooves and gives to the whole tooth the appearance of great strength.

The proximal surfaces are triangular; the broad base of the triangle is convex occlusally. Corresponding to the different position of the contact points, the mesial surface is higher than the distal one. The mesial surface is situated almost in the same plane as the mesial surface of the root, whereas the distal surface of the crown forms a definite angle with the distal surface of the root.

Frequently there is a secondary cusp on the distal slope of the occlusal edge. The accessory cusp is highly variable in its size and may sometimes almost reach the occlusal plane.

The root of the upper canine is the longest and strongest of the human dentition; the cross section of the root is triangularly oval, the labial border being broader and plumper than the lingual border. The mesial and distal surfaces of the root are well grooved. The root is bent distal to the crown, and, in addition to this slight divergence of coronal and radicular axes, the apical part of the root is often more abruptly curved distally, sometimes labiodistally.

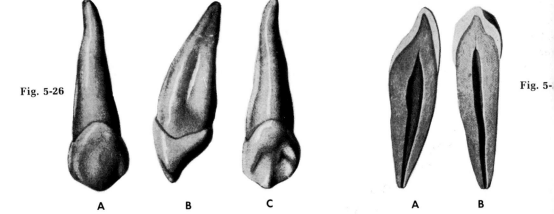

Fig. 5-26

Fig. 5-

A B C A B

Fig. 5-26. Right upper canine. **A,** Labial surface. **B,** Mesial surface. **C,** Lingual surface. (Sicher and Tandler: Anatomie für Zahnärzte.)

Fig. 5-27. Pulpal spaces of upper canine. **A,** Mesiodistal section. **B,** Labiolingual section. (Sicher and Tandler: Anatomie für Zahnärzte.)

The pulp cavity (Fig. 5-27) is spindle-shaped and slightly compressed in the mesiodistal direction. Its widest part corresponds to the cervical region of the tooth; in the crown the pulp chamber narrows to the one simple horn. Only if an accessory distal cusp is well developed may a slight diverticulum of the pulp chamber reach into its base.

The average measurements for the upper canine are as follows:

Overall length of tooth	27.0 mm.
Greatest mesiodistal diameter of crown between contact points	7.6 mm.
Length of crown	10.9 mm.
Cervical mesiodistal diameter	5.6 mm.
Cervical labiolingual diameter	81. mm.

Lower canine (Fig. 5-28). Contrasted with the upper canine, the lower canine is smaller and more slenderly built. Although it duplicates roughly the shape of the upper canine, the lower can be recognized by the relatively weak development of the longitudinal ridges both on the labial and lingual surfaces. The slenderness of the lower tooth is responsible for a less divergent position of the mesial and distal surfaces. The crown is also less asymmetrical than that of the upper canine; that is, the difference in length and inclination of the mesial and distal arms of the occlusal edge is less conspicuous in the lower than in the upper canine. Another characteristic difference between the upper and lower teeth is the fact that the enamel on the labial surface of the lower canine extends farther apically than that on the lingual surface. Finally, the labial surface of the crown is more inclined lingually than the corresponding surface of the upper canine, which is almost in a vertical position.

The root of the lower canine is not only shorter and weaker than that of the upper,

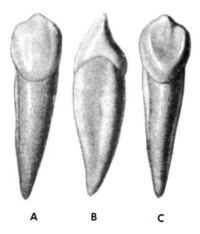

A   B   C

Fig. 5-28. Right lower canine. **A,** Labial surface. **B,** Mesial surface. **C,** Lingual surface. (Sicher and Tandler: Anatomie für Zahnärzte.)

but corresponding to the slenderness of the crown, it is also more flattened in the mesiodistal direction than that of the upper tooth. The longitudinal grooves are well developed, especially the one on the distal surface. Frequently the root of the lower canine shows a division of its apical part, which by transitions leads to an almost complete partition into a buccal and a lingual root. Such variations are almost unknown in the upper jaw.

The pulp cavity is simple, spindle-shaped, and often well compressed in the mesiodistal direction. The compression is most conspicuous in the root where, if it is deeply grooved, the canal may assume a dumbbell shape in a cross section. Fusion of the longitudinal prominences at the mesial and distal walls of the root canal may lead to a subdivision of the root canal for a variable distance. Such divisions lead gradually to the establishment of separate labial and lingual canals, a variation that can be regarded as the forerunner of the division of the root itself.

The average measurements of the lower canine are as follows:

Overall length of tooth	25.4 mm.
Mesiodistal diameter of crown between contact points	6.7 mm.
Length of crown measured on labial surface	11.4 mm.
Cervical mesiodistal diameter	5.3 mm.
Cervical labiolingual diameter	7.8 mm.

Upper first premolar (Figs. 5-29 and 5-30). The premolars are characterized by the development of a true occlusal surface, which is lacking in incisors and canines. The buccal surface of the upper first premolar is strikingly similar to that of the canine but is more nearly symmetrical. The buccal surface is traversed by a longitudinal, variably high ridge that terminates in the buccal cusp. The occlusal borders of the buccal surface meet at the cusp almost at a right angle. The lingual surface is slightly lower and much narrower than the buccal surface and continues into the corresponding surface of the lingual cusp. The proximal surfaces are roughly rectangular and slightly convex, the convexity of the distal surface being stronger. The height of the convexity, the contact point, is found on both proximal surfaces close to their occlusal border. On the distal surface it is slightly shifted, and on the mesial surface more conspicuously shifted, toward the buccal side. The line of the cementoenamel junction on the buccal and lingual surfaces is slightly convex toward the root, but on the proximal surfaces it is curved in the opposite direction, the convexity facing occlusally.

The contour of the occlusal surface is asymmetrically quadrilateral; the proximal surfaces converge lingually, but the distal margin curves strongly mesially. Thus the lingual cusp seems slightly shifted mesially when compared with the position of the buccal cusp.

The two cusps are roughly cone-shaped, the buccal cusp always being larger in circumference and higher than the lingual cusp. From the tip of each cusp a ridge runs toward the occlusal fissure. The two cusps are separated from each other by a sharp mesiodistal groove or fissure, which, however, does not reach either the mesial

Fig. 5-29

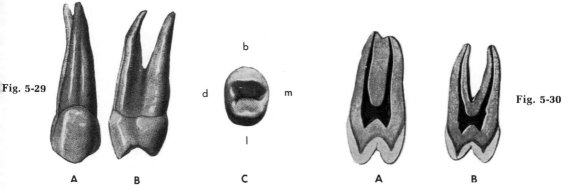

Fig. 5-30

Fig. 5-29. Right upper first premolar. **A,** Buccal surface. **B,** Mesial surface. **C,** Occlusal surface. (Sicher and Tandler: Anatomie für Zahnärzte.)

Fig. 5-30. Pulpal spaces of upper first premolar, buccolingual sections. **A,** Single-rooted tooth. **B,** Two-rooted tooth. (Sicher and Tandler: Anatomie für Zahnärzte.)

or the distal border of the occlusal surface. Here the two cusps are joined one to the other by marginal ridges. The mesial and distal ends of the occlusal fissure are frequently deepened, and from these small pits shallow grooves extend buccally and lingually. The two buccal and the two lingual grooves diverge from their origin in the mesiodistal fissure, buccally and lingually, respectively. The distobuccal groove is generally the deepest and longest and may even cut into the distal slope of the buccal cusp. This cusp then carries an accessory cusplet, thus increasing the similarity of the buccal surface of the first premolar to the labial surface of an upper canine.

In more than 50% of the examined teeth the root of the upper first premolar is divided into two roots. The division, starting at the apex, reaches variably far cervically. If the root is simple, it resembles that of the canine tooth, but it is always more flattened and more deeply grooved. The mesial and distal grooves may be so deep that the dentinal part of the root is divided; the two divisions, however, are still united by a common covering of cementum. This type is the transition to a true division of the root. If the upper first premolar is birooted, the two roots may diverge to a variable degree. The buccal root which is always thicker than the lingual one, may show a variably deep groove on its lingual surface. Eventually this groove may lead to a subdivision of the buccal root into a mesiobuccal and a distobuccal root. The division starts at the apex and is only rarely complete. The distal curvature of the apical part of the root or roots is well marked in most upper first premolars.

The pulp chamber, or coronal pulp cavity (Fig. 5-30), is, corresponding to the shape of the crown, narrow in the mesiodistal and wide in the buccolingual direction. Toward the two cusps, two pulpal horns extend from the common chamber. Of these, the buccal one, as a rule, is longer. The root canal of the upper first premolar is almost always divided into a buccal and a lingual canal even if the root is outwardly simple.

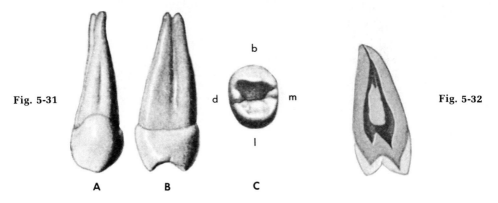

Fig. 5-31   Fig. 5-32

A   **B**   **C**

Fig. 5-31. Right upper second premolar. **A,** Buccal surface. **B,** Mesial surface. **C,** Occlusal surface. (Sicher and Tandler: Anatomie für Zahnärzte.)
Fig. 5-32. Buccolingual section through upper second premolar. (Sicher and Tandler: Anatomie für Zahnärzte.)

The average measurements of the first upper premolar are as follows:

Overall length of tooth	21.7 mm.
Greatest width of buccal surface of crown	6.8 mm.
Height of buccal surface	8.7 mm.
Height of lingual surface	7.5 mm.
Cervical mesiodistal diameter of crown	4.8-5.3 mm.
Cervical lingual diameter	8.5-9.3 mm.
Distance of tips of cusps	5.5 mm.

Upper second premolar (Figs. 5-31 and 5-32). The upper second premolar is, in most persons, somewhat smaller than the first. The crown pattern of the two upper premolars shows only small differences. The difference in the size of the two cusps in favor of the buccal one is less marked in the second premolar than in the first; this is caused by a decrease in volume of the buccal cusp in the second premolar. Seen from the occlusal surface, the crown of the second premolar is more symmetrically shaped than is that of its mesial neighbor. Collateral branches of the occlusal fissure are more frequent and better developed on the second than on the first premolar. Accessory cusps on the slope of the buccal cusp, especially on its distal slope, are therefore found in a greater percentage of second premolars.

Division of the root of the upper second premolar is rare; in about 85% of these teeth the root is simple but deeply grooved.

Although the pulp chamber of the second premolar duplicates that of the first (Fig. 5-32), the root canal of the second premolar is frequently an undivided space, wide buccolingually but narrow mesiodistally. Its mesial and distal walls often bulge prominently into its lumen, and fusion of these walls leads to a gradually progressing division of the single canal into a buccal and a lingual branch. The two canals may fuse at a variable distance from the apex of the root and may open in a single apical foramen.

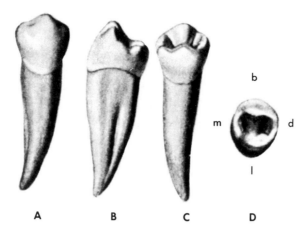

Fig. 5-33. Right lower first premolar. **A,** Buccal surface. **B,** Mesial surface. **C,** Lingual surface. **D,** Occlusal surface. (Sicher and Tandler: Anatomie für Zahnärzte.)

The average measurements of the upper second premolar are as follows:

Overall length of tooth	21.5 mm.
Greatest mesiodistal diameter of crown	6.5 mm.
Height of crown buccally	7.9 mm.
Height of crown lingually	7.5 mm.

Lower first premolar (Fig. 5-33). The most conspicuous difference between lower premolars and their upper antagonists is the more nearly circular perimeter of the occlusal surface of the lower teeth. There is also a more pronounced difference in the height of buccal and lingual cusps, which is especially striking in the lower first premolar.

The labial surface of the lower first premolar is so much inclined lingually that the tip of the buccal cusp lies almost above the center of the cervical cross section of the tooth. The lingual surface is slightly narrower and much lower than the labial surface because of the slight development of the lingual cusp. This may be reduced to not much more than a tubercle—thus it is not truly "bicuspid." The proximal surfaces are convex and are higher at their buccal margin than at the lingual border. The height of the convexity of the mesial surface is found farther buccally than that of the distal surface, which is a difference necessitated by the contact of the mesial surface of the first premolar with the canine.

Viewed from the occlusal surface, the circumference of the crown is almost circular but narrower on the mesial than on the distal side. The large, high buccal cusp may be separated from the small, considerably lower lingual cusp by a sharp mesiodistal fissure that ends at some distance from the mesial and distal borders of the occlusal surface at the marginal ridges. Often the cusps are united by a blunt enamel ridge, slightly saddled between the two cusps. In such teeth the occlusal fissure is broken up into a mesial and a distal pit. From the pits or from the deepened mesial and distal ends of the fissure, small sulci extend buccally and lingually. They may separate small mesial and distal accessory cusplets on the slopes of the main buccal and lingual cusps. The lingual groove, which arises from the mesial pit, often continues to the lingual surface of the tooth so that a mesial marginal ridge is separated from the larger part of the lingual surface. In such cases there is a striking similarity of the mesial half of the lower first premolar to the corresponding half of the lower canine. It is well to note that the mesial half of the crown of the lower first premolar occludes with the distal half of the upper canine.

The distolingual accessory cusp is variable in its size and may be almost as large and high, or just as large and high, as the lingual cusp itself. One can then describe this type of lower first premolar as tricuspid. The mesiolingual cusp, however, is clearly recognizable as the main lingual cusp because only this cusp is united with the buccal cusp by a slightly shifted buccolingual enamel ridge.

The cross section of the root is oval, but its mesiodistal diameter is often only slightly shorter than the buccolingual diameter. This fact is of importance because the extraction of this tooth is, in many individuals, possible by a rotating movement. The mesial and distal longitudinal grooves of the root are only rarely deepened to such an extent that the tip of the root is divided. If such a division is present, it reaches only occasionally to the cervical region of the tooth. Still rarer are examples of a division of the root into three roots, two of which are found buccally and one of which is found lingually.

The straight and simple root canal widens gradually into the pulp chamber. The buccolingual diameter of the latter is greater than its mesiodistal diameter. The coronal pulp is, as a rule, elongated only into one pulp horn, which corresponds to the buccal cusp. In a minority of teeth a small lingual diverticulum is found at the base of the lingual cusp.

The average measurements of the lower first premolar are as follows:

Overall length of tooth	18.5-27.0 mm.
Mesiodistal diameter of crown	6.0-8.0 mm.
Height of crown buccally	7.5-11.0 mm.
Height of crown lingually	5.0-5.8 mm.

Lower second premolar (Figs. 5-34 and 5-35). The crown of the lower second premolar is much larger than that of the first. It is characterized mainly by the greater development of the lingual cusp, although it never reaches the height of the buccal cusp. The shape and inclination of the buccal surface are similar to that of the first premolar, but the buccal cusp is blunter than that of its mesial neighbor. The lingual surface is slightly narrower and slightly lower than the buccal surface and is often asymmetrically shaped if the lingual cusp has shifted mesially.

The two cusps are separated from one another by a sharp fissure that only rarely is interrupted by a fusion of the enamel ridges on the opposing slopes of the two cusps. The deepened mesial and distal ends of the occlusal fissure send shallow branches buccally and lingually. Frequently the buccal grooves separate a mesial and a distal accessory cusp from the main buccal cusp. The lingual grooves are only rarely of equal depth, the mesial groove being, as a rule, shallow or even lacking. The distolingual groove, however, is almost always present and is often deep. Then a distolingual accessory cusp is formed, which, if it is well developed, causes a mesial shift of the lingual cusp. In a considerable percentage of persons the distolingual accessory cusp approximates or even reaches the size of the main lingual cusp, so that a *tricuspid* tooth develops. The buccal cusp in such teeth is placed opposite the groove separating the two lingual cusps.

The root of the lower second premolar is stronger than that of the first and, in cross section, still more nearly circular. Longitudinal grooves of the root are rarely well developed, and a division of the root is a great rarity.

The root canal (Fig. 5-35) is almost with exception simple, and the pulp chamber is

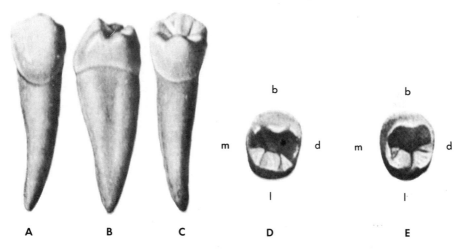

Fig. 5-34. Right lower second premolar. **A,** Buccal surface. **B,** Mesial surface. **C,** Lingual surface. **D,** Occlusal surface. **E,** Occlusal surface of three-cusped lower second premolar. (Sicher and Tandler: Anatomie für Zahnärzte.)

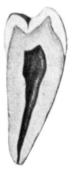

Fig. 5-35. Buccolingual section through lower second premolar. (Sicher and Tandler: Anatomie für Zahnärzte.)

spacious and only slightly narrowed in mesiodistal direction. The pulp chamber continues into two or three horns corresponding to the buccal and lingual cusps.

The average measurements of the lower second premolar are as follows:

Overall length of tooth	23.2 mm.
Greatest mesiodistal diameter of crown	7.3 mm.
Height of crown	8.5 mm.
Cervical mesiodistal diameter	5.5 mm.
Cervical buccolingual diameter	8.3 mm.

Upper first molar (Figs. 5-36 to 5-39). The occlusal surface of the upper first molar is diamond-shaped; the longer diagonal extends from the mesiobuccal to the distolingual corner; the shorter diagonal connects the distobuccal and mesiolingual corners. The four cusps of this tooth are separated from each other by an irregularly H-shaped arrangement of grooves. One of these grooves commences at about the midpoint of the buccal border of the occlusal surface between the two buccal cusps. It continues for a variable distance on the buccal surface of the crown. If one follows this fissure lingually, it gains in depth and ends in a pit near the center of the occlusal surface. From here it continued almost at a right angle by a second fissure that runs mesially but does not reach the mesial border of the occlusal surface. Behind the mesial border the fissure widens into a shallow mesial groove that is bordered by the low mesial marginal ridge connecting the two mesial cusps.

At about the center of the lingual surface of the crown another groove can be observed that reaches in an occlusal and slightly distal direction to the lingual border of the occlusal surface and then separates the larger mesiolingual from the slightly small distolingual cusp. On the occlusal surface this fissure curves buccodistally, to end mesial to the distal marginal ridge in a shallow groove. The convexity of the linguodistal fissure is connected with the angle at which the buccal and mesial fissures meet by an oblique groove that thus completes a crossbar of the letter H. The oblique furrow is always shallower than the other fissures and is often interrupted by a strong ridge that connects the distobuccal with the mesiolingual cusp.

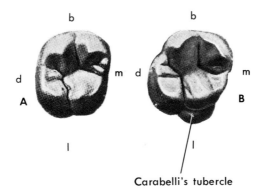

Fig. 5-36. Occlusal surface of two right upper first molars. **A,** Four-cusped type. **B,** With Carabelli's tubercle. (Sicher and Tandler: Anatomie für Zahnärzte.)

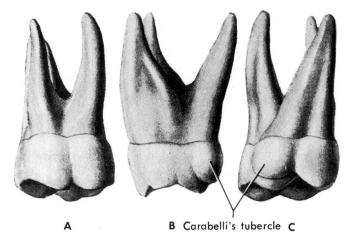

A   B Carabelli's tubercle C

Fig. 5-37. Right upper first molar. **A,** Buccal surface. **B,** Mesial surface. **C,** Lingual surface. (Sicher and Tandler: Anatomie für Zahnärzte.)

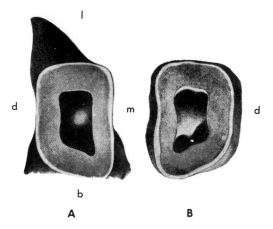

Fig. 5-38. Upper first molar bisected at cervical plane. **A,** Floor of pulpal chamber. **B,** Roof of pulpal chamber. (Sicher and Tandler: Anatomie für Zahnärzte.)

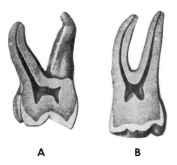

Fig. 5-39. Buccolingual sections through upper first molar. **A,** In plane of mesiobuccal root. **B,** In plane of distobuccal and lingual roots. (Sicher and Tandler: Anatomie für Zahnärzte.)

The two buccal cusps are almost equal in circumference and height, but the mesial cusp is sometimes slightly larger than the distal one. Of the two lingual cusps the mesial is not only considerably larger than the distal, but it is the largest cusp of the tooth. This cusp is connected with the distobuccal cusp by a bulky, oblique, slightly saddled enamel ridge. The two mesial cusps and the two distal cusps are connected by the marginal ridges. The mesial ridge is always wider and higher than the distal ridge and is often subdivided into two or three small marginal cusplets.

The buccal surface of the upper first molar is, on the whole, convex, its occlusal half divided by the continuation of the fissure between the two buccal cusps. The convex lingual surface decreases in height distally, corresponding to the smaller size of the distolingual cusp. The groove that reaches the lingual surface as a continuation of the fissure between the two lingual cusps is directed cervically and mesially, sometimes traverses the entire height of the lingual surface, and may even continue into the lingual groove of the lingual root.

An accessory cusp may develop on the mesial half of the lingual surface, which is known as Carabelli's tubercle (Fig. 5-36, *B*). If this accessory cusp is well developed, it is separated from the mesiolingual cusp by a curved groove that starts at the middle of the lingual surface and ends where the mesial and lingual surfaces meet. Carabelli's tubercle, or cusp, is sometimes so large that the upper first molar seems to possess five cusps; Carabelli's tubercle, however, never reaches the occlusal plane. A well-developed Carabelli's tubercle is found in from 10% to 15% of all upper first molars. From the stage of full development, transitional stages lead to the final disappearance of the accessory cusp. A small pit, the remnant of the groove between Carabelli's cusp and the base of the mesiolingual cusp, is the last evidence of this accessory element of the upper first molar. Such pits on the mesial half of the lingual surface are found in about 40% of all upper first molars.

The proximal surfaces on most molars are convex; the distal surfaces are usually more strongly convex than the mesial. The cervical part of the latter may be flat or even concave. The greatest convexities of the proximal surfaces, that is, the contact points, are always close to the occlusal third of the tooth and about midway between the buccal and lingual corners.

The three roots of the upper first molar, two buccal roots and one lingual root, arise from a common root stock, or base, and diverge considerably. The root stock itself differs in its cross section from the rhomboid cross section of the crown. It is more nearly triangular because of a reduction in volume at the corner that corresponds to the mesiolingual cusp of the crown. This part of the crown, therefore, forms a pronounced overhang. The difference of the cross sections of crown and root stock is caused by the fact that the lingual root is not placed opposite to the bifurcation of the two buccal roots but is shifted distally. It is almost in the same frontal plane as the distobuccal root. The lingual root is always the strongest of the three and often also the longest. It is almost circular in cross section, only slightly compressed in buccolingual direction. The lingual surface of the lingual root is often grooved, especially in its cervical two thirds. In most teeth the lingual root diverges from the axis of the crown more than do the buccal roots.

The mesiobuccal root is wider in the buccolingual direction than is the distobuccal root and in cross section is oval, the longer diameter of the oval being placed buccolingually. In other words, the mesiobuccal root is considerably compressed in the mesiodistal direction. The distobuccal root is more rounded, although a mesiodistal compression is also apparent. The buccal roots diverge only slightly from the axis of the tooth buccally, but often considerably from each other. The tips of the buccal roots, however, sometimes are curved toward each other. A reduction in number of the roots of the upper first molar is fairly rare. In such teeth the two buccal roots may be fused for a variable distance, or a fusion may occur between the lingual and the distobuccal roots.

The pulp chamber of the upper first molar (Figs. 5-38 and 5-39) is partly contained in the common root stock, partly in the crown itself. From its spacious central part four horns extend into the base of each of the four cusps of the tooth. Generally speaking, the pulp chamber can be compared with a slightly irregular cube except that the walls bulge convexly into the space. The strongest convexities are at the floor and roof of the chamber.* Corresponding to the change in the cross section of the root stock, the shape of the floor of the pulp chamber differs slightly from that of the roof. The lingual border of the floor is considerably shorter than its buccal border and is also shifted distally. The points of entrance into the root canals are arranged in such a way that the widest canal is found in the rounded lingual corner of the floor, whereas its two buccal corners mark the entrance into the more rounded distobuccal and into the slit-shaped mesiobuccal canal. In about half of all the examined teeth the mesiobuccal canal is, for a variable length and sometimes entirely, divided into a buccal and a lingual branch.

The average measurements of the upper first molar are as follows:

Overall length of tooth	21.3 mm.
Greatest mesiodistal diameter of crown	10.1 mm.
Greatest buccolingual diameter	11.7 mm.
Height of buccal surface	7.7 mm.

Upper second molar (Figs. 5-40 and 5-41). The crown of the upper second molar may duplicate that of the first, but it shows a great number of variations. The upper second molar may be described as presenting three typical patterns that, however, are linked by transitional forms. As was mentioned, the first type duplicates the pattern of the first molar of the upper jaw, but the distolingual cusp shows, as a rule, a more pronounced reduction in size than that of the first molar. The reduction leads finally to the complete disappearance of this cusp and the resulting second type of the upper second molar is thus tricuspid. The single lingual cusp is shifted distally and placed opposite the notch that separates the two buccal cusps. The system of fissures on the occlusal surface of this tooth almost resembles a T. One of the fissures begins on the buccal surface near its occlusal border. Cutting across the buccal border of the occlusal surface this fissure separates the two buccal cusps. Toward the center of the

---

*It is convenient to call the occlusal wall of the pulp chamber the roof and to call the opposite wall the floor, regardless of the position of the tooth in the upper or lower jaw.

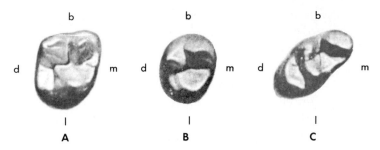

Fig. 5-40. Three types of crown of upper second (right) molar **A,** Four-cusped type. **B,** Three-cusped reduction type. **C,** Three-cusped compression type. (Sicher and Tandler: Anatomie für Zahnärzte.)

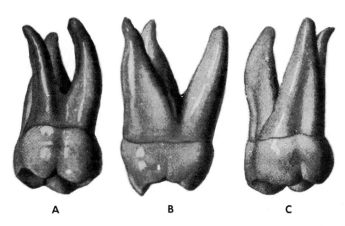

Fig. 5-41. Upper right second molar. **A,** Buccal surface. **B,** Mesial surface. **C,** Lingual surface. (Sicher and Tandler: Anatomie für Zahnärzte.)

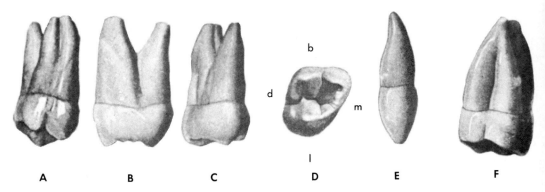

Fig. 5-42. Right upper third molars. **A,** Buccal surface. **B,** Mesial surface. **C,** Lingual surface. **D,** Occlusal surface. **E,** Peg-shaped tooth. **F,** Fusion of the three roots. **A, B, C,** and **D** are from same tooth of an 18-year-old man; root tips were not fully developed. (Sicher and Tandler: Anatomie für Zahnärzte.)

occlusal surface it deepens and ends in the central fovea. From this point two other fissures reach mesially and distally, separating the two buccal cusps from the large lingual cusp. These two fissures are almost in a straight mesiodistal line. They extend toward the mesial and distal borders of the occlusal surface but remain separated from the borders by marginal ridges.

The third type of upper molar looks as if it had been formed from the first four-cusped type by a compression of the crown in the direction of the short diagonal, which connects the mesiolingual and distobuccal corners. The crown assumes in occlusal view the shape of a long oval, the long diameter of which runs in mesiobuccal-distolingual direction. The distobuccal and the mesiolingual cusps approach each other and finally fuse. The fusion is initiated by a heightening of the oblique ridge that connects the mesiolingual and distobuccal cusps. An upper second molar of the pure third type is, therefore, also tricuspid. The three cusps however do not correspond to those of the other tricuspid type in which the distolingual cusp is lost. In a molar of the third type the three cusps are lined up in a straight line with the mesiobuccal cusp followed by the middle cusp, which is derived from a fusion of the distobuccal with the mesiolingual cusp. The middle cusp is then followed by the well-developed dis-tolingual cusp.

The third type of upper second molar is the rarest and is found in about 5% to 10% of the examined teeth. The most frequent type is the second type, which develops by reduction of the distolingual cusp. This type is found in 50% to 55%. The second molar may show a Carabelli's tubercle, but its presence is rare.

The roots of the upper second molar may also duplicate those of the first. However, the divergence of the roots is usually not as pronounced as on the first molar. Fusion between two roots is also more frequent in the second than in the first molar. It is interesting that in the second molar the fusion most frequently occurs between the lingual and mesiobuccal roots, in contrast to the first molar, where a fusion between the lingual and distobuccal roots seems to be the rule. The distal shift of the lingual root into the plane of the distobuccal root is still more pronounced in the second molar than in the first.

In an upper second molar of the first type, the pulp chamber and root canals show the same details as were described for the first molar. However, a division of the mesiobuccal canal is an exception. In teeth of the second or third type the pulp chamber conforms to the changed shape of the crown.

The average measurements of the upper second molar are as follows:

Overall length of tooth	21.2 mm.
Mesiodistal diameter of crown	9.8 mm.
Buccolingual diameter	11.5 mm.
Height of crown	7.7 mm.

Upper third molar (Fig. 5-42). The upper third molar, or upper wisdom tooth, is the most variable tooth of the human dentition. The most common type resembles the tricuspid crown of a second molar. The third molar may also duplicate the four-

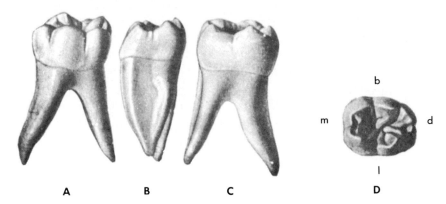

Fig. 5-43. Right lower first molar. **A,** Buccal surface. **B,** Mesial surface. **C,** Lingual surface. **D,** Occlusal surface. (Sicher and Tandler: Anatomie für Zahnärzte.)

cusped type or the compression type of its mesial neighbor. In addition, a further reduction of the crown may lead through many transitional forms to a peg-shaped tooth with a small cone-shaped crown. On the other hand, complications in the pattern of the crown of the upper third molar are fairly frequent and lead to the formation of one or more accessory cusps. No definite rule can be given for the site and size of such accessory cusps.

The upper third molar may possess three roots; more often, however, a fusion of roots can be observed. The first indication of a fusion is a heightening of the common root stock. Other teeth show a complete fusion of two or all three roots. Peg-shaped teeth have, as a rule, a simple and cone-shaped root. Irregular curvature of one or more of these roots is also frequent. Just as the crown and roots vary in an almost unpredictable way, nothing specific can be said about the many variations of the size and shape of the pulp chamber or of the number and position of root canals.

Lower first molar (Figs. 5-43 and 5-44). The lower first molar is, in the great majority of examined teeth, characterized by the presence of five cusps, three of which occupy the buccal and two the lingual moiety of the tooth. The five-cusped pattern is reduced to a four-cusped pattern in only 5% to 6%. The arrangement of the four main cusps of the tooth varies. Two typical patterns can be distinguished. In one type the mesiobuccal and the mesiolingual cusps are of about the same length in mesiodistal direction, although the lingual cusp is stronger and higher than its buccal counterpart. In the second type the mesiodistal length of the mesiolingual cusp is greater than that of the mesiobuccal cusp (Fig. 5-43, *D*).

The pattern of the grooves separating the cusps from one another varies with the relative size of the cusps. In the first type a sharp groove begins on the buccal surface of the tooth, separates the mesiobuccal cusp from its distal neighbor, and, deepening, runs in a lingual direction to about the center of the crown. From there it continues, separating the two lingual cusps, toward the lingual border of the occlusal surface, across which it can be followed for some distance on the lingual surface of the crown.

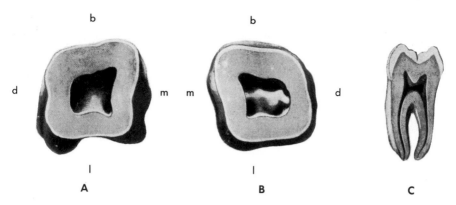

Fig. 5-44. Sections through lower first molar. **A,** Floor of pulpal chamber. **B,** Roof of pulpal chamber. **C,** Mesiodistal section. (Sicher and Tandler: Anatomie für Zahnärzte.)

From the anterior fossa of the occlusal surface behind the mesial marginal ridge begins the mesiodistal fissure separating the two mesial cusps. It crosses the central fovea, the deepest point of the buccolingual groove, and continues distally to split into two branches in the shape of an irregular Y. One branch continues almost straight distally, only slightly deviating lingually; it ends in front of the distal marginal ridge, slightly widening to form the distal fovea. The second branch of the mesiodistal fissure turns buccodistally, reaches the buccal border of the occlusal surface distal to the distobuccal cusp, and continues on the buccal surface just in front of the line angle between the buccal and distal surfaces. The two arms of the Y-shaped sulcus enclose the small fifth cusp of the lower first molar, which occupies the most distal part of the buccal half of the tooth. Since it projects farthest distally, it is commonly referred to as the distal cusp.

The second type of crown pattern of the lower first molar is characterized by a distal shift of the lingual half of the buccolingual fissure (Fig. 5-43, *D*). In such teeth the fissure separating the mesiobuccal from the mesiodistal cusp does not continue to the lingual border across the mesiodistal fissure. Instead it ends at the mesiodistal fissure, and the lingual half of the buccolingual furrow arises from the mesiodistal fissure at a point distal to its junction with the buccal arm of the transverse fissure.

The second pattern, in which the mesiolingual cusp is in all its dimensions larger than the other cusps, seems to be the more primitive pattern and is often referred to as a dryopithecus pattern. This term is derived from the genus *Dryopithecus,* an extinct anthropoid ape, which in all probability was related to the common ancestor of man and the living great apes.

The buccal surface of the lower first molar is longer than it is high and continues without a sharp boundary into the strongly convex distal surface. This relation is caused by the presence of the distal cusp. It has been mentioned that the two fissures that separate the three buccal cusps from each other continue as grooves over the occlusal half of the buccal surface. The mesial groove, always deeper and longer, may end in a small blind pit, the foramen cecum, which often is a site of a carious lesion. At the cervical line the enamel is sometimes elongated into a pointed tonguelike extension, reaching toward the bifurcation of the roots. The occlusal half of the buccal surface is strongly inclined lingually.

The lingual surface of the crown is evenly convex and its occlusal part is only slightly grooved by a continuation of the fissure that separates the two lingual cusps. Of the two proximal surfaces, the distal one is always more strongly convex than the mesial, a difference which is also caused by the presence of the distal cusp.

If the distal cusp is missing, the crown of the first molar assumes an almost cubic shape with the four cusps symmetrically arranged and separated by a cross-shaped system of grooves. In all types of the lower second molar the lingual cusps are higher than the buccal cusps.

The two roots of the first molar, arising from a common root stock, are arranged in mesiodistal order. Both the mesial and distal roots are strongly compressed in mesiodistal direction. The compression usually is more pronounced in the mesial root. Both roots may show a distal curvature, which, in the mesial root, is often so strong that its apex tends to approach the apex of the distal root. The distal root, in buccolingual direction narrower and in mesiodistal direction thicker than the mesial root, is often slightly shorter and in most teeth fairly straight. Both roots carry longitudinal grooves that are deeper on the mesial root than on the distal root. The groove on the distal surface of the distal root is, in turn, shallower than that on its mesial surface.

The pulp chamber (Fig. 5-44) corresponds in its general shape to that of the crown. Depending on the number of the cusps, its roof is raised into five horns, or more rarely into four, which reach into the base of the cusps. The root canals begin at the mesial and distal borders of the pulpal floor. The distal root contains a single wide canal; the mesial root contains two narrow canals that develop from the longitudinal partition of a simple slitlike canal. The partition begins to form at about the fourteenth year of life.

The average measurements of the lower first molar are as follows:

Overall length of tooth along mesial root	22.8 mm.
Greatest mesiodistal diameter of crown	11.5 mm.
Buccolingual diameter	10.4 mm.
Height of crown	8.3 mm.

Lower second molar (Fig. 5-45). The lower second molar typically carries four cusps. The occlusal surface is almost square. The four cusps, of which the lingual two are higher, are symmetrically arranged. A groove beginning on the buccal surface of the crown, traversing the occlusal surface in a buccolingual direction, and continuing for a short distance onto the lingual surface divides the tooth into a mesial and a distal half. A second, mesiodistal, groove starts behind the mesial marginal ridge in a shallow fossa and ends in a similar depression in front of the distal marginal ridge. This

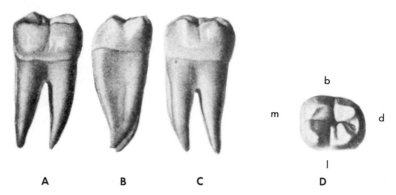

Fig. 5-45. Lower right second molar. **A,** Buccal surface. **B,** Mesial surface. **C,** Lingual surface. **D,** Occlusal surface. (Sicher and Tandler: Anatomie für Zahnärzte.)

groove separates the buccal from the lingual cusps. The buccolingual groove ends on the buccal surface frequently with a blind pit, the foramen caecum. The point where the mesiodistal and buccolingual fissures meet is the deep central pit. Nothing about the other surfaces of this tooth deserves special mention.

Roots and pulpal spaces resemble those of the first molar. The roots of the second molar are generally shorter and weaker than those of the first and not too rarely partially fused. It is also noteworthy that in about a third of the teeth the canal of the mesial root remains undivided. It shows in such teeth a dumbbell-shaped cross section. If the mesial canal is divided, the two branches often join close to the apex of the root to open in a single apical foramen.

The average measurements of the lower second molar are as follows:

Overall length of tooth at mesial root	22.8 mm.
Mesiodistal diameter of crown	10.7 mm.
Buccolingual diameter	9.8 mm.
Height of crown	8.1 mm.

Lower third molar (Fig. 5-46). The lower third molar, or lower wisdom tooth, is a variable element of the human dentition, but the range of variation is not so wide as that of the upper third molar. In particular its variations in size are restricted and it seems to follow more nearly an all-or-none proposition, the tooth being either fairly well developed or entirely missing. Half of the number of lower wisdom teeth are characterized by the presence of four cusps. About 40% show five cusps, and the remaining 10% are either tricuspid or show a higher number of sometimes irregularly arranged cusps. The lower wisdom tooth is in most persons the smallest of the lower three molars; sometimes, however, it is smaller than the first but larger than the second molar. Normally its mesiodistal diameter is longer than that of the upper third molar. By this distal elongation of the lower arch a locking of the occlusion at the distal end of the dental arches is achieved.

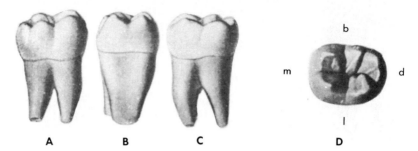

Fig. 5-46. Lower right third molar, root tips not fully developed. **A,** Buccal surface. **B,** Mesial surface. **C,** Lingual surface. **D,** Occlusal surface. (Sicher and Tandler: Anatomie für Zahnärzte.)

The crown of the lower wisdom tooth may resemble either the first or the second molar, but it shows irregularities in many cases, especially in the size of the different cusps. Its roots may be similar to those of the second molar, but fusion is frequent. It leads sometimes to the formation of a simple cone-shaped root. In such teeth the root canal may be wide and funnel-shaped. Most lower third molars have only two root canals, a mesial and a distal.

Special description of deciduous teeth

Deciduous incisors. The deciduous incisors closely resemble their permanent successors. However, they are not only smaller than the teeth of the permanent dentition, but they also appear to be plumper, their transverse diameters being accentuated in comparison with their longitudinal measurements.

Upper first (central) deciduous incisor (Fig. 5-47). The upper central deciduous incisor shows clearly the difference of the mesial and distal angles at the incisal edge, the mesial corner being sharp and almost a right angle, whereas the distoincisal corner is well rounded. The labial surface, almost always uniformly convex, bulges prominently near its cervical border. Thus the indication of a labial cingulum develops, a formation that is characteristic for all deciduous teeth, although its development is variable. The lingual surface shows fewer variations than the corresponding surface of the permanent tooth. This greater constancy in shape is characteristic of all the elements of the deciduous dentition. The lingual tubercle is almost always well developed, occupying a rather large area of the lingual surface. It continues along the proximal borders toward the incisal edge in the shape of rather low and often indistinct marginal ridges. The central part of the lingual surface is simply concave.

The root of the upper central deciduous incisor is slightly compressed in labiolingual direction. The axis of the root forms an angle with the axis of the crown that opens distally. This causes a divergence of the roots of the right and left teeth, which is often pronounced. In addition, the root and crown are bent against each other in the labiolingual plane with the angle opening labially, as if to give more space to the crown of the permanent incisor, which lies lingual to the root of the deciduous tooth.

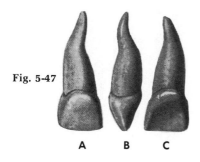

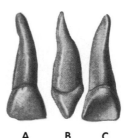

Fig. 5-47

Fig. 5-48

A B C

A B C

Fig. 5-47. Upper right first deciduous incisor. **A,** Labial surface. **B,** Mesial surface. **C,** Lingual surface. (Sicher and Tandler: Anatomie für Zahnärzte.)
Fig. 5-48. Upper right second deciduous incisor. **A,** Labial surface. **B,** Mesial surface. **C,** Lingual surface. (Sicher and Tandler: Anatomie für Zahnärzte.)

As in all other deciduous teeth, the pulp cavities are relatively wide but their shape closely corresponds to that of the permanent incisor.

The average measurements of the upper central incisor are as follows:

Overall length of tooth	17.0-19.0 mm.
Mesiodistal diameter of crown	6.0-7.15 mm.
Height of crown	6.0-7.3 mm.

Upper second (lateral) deciduous incisor (Fig. 5-48). The upper lateral incisor duplicates the shape of its mesial neighbor much more closely in the deciduous dentition than in the permanent dentition. Again it has to be stressed that variations of the crown in general and especially of its lingual surface are relatively rare, though they are frequent in the upper second incisor of the permanent arch.

The average measurements of the upper lateral incisor are as follows:

Overall length of tooth	14.5-17.0 mm.
Mesiodistal diameter of crown	4.2-6.6 mm.
Height of crown	5.5-6.8 mm.

Lower first (central) and second (lateral) deciduous incisors (Figs. 5-49 and 5-50). The lower central and lateral deciduous incisors differ mainly in size, the lateral being larger than the central. The difference in size of the two teeth is, in most persons, more pronounced in the deciduous than in the permanent dentition. The lower lateral deciduous incisor often shows a well-rounded distoincisal corner and thus sometimes is similar to the corresponding tooth in the upper jaw. Compared with the permanent teeth, the roots of the deciduous mandibular incisors are far less flattened in the mesiodistal direction so that their cross section approaches a more nearly circular form.

The average measurements of the lower central incisor are as follows:

Overall length of tooth	15.0-19.0 mm.
Mesiodistal diameter of crown	3.6-5.5 mm.
Height of crown	5.0-6.6 mm.

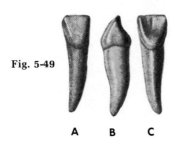
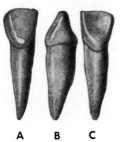

Fig. 5-49

Fig. 5-50

A   B   C   **A   B   C**

Fig. 5-49. Lower right first deciduous incisor. **A,** Labial surface. **B,** Mesial surface. **C,** Lingual surface. (Sicher and Tandler: Anatomie für Zahnärzte.)

Fig. 5-50. Lower right second deciduous incisor. **A,** Labial surface. **B,** Mesial surface. **C,** Lingual surface. (Sicher and Tandler: Anatomie für Zahnärzte.)

The average measurements of the lower lateral incisor are as follows:

Overall length of tooth	15.0-19.0 mm.
Mesiodistal diameter of crown	3.8-5.9 mm.
Height of crown	5.6-7.0 mm.

Deciduous canines (Figs. 5-51 and 5-52). The deciduous canines also show the exaggeration of their mesiodistal measurements. The crown of the deciduous upper canine (Fig. 5-51) is, in contrast to that of its permanent successor, often fairly symmetrical. If an asymmetry is pronounced, then it is a reversal of that of the permanent canine. In the deciduous tooth, not the distal but the mesial contact point is shifted cervically.

The labial surface is strongly convex, the convexity being strongest at the cervical border. A longitudinal ridge almost always connects the labial cingulum with the tip of the crown; the ridge is flanked mesially and distally by shallow grooves. The tubercle on the lingual surface is, as a rule, well developed. The occlusal part of the lingual surface is often divided into a mesial and a distal half by a longitudinal ridge that is terminated by the dental tubercle. The root of the upper deciduous canine is approximately triangular in cross section. The labial, the mesiolingual, and the distolingual surfaces are separated by well-rounded edges.

The lower deciduous canine (Fig. 5-52) is, as a whole, narrower and therefore appears to be more slender than its antagonist. Furthermore, the concavity of the lingual surface is but rarely interrupted by a longitudinal ridge.

The average measurements of the upper deciduous canine are as follows:

Overall length of tooth	17.5-22.0 mm.
Mesiodistal diameter of crown	6.2-8.0 mm.
Height of crown	6.5-7.8 mm.

The average measurements of the lower deciduous canine are as follows:

Overall length of tooth	17.5-22.0 mm.
Mesiodistal diameter of crown	5.2-7.0 mm.
Height of crown	6.5-8.1 mm.

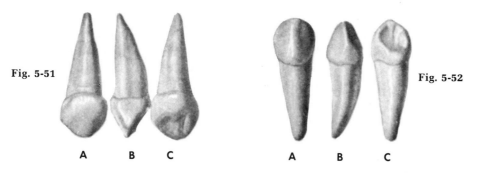

Fig. 5-51

Fig. 5-52

A   B   C   A   B   C

Fig. 5-51. Upper right deciduous canine. **A,** Labial surface. **B,** Mesial surface. **C,** Lingual surface. (Sicher and Tandler: Anatomie für Zahnärzte.)
Fig. 5-52. Lower right deciduous canine. **A,** Labial surface. **B,** Mesial surface. **C,** Lingual surface. (Sicher and Tandler: Anatomie für Zahnärzte.)

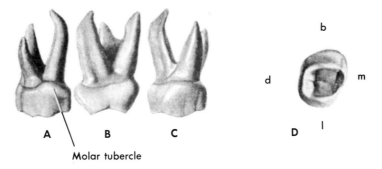

b

d   m

A   B   C   D   l

Molar tubercle

Fig. 5-53. Upper right first deciduous molar. **A,** Buccal surface. **B,** Mesial surface. **C,** Lingual surface. **D,** Occlusal surface. (Sicher and Tandler: Anatomie für Zahnärzte.)

Upper first deciduous molar (Fig. 5-53). The first deciduous molars in both upper and lower jaws are built according to a special pattern that cannot easily be compared with that of any other tooth in the deciduous or permanent dentition.

The occlusal surface of the upper first deciduous molar is irregularly quadrilateral. The distal border runs in a straight buccolingual direction and therefore joins the buccal and lingual borders at right angles. The mesial border, however, is oblique in a mesiobuccal to distolingual direction. This is caused by the relative shortness of the lingual border and the relative narrowness of the lingual surface of the crown.

The occlusal surface is divided into a buccal and a lingual part by a deep mesiodistal groove. This groove does not extend to the mesial or distal borders, which are elevated by marginal ridges. The lingual half of the crown is heightened into a cone-shaped cusp. The buccal half of the crown can be described as a long cutting crest, compressed in buccolingual direction. The middle part of the crest is more or less clearly pointed. Sometimes the highest elevation of the buccal crest is flanked at the distal end, and more rarely on the mesial end, by a small secondary cusplet.

The buccal surface of the upper first deciduous molar is wider in its mesial than in its distal part because the enamel in the mesial part of the tooth reaches farther toward the root than distally. A buccal cingulum is rarely absent. This cervical ridge is especially accentuated in the mesial half of the tooth and is here sometimes developed to a hemispheric tubercle, the molar tubercle of Zuckerkandl. A cingulum is also present at the cervical border of the lingual surface.

The upper first deciduous molar has three roots that are in a position similar to that found in the permanent molars of the upper jaw. Their shape is comparable to that of the roots of the permanent molars: the mesiobuccal root is wide in the buccolingual direction and compressed in the mesiodistal direction; the distobuccal root is often the shortest root of this tooth, and in cross section it is more nearly circular but still somewhat flattened in the mesiodistal direction. The largest and longest root is the lingual root with an almost circular cross section. It is placed in the frontal plane of the distobuccal root. As a rule the divergence of the three roots is conspicuous in adaptation to the interradicular position of the germ of the first permanent premolar. The lingual and distobuccal roots are sometimes found fused.

The average measurements for the upper first deciduous molar are as follows:

Overall length of tooth	14.0-17.0 mm.
Mesiodistal diameter of crown	6.6-9.8 mm.
Height of crown	5.8-6.5 mm.

Lower first deciduous molar (Fig. 5-54). The occlusal surface of the lower first deciduous molar is oval with a longer mesiodistal diameter. The buccal half of the crown is elevated into two buccolingually compressed cusps, which are often separated from one another by only a shallow notch. The mesial cusp is always larger than the distal one. The two buccal cusps are separated from the lingual part of the crown by a zigzagging mesiodistal groove that ends at the mesial and distal marginal ridges. The lingual half of the tooth is narrower than the buccal half and carries, in most teeth, two approximately cone-shaped cusps, which are well separated from each other; the distolingual cusp is always smaller than the mesiolingual cusp and sometimes is reduced to an insignificant prominence. An enamel ridge frequently connects

Molar tubercle

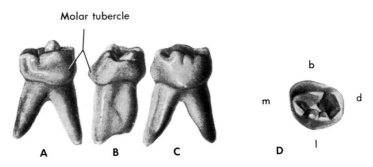

Fig. 5-54. Lower right first deciduous molar. **A,** Buccal surface. **B,** Mesial surface. **C,** Lingual surface. **D,** Occlusal surface. (Sicher and Tandler: Anatomie für Zahnärzte.)

the mesiobuccal with the mesiolingual cusp, interrupting the mesiodistal central fissure in the mesial half of the tooth. The fissure then is divided into a small fovea between the mesial marginal ridge and the transverse, or buccolingual, crest and a wider fovea between this crest and the distal marginal ridge.

The labial surface of the tooth is steeply inclined lingually, which accounts for the relative narrowness of the occlusal surface in the buccolingual direction. The buccal cingulum is well developed also on the lower first deciduous molar, and here, too, a molar tubercle may be present in the mesiocervical part of the labial surface.

The two roots of this tooth, the mesial and distal roots, are flat in mesiodistal direction, especially the mesial root. The two roots diverge strongly to make room for the germ of the lower first permanent premolar. The apical parts of the root are sometimes bent toward each other and may partly embrace the crown of the developing successor. In such a case, if the extraction of the deciduous molar is attempted while its roots still have their full length, the germ of the permanent premolar may be removed with the deciduous molar.

The average measurements for the lower first deciduous molar are as follows:

Overall length of tooth	14.0-17.0 mm.
Mesiodistal diameter of crown	7.5-8.5 mm.
Height of crown	6.6-7.0 mm.

Upper second deciduous molar (Fig. 5-55). The crown of the upper second deciduous molar is smaller than that of the first permanent molar, but otherwise it is almost an exact duplicate in all details, even the smallest. The only exception is the slightly stronger prominence of the buccal surface in its cervical part. The buccal cingulum, however, never develops a molar tubercle as in the first deciduous molar. A Carabelli's tubercle may also be found on the mesial half of the lingual surface; in fact, it is more frequent in this tooth than in the first permanent molar. In rare cases the distolingual cusp may be slightly reduced and only in exceptional cases is this element missing.

The roots of this tooth also resemble closely those of the first permanent molar, but their divergence is, as a rule, more pronounced. This is related to the fact that the

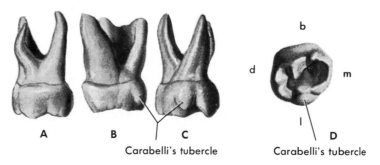

Fig. 5-55. Upper right second deciduous molar. **A,** Buccal surface. **B,** Mesial surface. **C,** Lingual surface. **D,** Occlusal surface. (Sicher and Tandler: Anatomie für Zahnärzte.)

second permanent premolar develops between the roots of its predecessor. Sometimes lingual and distobuccal roots are fused.

The average measurements of the upper second deciduous molar are as follows:

Overall length of tooth	17.5-19.5 mm.
Mesiodistal diameter of crown	8.3-9.3 mm.
Buccolingual diameter of crown	9.0-10.2 mm.
Height of crown	6.0-6.7 mm.

Lower second deciduous molar (Fig. 5-56). The lower second deciduous molar is a slightly reduced replica of the first permanent molar. The only significant differences between these two teeth are the greater prominence of a buccal cingulum and a stronger convexity of the proximal surfaces, which cause a conspicuous constriction of the cervical part of the deciduous tooth. The roots are always strongly divergent in their cervical half; however, their apices sometimes converge. In this point the roots of the second resemble those of the lower first deciduous molar, and the consequences as to a possible accidental removal of a lower second premolar have to be stressed again. The mesial root often shows an indication of a division into a buccal and a lingual part.

The average measurements of the lower second deciduous molar are as follows:

Overall length of tooth	17.5-19.5 mm.
Mesiodistal diameter of crown	10.0-11.5 mm.
Buccolingual diameter of crown	8.5-9.2 mm.
Height of crown	6.5-7.2 mm.

Age changes and anomalies of the pulpal spaces

The pulp chamber as well as the root canals are wide in young teeth. Since dentin formation continues, though at a diminishing rate, throughout the life of a tooth, the pulpal spaces gradually narrow. The restriction of these spaces does not occur, however, at an even rate on all surfaces, a fact that is especially pronounced in the molars. Here, the pulp chamber narrows concentrically for some time; later dentin apposition on the mesial, buccal, distal, and lingual walls slows down, while on the floor and on the roof of the pulp chamber dentin is formed in great volume. Thus in later years the height of the pulpal chamber decreases faster than its width. The dentin apposition is greatest at the roof, or occlusal wall, of the chamber. This can be explained as an adaptation to the progressive attrition of the teeth: the occlusal wall of the pulpal chamber is maintained at a certain safe thickness. However, the irregularity of attrition in the human dentition accounts for many variations in the progressive narrowing of the pulpal spaces. To present a clinically useful diagram of the apposition of dentin correlated to age or to the amount of attrition is therefore impossible. Only individual radiographs can reveal the individual variations.

Abnormalities of the pulp chamber are frequent. The most frequent anomalies are the accessory root canals (Figs. 5-57 and 5-58). These abnormal connections of the

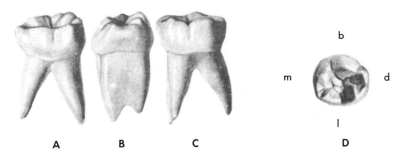

Fig. 5-56. Lower right second deciduous molar. **A,** Buccal surface. **B,** Mesial surface. **C,** Lingual surface. **D,** Occlusal surface. (Sicher and Tandler: Anatomie für Zahnärzte.)

pulp chamber or the root canal with the surface of the tooth, and thus connections of the pulp with the periodontal tissue in the living, can be divided into three types.

Some roots primarily contain one slit-shaped canal. Later this canal is divided into two canals by fusion of the protruding walls, as in the mesial root of lower molars and in some single-rooted upper first and, less frequently, upper second premolars. In such roots transverse, or horizontal, canals may persist and may connect the two regular canals at any level. Accessory canals of this type have little practical significance. They may owe their development to the presence of transverse blood vessels or nerves in the primary wide pulp canal.

Accessory pulp canals of the second type are limited to the apical end of the root and are characterized by the fact that they are bounded and divided from each other by cementum only (Fig. 5-57, A). These canals cause the presence of accessory apical foramina. Their development is caused by irregularities in the apposition of cementum at the root tip. Apposition of cementum in this area is always considerably greater than on the circumference of the root, a fact that is correlated to the continual eruption of the teeth. If cementum is formed at a higher rate of speed, periapical branches of the pulpal artery, vein, or nerve may be surrounded separately by the cementum. Formation of such accessory canals is normal in some animals, for instance, the dog.

Accessory root canals of the third type (Figs. 5-57, B and C, and 5-58), sometimes referred to as lateral canals or, unfortunately, as pulpoperiodontal fistulas, are characterized by the fact that these canals perforate the dentin and cementum of the root. They can develop at any level and on any surface of the root. If they are found in the furcation of two- or three-rooted teeth, they start at the pulpal floor and open between the roots. It has been incorrectly maintained that lateral canals are found only on root surfaces that face the furcation.

The accessory canals of the third type can be considered as developmental defects of the root. The shape of the root is molded by the proliferating epithelium of the enamel organ, the epithelial root sheath of Hertwig. The cells of the primary pulp are induced to differentiate into odontoblasts where they come into contact with the inner layer of the epithelial sheath. Where the continuity of the root sheath is inter-

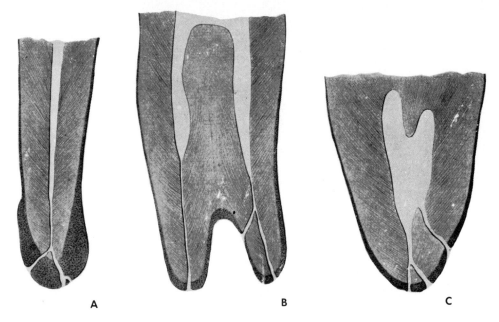

Fig. 5-57. Semidiagrammatic drawings of different types of accessory root canals. **A**, Lower premolar. **B** and **C**, Upper premolars. (Sicher and Tandler: Anatomie für Zahnärzte.)

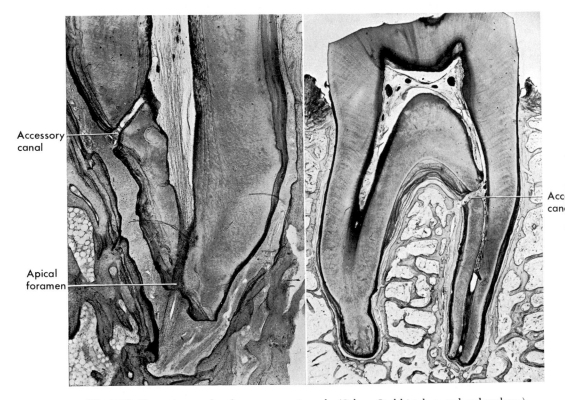

Accessory
canal

Apical
foramen

Acc
can

Fig. 5-58. Photomicrographs of accessory root canals. (Orban: Oral histology and embryology.)

rupted, the stimulus for the differentiation of odontoblasts is lacking, and, consequently, no dentin will be produced in the area of the defect. While the dentin
increases in thickness, the primary defect is transformed into a narrow canal. The
complicated events that lead to the division of the common root stock into two or
three roots make it understandable that the furcation is a frequent site of accessory
canals of the third type. Here, the epithelium at the cervical end of the developing
root forms horizontal tonguelike projections that grow toward each other and finally
fuse. Thus the primarily single opening of the epithelial sheath is divided into two or
three openings. Defects in the epithelium at the sites of fusion of these flaps may
readily occur. In some animals, for instance the rat, such defects are almost a normal
feature.

Accessory canals of the second and third types are of importance in dental practice
because they form an almost unsurmountable difficulty during root canal treatment.
Canals of the third type that are situated at some distance from the apical end of the
root may also be considered as potential points of entrance of bacteria from a periodontal source into the pulp. This means that a progressive periodontal disease,
characterized by formation of a pocket between root and surrounding tissues, may
cause a secondary pulpal infection at the time when the deepest point of the infected
pocket reaches the opening of an accessory canal. Even a fairly shallow pocket may
cause a pulpal infection if a lateral canal opens at the bifurcation or in the cervical
region of a root.

Attachment of the tooth

The tooth is attached to the bone of its socket by connective tissue that is known as
the periodontal ligament. This type of attachment is also termed a gomphosis, originally derived from the picture of a nail or peg driven into wood. Gomphosis is now
defined as a type of suture, namely, a peg-and-socket suture. It is, like sutures, a
syndesmosis.

The term periodontal membrane, so widely used in dental literature, is misleading. The connective tissue between the root and bone cannot be compared with any
type of anatomic structure other than a ligament.

The functional elements of the periodontal ligament, the principal fibers, are fiber
bundles that were thought to be anchored as Sharpey's fibers in the cementum on one
side, in the bone on the other side. The bundles consist of white or collagenous
nonelastic fibers. The arrangement of the fibers is, as in all ligaments, correlated to
the functional stresses, and their existence is largely dependent on normal function.

In the group of principal fibers of the periodontal ligament are also included fibers
that, in a strict sense, are not contained in the periodontal space. These fibers, however, are also anchored on one side in the cementum of the root and can be divided
into two groups. From the most cervical part of the cementum of the root, fibers
radiate into the gingiva and thus serve to attach the gingiva to the tooth itself. The
second group of fibers, found only in the interdental spaces, run across the interden-

tal septum from tooth to tooth and serve to unite all the teeth of one arch into a functional unit.

If we accept the definition of the periodontal ligament as including all fibers that are anchored in the cementum of the root, then it can be divided into three ligaments: (1) gingival ligament, (2) transseptal, or interdental, ligament, and (3) alveolodental ligament, or alveolar ligament.

The bundles of the alveolodental ligament in turn can be classified according to their arrangement. The most cervical bundles connect the cementum of the root with the crest of the alveolar process. The fibers have a horizontal course or they are attached to the root at a level occlusal to that of the alveolar crest. The next bundles are characterized by their horizontal arrangement. The deeper fibers assume a more and more oblique course. The oblique fibers are attached to the tooth at a level apical to that of their attachment to the bone. Finally, there are fibers that are attached to the apical cementum and from here radiate in all directions toward the bone at the fundus of the socket. The alveolodental ligament is conventionally subdivided into (1) alveolar crest fibers, (2) horizontal fibers, (3) oblique fibers, and (4) apical fibers.

The function of the alveolar fibers, which together can also be called the alveolodental ligament or the suspensory dental ligament, is to resist the forces of mastication. Pressure on the tooth will lead to a stretching of all or of some of the fiber bundles, and thus the *masticatory pressure* is transformed into *tension* action *on cementum and bone*. This transformation of forces is absolutely essential for the normal functional life of a tooth. In the section on tooth eruption it will be shown that there is appositional growth at the entire surface of the cementum and in wide areas of the alveolar bone throughout the life of a tooth. Growth of bone or cementum cannot and does not occur if the growing surface is under pressure.

The arrangement of the alveolar fibers is a clear indication that vertical forces, that is, forces acting in the direction of the axis of the tooth, are best resisted by the suspensory fibers. Under a vertical force nearly all the alveolodental fibers are evenly stretched. Any lateral force will stretch only part of the alveolar fibers, and therefore the resistance to a lateral force is lower than that to a vertical force. Normally this will not lead to serious damage to the tooth because the lateral forces are only components of an oblique masticatory pressure. However, if the lateral forces are exaggerated, for instance, by persistence of high cusps in persons of advanced age, damage to the supporting tissues can be expected. The alveolodental ligament also *limits* the masticatory movements of a tooth, thus *protecting* the tissues on the side toward which the tooth is moved during mastication.

The alveolar group of the principal fibers of the periodontal ligament, arranged in strong bundles, represent the alveolodental, or suspensory, ligament of the tooth. Embedded with one end in the alveolar bone proper and with the other end in the cementum, the single fibers of the bundles were believed to extend uninterrupted through the entire width of periodontal space. This concept is untenable. In continually erupting teeth with a high rate of daily or weekly eruption, a continual rearrangement of the periodontal fibers must occur without at any time lowering the

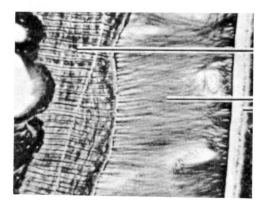

Alveolar bone

Intermediate plexus
cementum

Fig. 5-59. Intermediate plexus of human periodontal ligament. (Sicher: The periodontal ligament. In Kraus and Riedel, editors: Vistas in orthodontics, Philadelphia, 1962, Lea & Febiger.)

functional efficiency of the suspensory dental ligament. In the molars of the guinea pig and in the incisors of the rat the site of this continual rearrangement of the periodontal ligaments was found to be an intermediate plexus. The fibers arising in the bone and those inserted in the cementum are joined and interwoven in a rather broad zone of irregularly arranged argyrophil fibers, the intermediate plexus. Dissolution of fiber connections occurs in this zone, along with the production of new fibers and the formation of new functionally adapted fiber connections. The great number of mitoses in the fibroblasts indicates the high activity in the intermediate plexus, and the argyrophilia of the fibers reveals them as young collagenous fibers (Fig. 5-59).

In human and all other mammalian teeth there is also need for a constant rearrangement of the principal fibers of the periodontal ligament in correlation to the continued vertical eruption and mesial drift. Vertical eruption of the functioning tooth is fast during the period of growth but continues later, though slowly, in compensation for occlusal attrition; mesial drift is, of course, also continual as compensation of continual wear at the contact surface. Rearrangement of the alveolodental ligament includes among other changes a lengthening of the fibers in the distal part of the periodontal membrane to allow a mesial movement of the tooth.

A study of good silver-impregnated sections through human teeth shows that no single principal fiber can ever be traced from bone to cementum. Instead they all seem to end or begin somewhere in a middle zone of the periodontal ligament. In other words, the single fiber bundles consist of shorter fibers that seem to be "spliced" in their middle. However, it is more correct to state that the human periodontal ligaments consist of alveolar fibers, dental fibers, and an intermediate plexus. The existence of this plexus in man escaped notice for so long because it is inconspicuous. This in turn is the consequence of the slow rate of movements in human teeth compared with the fast rate of eruption in rodent incisors and molars.

The ligamentous principal fibers are only one, although the most important, structural element of the periodontal ligament. Between the fiber bundles a moderate amount of loose connective tissue is found that surrounds the branches of the periodontal blood vessels, lymph vessels, and nerves. These accumulations of loose connective tissue appear in sections as round or oval areas between the bundles of the principal fibers.

The blood vessels in these "spaces" consist of glomi, that is, convolutions of veins and of arteriovenous junctions. During masticatory movements of a tooth the veins on the side of compression, that is, the side toward which the tooth moves, are speedily emptied, the blood leaving through the communications with septal veins. Thus any pressure that might otherwise damage the tissue is aborted. One should, therefore, not speak of a *tension* and a *pressure* side, but rather of a side of *tension* and a side of *compression*. The arteriovenous anastomoses serve for a speedy refilling of the venous convolutions during the rebounding movement of a tooth, when the masticatory forces cease their action. Thus the protection of periodontal tissues is due to the limitation of masticatory movements by the alveolodental ligament and the presence of the venous convolutions.

Remnants of the epithelial root sheath, the epithelial rests of Malassez, are a regular feature of periodontal ligament. The epithelial remnants form a more or less continuous network of epithelial cords around the entire surface of the root, situated closer to the root surface than to the bone of the socket. In sections they appear as round or oval islands of epithelial cells. They gain importance if they proliferate under the stimulus of an inflammation, and may then form the epithelial lining of a radicular cyst.

The periodontal space is normally narrow, its width varying from 0.1 to 0.2 mm. The width is smallest in the middle third of a root and slightly greater apically and cervically. This behavior of the periodontal ligament has been correlated to the movement of the tooth under lateral pressure. The tooth seems then to swing or to rotate minutely around a horizontal axis, passing somewhere through the middle third of the root. It follows that pressure on the lingual surface of an incisor, for instance, will stretch the principal fibers on the lingual side of the tooth in the cervical half of the root and the labial fibers in the apical half of the root. Under this force the crown will move slightly labially, the apex of the root slightly lingually. This explanation is questionable and has been opposed by some authors who believe that the apex of the root remains fairly stable when a lateral force acts on the tooth.

Eruption of teeth

Introductory remarks. Too many crude or gross mechanical factors still are adduced to explain the "forces" of tooth eruption. The following analysis may be helpful to see the difference between mechanics in the living and in the nonliving world.*

A tooth germ grows in the confined space of its bony crypt and, after due time, erupts into the oral cavity, cutting through the dense tissue of the gingival ridge. For a long time anato-

---

*From Sicher: Biomechanics, Bur **63**:18, 19, March, 1962.

mists have sought—and "found"—a force of eruption. They described the final emergence of the tooth through the soft tissues by using the colloquial expression of the tooth "cutting" the gingiva. Such gross mechanical interpretations have, by no means, disappeared from the scientific literature.

In describing the influence of the growing brain on the growth of its bony capsule, again the brain is seen as "spreading" the cranial bones apart.

In describing a rapid growth of the intestinal tube, it has been said that the narrow mesentery is pulled into the fan-shaped mesentery of jejunum and ileum.

Examples of such mechanistic descriptions and interpretations could easily be multiplied.

It is, of course, true that the growing tooth germ or the growing brain do exert pressure upon the surrounding and confining tissues. What, then, is the difference between a root growing in the cleft of a rock and finally splitting it, or a bean sprout piercing a covering aluminum foil, and the action of the growing tooth germ or the growing brain?

The answer to this question is superbly simple. The forces generated by the growing plant are exerted against inert material, they increase and, finally, the rock splits, the foil is perforated. The forces generated by the growing tooth or brain are directed against living tissues that can and do react. And their reaction is in principle always the same, namely, to reduce the developing pressure—or pull—and to eliminate it.

This is accomplished in different ways. When the tooth grows, the slight rise in pressure within the crypt leads to the differentiation of osteoclasts and bone resorption, but also to proliferation of connective tissue and enlargement of the dental sac. In the "cutting" of the tooth through the oral tissues the pressure of the crown against the overlying connective tissue leads to the elaboration—or activation—of desmolytic enzymes, collagenases and/or hyaluronidases, most probably by the cells of the united enamel or dental epithelium that covers the crown to the moment of the emergence of the tooth. That this epithelial covering remains intact while the tooth "cuts" or "pierces" the soft tissues is absolute evidence against crude mechanical interpretations.

When the brain grows in its bony capsule the attending pressure is but the stimulus for the growth of the derivatives of the brain capsule: cartilage at the cranial base and fibrous tissue elsewhere. Thus the capsule grows between the bony parts of the cranium or, to use a more orthodox term, between the cranial bones. And, again, this growth immediately eliminates intracranial pressure.

The growing small intestine certainly exerts some traction on its mesentery. But the latter responds immediately by its surface growth and the mechanical force is eliminated.

Briefly summarized, the forces in living organisms are acting as stimuli to set in motion changes that will recover balance of forces. Forces of pressure or traction do indeed play a role in development and growth. But they are, in truth, self-eliminating. And this is the basis of biomechanics.

The tooth germs, developing and growing in the growing jaws, undergo changes of their position long before the actual eruption commences. These movements are mostly spreading movements; that is, the growing teeth grow into the widening space of the arches of maxilla and mandible. The enlargement of the teeth is directed mainly buccally, but they expand also in all other directions. There is at this time no fixed plane in the "cervical" parts of the tooth germ. During the preeruptive period, the inner surface of the bony crypt of the tooth, always wide open toward the surface of the jaw, rarely shows signs of apposition anywhere; there is, as a rule, resorption on all bony walls, which is proof of the eccentric growth of the tooth germs. In this phase of tooth development the movements of the teeth serve to keep the growing germs of the deciduous teeth in an even arrangement.

The preeruptive movements of the permanent teeth are in principle similar to those of the deciduous teeth; in other words, the teeth *grow* into their preeruptive positions. The changes in the relation of the permanent tooth germs to their deciduous predecessors are the result not only of the eccentric growth of the permanent germs, but also of the simultaneous eruptive movements of the deciduous teeth.

The large size of the crown of some permanent teeth causes their crowded position in the relatively small jaw. Thus the germs of the permanent incisors are often rotated around a longitudinal axis or they are found in a staggered position. The first arrangement is the rule in the lower jaw, and the second type of crowding is more frequent in the upper jaw, where the germ of the second permanent incisor often is situated lingual to the distal half of the first incisor. The large canine crowns are displaced downward in the lower jaw and upward in the upper jaw. The germ of the lower permanent canine is almost in contact with the lower border of the mandible, whereas that of the upper is found immediately below the infraorbital rim.

The permanent premolars, which are smaller than their predecessors, grow between the roots of the deciduous molars where they find enough space to develop to their final size.

The position of the permanent molars is dependent on the gradual lengthening of the alveolar process behind the last deciduous tooth. When they start their development, the lower molars are in the base of the ascending ramus of the mandible, the upper molars in the lower bulging part of the tuberosity of the maxilla (Fig. 5-60). The molars are obliquely placed, the occlusal surface of the lower molars facing forward and upward. The tilt of the upper molars is in the opposite direction, their occlusal

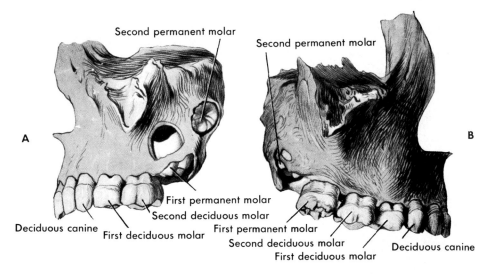

Fig. 5-60. Position of developing molars in maxillary tuberosity. **A,** 5 years of age. **B,** 7 years of age. (Sicher and Tandler: Anatomie für Zahnärzte.)

surface facing backward and downward. Gradually and successively the molars gain a more or less upright position while the jaws expand posteriorly.

Actual eruption starts when the teeth begin to move toward the surface of the jaws. In human teeth, this moment coincides with the start of root development. The eruption leads to the "cutting" of the teeth, that is, to their appearance in the oral cavity. Although the cutting is of clinical importance, it is but a transitory stage in the eruptive movement of the tooth. When the tooth comes into contact with its antagonist or antagonists and commences its function, the first, or prefunctional, phase of eruption ends, but not eruption itself. In fact, the eruptive movements continue during the functional period until the tooth is lost or the individual dies. The movements of the teeth in the functional period of eruption are correlated to the continued growth of the jaws, especially in vertical dimension, and to the loss of tooth substance by attrition at the occlusal surfaces and at the contact points. Summarizing, the movements of the teeth can be classified as follows:

Preeruptive movements

Eruptive movements

    Prefunctional period

    Functional period

The movements of the teeth in the eruptive period can also be classified according to their direction. The movement along the long axis of a tooth can be called *axial*, or *vertical*, movement. It is, of course, the most conspicuous component of the complicated movements of the erupting tooth. The movement around one of the transverse labiolingual or buccolingual axes of a tooth is a *tilting*, or *tipping*, movement. It is most pronounced in the erupting molars when they turn from a nearly horizontal to a nearly vertical position. The movement of a tooth around one of its longitudinal axes may be termed a *rotatory* movement. The crowded lower permanent incisors, for instance, rotate to find their normal position in the growing jaw. Finally, a tooth may move bodily, that is, parallel to itself. This movement is the *drifting* movement. It is conspicuous in the labial movement of the erupting permanent incisors, which develop lingual to the roots of the deciduous incisors.

Chronology of human dentition (Figs. 5-61 to 5-68). The development, especially the eruption, of the human teeth varies considerably in time. It is, therefore, impossible to give more than the range of these variations; only deviations considerably outside this range can be considered as pathologic. Table 1 summarizes the data.

Biology of tooth eruption. The eruptive movements of a tooth are the effect of differential growth. One speaks of differential growth if two topographically related organs or two parts of an organ grow at different rates of speed. Changes in the spatial relations of such organs or of parts of an organ are the inevitable consequence of differential growth. The ontogenesis of almost any organ and of the whole embryo proves that differential growth is one of the most important factors of morphogenesis. In the jaws it is the differential growth of tooth and bone that leads to the movements of a tooth.

The most obvious eruptive "force" is generated by the longitudinal growth of the

Text continued on p. 289.

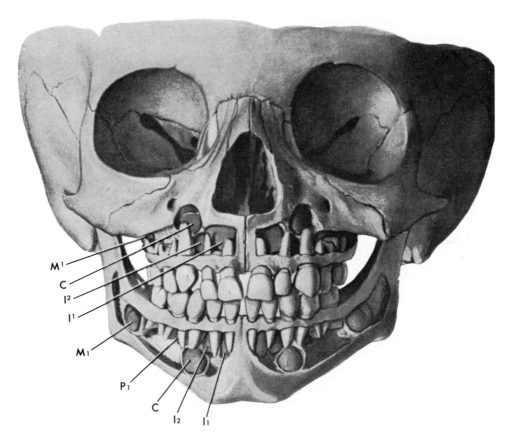

Fig. 5-61. Skull of child 2½ years of age. Roots of deciduous teeth and developing crowns of permanent teeth are exposed. Here and in following seven figures (to Fig. 5-68) inclusive), permanent teeth are darkly shaded. (Sicher and Tandler: Anatomie für Zahnärzte.)

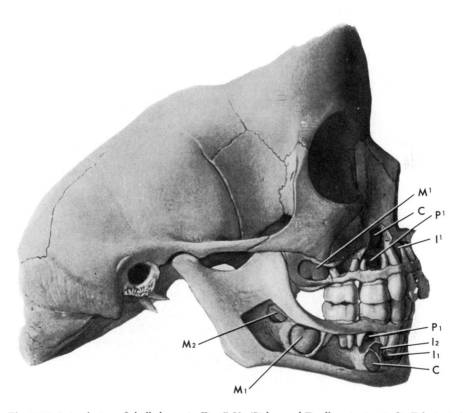

Fig. 5-62. Lateral view of skull shown in Fig. 5-61. (Sicher and Tandler: Anatomie für Zahnärzte.)

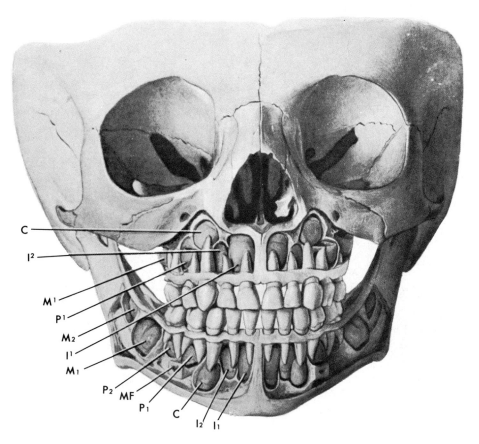

Fig. 5-63. Skull of 4-year-old child. (Sicher and Tandler: Anatomie für Zahnärzte.)

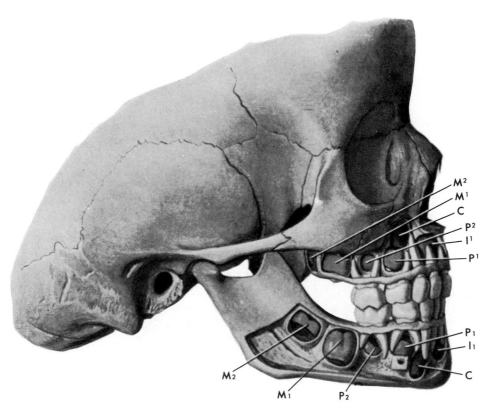

Fig. 5-64. Lateral view of skull shown in Fig. 5-63. (Sicher and Tandler: Anatomie für Zahnärzte.)

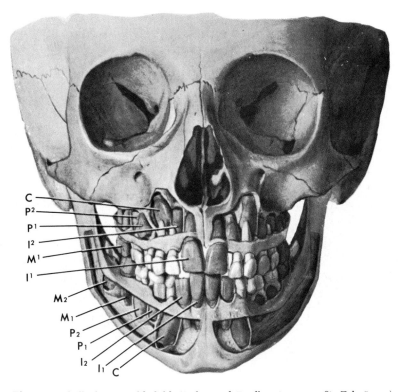

Fig. 5-65. Skull of 8-year-old child. (Sicher and Tandler: Anatomie für Zahnärzte.)

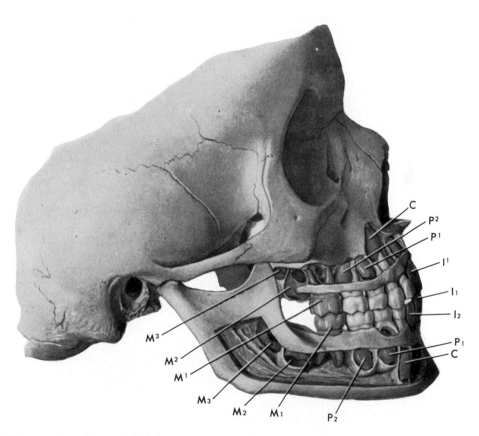

Fig. 5-66. Lateral view of skull shown in Fig. 5-65. (Sicher and Tandler: Anatomie für Zahnärzte.)

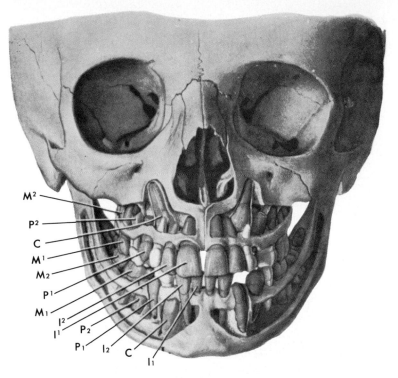

Fig. 5-67. Skull of 10-year-old child. (Sicher and Tandler: Anatomie für Zahnärzte.)

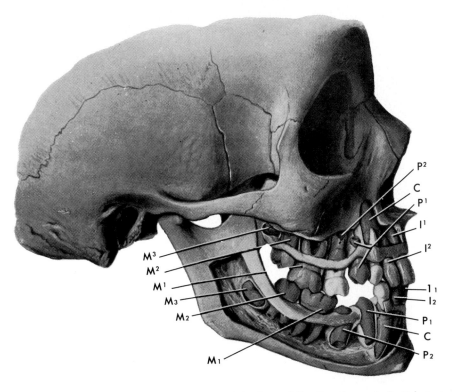

Fig. 5-68. Lateral view of skull shown in Fig. 5-67. (Sicher and Tandler: Anatomie für Zahnärzte.)

root of the tooth. However, the different movements of an erupting tooth cannot be explained by the development of its root alone. We know that some teeth, even while their roots develop, travel a distance that is longer than the fully developed root. Only an auxiliary factor can account for the additional distance. We know also that teeth move in different directions, for instance, by tilting, rotating, or drifting, but the growth of the root can account only for the axial, or vertical, movement. Therefore one has to look for an additional moving force to explain the variety of eruptive movements. It will be shown that the additional "force" is generated by the growth of bone in the neighborhood of the tooth germ.

Table 1. Chronology of human dentition*

Tooth	Hard tissue formation begins	Amount of enamel formed at birth	Enamel com-pleted	Eruption	Root com-pleted
Deciduous dentition					
Maxillary					
Central incisor	4 mo. in utero	Five sixths	1½ mo.	7½ mo.	1½ yr.
Lateral incisor	4½ mo. in utero	Two thirds	2½ mo.	9 mo.	2 yr.
Canine	5 mo. in utero	One third	9 mo.	18 mo.	3½ yr.
First molar	5 mo. in utero	Cusps united	6 mo.	14 mo.	2½ yr.
Second molar	6 mo. in utero	Cusp tips still isolated	1 mo.	24 mo.	3 yr.
Mandibular					
Central incisor	4½ mo. in utero	Three fifths	2½ mo.	6 mo.	1½ yr.
Lateral incisor	4½ mo. in utero	Three fifths	3 mo.	7 mo.	1½ yr.
Canine	5 mo. in utero	One third	9 mo.	16 mo.	3¼ yr.
First molar	5 mo. in utero	Cusps united	5½ mo.	12 mo.	2¼ yr.
Second molar	6 mo. in utero	Cusp tips still isolated	10 mo.	20 mo.	3 yr.
Permanent dentition					
Maxillary					
Central incisor	3-4 mo.	—	4-5 yr.	7-8 yr.	10 yr.
Lateral incisor	10-12 mo.	—	4-5 yr.	8-9 yr.	11 yr.
Canine	4-5 mo.	—	6-7 yr.	11-12 yr.	13-15 yr.
First premolar	1½-1¾ yr.	—	5-6 yr.	10-11 yr.	12-13 yr.
Second premolar	2-2¼ yr.	—	6-7 yr.	10-12 yr.	12-14 yr.
First molar	At birth	Sometimes a trace	2½-3 yr.	6-7 yr.	9-10 yr.
Second molar	2½-3 yr.	—	7-8 yr.	12-13 yr.	14-16 yr.
Third molar	7-9 yr.	—	12-16 yr.	17-21 yr.	18-25 yr.
Mandibular					
Central incisor	3-4 mo.	—	4-5 yr.	6-7 yr.	9 yr.
Lateral incisor	3-4 mo.	—	4-5 yr.	7-8 yr.	10 yr.
Canine	4-5 mo.	—	6-7 yr.	9-10 yr.	12-14 yr.
First premolar	1¾-2 yr.	—	5-6 yr.	10-12 yr.	12-13 yr.
Second premolar	2¼-2½ yr.	—	6-7 yr.	11-12 yr.	13-14 yr.
First molar	At birth	Sometimes a trace	2½-3 yr.	6-7 yr.	9-10 yr.
Second molar	2½-3 yr	—	7-8 yr.	11-13 yr.	14-15 yr.
Third molar	8-10 yr.	—	12-16 yr.	7-21 yr.	18-25 yr.

*Compiled by Logan and Kronfeld; slightly modified by McCall and Schour.

It is also a fact that the teeth move extensively after their dentinal roots have been fully formed. The continued growth of the cementum covering the root and the growth of the surrounding bone cause the movements of the tooth in this period.

Before development of the root begins, the outer and inner enamel epithelia extend apically from the region of the future cementoenamel junction as a double epithelial layer called *Hertwig's epithelial root sheath.* This band forms a ring, in three dimensions, which ends at an approximately right-angled inward bend. The horizontal inward extension narrows the cervical opening into the developing crown. This extension is thus known as the epithelial diaphragm (Figs. 5-69 to 5-73). The

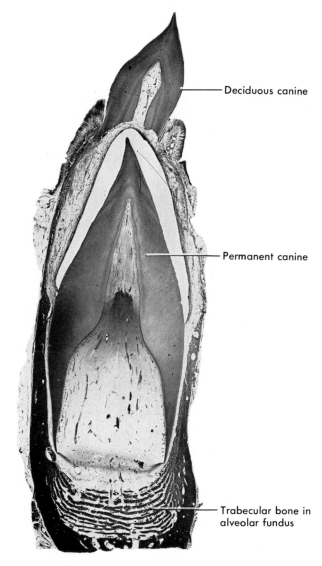

Deciduous canine

Permanent canine

Trabecular bone in alveolar fundus

Fig. 5-69. Labiolingual section through lower deciduous and permanent canine from 8-year-old child. (R. Kronfeld.) (Weinmann and Sicher: Bone and bones.)

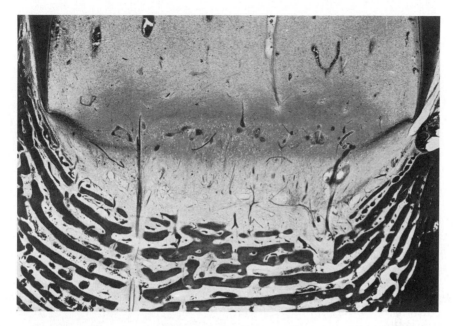

Fig. 5-70. High magnification of root end and bone in fundus of socket of permanent canine shown in Fig. 5-69.

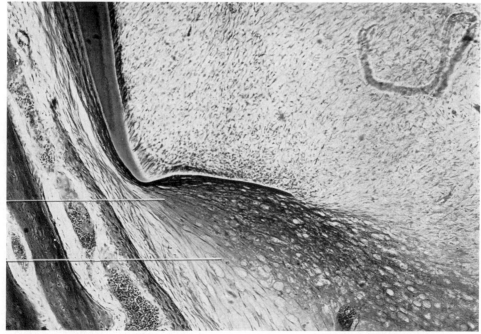

ammock
gament

Fluid in
gament

Fig. 5-71. Part of root end of permanent canine shown in Figs. 5 69 and 5-70, high magnification. Note "diaphragm" above hammock ligament.

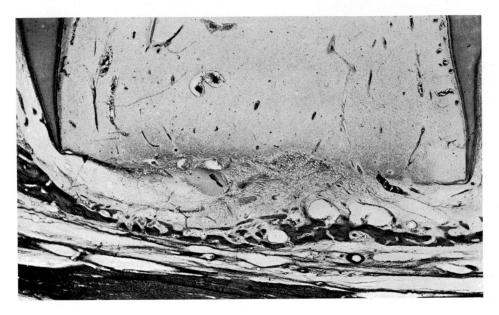

Fig. 5-72. Mesiodistal section through root end of erupting lower second molar from child 8 years of age.

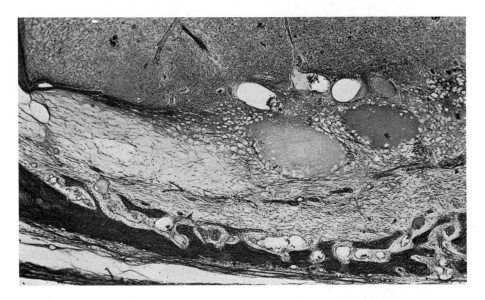

Fig. 5-73. Part of root end of specimen shown in Fig. 5-72, under high magnification.

epithelial diaphragm forms a definite boundary between the growing pulp of the tooth germ and the adjacent connective tissue that intervenes between the tooth germ and bony wall of the crypt. Thus growth and development of the root are possible only by active proliferation of the pulpal tissue itself. The active interstitial growth creates the tissue pressure that contributes to tooth eruption.

The pressure generated by the increase in volume of the pulp in the restricted space of the dental crypt would act against the bone in the bottom of the crypt and cause resorption of the bone; in other words, the root would grow into the jaw. Growth of the pulp could not cause an eruptive movement of the tooth germ without the presence of an auxiliary structure. The auxiliary structure that protects the bone at the bottom of the crypt from pressure, prevents resorption of the bone, and causes the tooth to grow or move away from the bottom of the crypt is a ligament. It is anchored in the bone above the bottom of the crypt and lies immediately apical to the developing root and the epithelial diaphragm. The tooth rests on this suspensory ligament, and therefore the ligament was called a "hammock ligament" (Figs. 5-71 to 5-73). If tissue pressure increases by the proliferation of the growing pulp, this ligament is tensed, the pressure is transmitted as tension to the bone to which the ligament is anchored, and no pressure is directed against the bone at the bottom of the crypt. Thus the hammock ligament is the fixed base, or plane, from which the tooth grows and erupts because elongation of the *suspended* tooth can only result in growth toward the surface of the jaw.

As previously mentioned, the growth of the root alone cannot move a crown as far as is necessary to reach the occlusal position because some teeth develop so far from the surface of the jaw that root growth alone cannot account for their total vertical movement. In addition, it has to be remembered that the jaws grow rapidly at the alveolar crests while the teeth erupt. During the period of eruption the distance of the tooth from the surface of the jaw increases considerably. Growth of the root is therefore not sufficient to let the tooth grow out of the jaw. The erupting movement of most teeth is aided by growth of bone at the bottom of the crypt, lifting the growing tooth with the hammock ligament toward the surface. The formation of bone at the bottom of the crypt, preceded, of course, by the proliferation of "osteogenic" loose connective tissue, occurs in different teeth at different rates of speed. Where the production of new bone is slow, new layers of bone are laid down on the old bone, and a more or less compact bone results. Where growth of bone is rapid, spongy bone is formed in the shape of a framework of trabeculae (Figs. 5-69 and 5-70). These trabeculae develop by the growth of small projections of bone from the old surface; at some distance these sprouts seem to mushroom and to form a new trabecula parallel to the old surface. In this way, tier after tier of bone tissue develops in the deepest part of the socket.

The increased tissue pressure, which is inevitably linked with the proliferation of connective tissue before the formation of bone in the crypt, would tend to compress the hammock ligament and thereby destroy the fixed base that is essential for the normal eruption of a tooth. Finally the bone would encroach on tooth and pulp and thus bring the eruption to a standstill. These consequences are prevented by a peculiar structural differentiation of the hammock ligament that, teleologically speaking, renders the hammock ligament relatively incompressible. The hammock ligament is changed into what may be called the "cushioned hammock ligament." Histologically, the change consists of the accumulation of a fluid or a semifluid substance between the fibers of the hammock ligament (Figs. 5-71 to 5-73). The fluid is distributed throughout the ligament in small round droplets. Sometimes the small droplets of fluid in the connective tissue fuse and thus form rather large round drops. In such specimens it can be shown that this fluid coagulates under the influence of the fixing reagent (Fig. 5-73). The presence of fluid in confined spaces is, of course, the cause of the relative incompressibility of the hammock ligament. The incompressibility is relative but it evidently gives sufficient protection against the pressure forces of low intensity generated during tooth eruption. That this pressure normally never reaches any higher intensity is explained by the simple fact that reactive tissue changes immediately follow the increase of tissue pressure and relieve it. The cushioned hammock ligament therefore serves a twofold function. Its fibers, anchored in the bone on the lateral walls of the crypt, protect the tissue at the bottom of the crypt from pressure and direct the growth of the tooth toward the surface of the jaw. The fluid contained in the ligament prevents its compression by the bone growing at the bottom of the crypt and at the same time distributes the pressure exerted by the growth of bone evenly to the entire apical end of the growing root.

While in this way hammock ligament and teeth are lifted toward the surface, the

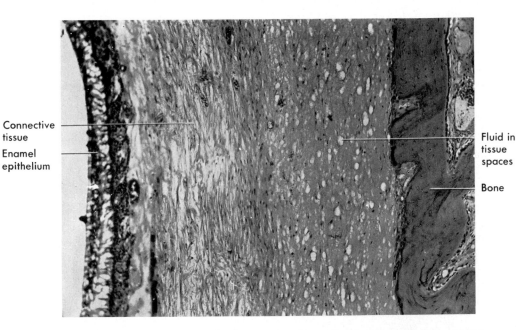

Fig. 5-74. Pericoronal tissue of upper first deciduous molar of 4-month-old child. (Weinmann and Sicher: Bone and bones.)

anchoring fibers of the hammock ligament have to be continually reconstructed. In other words, the hammock ligament has to shift its anchoring plane toward the surface of the jaws. The mechanism of this shift must be similar to that occurring in the intermediate plexus of the periodontal ligament during movements of a functioning tooth, movements that occur without disrupting the normal function of the erupting tooth.

The structure of the cushioned hammock ligament seems to be almost unique. It is duplicated only in the pericoronal tissue of growing and shifting tooth germs (Fig. 5-74). The shift of such germs is caused by the growth of bone in certain areas of the inner surface of the crypt. The pressure exerted on the tooth germ by the proliferation of loose connective tissue preceding bone formation causes it to move. Movement of the developing tooth in turn causes resorption of bone on the surface toward which it moves. During this phase of development a protective structure has to be postulated that prevents the encroachment of the growing bone on the tooth germ but permits growth and differentiation of the tooth germ while it is being moved. This protective structure may be called the "cushioned," or "incompressible," dental capsule. In this stage the crypt of the tooth germ is wide, and a rather thick layer of connective tissue is interposed between the epithelial enamel organ and the bony crypt. This connective tissue is clearly differentiated into two layers (Figs. 5-74 and 5-75). The inner layer, immediately surrounding the tooth germ, is simple loose connective tissue that allows changes in size and shape of the developing tooth. The outer layer, which is in contact with the bone of the crypt, contains a great volume of a fluid or a semifluid substance, rendering the outer layer incompressible to the limited forces generated during normal tooth development. The fluid is distributed in the connective tissue in the shape of innumerable small droplets. Thus the structure of the cushioned capsule is almost identical to that of the cushioned hammock ligament.

Any increase in tissue pressure by the proliferation of connective tissue and the consecutive formation of new bone, which as a rule occurs slowly, acts primarily on the capsule, and by a shift of the capsule and its contents the pressure is transmitted to the opposite side of the crypt, where it causes osteoclastic resorption of the bone. The resorption opens the way for a shift of the entire content of the crypt and at the same time relieves the pressure as the sequence of actions and reactions repeats itself.

Enlargement of the root does not cease when the dentinal root is fully formed. By continuous apposition of cementum the root grows slightly in its transverse diameters and more rapidly in length. The growth of cementum is not only increased in the apical area of the roots, but the furcation of two- or three-rooted teeth is also a site of slightly increased growth of cementum. There is continuous growth of bone at the fundus of the socket and at the crests of the alveolar process. The bone growth at the fundus and at the free border of the alveolar process is rapid in young persons; it slows down in the thirties, but in the healthy dentition it never ceases entirely. Growth at the alveolar crest, especially, is found only when the covering soft tissues are normal.

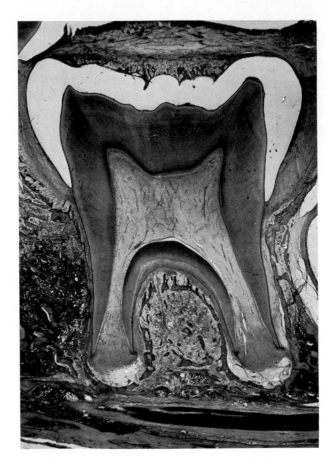

Fig. 5-75. Mesiodistal section through lower first molar of child 4½ years of age.

The frequency of inflammatory changes at the dentogingival junction, preventing growth of bone or even causing its destruction, accounts for the fact that this site of bone growth has been overlooked for a long time. There is also constant growth of bone on the distal wall of each socket, whereas the mesial wall shows resorption of the bone alternating with localized reparative apposition.

Elongation of the root and growth of bone at the fundus of the socket are correlated with a continued vertical eruption of the tooth during its functional period. The changes on the mesial and distal alveolar walls are correlated to a movement of all teeth toward the midline, or mesial drift. The continued occlusomesial movement is necessary to compensate for the loss of tooth substance at the occlusal and contact surfaces, in other words, for a gradual loss of tooth substance by incisal, occlusal, and contact attrition. However, the vertical or axial component of eruption during the earlier years of the functional period is far more extensive than could be accounted for by the still-restricted attrition. In this period the teeth have to erupt fast enough to keep out of the alveolar processes, which grow rapidly at their free borders.

Mesial drift, the mesial component of the physiologic movement of the teeth, occurs in adaptation to the loss of tooth substance at the contact surfaces. If the teeth are to keep contact with each other, the loss in mesiodistal dimension must be compensated for by a mesial movement of all teeth. The extent of this movement is least for the central incisors and increases for each tooth in distal direction.

Although the correlation of bone changes and movement of teeth is self-evident, the question has to be examined as to whether the bone changes are primary and thus the cause of the movement of the teeth. The impossibility of finding any internal or external "forces" that would account for the continuous vertical eruption and mesial drift is already an indication that growth of bone and cementum plays the same role in the functional period that can be ascribed to it in the pre-eruptive and prefunctional eruptive movements.

That the differential growth of alveolar bone and cementum, preceded by growth of loose "osteogenic and cementogenic" connective tissue, causes the eruptive movements of a tooth in its functional period is confirmed by the following findings: When the roots of two- or three-rooted teeth are developed to a certain length and cementum formation at the furcation has progressed for a time, the cushioned hammock ligament disappears, the epithelial diaphragm is bent outward and loses its relation to the growing pulp, and the pulp itself seems to protrude from the wide-open apical end of the root (Fig. 5-75). The bone at the crest of the interradicular septum is in rapid proliferation, forming spicules and trabeculae opposite to the growing cementum of the furcation. In such a tooth it is the growth of interradicular septum and cementum that "lifts" the tooth toward the surface of the jaw and out of its socket, and the complicated structures at the root end, especially the hammock ligament, become nonfunctional and therefore disappear.

In the life of every tooth there comes a time in which the "forces" of eruption undergo a radical change. It is, of course, the time at which the pulp has fully grown and the dentinal root is fully formed. From then on it is the differential growth of bone and cementum and not that of pulp and bone that causes the continued eruptive movement of the tooth. The mechanism of eruption of two- or three-rooted teeth differs only in one point, namely, in the much earlier shift from one mechanism of eruption to the other. When the furcation is fully formed, this shift can occur although the roots are still growing.

The mesial drift, mesial component of tooth movement (Fig. 5-76), is caused in principle by similar changes of bone and tooth. However, this movement is greatly complicated by the fact that extensive bone resorption at the mesial alveolar walls has to open a space into which the teeth move while the vertical component of tooth movement is not opposed by bone.

Growth of bone on the distal (Fig. 5-77) surface of the socket leads to an increase of the intra-alveolar pressure, which is relieved by resorption of bone at the mesial wall of the socket (Fig. 5-78). The rapid release of the minimal pressure caused by the prliferation of osteogenic tissue is, in all probability, the reason for an orderly pattern of bone resorption. Growing and cell-covered areas of bone and cementum are thus "protected."

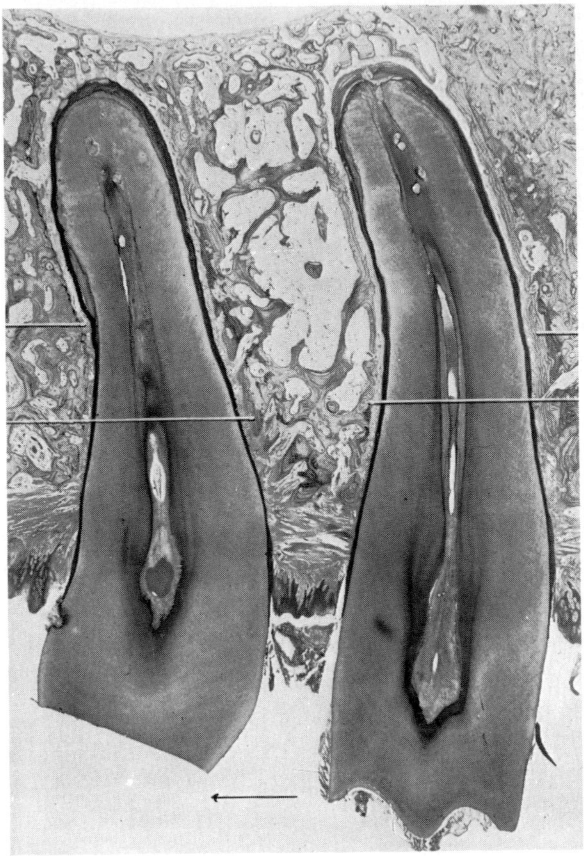

Fig. 5-76. Mesial drift. Mesiodistal section through upper first and second premolars. Arrow indicates direction of mesial movement. (Weinmann and Sicher: Bone and bones.)

In both the vertical and mesial components of the movements of functioning teeth a continual rearrangement of the principal fibers of the periodontal ligament has to be postulated. This rearrangement occurs in the intermediate plexus of the periodontal ligament. Of special interest are the changes the prevent a disruption of the ligamentous anchorage of the tooth on its mesial surface during the continuous mesial drift. To understand these readjustments it is necessary to take cognizance of the peculiar reaction of bone to pressure or during modeling resorption, which could be called the law of excessive resorption. Resorption of bone under pressure is always more extensive than would be necessary to relieve the pressure. If a bony surface, adapted to the functional needs of the particular area, is destroyed during a period of resorption, the newly exposed surface lacks these adaptational qualities. Therefore the resorption continues until space is provided for a reconstruction of a functionally adequate new surface. This is the reason that under normal circumstances resorption is almost never a continuous process but instead occurs in waves, with periods of resorption alternating with periods of reparative or reconstructive apposition.

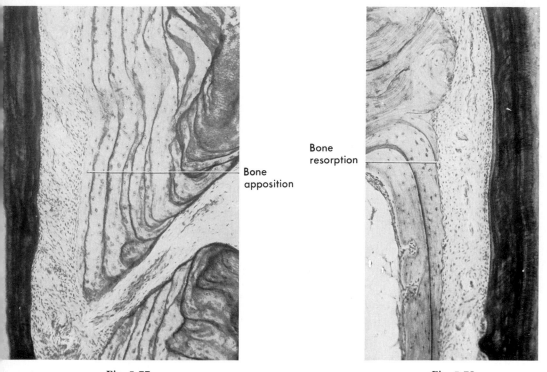

Bone apposition

Bone resorption

Fig. 5-77   Fig. 5-78

Fig. 5-77. Distal alveolar wall and periodontal ligament of second premolar. Detail of specimen shown in Fig. 5-76. (Weinmann and Sicher: Bone and bones.)
Fig. 5-78. Mesial alveolar wall and periodontal ligament of a second premolar. Detail of specimen shown in Fig. 5-76. (Weinmann and Sicher: Bone and bones.)

This sequence of events can be observed clearly during the mesial drift of a tooth. Some principal fibers lose their attachment during the period of bone resorption and are then reattached or replaced by new fibers during the period of repair. Furthermore, it can be observed that the bone resorption does not occur on the entire extent of the mesial alveolar surface at the same time. Instead, at a given moment, areas of resorption alternate with areas of reparative apposition. It seems that the tooth moves mesially in a complicated "wriggling" movement. Thus resorption occurs only in restricted areas in one period and reconstruction occurs in the same area while the moving tooth, minutely tilting or rotating, causes resorption in another area. Only this can account for the fact that the functional integrity of the tooth is maintained despite its continued movements.

Signs of this complicated process can be seen not only in the simultaneous presence of areas of resorption and apposition of bone in the mesial wall of the socket, but also in the periodontal membrane itself if the movement of the tooth is fairly rapid. Until now it was only possible to see these changes in the rat, whose molars drift distally and, in the young animals, move at a considerable rate of speed. Here the bundles of the distal periodontal ligament can be seen in a state of disorganization in those areas that correspond to areas of resorption of the distal alveolar wall. In other areas in which the reconstructive apposition of bone has begun, the periodontal ligament shows a gradual reorganization to a fully normal arrangement.

Arrangement of the teeth

The examination of dental arches has to consider the arrangement of the teeth in each arch and the relations of the upper and lower arches to each other. The position of the masticatory apparatus to the skull as a whole has been discussed under anthropology.

The teeth of a normal dentition are arranged in close sequence; that is, each tooth is in firm contact with its neighbors or neighbor. The contact occurs first at *points* of contact. The wear at the contact points, caused by the individual masticatory movements of the teeth, leads soon to the establishment of areas, or *facets*, of contact, which gradually increase in size. The contact points are the points of highest convexity on the proximal surfaces. The incisors touch each other at a point approximately between the middle and incisal thirds of their proximal surfaces. Attrition at the incisal edges leads to an apparent incisal shift of the contact point. The contacts of the canines are of interest. Since the convexity of the approximal surfaces in the incisors is situated far labially, the contact of the canine and lateral incisor is similar to that between two incisors. The position of the highest point of the distal convexity of the canine close to its labial surface necessitates an asymmetrical curvature of the mesial surface of the first premolar; the highest point of the convexity of its mesial surface is shifted buccally, whereas the distal surface culminates midway between its buccal and lingual borders. From here on distally the contact points are almost in the middle of the buccolingual width of the crown.

The buccal and lingual embrasures, that is, the spaces between two neighboring teeth buccally and lingually to the contact area, are, in the molar and premolar regions, of fairly equal depth on the two sides of the contact point. In the space between the first premolar and canine, however, the lingual embrasure is much deeper than the buccal embrasure. The interdental spaces (Figs. 5-79 and 5-80), in a strict sense, are the spaces between the two opposing surfaces of a tooth cervical to the contact point or the contact facet and between the latter and the crest of the interdental or interalveolar septum. The spaces, filled by the interdental papillae of the gingiva, are roughly comparable to a gabled tent, with the labial or buccal and the lingual corners elevated and the ridge of the tent concave.

The shape of the dental arches varies considerably. In a normal or, rather, in an average individual, the upper arch can be described as elliptic, the lower arch as parabolic. This means that the divergence of the premolar and molar regions decreases steadily in the upper arch and increases in the lower arch. Of the many variations of the dental arches only the so-called U-shaped arch, or rectangular arch, may be mentioned here. In this type the front teeth are aligned in an almost frontal plane and there is a sharp, almost angular bend at the canines. The side teeth are then arranged roughly parallel to each other in an almost sagittal plane. An arrangement of

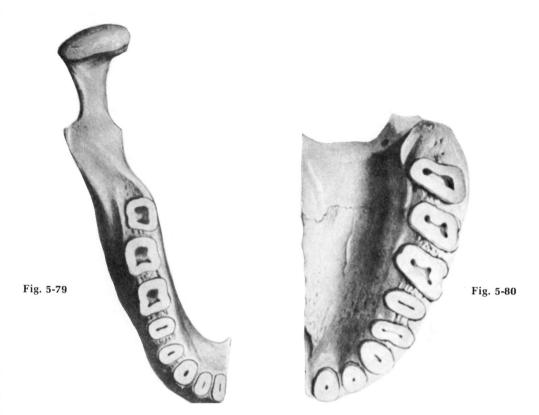

Fig. 5-79

Fig. 5-80

Fig. 5-79. Horizontal section through lower teeth in cervical plane. (Sicher and Tandler: Anatomie für Zahnärzte.)

Fig. 5-80. Horizontal section through upper teeth in cervical plane. (Sicher and Tandler: Anatomie für Zahnärzte.)

the teeth in a U-shaped arch has been described as a primitive, or anthropoid, characteristic.

The biting surfaces of the teeth are, as a rule, not situated in one horizontal plane. Instead, observation in profile view shows that the occlusal plane is downwardly convex (Fig. 5-81). Sometimes the occlusal plane is inclined slightly downward from the canine to the first molar to rise again in the region of the molars; in other individuals the occlusal plane in front of the first molar is more nearly horizontal. The curve is known as the curve of Spee. Only in a minority of persons is the curve of Spee well pronounced; more often it is just indicated, and in some it is lacking. The curve of Spee is explained by some as an adaptation to secure a balanced articulation. This seems, to say the least, improbable. The curve of Spee is caused by the tendency of the single individually attached and movable tooth to assume that position in the jaw in which its longitudinal axis coincides with the direction of the resultant masticatory force at this point. This position gives to each tooth the optimal resistance under the maximal force of the elevators of the mandible—masseter, temporal, and medial

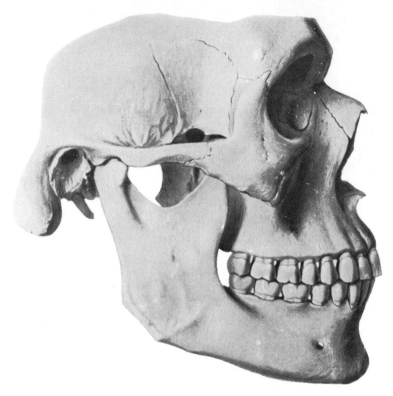

Fig. 5-81. Normal occlusion of permanent dentition, lateral view. (Sicher and Tandler: Anatomie für Zahnärzte.)

pterygoid muscles. The obliquity of the resultant force causes the oblique position of the tooth. The forces in the molar region are increasingly inclined anteriorly, and the corresponding position of the molars leads to the formation of the curve of Spee.

The relation of upper and lower teeth to each other after closure of the jaws is called *occlusion*. The relations of upper and lower teeth to each other during movements of the lower jaw are called *articulation*. Occlusion should not be regarded as a *static* relation between maxillary and mandibular teeth, since there is a constant adaptive movement of the teeth in mesio-occlusal direction. These movements are of course, in adaptation to the occlusal or incisal and contact attrition. Occlusion is, therefore, a *dynamic* state.

The normal relations of the two arches in occlusion (Fig. 5-81 to 5-84) are characterized by the maxillary overbite, which is caused by the greater diameter of the upper arch. The incisors and canines of the upper jaw bite labial to the lower teeth; premolars and molars of the upper jaw are shifted buccally to such an extent that the buccal cusps of the lower teeth occlude with the grooves between the buccal and lingual cusps of the upper teeth or, to reverse the description, that the lingual cusps of the upper teeth are in contact with the grooves between the buccal and lingual cusps of the lower teeth.

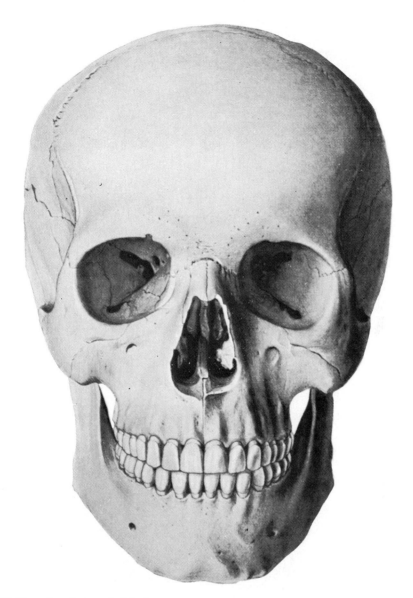

Fig. 5-82. Normal occlusion of adult dentition, anterior view. (Sicher and Tandler: Anatomie für Zahnärzte.)

On the average, the upper incisors cover in occlusion the incisal third of the lower teeth. Distally the overbite decreases and with it also the overjet, that is, the distance between the incisal edge of the lower and the incisal edge of an upper tooth, or the corresponding distance between cusps.

The differences in the mesiodistal diameters of the upper and lower first incisors also cause a distal position of the upper to the lower teeth. The upper first incisor

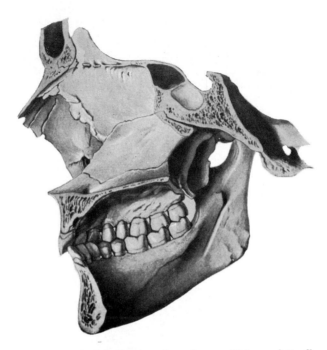

Fig. 5-83. Normal occlusion of adult dentition, lingual view. (Sicher and Tandler: Anatomie für Zahnärzte.)

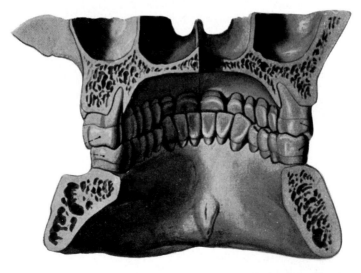

Fig. 5-84. Normal occlusion of adult dentition, posterior view. (Sicher and Tandler: Anatomie für Zahnärzte.)

occludes with the lower first and the mesial half of the lower second incisor. The upper second incisor is in contact with the distal half of the lower second incisor and the mesial half of the lower canine. The upper canine bites distal to the lower canine, occluding with the distal half of the latter and the mesial half of the lower first premolar. The first upper premolar is interposed between the two lower premolars and is in contact with the distal half of the first and the mesial half of the second lower premolar. Its buccal cusp overlaps the buccal cusps of the lower premolars buccally. The distal slope of the first and the mesial slope of the second lower premolar fit into the mesiodistal groove of the upper first premolar. The lingual cusp of the upper first premolar is in contact with the distal occlusal fovea of the first and the mesial occlusal fovea of the second lower premolar, whose lingual cusps protrude lingual to that of the upper first premolar. The upper second premolar is in a similar relation to the lower second premolar and the mesial half of the lower first molar.

The occlusal relations between the molars are variable, depending on the presence or absence of a fifth, or distal, cusp on the lower first molar. It should be remembered that this cusp is situated at the distobuccal circumference of the crown. If a fifth cusp is well developed, the molar relations are as follows: The mesiobuccal cusp of the upper first molar occludes, projecting buccally, with the groove between the mesiobuccal and distobuccal cusp of the lower first molar; the distobuccal cusp of the upper first molar fits into the triangle between the distobuccal and distal cusp of the lower first and the mesiobuccal cusp of the lower second molar. The diamond shape of the occlusal surface of the upper molar causes a distal shift of the mesiolingual cusp compared with the mesiobuccal cusp. The mesiolingual cusp occludes with the central groove between the four main cusps of the lower first molar; the distolingual cusp of the upper first molar is in contact with the distal marginal ridge of the first and the mesial marginal ridge of the second lower molar. The small distal cusp of the lower first molar is in contact with the mesial surface of the distal marginal ridge of the upper first molar.

Similar relations exist between the upper second molar and its antagonists, but the pattern is less complicated because of the more regular shape of the lower second molar.

In a normal dentition the distal overlapping of the upper tooth over the lower is almost evened out at the distal end of the arches by the difference in the mesiodistal diameters of the upper and lower third molars. The greater dimension of the lower wisdom tooth causes the distal surfaces of the upper and lower wisdom teeth to fall almost into the same plane.

And end-to-end bite, rare in young persons, is sometimes established in older persons if the attrition of the teeth is extensive and regular.

The occlusal relations of the temporary dentition (Figs. 5-85 and 5-86) are in principle similar to those of the permanent dentition. It is especially important to note that the difference in mesiodistal dimension of the upper and lower second deciduous molars causes the distal surfaces of the upper and lower second molars to fall into the same frontal plane.

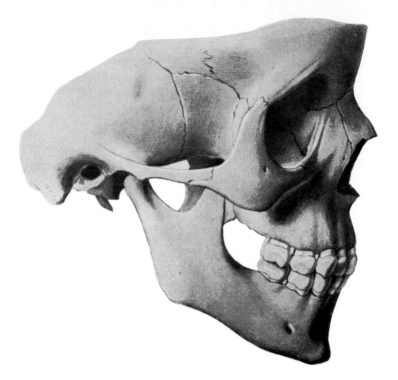

Fig. 5-85. Normal occlusion of deciduous dentition, lateral view. (Sicher and Tandler: Anatomie für Zahnärzte.)

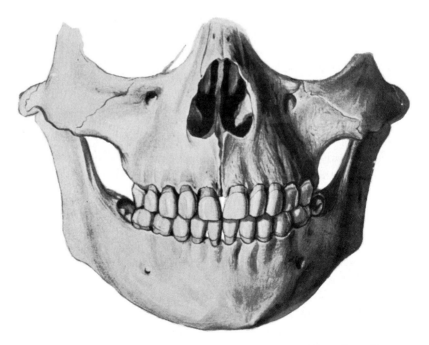

Fig. 5-86. Normal occlusion of deciduous dentition, anterior view. (Sicher and Tandler: Anatomie für Zahnärzte.)

Anomalies of teeth and dentition

The most frequent variations of single teeth have been mentioned earlier in this chapter. They consist in the reduction or loss of some cusps or in the development of supernumerary cusps. The latter may sometimes give rise to isolated supernumerary elements. The next category of dental anomalies is the absence of some teeth or the presence of supernumerary teeth.

Simplification of the pattern of a tooth is mainly restricted to the molars and most frequently observed in the third molar. The lack of some of the typical cusps in such teeth is often combined with a reduction in the number of roots and their size. Supernumerary elements are occasionally found on all teeth. One deals here either with the overdevelopment of a normally inconspicuous part of a tooth or with the appearance of new elements. In the incisors, especially in the upper jaw, and in the canines the dental tubercle on the lingual surface of the tooth can grow to such prominence that the tooth resembles a premolar. A prominent dental or lingual tubercle may be separated from the labial part of the crown by a deep groove that may continue to the root. In extreme cases, grooving of the root leads to the separation of an accessory root and the abnormal tooth appears as if it had formed from fusion of two teeth, one labial and one lingual.

In the molars, and almost exclusively in the second and third molars, a supernumerary cusp may develop on the mesial half of the buccal surface (Fig. 5-87). The relation of this supernumerary cusp to the mesiobuccal cusp of the molar is similar to that between Carabelli's cusp and the mesiolingual cusp of a molar. The buccal supernumerary cusps are called paramolar tubercles and may develop progressively to independent small peglike or irregularly patterned teeth, the paramolars (Fig. 5-88).

The third molar sometimes carries a single or divided tubercle on its distolingual circumference (Figs. 5-88 and 5-89). These tubercles have been called distomolar tubercles. These cusps also are variable in their size and may even separate from the third molar and then represent a distomolar, or fourth molar.

Absence of all the teeth or of some of the teeth has been observed as an isolated anomaly or in combination with other developmental defects. For instance, anodontia, total lack of teeth, is often combined with lack of sweat glands, persistence of the fetal hair, lanugo, and defects of the nails. Such individuals suffer from a generalized deficient development of the ectodermal derivatives, anhidrotic ectodermal dysplasia.

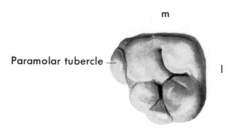

Fig. 5-87. Paramolar tubercle on left lower third molar. (Sicher and Tandler: Anatomie für Zahnärzte.)

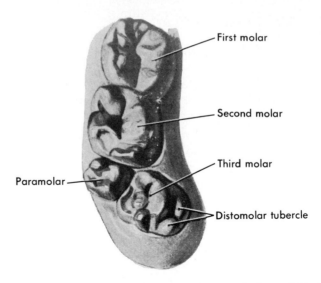

Fig. 5-88. Paramolar tooth and distomolar tubercles in same jaw. (Sicher and Tandler: Anatomie für Zahnärzte.)

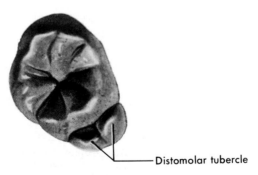

Fig. 5-89. Distomolar tubercle on upper right third molar. (Sicher and Tandler: Anatomie für Zahnärzte.)

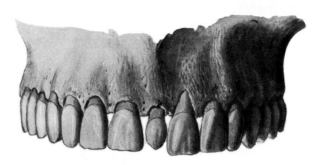

Fig. 5-90. Peg-shaped supernumerary incisor, or mesiodens. (Sicher and Tandler: Anatomie für Zahnärzte.)

Lack of one or of all of the third molars or lack of one or both upper second incisors is frequent. The absence of a permanent second premolar and the retention of the second deciduous molar, sometimes throughout life, is also a typical anomaly of the human dentition.

Supernumerary teeth can be found in any location in the dental arch. Most frequent are supernumerary molars, incisors, and premolars. Much rarer is the presence of a supernumerary canine. It has been mentioned that supernumerary molars may be found in two locations, namely, mesiobuccal to the second and third molars and distal or distolingual to the third molar. For descriptive reasons the terms paramolars for the former and distomolars for the latter are well chosen. Supernumerary molars are either peg-shaped or have a larger crown with an irregular pattern of their cusps. Only rarely does a distomolar, or fourth molar, resemble a normal human molar.

Supernumerary premolars are more often shaped like a normal premolar but sometimes are reduced in size and pattern to a peg-shaped element.

Supernumerary incisors are of three types. The development of a lingual tubercle can progress so far that it becomes separated from the tooth and forms a peg-shaped supernumerary tooth with a thin root, situated, as a rule, lingually and in close proximity to the tooth from which it was derived.

A second type of supernumerary incisor is found at or close to the midline (Fig. 5-90). It may be present on one or on both sides. The supernumerary tooth may be situated between the two central incisors or lingually to these teeth or, rarely, on their labial side. This type of supernumerary incisor has been called a mesiodens because of its position mesial to the first incisor.

Finally, there is a type of supernumerary incisor resulting from a doubling of one incisor, more frequently of the second incisor. Such supernumerary teeth may equal a normal incisor in shape as well as in size or may be reduced to a varying degree.

In the rare instances of a supernumerary canine the abnormal tooth is of canine pattern.

In connection with supernumerary teeth the twinning of teeth has to be mentioned. It should not be confused with the fusion of two neighboring teeth; it is a transitional stage in the development of a supernumerary tooth. The most frequent localization of twinning is the incisal region.

Supernumerary teeth have often been regarded as atavistic, that is, a reversion to an ancestral pattern. For the great majority of supernumerary teeth this explanation does not seem tenable. The appearance of a third premolar or a fourth molar, however, could be considered a remutation.

If one remembers that tooth germs develop and that the pattern of the crown and root is formed by differential growth of the epithelial organ, in other words, by folding and refolding of the derivatives of the oral epithelium, then anomalies of crown pattern and formation of supernumerary cusps and teeth can be understood as consecutive stages of an excessive growth of the epithelial tooth matrix.

Lack of third molars and second incisors is often regarded as pointing to a more

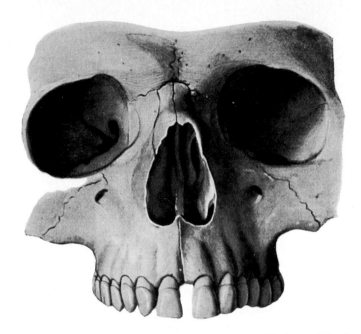

Fig. 5-91. Median diastema, or trema; lateral incisors are missing. (Sicher and Tandler: Anatomie für Zahnärzte.)

reduced dentition of the future human race. Though the mutation leading to the loss of these teeth is in the line of progressive reduction of dentition, so conspicuous in the ancestry of man, the conclusion is not warranted that this new and further reduced type of dentition will sooner or later become characteristic of the entire human species. Since lack of second upper incisors or third molars does not influence selection of a mate, mating occurs at random as far as this physical characteristic is concerned. Under the present nutritional habits of human civilization the reduction of the dentition cannot have and positive survival value, so that no pressure of natural selection will influence the spread of the mutation. If there should not be a considerable increase in the frequency of the mutation or the mutations, leading to loss of second upper incisors and wisdom teeth, this type of the human dentition will, in all probability, remain a variation.

Variations in the position of the teeth that cannot be interpreted as the result of disturbed growth or disturbed harmony in the facial skeleton are mainly the presence of a variably wide space between the first incisors or between upper second incisor and canine. The first type, spacing of the normally closed dental arch in the midline, the median diastema, or trema (Fig. 5-91), is more frequently observed in the upper jaw. The second type, the lateral diastema (Fig. 5-92), is found only in the upper jaw. The median diastema is sometimes combined with lack or a reduction in size of the second incisors. In cases of trema, the superior labial frenum is attached to the free border of the alveolar process, and in the upper jaw it is often continuous with the incisive, or palatine, papilla. The labial frenum then repeats a condition that is normal

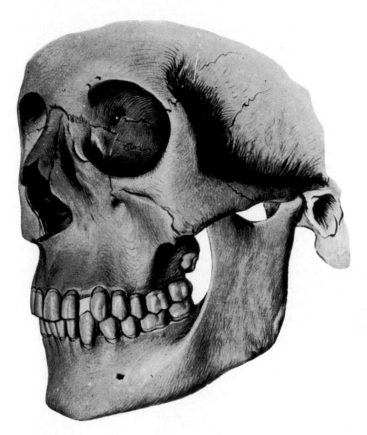

Fig. 5-92. Lateral diastema between lateral incisor and canine. (Sicher and Tandler: Anatomie für Zahnärzte.)

in the fetus and is known as tectolabial frenum. Whether the persistence of tectolabial frenum causes the trema or whether the spacing of the first incisors is primary and the persistence of the fetal relation of the frenum secondary has not yet been decided.

The lateral diastema resembles the relations in anthropoid apes and some fossil specimens of human skulls where the large lower canine necessitates a diastema between the upper second incisor and upper canine. The interpretation of a lateral diastema as a reversion to an ancestral pattern is, despite this resemblance, questionable.

Attrition

Wear of the teeth is, in most mammals, a physiologic and regular occurrence. In fact, the teeth of many species are not well adapted to mastication before attrition has removed the smooth enamel-covered cusps. This is especially apparent in herbivorous animals, cattle, sheep, horses, and many rodents. The attrition of the enamel exposes the dentin, and from then on mastication will wear the different tissues of the tooth to different degrees so that the masticatory surfaces consist of ridges of hard enamel separated by grooves worn in the softer dentin. If cementum participates in the formation of the crown, three tissues of different hardness are present. Regular attrition in modern man can be regarded as an ideal condition that is no longer found as a "normal" occurrence. The human habits of preparing food and the frequent diseases of the teeth contribute to irregularities of attrition. Attrition is not confined to the masticatory surfaces and edges of the teeth but it also occurs at the contact points. Occlusal and incisal attrition are compensated for by the continued vertical component, and contact attrition is compensated for by the mesial component of the mesio-occlusal movements of the teeth. The vertical active eruption in turn is combined with a correlated passive eruption, that is, a progressive exposure of the crown.

Extreme wear, but still within normal limits, leads in some persons to the establishment of an almost horizontal occlusal plane, loss of incisal overbite, and establishment of an edge-to-edge bite (Fig. 5-93). The mechanism of the change from overbite to edge-to-edge bite in severely worn dentitions is not yet understood.

The timing of eruption of the permanent molars in man is responsible for a phenomenon that has been described as "high position" of the first molar. Frequently the apices of the roots of the first molar are found at a more occlusal level than those of the second premolar and second molar. The cause of this irregularity is the early eruption

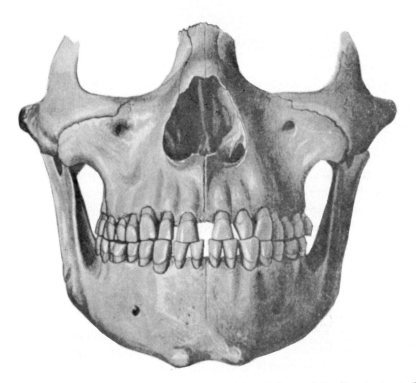

Fig. 5-93. End-to-end bite combined with severe attrition. (Sicher and Tandler: Anatomie für Zahnärzte.)

of the first molar and, therefore, its advanced wear compared with that of the much later erupting neighboring teeth (Figs. 5-94 and 5-95). Because the first molar has lost more substance at the occlusal surface than its neighbors, the first molar has erupted farther than the neighboring teeth.

The interval between the eruption of each molar tooth in man (6 years) is double that of the apes (3 years). Hence the degree of attrition of each tooth is markedly different in hominids (Fig. 5-94) and much less different in pongids. This pattern was genetically established early in the hominid line, as can be clearly seen in the australopithecine fossils (more than 3 million years ago).

The molars, especially the first molars, and sometimes also the premolars, often show an irregular attrition insofar as in the upper jaw the lingual and in the lower jaw the buccal cusps are worn considerably faster (Fig. 5-95). This phenomenon may be favored by the different position of these teeth in the upper and lower jaws, the upper teeth being inclined buccally, the lower lingually.

Normal attrition is accompanied by a progressive retraction of the pulp from the biting surfaces. The formation of secondary and irregular dentin, which causes the retraction, is stimulated by the exposure of dentin and processes of odontoblasts in the dentinal tubules. If attrition occurs abnormally fast, formation of dentin may lag, and exposure of the pulp may be the consequence. Many primitive races of mankind, especially in prehistoric times, suffered from the consequences of abnormal attrition because of the admixture of sand from soft millstones to their food. Though these

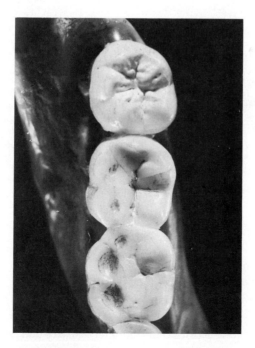

Fig. 5-94. Marked differential in wear of first, second, and third molar teeth.

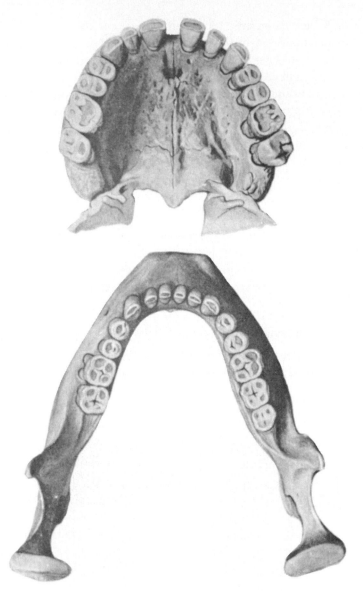

Fig. 5-95. Occlusal views of upper and lower jaws of skull shown in Fig. 5-93. (Sicher and Tandler: Anatomie für Zahnärzte.)

populations were immune to caries or showed a low incidence of caries, the destruction of their dentitions by exposure and infection of the pulp, with all their consequences, was severe. In such dentitions, contact between the teeth of each arch was lost because the crowns were quickly worn to a level cervical to the contact areas. Ensuing food impaction then caused periodontal diseases that added their destructive influence to the ravages of pulp exposure and its consequences.

Despite the claim of some authors that attrition in man is to be considered a pathologic process, it has to be understood that slowly progressing attrition is not only a normal process but, indeed, a process necessary for the total health of the human dentition. To maintain the functional integrity of any tooth, continual cementum apposition is of prime importance. Periodic growth of the cementum, however, needs a gradual widening of the periodontal space that is in turn possible only by continual eruptive movement of the teeth, since widening by resorption is, of course, impossible. Restriction or lack of occlusal attrition might possibly be more damaging to the human dentition if it were not for the *ever-present* contact point attrition.

Correlation of active and passive eruption

Active vertical eruption during the functional period of the tooth, that is, after complete formation of its dentinal root, occurs by a combination of growth of the apical cementum and the alveolar bone at the fundus of the socket. Passive eruption, after full eruption of the anatomic crown, is determined and, in all probability, initiated by the downgrowth of the epithelial attachment along the surface of the root. Correlated to the downgrowth of the epithelium is a peeling off of the epithelium below the gingival sulcus and an atrophy of the marginal gingiva. The downgrowth of the epithelium can occur only when the most cervical principal fibers of the periodontal ligament degenerate and simultaneously detach from the cementum. Whether the fibers detach and degenerate because of the primary degeneration of the cementum or whether the epithelium actively contributes to the dissolution of the fibers is still controversial. The latter concept seems to be better founded biologically because passive eruption is but one phase of tooth eruption as a whole, which, in turn, is the result of processes of growth. To assume that bacterial toxins, diffusing into the tissues from the gingival sulcus, lead to a degeneration of the cementum before the epithelium can proliferate into the depth would introduce a pathologic factor into the mechanism of normal correlated growth. (This should not be interpreted as excluding or ignoring this mechanism in pathologic cases.)

Although the relations between attrition and continuous eruption and between active and passive eruption are obvious and have been recognized as such, no attempt has been made to fit the various known facts into one complete picture. Active eruption during the functional period (after the tooth has reached the occlusal plane) and passive eruption (the age changes of the epithelial attachment occurring at the same time) are generally treated separately. Thus the student receives the impression that there is a progressing exfoliation of the human tooth. The picture is entirely pessimistic and leads to a distorted interpretation of the physiologic changes that can be expected to be useful and adaptive under ideal conditions. The reason for the misconception is twofold: the prevalence of pathologic conditions in man and the lack of close correlation of the observed facts.

From the known facts, the following conclusions can be drawn:
1. Under ideal conditions the attrition on the incisal edges and occlusal surfaces progresses at an even rate of speed.

2. The active eruption of a tooth is, under ideal conditions and after facial growth had ceased, equal to the loss of substance on its occlusal surface; thus the facial height is kept constant.

3. The active eruption is achieved by apposition of cementum at the root apices (and in the furcations) and apposition of bone at the alveolar fundus (and at the crests of interradicular septa). Under ideal conditions the amount of cementum and bone formed is approximately equal.

4. Under ideal conditions apposition of bone at the free borders of the alveolar process is active even in old persons. The amount of bone formed at the alveolar crest seems to be smaller than that at the alveolar fundus.

5. Under ideal conditions the distance between the alveolar crest at any point of the circumference of the tooth and the deepest point of the epithelial attachment is constant, to allow the passage of the gingival and, in the interdental spaces, of the transseptal fibers. The fact that the deepest point of the epithelial attachment is found at about an equal distance from the alveolar crest can also be expressed by stating that the apposition of bone at the alveolar crest checks the downward growth of the epithelial attachment.

6. In ideal cases the length of the epithelial attachment from the gingival sulcus to the deepest point of the epithelium remains constant once the attachment has crossed the cementoenamel junction.

To arrive at a true interpretation of the age changes of the human tooth, all of the preceding points must be considered. Fig. 5-96 summarizes the changes of a tooth and its supporting structures in a buccolingual section through an upper premolar. The right half of the illustration shows the tooth at the beginning of the functional period. The arrow indicates the level to which the crown will be abraded until the stage represented in the left half of the picture is reached. In this later stage attrition has been compensated for by active eruption. Cementum and bone have contributed equally to this movement. At the same time there has been apposition of bone at the alveolar crest, the amount of which has been assumed to be half of that formed at the alveolar fundus. The epithelial attachment has moved onto the cementum from its position on the enamel. The downward growth has been equal to three quarters of the extent of active eruption; thus the distance between the deepest point of the epithelial attachment and the highest point of the alveolar crest has remained constant.

The most important point is that passive eruption under ideal conditions lags behind active eruption. As a consequence, the relation between height of the clinical crown and length of the clinical root changes to the advantage of the root. Since active eruption, compensating for occlusal attrition, occurs only half by an elongation of the root (apposition of cementum), the entire length of the tooth and that of its clinical root have actually been diminished. Shortening of the root, of course, amounts to a decrease in the absolute firmness of the tooth. The loss in firmness is compensated for, however, by the improvement in the leverage of the tooth due to the change in the ratio between clinical crown and clinical root.

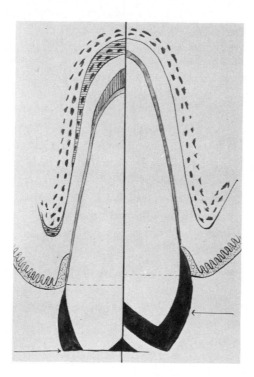

Fig. 5-96. Diagrammatic reconstruction of changes correlated to occlusal attrition. *Horizontal hatching,* newly formed bone; *vertical hatching,* newly formed cementum. Further explanation is included in text. (Weinmann and Sicher: Bone and bones.)

In this light the passive eruption appears to be part of a well, but delicately, balanced mechanism that compensates for the inevitable shortening of the teeth by attrition. Seen in this light, the downgrowth of the epithelium is, under ideal conditions, certainly not to be considered as an attempt of the organism to exfoliate a degenerating tooth.

The maintenance of the balance of active and passive eruption can be said to center in the undisturbed continuous apposition of bone at the alveolar crest.

It has been stressed repeatedly that the changes sketched in the preceding paragraphs occur only under ideal conditions. Such ideal conditions are realized so rarely that they no longer appear to be the "normal" conditions. The reason for this has often been sought in the departure of human living conditions from the "natural" conditions; in other words, in what has been called the self-domestication of man. It is probably the inhibition of bone apposition at the alveolar crest or even the reversal of apposition into degenerative resorption by inflammatory conditions that is responsible for the disturbance of the delicately balanced age changes of the dentition.

Despite the fact that even in "normal" jaws ideal conditions of the human masticatory apparatus are rarely realized, their analysis seems indispensable for a true understanding and evaluation of this complex system of tissues and organs.

One more important aspect of attrition should once more be considered. Cementum, like bone, ages and finally degenerates. In bone this process leads to resorption of the old and its replacement by new bone. In the cementum such turnover is impossible. Instead, the aging cementum is covered by the formation of an additional young layer of cementum. This continuous apposition of new cementum occurs, in all probability, in waves separated by periods of rest. Growth of cementum is evidently indispensable for the integrity of the dentition. Continued growth of the cementum, however, needs space, and space is provided by the continued active eruption of the teeth. The latter, in turn, depends on continued occlusal and incisal wear. Thus attrition as the prerequisite of compensatory active eruption is itself a necessary factor for the health of the teeth. The often-claimed "degeneration" of the dentition of modern man, with its susceptibility to periodontal diseases, may well be caused in part by the common lack of regular attrition.

CHAPTER 6

The oropharyngeal system

The oral apparatus is the "gateway to the gut." As such, it is in unbroken continuity with the pharynx, which funnels directly into the esophagus. The structure of this food channel is complicated by the peculiar crossing of the airway at the larynx. Since the oral apparatus not only prepares food but also initiates swallowing, it is designed to function in close coordination with the pharynx. Furthermore, the oropharyngeal system is tightly integrated in the production of speech. The pharynx and larynx will be described in that order, and then their activities in conjunction with the oral complex will be dealt with in some detail.

PHARYNX

The pharynx (Figs. 6-1 and 6-2) is a funnel-shaped space that is slightly compressed in an anteroposterior direction. Its roof is situated immediately below the cranial base; its inferior end continues into the esophagus. Its posterior wall lies immediately in front of the vertebral bodies; its lateral walls converge downward. The anterior wall is incomplete because, through it, the nasal cavities open into the upper part and the oral cavity into the middle part of the pharynx, whereas from the lower part of the pharynx the entrance into the larynx is accessible. According to the communication with the three cavities the pharynx is arbitrarily divided into a nasal, an oral, and a laryngeal part.

The roof of the pharynx, below the sphenoid and occipital bones, contains the pharyngeal tonsil, an oval body of lymphatic tissue, the surface of which is irregularly grooved by variably deep fissures. Like the other parts of the lymphatic system, for instance palatine and lingual tonsils, the pharyngeal tonsil is rather voluminous in childhood and diminishes in size after puberty, to become atrophic in late adulthood. The posterior wall of the pharynx is smooth, and through it one can palpate the anterior surfaces of the upper four or five cervical vertebrae.

The lateral wall of the superior, or nasal, division of the pharynx contains the opening of the auditory, or Eustachian, tube. The pharyngeal ostium of the tube is situated in the horizontal plane of the attachment of the lower concha to the lateral nasal wall. The cartilage of the tube bulges into the pharyngeal cavity; the bulge, the tubal elevation, or tubal torus, flanks the opening of the tube on its upper and posterior circumference (Fig. 6-1). From the anterior end of this C-shaped prominence a small fold, the salpingopalatine fold, can be followed toward the root of the soft palate.

A much more prominent and sharper fold arises from the posteroinferior end of the tubal torus and continues downward on the lateral wall of the pharynx itself. This fold, the salpingopharyngeal fold, contains the salpingopharyngeus muscle.

Behind the prominence of the cartilage of the tube, a deep and narrow recess of the pharyngeal cavity, the pharyngeal, or Rosenmüller's recess, leads laterally and posteriorly. Its blind end is in relation to the internal carotid artery at its entrance into the carotid canal. Below the opening of the tube and at the root of the soft palate the elevator of the soft palate bulges the mucous membrane to a low, wide ridge, the ridge, or torus, of the levator palati muscle.

The surface of the walls of the oral part of the pharynx is simple. From the soft palate, which marks the boundary between the nasal and oral pharynx, the palato-pharyngeal fold extends downward and slightly backward over the entire height of the oral part and, especially in children, even into the laryngeal part of the pharynx (Fig. 6-2). The fold is elevated by the palatopharyngeus muscle. The anterior wall of the oral pharynx is incomplete; here the communication with the oral cavity, the fauces, the narrowest part of which is the isthmus faucium, is established between the glossopalatine arches. The base of the tongue, with its vertical pharyngeal surface, is

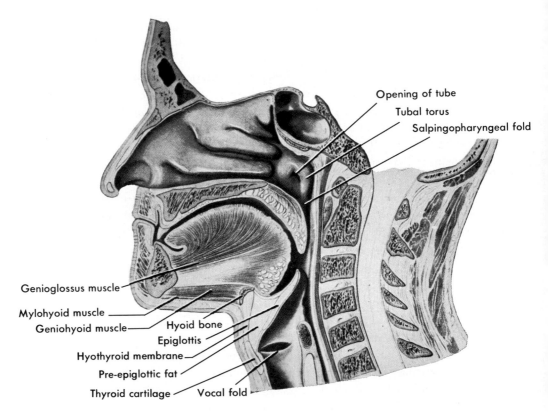

Fig. 6-1. Median section through head and neck of adult. (Sicher and Tandler: Anatomie für Zahnärzte.)

visible below the soft palate if the pharynx is opened from behind (Fig. 6-2) or inspected by the use of a mirror. Posterior to the base of the tongue and separated from it by the epiglottic valleculae, the epiglottis forms the anterior superior boundary of the laryngeal entrance (see Fig. 5-7). From the epiglottis, two folds, the lateral glossoepiglottic folds, one on either side, can be followed laterally to the lateral wall of the base of the tongue. They bound laterally the epiglottic valleculae that are separated from one another by the median glossoepiglottic fold.

The laryngeal part of the pharynx is narrowed by the larynx protruding into its space. The entrance into the larynx, a pear-shaped opening, is in an almost vertical plane. The upper, rounded border is the free protruding border of the epiglottis, the apex of the opening points downward and is situated between the tips of the arytenoid cartilages. The lateral boundaries are two plump and soft folds, the aryepiglottic folds, connecting the epiglottis with the arytenoid cartilages. The protrusion of the laryngeal entrance into the space of the pharynx causes a deep groove on each side, the piriform recess, or piriform sinus, between the aryepiglottic fold and the lateral pharyngeal wall. The recess is accessible from above through the isthmus faucium. At its lower end the piriform recess flattens and leads between the cricoid and thyroid

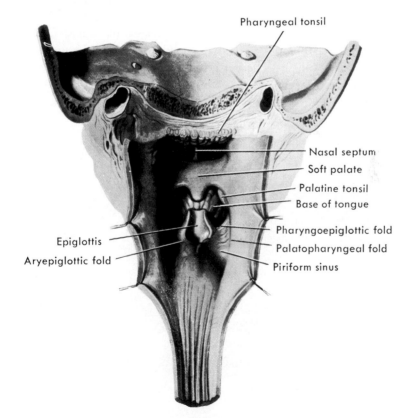

Fig. 6-2. Child's pharynx, exposed and opened from behind. (Pharyngoepiglottic fold is correctly called the lateral glossoepiglottic fold.) (Sicher and Tandler: Anatomie für Zahnärzte.)

plates into the lowest part of the pharynx. An oblique fold in the piriform recess, Hyrtl's fold, owes its existence to the internal branch of the superior laryngeal nerve. Below the piriform recess and the laryngeal prominence the pharyngeal space narrows rather abruptly and continues into the esophagus.

Muscles of the soft palate and pharynx

The muscles of the soft palate and pharynx will be discussed jointly because they are, anatomically and functionally, hardly separable. Anatomically, some of the pharyngeal muscles arise in the soft palate from the tendinous expansion of one of the palatine muscles. Functionally, palatal and pharyngeal muscles act together during deglutition.

MUSCLES OF THE SOFT PALATE

The palatine muscles are (1) the tensor palati muscle, (2) the levator palati muscle, and (3) the uvular muscle.

Tensor palati muscle. This muscle (Figs. 6-3 and 6-17) arises from the greater wing of the sphenoid bone immediately in front of and lateral to the sphenopetrosal fissure, to which the auditory tube is attached, and from the scaphoid fossa at the root of the pterygoid process. Furthermore, the muscle receives fibers from the anterolateral membranous wall of the tube. The tensor palati muscle is flat and occupies the narrow space between the origin of the medial pterygoid muscle and the medial plate of the pterygoid process. Downward, the muscle narrows considerably and continues into a strong tendon just above the level of the pterygoid hamulus. The tendon then winds around the hamulus in the deep notch on its lateral side and bends sharply from a

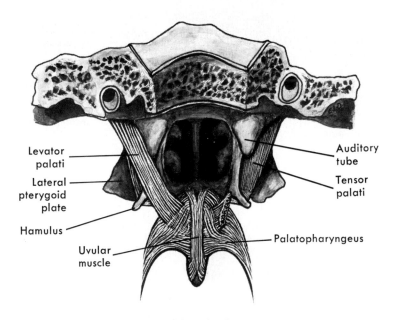

Fig. 6-3. Muscles of the soft palate, posterior view.

vertical into a horizontal plane. Where it curves around the hamulus the muscle is separated from it by a synovial bursa. The horizontal part of the tendon of the tensor palati muscle expands in a fanlike fashion and is known as the palatine aponeurosis. The anterior border of this thin but firm connective tissue plate is attached to the posterior border of the hard palate. Medially, it fuses with the aponeurosis of the other side; the posterior border is not well marked and continues into the connective tissue of the soft palate. The palatine aponeurosis has been termed the fibrous skeleton of the soft palate. This term is well founded because the tendon fulfills two important functions. When the tensor palati muscles contract, the aponeurosis not only becomes taut, but, since the hamular notch is *below* the level of the hard palate, the aponeurosis is *lowered,* causing a downward bulge of the anterior portion of the soft palate. The simultaneous action of the levator palati muscles lifts the posterior part of the soft palate and transforms it into a rigid, S-curved, horizontal plate that effectively seals the oral from the nasal pharynx (see Fig. 6-15, A). Moreover, the palatine aponeurosis serves as the origin for pharyngeal muscles and is, in this sense, a skeletal supplement.

The tensor palati muscle has, however, a functional influence not only on the soft palate, but also on the auditory tube. The fibers that arise from the anterolateral membranous wall of the tube pull this wall away from the cartilaginous posteromedial wall and thus open the tubal canal. In this way, the tensor palati muscle allows a refilling of the tympanic cavity with air and an equalization of the pressure in the middle ear and the outside pressure. This can easily be verified by observing the dull tension in the middle ear that one experiences, for instance, in riding up or down in a fast elevator and its relief during the act of swallowing.

The motor nerve supply of the tensor palati muscle is provided by the mandibular nerve, the third division of the trigeminal nerve.

Levator palati muscle. This muscle (Fig. 6-3) arises from the lower surface of the apical part of the petrosal bone anteromedial to the entrance into the carotid canal and posteromedial to the cartilaginous wall of the tube from which some fibers of this muscle arise. The muscle, in cross section almost circular, runs downward, medially, and forward and enters the soft palate just below the pharyngeal orifice of the auditory tube. It is here that the belly of the muscle creates the ridge of the levator palati. In the palate the levator muscle is situated above and slightly behind the palatine aponeurosis, the tendon of the tensor palati muscles. Toward the midline the levator spreads slightly and flattens; its divergent bundles interlace with those of the contralateral muscle. Thus the two muscles form a sling in the movable part of the soft palate, at a considerable distance behind the posterior end of the hard palate.

The action of the levator palati muscles is to elevate the almost vertical posterior part of the soft palate into a horizontal position and to pull it slightly backward. In this position the soft palate is made rigid by the simultaneous action of the tensor muscles, and, touching the posterior wall of the pharynx, the soft palate closes the oral from the nasal pharynx. The levator muscle has no influence on the auditory tube.

The levator palati muscle is supplied by a branch of the vagus nerve via the pharyngeal plexus.

Muscle of the uvula. The uvular muscle is apparently a paired structure, the two sides being separated at their origins and terminations at the uvular tip. The uvular muscle can be separated only arbitrarily along most of its length (Fig. 6-3). The fibers arise from the dorsal surface of the palatine aponeurosis, run the length of the soft palate, and insert under the mucous membrane of the pendant elongate uvula. Upon contraction, the muscle shortens and thickens the uvular mass. With the contraction of the palatopharyngeal sphincter in closing off the nasal space when swallowing, the uvula is pulled up to complete the seal like a cork in a bottle (see Fig. 6-15, A).

MUSCLES OF THE PHARYNX

Three of the pharyngeal muscles can be compared with the circular muscles of the digestive canal and are known as the constrictors of the pharynx. Two other muscles are longitudinally arranged. They are the stylopharyngeus, which broadens the pharyngeal space, and palatopharyngeus muscles. A part of the latter is designated as the

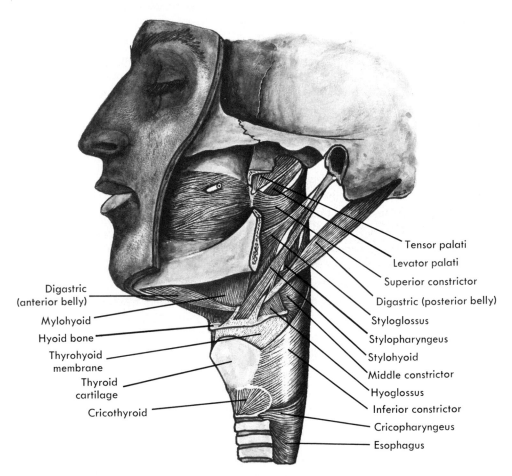

Digastric (anterior belly)
Mylohyoid
Hyoid bone
Thyrohyoid membrane
Thyroid cartilage
Cricothyroid

Tensor palati
Levator palati
Superior constrictor
Digastric (posterior belly)
Styloglossus
Stylopharyngeus
Stylohyoid
Middle constrictor
Hyoglossus
Inferior constrictor
Cricopharyngeus
Esophagus

Fig. 6-4. Muscles of the pharynx, lateral view. The ramus of the mandible and the lower part of the lateral pterygoid plate have been cut away.

salpingopharyngeus muscle. The last muscle of this group, forming the substance of the palatoglossal arch, the palatoglossus muscle, is described by some authors as a pharyngeal muscle, by others as a palatine muscle, and by others as a muscle of the tongue. A controversy on this point seems futile.

Pharyngeal constrictors. These three muscles (Figs. 6-4 and 6-5) arise on each side in a broken line that begins at the medial plate of the pterygoid process and ends on the cricoid cartilage of the larynx. Their relations are well expressed in the old terms: cephalopharyngeus muscle for the superior constrictor because of its origin in the head; hyopharyngeus muscle for the middle constrictor, which arises from the hyoid bone; and the laryngopharyngeus muscle for the inferior constrictor, whose origin is confined to the larynx. The muscle fibers on either side surround the lateral and posterior walls of the pharynx and join the corresponding fibers of the other side in a tendinous strip, the pharyngeal raphe, which runs in the midline of the posterior wall from the pharyngeal tubercle of the occipital bone throughout the entire length of the

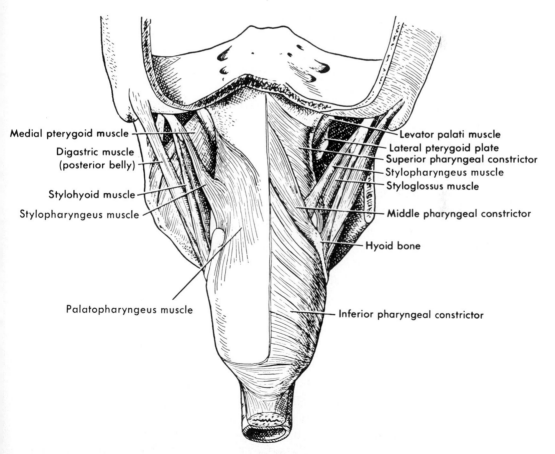

Fig. 6-5. Muscles of the pharynx, posterior view. The constrictors have been removed on the left side of the specimen. (Modified and redrawn from Sicher and Tandler: Anatomie für Zahnärzte.)

pharynx. The fibers of the constrictors overlap so that in a posterior view the middle constrictor covers part of the superior constrictor and is, itself, partly covered by fibers of the inferior constrictor.

The superior constrictor of the pharynx can, according to its origin, be separated into four subdivisions. The uppermost fibers arise from the lower third or fourth of the medial pterygoid plate at its posterior border, from the small ligament that bridges the hamular notch, and from the tip of the hamulus itself. This part of the muscle is designated the pterygopharyngeus muscle. The next section of the upper constrictor takes its origin from the pterygomandibular raphe (Fig. 6-4), the tendinous band stretching from the tip of the pterygoid hamulus to the retromolar triangle of the mandible. Since, anteriorly, fibers of the buccinator muscle arise from the raphe, the second part of the upper constrictor is called the buccopharyngeus muscle.

The third part of the superior constrictor is the mylopharyngeus muscle. Its name indicates its origin from the lower jaw. However, the muscle fibers themselves do not originate from the bone but arise from the membranous floor of the oral cavity and are, by the intervention of this membrane, indirectly attached to the mandible.

The fourth (lowest) part of the superior constrictor consists of a variable number of muscle bundles that are the continuation of some longitudinal and transverse fibers of the tongue. This part of the superior constrictor is, therefore, designated the glossopharyngeus muscle.

The most superior fibers of the superior constrictor ascend from the lower part of the pterygoid plate in superiorly concave curves toward the pharyngeal tubercle. Because of this arrangement an area of the lateral and posterior pharyngeal walls immediately below the base of the skull lacks a muscular coat. The wall of the pharynx is here formed by a connective tissue membrane only, the pharyngobasilar, or craniopharyngeal, membrane, which is lined on the inside by the mucous membrane. The membranous wall of the pharynx corresponds to the uppermost part of the nasopharynx, which serves as an air passage and does not change its lumen.

The levator palati muscle enters the pharyngeal space above the superior constrictor to proceed into the soft palate, which it reaches at its lateral root. The flat muscle belly of the tensor palati is also situated outside the pharynx. Its tendon enters the pharynx and the soft palate by passing through the small opening between the hamular notch and its bridging ligament.

The origin of the middle constrictor is from the hyoid bone and often from the adjacent stylohoid ligament. The muscle consists of two parts: the fibers that arise from the greater horn are designated the ceratopharyngeus muscle; the other, the chondropharyngeus muscle, takes its origin from the lesser horn of the hyoid bone. It is sometimes reduced to a few bundles.

The fibers of the middle constrictor of the pharynx diverge from their origin so that the uppermost fibers course steeply upward, whereas the lowermost fibers descend toward the midline. Thus muscles of the two sides form a large diamond-shaped plate. The upper part of it covers the lower part of the superior constrictor, and the upper point of the diamond is found not far below the occipital bone. The lower part of the middle constrictor is, in turn, covered by the inferior constrictor. Between the superior and middle constrictors there is, on the lateral wall of the pharynx, a distinct cleft that is used by the stylopharyngeus muscle to gain entrance into the pharynx.

The lower constrictor of the pharynx originates from the skeleton of the larynx. Its upper part, the thyropharyngeus muscle, originates from the oblique line of the thyroid cartilage; the lower part, the cricopharyngeus muscle, arises from the lateral circumference of the cricoid cartilage. The uppermost fibers turn obliquely upward, thus covering the lower parts of the middle constrictor. Most of the lower fibers are horizontal; the most inferior fibers descend slightly. The inferior constrictor is continuous downward with the striated circular musculature of the upper part of the esophagus.

The action of the constrictor muscles is the narrowing of the pharyngeal space. In deglutition, the contraction simulates a peristaltic wave, that is, a successive contraction of the fibers from above downward. The act of swallowing can be initiated voluntarily but, once started, it rolls off automatically.

The nerve supply to the pharyngeal constrictors is provided by the pharyngeal plexus, to which the glossopharyngeal and vagus nerves contribute branches.

Stylopharyngeus muscle. This muscle (Fig. 6-5) is a longitudinal muscle that widens the pharynx. Like the other longitudinal muscles, it spreads its fibers on the inside of the constrictors, between the latter and the mucous membrane. It originates from the posteroinferior surface of the styloid process. The slender muscle runs downward and medially and reaches the lateral pharyngeal wall between the upper and middle pharyngeal constrictors. After passing between these muscles, the bundles of the stylopharyngeus muscle continue downward on the inner side of the middle constrictor, diverge in their course downward, and extend over the lateral and posterior walls of the lower half of the pharynx.

The stylopharyngeus muscle is supplied by a branch of the glossopharyngeal nerve.

Palatopharyngeus muscle. This muscle (Fig. 6-6) is the second longitudinal muscle of the pharynx. Its origin in the palate extends from the midline to the lateral wall of the pharynx. The most medial fibers arise from the upper surface of the palatine aponeurosis at and behind the posterior nasal spine. Following the line of origin laterally, the bundles of the palatopharyngeus muscle arise from the palatine aponeurosis at some distance from the posterior border of the hard palate. The most lateral fibers arise in the neighborhood of the pterygoid hamulus and, finally, from the cartilage of the auditory tube. The bundles arising from the tubal cartilage constitute the salpingopharyngeus muscle. Laterally and downward the fibers of the palatopharyngeus muscle converge in the palatopharyngeal fold and then spread in the lateral pharyngeal wall, forming part of the longitudinal inner muscular layer of the lower half of the pharynx, anterior to the fibers of the stylopharyngeus muscle.

The most posterior fibers of the palatopharyngeus muscle reach the midline,

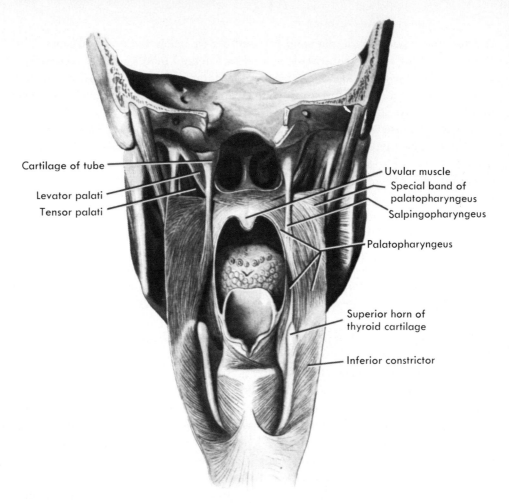

Cartilage of tube

Levator palati

Tensor palati

Uvular muscle

Special band of
palatopharyngeus

Salpingopharyngeus

Palatopharyngeus

Superior horn of
thyroid cartilage

Inferior constrictor

Fig. 6-6. Longitudinal muscles of the pharynx dissected from within; the pharynx has been opened from behind. (Sicher and Tandler: Anatomie für Zahnärzte.)

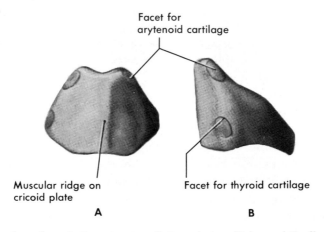

Facet for
arytenoid cartilage

Muscular ridge on
cricoid plate

Facet for thyroid cartilage

A

B

Fig. 6-7. Cricoid cartilage. **A,** Posterior view. **B,** Lateral view. (Sicher and Tandler: Anatomie für Zahnärzte.)

where they are attached to the pharyngeal raphe. The lateral fibers end in the mucous membrane of the lateral wall of the pharynx; some of the anteriormost fibers may find an attachment on the upper horn and the posterior border of the thyroid cartilage.

The palatopharyngeus muscle is supplied by the pharyngeal plexus.

Palatoglossus muscle. See Chapter 5, p. 225 and Figs. 6-16 and 6-17.

LARYNX

The larynx, as the entrance to the deeper air passages, serves mainly as a valve for the protection of the lung. At the same time it is able to produce vocalization. It is accessible from the inferior part of the pharynx and continues into the trachea. It has its own skeleton consisting of cartilage. The single cartilaginous parts are movably linked together, partly by ligaments, partly by true joints. A series of muscles serves the coarser and finer adjustment of the laryngeal spaces.

The major laryngeal cartilages are the unpaired cricoid cartilage, thyroid cartilage, epiglottic cartilage, and the paired arytenoid cartilages. The cricoid cartilage consists of hyaline cartilage only, and the thyroid cartilage consists of two symmetrical plates of hyaline cartilage joined by a narrow median strip of elastic cartilage. The epiglottis is formed of elastic cartilage. The main body of the paired arytenoid cartilage is composed of hyaline cartilage, its vocal process of elastic cartilage.

The *cricoid cartilage* (Fig. 6-7) resembles a signet ring. The narrow part of the ring, the cricoid arch, faces anteriorly; the wide plate, the cricoid lamina, faces posteriorly. The lamina carries a median vertical crest. At the upper corners of the plate an oval articulating facet serves as the articulation with the arytenoid cartilage on either side. Below this facet and close to the lower border of the cartilage, a smaller,

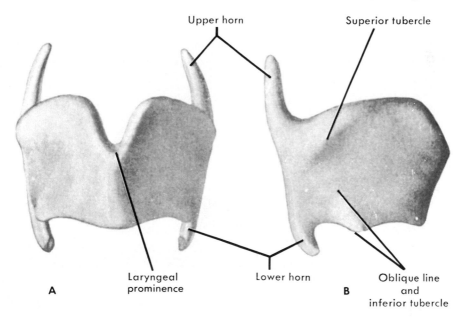

Fig. 6-8. Thyroid cartilage. **A,** Anterior view. **B,** Lateral view. (Sicher and Tandler: Anatomie für Zahnärzte.)

more circular facet serves as the junction with the lower horn of the thyroid cartilage.

The *thyroid cartilage* (Fig. 6-8) consists of two roughly rectangular plates, which are joined in an angle at the midline. The posterior border of each plate extends superiorly into the longer superior horn, inferiorly into the shorter inferior horn. The latter articulates with the lower facet on the cricoid cartilage. The outer surface of the thyroid plate is traversed by a muscular crest, the oblique line. The upper border of the thyroid cartilage is notched in the midline by the thyroid notch, below which the laryngeal prominence protrudes. This prominence is far more pronounced in the male and is colloquially known as the Adam's apple. The female thyroid cartilage differs from the male in two respects: the angle between the right and left plates is wider in the female, and a strong laryngeal prominence is lacking.

The *arytenoid cartilage* (Fig. 6-9) is a small, irregular three-sided pyramid. The base carries the concave articular surface for articulation with the cricoid cartilage; the posterior surface is slightly concave, and the medial surface is flat. The third side of the pyramid faces anterolaterally and is excavated by a shallower inferior and a deeper superior fovea. The former serves as the attachment of muscles, the latter contains aggregated glands. The anteroinferior corner of the arytenoid cartilage extends into the slender and pointed vocal process; the posteroinferior corner protrudes laterally and posteriorly as the plump and short muscular process. To the apex of the arytenoid cartilage is joined a small elastic cartilage, the *corniculate cartilage* of Santorini.

The *epiglottic cartilage* (Fig. 6-10) is a thin, spoon-shaped elastic cartilage. The short handle of the spoon, the petiolus, extends inferiorly. The epiglottic cartilage is concave posteriorly in transverse direction. In longitudinal direction, however, it is doubly curved; its upper part is posteriorly concave, and its lower part is posteriorly convex. The convexity protrudes as the epiglottic tubercle.

The parts of the cartilages that consist of hyaline cartilage calcify with advancing age and later are replaced by bone. The ossification occurs in women at a much later age than in men.

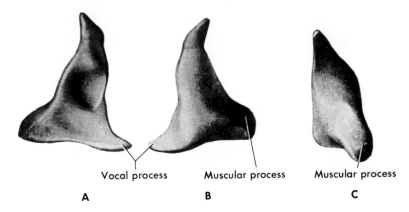

Vocal process   Muscular process   Muscular process

A   **B**   **C**

Fig. 6-9. Arytenoid cartilage, greatly enlarged. **A,** Lateral view. **B,** Mesial view. **C,** Posterior view. (Sicher and Tandler: Anatomie für Zahnärzte.)

The laryngeal cartilages are partly connected by ligaments and partly joined to each other by true articulations. The laryngeal skeleton is suspended from the hyoid bone by the thyrohyoid membrane; inferiorly the larynx is connected with the trachea (see Fig. 3-11).

The paired cricothyroid articulation permits a hingelike rotation of the cricoid cartilage around a transverse axis. The cricoarytenoid articulation permits rather extensive movements of the arytenoid cartilage. In a sliding movement the two cartilages can approximate each other or move away from each other. Moreover, the arytenoid cartilage can rotate around a vertical axis. In rotating, the vocal process and the muscular process move in opposite directions. If the muscular process is pulled medially, the vocal process deviates laterally and vice versa.

The stalk of the epiglottic cartilage is joined to the inner surface of the thyroid cartilage just below the thyroid notch by the thyroepiglottic ligament. A second ligament, the hyoepiglottic ligament, binds the anterior surface of the epiglottis to the posterior surface of the body of the hyoid bone.

The thyrohyoid membrane connecting the thyroid cartilage with the hyoid bone is attached to the upper border of the thyroid cartilage and to the tips of the upper horns. The middle part and the lateral edges of the membrane are strengthened to form middle and lateral thyrohyoid ligaments. A small accessory cartilage, the cartilago triticea, is enclosed in the lateral ligament.

In the lower parts of the larnyx, the submucous layer is developed to a firm elastic membrane, the elastic cone. It commences at the inner surface of the cricoid cartilage and extends from its upper border as a medially inclined membrane that ends with a free strengthened edge, the vocal ligament. The latter is attached posteriorly to the vocal process of the arytenoid cartilage and anteriorly to the inner surface of the thyroid cartilage close to the midline. The anterior part of the elastic cone is visible in

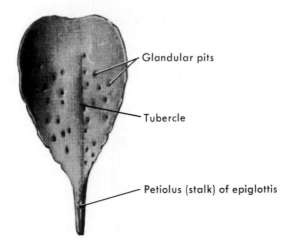

Glandular pits

Tubercle

Petiolus (stalk) of epiglottis

Fig. 6-10. Epiglottic cartilage. (Sicher and Tandler: Anatomie für Zahnärzte.)

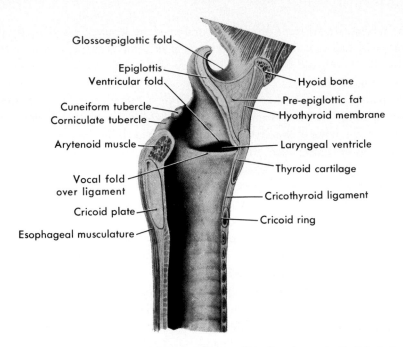

Fig. 6-11. Median section through larynx. (Sicher and Tandler: Anatomie für Zahnärzte.)

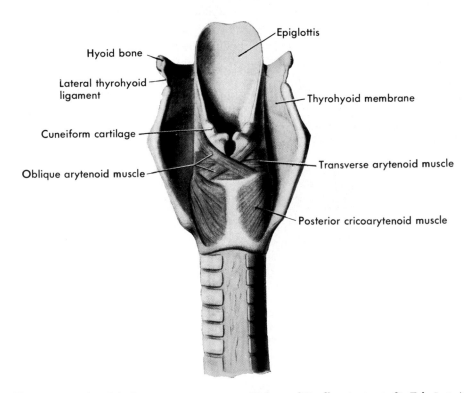

Fig. 6-12. Muscles of the larynx in posterior view. (Sicher and Tandler: Anatomie für Zahnärzte.)

front, between the thyroid and cricoid cartilages, and is called the cricothyroid, or conic, ligament (Fig. 6-11).

The muscles that move the cartilages of the larynx (Figs. 6-12 and 6-13) can be subdivided into an extrinsic and an intrinsic group. The muscles of the first group connect the thyroid cartilage with the hyoid bone above and with the sternum below (pp. 159-161). Most of the intrinsic muscles of the larynx are attached to the arytenoid cartilages. Their main function is to change the shape and tension of the vocal ligaments and folds and the width and shape of the glottis, the gap between the vocal folds.

The *cricothyroid muscle* (see Figs. 3-11 and 3-12) arises from the lower border and the inferior horn of the thyroid cartilage and from the inner surface of this cartilage close to the inferior border and inserts on the anterior surface of the cricoid cartilage. A triangular space between the two muscles has its base above and its apex below. The floor of this triangular depression is formed by the cricothyroid, or conic, ligament. The cricothyroid muscles lift the anterior part of the cricoid cartilage toward the thyroid cartilage. In this movement the cricoid cartilage rotates around a transverse axis running through the cricothyroid articulations. In so doing, the upper border of the cricoid plate swings posteriorly and carries with it the arytenoid cartilages, which are joined to the upper corners of the cricoid plate and are held by the cricoarytenoid muscles. Thus the distance between the arytenoid cartilages and the

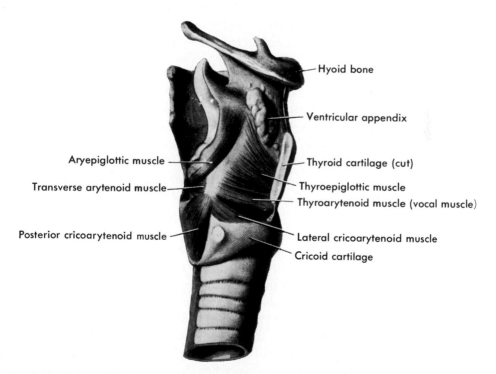

Hyoid bone

Ventricular appendix

Aryepiglottic muscle

Transverse arytenoid muscle

Posterior cricoarytenoid muscle

Thyroid cartilage (cut)

Thyroepiglottic muscle

Thyroarytenoid muscle (vocal muscle)

Lateral cricoarytenoid muscle

Cricoid cartilage

Fig. 6-13. Muscles of the larynx in lateral view after removal of the right half of the thyroid cartilage. (Sicher and Tandler: Anatomie für Zahnärzte.)

angle of the thyroid cartilage is increased, and the vocal ligaments extending between these cartilages are stretched and made tense. The muscle can be called the coarse adjustor of the vocal ligaments. Its action is preparatory to vocalization. The crico-thyroid muscle is supplied by the external branch of the superior laryngeal nerve.

There are two *cricoarytenoid muscles* on either side. The posterior cricoarytenoid muscle (Fig. 6-12) arises from the posterior surface of the cricoid plate, and its fibers converge superiorly and laterally to attach to the muscular process of the arytenoid cartilage. The lateral cricoarytenoid muscle (Fig. 6-13) arises from the upper border and the lateral surface of the cricoid cartilage and runs to the muscular process of the arytenoid cartilage in a posterosuperior direction. These two muscles are rotators of the arytenoid cartilage. The posterior cricoarytenoid muscles pull the muscular pro-cesses backward and inward so that the vocal processes of the arytenoid cartilages rotate laterally. Thus the slit between the two vocal folds, the glottis, is opened and widened. The lateral cricoarytenoid muscles pull the muscular processes forward and outward; the vocal processes then rotate medially, and the glottis is narrowed or closed. (For details see section on swallowing.)

The *arytenoid*, or *interarytenoid*, *muscle* (Fig. 6-12) consists of transverse and oblique fibers. The transverse fibers connect the posterior surfaces of the arytenoid cartilages horizontally. The oblique fibers are superficial and arise from the base of the muscular process on one side and ascend to the apex of the arytenoid cartilage of the other side. Some of the fibers continue in the aryepiglottic fold to reach the lateral border of the epiglottis. The interarytenoid muscle pulls the arytenoid cartilages toward the midline and toward each other. It is a closer of the glottis. All the muscles act as a group.

The *thyroarytenoid muscle* (Figs. 6-13 and 6-14) is incompletely divided into an outer and an inner part. The latter forms the substrate of the vocal fold. The muscle arises from the inner surface of the thyroid cartilage close to the midline and down to its lower border and is inserted on the vocal process and the lower part of the lateral surface of the arytenoid cartilage. In frontal section the muscle is triangular (Fig. 6-14). The outer surface is vertical, the upper surface is horizontal, and the third surface faces obliquely downward and inward. The inner edge of the muscle, at the level of its upper surface, juts into the laryngeal space and thus forms the substance of the vocal fold. The thyroarytenoid muscle serves as the fine adjustor of the vocal fold and ligament by changing its shape and tension. Because of the importance of the thyroarytenoid muscle for vocalization, it also has been called the vocal muscle.

All the intrinsic muscles of the larynx, with the exception of the cricothyroid muscle, are supplied by the inferior or recurrent laryngeal nerve. It should be under-stood that in vocalization or singing all of these muscles operate in a delicate bal-ance.

The laryngeal space is accessible from the pharynx through the laryngeal entrance, or laryngeal aditus. The plane of this opening is almost vertical and steeply inclined posteriorly and inferiorly. The entrance into the larynx is bounded anteriorly by the upper edge of the epiglottis and laterally by the plump aryepiglottic folds,

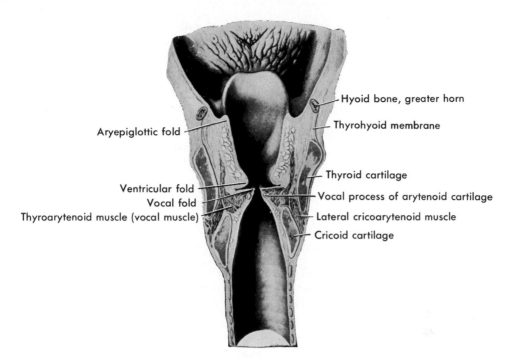

Fig. 6-14. Frontal section through the larynx. (Sicher and Tandler: Anatomie für Zahnärzte.)

connecting the epiglottis with the apex of the arytenoid cartilage (see Figs. 5-7 and 6-11). The posteroinferior end of this fold is slightly elevated by the corniculate cartilage. Above the corniculate tubercle, a second prominence is caused by the enclosure of another small accessory cartilage, the cuneiform cartilage (Fig. 6-11). Between the apices of the arytenoid cartilages, the border of the laryngeal aditus forms the shallow and narrow interarytenoid notch.

The laryngeal space is divided into three compartments by two folds protruding on each side from the lateral wall of the larynx (Figs. 6-11 and 6-14). The superior ventricular fold, sometimes called the false vocal fold, is loose and plump, its edge rounded. Below the ventricular fold, the vocal fold protrudes as a firm fold with a sharp edge (Fig. 6-14). Its upper surface is horizontal; its lower surface slopes downward and outward.

The ventricular fold contains loose connective tissue and mucous glands. The substance of the vocal fold is formed by the thyroarytenoid, or vocal muscle; its edge contains in its posterior part the tip of the vocal process of the arytenoid cartilage; in its longer anterior part it contains the elastic vocal ligament.

The upper laryngeal space, the laryngeal vestibule, is situated above the ventricular folds. Its anterior wall, formed by the epiglottis, is high; its posterior wall, formed by the upper parts of the arytenoid cartilages, is low. The lateral walls of the vestibule are the aryepiglottic folds.

The middle laryngeal space, the laryngeal ventricle, is narrow, extending from the level of the vestibular to that of the vocal folds. Laterally it extends between the two folds to the inner surface of the thyroid cartilage. It continues anteriorly into a variably large ventricular pouch, a vestige of the resonating sound pouch, so prominent in some monkeys and apes, such as the orangutan.

The middle laryngeal space communicates with the lower, infraglottic laryngeal space through the glottis, the slit between the two vocal folds, which is the narrowest point of the larynx. The lower laryngeal space widens gradually inferiorly and continues without sharp boundary into the lumen of the trachea. Its anterior wall is the cricothyroid, or conic, ligament; through this superficially located ligament the lower laryngeal space can be entered surgically.

The relations of the larynx to the tongue on one side and to the pharynx on the other, although already mentioned, merit once more a short description. Between the base of the tongue and the anterior surface of the epiglottis are located the paired depressions called the epiglottic valleculae. Cricoid plate and arytenoid cartilages with their muscles, and epiglottis with the aryepiglottic folds, protrude into the lumen of the pharynx, and the lateral wall of the pharynx is situated in the plane of the thyroid cartilage. Between thyroid cartilage laterally, and cricoid cartilage and aryepiglottic folds medially, there is on either side a deep recess, the piriform sinus, or piriform recess, of the pharynx. Its lateral wall is formed by the thyroid cartilage and the thyrohyoid membrane, and its medial wall is formed by the lateral surface of the cricoid and arytenoid cartilages and the aryepiglottic fold (Figs. 6-2 and 6-12).

The mucous membrane of the larynx is covered by a stratified or pseudostratified ciliated columnar epithelium. It is replaced by stratified squamous epithelium only at the sharp edge of the vocal fold. The structure of the submucosa that attaches the mucous membrane to the underlying structures is of great clinical importance. The mucous membrane is tightly bound to the posterior surface of the epiglottis, the vocal folds, and to the elastic cone in the infraglottic laryngeal space. In all other areas the mucous membrane is loosely attached to the deeper structures by a variably thick, loosely textured submucosa.

The submucous layer is especially voluminous in the aryepiglottic and ventricular folds. From the laryngeal entrance the loose submucosa extends into the epiglottic valleculae and from there into the palatine arches. Where the submucosa is loosely textured, in other words, where the mucous membrane is loosely attached, edematous fluid can accumulate and lead to a considerable swelling. An edema of the laryngeal and perilaryngeal submucosa is known as glottis edema. This term is misleading because the area of the glottis itself, that is, the vocal folds, remains practically free of edema, since the mucous membrane in this zone is tightly attached and a submucous layer is not only reduced in width but is also densely textured (see Chapter 15).

MECHANISMS OF THE SYSTEM

The human oral apparatus is a special complex built to perform two crucial functions, one of which is peculiar to man. It is a food processing device in feeding and a major part of a sound processing device in the specific form of communication called speech.

Swallowing

For feeding, three essential features have been incorporated into local design: an input device, a processing mechanism, and an output device. Thus three separate performances can be distinguished in normal feeding: movements of taking food into the mouth, movements for the preparation of the bolus, and movements of swallowing. These activities are so integrated, however, as to overlap within the oral cavity. Movements for taking food into the mouth depend on the consistency of the food. Liquids are brought in by sucking, which is separable into infantile suckling and adult drinking. Solids are pulled in by plucking from fingers or feeding utensils. Since little preparation is needed for the passing of liquids through the oral cavity, the processing activities for liquids and solids are different. Swallowing activities for liquids and solids also show differences and swallowing behavior is further influenced by the size of the bolus. The conspicuous feature of the entire swallowing system is the extraordinary crossing of air and food channels. Around this critical location precisely timed valvular devices have been installed (see Figs. 6-1 and 6-17).

Normally the act of swallowing moves a bolus from the front of the mouth to the esophagus in a swift, distinctive pattern of smooth flow interrupted by intervals of momentary hesitation at security checkpoints along the food channel. Swallowing is begun by voluntary movements that manipulate the food in the oral cavity back to the entrance of the pharynx at the palatoglossal arches (anterior pillars of the fauces). From this exit onward the activity is involuntary. The consistently observed sequences for normal swallowing will be described for liquids, first in the suckling of nursing infants and next for drinking in adults. Finally, the more complicated swallowing of solid foods will be analyzed in greater detail.

SUCKLING

The nursing infant first takes the nipple into the mouth by sucking, which elongates it and includes part of the areola. The neck of the nipple is held firmly between the upper gum above and the tip of the tongue resting on the gum pad of the lower jaw below. The pursed lips seal the oral cavity against the areola in front. The orifices of the nipple are held near the junction of hard and soft palates. The oral cavity is closed behind by the soft palate, which is drawn forward in tense, close apposition with the base of the tongue. Food is taken in by lowering the jaw, which creates a further negative pressure to fill the nipple and elongate it to about three times its resting length. The jaw is then moved upward and forward so that the neck of the nipple is pinched to about half its normal width between the upper gum and the tongue tip backed by the lower jaw.

In swallowing, the tongue, beginning at the tip, is pressed along the nipple from before backward to squeeze the milk into the grooved midline portion of the dorsum of the tongue. Tongue base and soft palate then separate to move the milk bolus down the increasingly slanting tongue base in the direction of the pharynx. The fluid is momentarily checked at the anterior pillars of the fauces to allow the back of the soft palate to rise and press firmly against the spongy adenoidal pad at the roof and posterior wall of the pharynx. The upper posterior wall of the pharynx above moves forward toward the base of the tongue, and together they squeeze the bolus down from the back of the mouth. At the same time the larynx is raised and arched backward. The epiglottis is turned back, the glottis is closed, and the lower food channels are opened. The fluid is expressed from the pharynx by a peristaltic wave of the pharyngeal walls beginning against the tongue base above. The fluid then clears the pharynx along the lateral food channels below the tonsils, after which the streams join to enter the esophagus. Apparently the spongy consistency of adenoidal and tonsillar pads has a distinct biomechanical function in feeding in infants. As soon as the last of the bolus has passed into the esophagus, the airway is opened and the sequence is repeated until feeding is finished. It is obvious that design and construction of artificial devices, such as bottle feeders, to substitute for normal breast feeding, must depend wholly on an understanding of normal suckling mechanisms.

DRINKING

The adult takes liquid into the mouth first by gripping the lower edge of the container with protruded lips. The cup is then tilted until the fluid reaches the lips with the upper lip rim below liquid level. At this time the dorsum of the tongue rests against hard and soft palates to obliterate the oral cavity. The bolus is sucked into the mouth by withdrawing the tongue from the palate from before backward as the jaw is lowered, which creates the negative pressure that pulls in the liquid. Spill over the back and sides of the tongue is prevented by close contact of the base of the tongue with the forwardly bulged soft palate and by contact of the sides of the tongue with the upper teeth and gums. This contact continues back across the junction of the buccinator and the pharyngeal sphincter at the raphe and along the isthmus of the fauces from anterior to posterior pillars. When the mouth is full the fluid is trapped fore-and-aft in a hollow caused by the vertically raised tongue tip against the alveolar ridge in front and the raised tongue base behind.

Swallowing begins by increasing the palatal contact of the tongue from before backward as the back of the tongue is lowered in the same sequence. This is exactly the reverse of the wave of movement used to draw the fluid into the mouth. The mandible has risen into occlusion, which establishes a fixed base from which the muscles anchored to the body of the jaw can work. When the moving front of the bolus reaches the back of the mouth, it is held up momentarily at the anterior faucial pillars while the soft palate shortens, thickens, and rises toward the posterior pharyngeal wall. In being pulled up and back the palate is bent sharply by the tug of the transversely interlacing fibers of the opposite levator palati muscles (Fig. 6-15, A). At this instant the pharynx and soft palate close as a sphincter to shut off the nasal channel above. When the bolus has passed the pillars, the mouth is shut off by sphincteric contraction of the palatoglossus muscles, which constricts the oral outlet considerably. The remaining gap is finally plugged by the backwardly jammed base of the tongue. The entire activity thus far has been impelled by the wave along the dorsum of the tongue, which has swept the fluid backward toward the cataract down

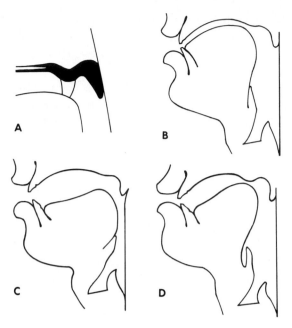

Fig. 6-15. A, Closure of nasopharynx; soft palate in solid black. Note: 1, Downward dip of soft palate from contraction of tensor palati occurs just behind hard palate at level of palatoglossal arch and junction of middle and posterior thirds of tongue. 2, "Footlike" appearance caused by upward tug of levator palati and down-bent uvula. 3, Forward position of posterior pharyngeal wall caused by special horizontal band of palatopharyngeus. **B,** Forming vowel sound /i/. Note that oral resonator is constricted and pharyngeal resonator is expanded. **C,** Forming vowel sound /a/. Note that oral resonator is expanded and pharyngeal resonator is constricted. **D,** Forming vowel sound /u/. Note that both oral and pharyngeal resonators are expanded. A strong constriction between these coupled resonators is produced by contraction of tensor palati, palatoglossus, and styloglossus muscles. (Tracings of radiographs.)

the pharynx. When the bolus spills into the valleculae, it is again checked momentarily by the epiglottis, which has begun to swing back against the posterior pharyngeal wall. Above this, the base of the tongue moves farther back to meet the posterior pharyngeal wall as a peristaltic wave of the pharyngeal sphincters moves down toward the esophagus. The larynx rocks back, which causes the fluid to surge over the lateral glossoepiglottic folds into the lateral food channels and then to spurt down each side of the walls of the raised, backbent, tightly closed larynx. The two streams join just below the larynx to meet at the cricoesophageal sphincter, which opens as the pharyngeal constrictors squirt the fluid into the esophagus.

SWALLOWING SOLIDS

When one sits at ease in the upright position, the airway is wide open, patent from external nares to trachea. The soft palate hangs down from above, in close contact with the tongue base, and the epiglottis stands erect from below in close contact with the tongue base. This leaves a broad, uninterrupted deep channel between anterior and posterior boundaries of the pharynx. The hyoid bone lies below and approximately parallel to the lower border of the jaw at rest, suspended in this position by the balance of normal tonus between suprahyoid, infrahyoid, and pharyngeal musculature. Thus the ends of the greater cornua lie a bit above the level of the hyoid body.

From this starting posture solid food is taken into the mouth by prehension with lips or anterior teeth or both. When food is taken from a portion in the hand, the lips are drawn from the dental cutting edges, which pinch and then shear off morsels in convenient bite sizes of some 1.5 cc. or more. When taken from a table utensil, the implement is put into the mouth and the lips and teeth are closed on it. The food is scraped off by pulling out the implement. The morsel is then manipulated farther into the oral cavity by the tongue tip and positioned properly for chewing. At this time the food is processed to an amorphous pulp. This is accomplished by some 60 to 70 masticatory strokes for resistant food, but the number of strokes varies greatly depending on the food's original consistency (Chapter 4). The crushed mass is continually mixed and lubricated with saliva during this process by the tongue, which ultimately molds it into a more or less solid spheroidal bolus. The biomechanical purpose of this process is to present a plastic streamlined form of least resistance for a monitored, smooth flow through a closely fitting, flexible tube.

When the preparation of the bolus is complete, it is closely encompassed between palate and tongue on all sides. At this time the mandible normally rises into dental occlusion. From this stable base, oral and pharyngeal outlets are sealed by the lips and by the soft palate pressed firmly forward against the tongue base. This last effect is accomplished mainly by the tensor palati muscles, whose tendons, turning horizontally in the hamular grooves, lie well below the level of the hard palate, assisted in this downward and forward traction by the palatoglossus muscles (Figs. 6-16 and 6-17).

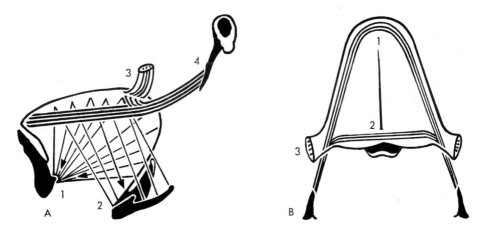

Fig. 6-16. Diagrammatic representation of extrinsic muscles of the tongue. **A,** Lateral view: *1*, genioglossus muscle; *2*, hyoglossus muscle; *3*, cut stump of palatoglossus muscle; and *4*, styloglossus muscle. **B,** Dorsal view: *1*, anterior "sling" formed by styloglossus muscle; *2*, posterior "sling" formed by styloglossus muscle; and *3*, cut stumps of palatoglossus muscle. (Modified from DuBrul, E. L., Ann. N.Y. Acad. Sci. **280,** 1976.)

Swallowing begins at the highly mobile tongue tip, which presses against the palate from before backward, thus squeezing the bolus back to the entrance of the pharynx at the palatoglossal arches. This smooth, voluntary wave of contraction is closely controlled by neuromuscular spindles strategically disposed within the intrinsic musculature of the tongue. The greatest concentration of these organs appears to be in the superior longitudinal, transverse, and vertical muscles around the area of junction between the free and deftly mobile anterior third and the more stably based middle third of the tongue. Only the vertical fibers are serviced by the spindles within the anterior third. This arrangement seems functionally most suitable for controlling the swift shifts in tongue tip shapes, which are essential for food manipulation and speech. Fast-firing signals from the spindles dart up the hypoglossal nerve, leaving it near the skull base to enter the central nervous system via fibers in the dorsal roots of the first and second cervical nerves. The fibers continue, uninterrupted, to

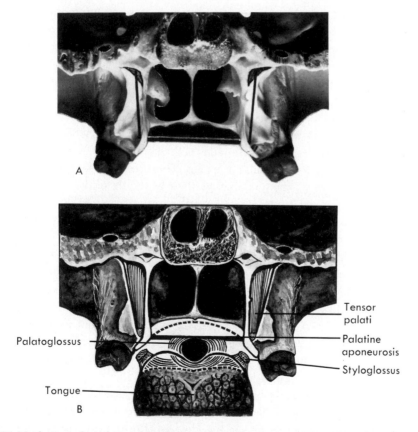

Fig. 6-17. Mechanism of oropharyngeal sphincter. **A,** Transverse section through skull. Note: darkened origins of tensor palati muscles in scaphoid fossae; lines drawn to show tensing of palatine aponeurosis *below* level of hard palate. **B,** Dissection superposed on tracing of skull. Note: dashed lines indicate resting positions of aponeurosis and tongue; tensor palati muscles lower aponeurosis, styloglossi (cut stumps) raise angle of tongue, both aid action of palatoglossi to complete oropharyngeal sphincter at center. (Modified from DuBrul, E. L., Ann. N.Y. Acad. Sci. **280,**1976.)

synapse directly on the motor neurons in the hypoglossal nucleus. As with all pro-prioceptors except those of the fifth nerve, their cell bodies lie in ganglia outside of the central nervous system, in this instance in the dorsal root ganglia of C1 and C2. In this way information about the rate, extent, and direction of movement is supplied by the spindles, which are arranged in three planes of space parallel to the somatic musculature of the tongue. In the absence of movable joints within the tongue, infor-mation ordinarily coming from end organs in joint capsules and ligaments, etc., which tells of orientation and positions in space of a moving bone, is substituted by infor-mation from end organs of touch and pressure in the tongue surface. These tell, by contact, of the locations, postures, and relations of various segments of the tongue within the oral space, and they signal along the lingual nerve to centers in the brain-stem.

Up to this point, firm closure of the isthmus of the fauces has been essential in preventing premature penetration of the bolus into the unalerted pharynx. When the moving bolus butts against the anterior faucial pillars, it is held up momentarily until the pressure of this contact rises to the threshold that triggers the release of the oropharyngeal gate, which sets off the ensuing rapid, involuntary swallowing sequence. End organs of touch and pressure concentrated in the mucosa of these especially sensitive strips signal this information up the glossopharyngeal nerve to the nucleus ambiguous in the brainstem.

Impelled by the first of these signals, the soft palate, or velum, begins to rise backwardly in conjunction with a forward rise and inward constriction of the walls of the upper pharynx. In so doing, the soft palate is thickened and bent to a right angle at the level of the tug of the levator palati muscles. This creates a "footlike" appearance in lateral radiographic view, the toe hanging down as the tip of the uvula (Fig. 6-15, A). Thus a thick, firm seal shuts out the nasal passages completely. Bands of the palatopharyngeus muscles, running around the lateral sides of the levator palati mus-cles and meeting at the median raphe in the posterior pharyngeal wall, are especially effective in this sphincteric action (see Figs. 6-3 and 6-6). They are raised into an almost horizontal ring with the pulling up of the whole pharynx by the converging vertical fibers of the palatopharyngeus. As the pharynx is thus pulled up over the bolus, the mass is thrust swiftly down and back by the base of the tongue, which meets and assists the descending wave of pharyngeal constriction to squeeze out further contact between bolus and soft palate. At all times and on all sides the bolus is closely contained within the form-fitting pharyngeal mucosa, which thus normally excludes any entrapment of air around the bolus.

As the bolus moves into the pharynx it bulges the base of the tongue slightly forward and the epiglottis bends back to the posterior pharyngeal wall. This action has two crucial effects. It raises and tenses the glossoepiglottic ligament and fold into a rigid midline partition, which begins shunting the bolus to either or both sides of the epiglottis. At the same time it spreads the valleculae widely to accommodate the oncoming bolus. But the vestibule of the larynx is still slightly open. Thus here, in the vallecular pockets, the bolus is momentarily stalled for a second time as the final protective mechanisms of the larynx are shifted into play. The larynx then rocks back and spills the bolus out of the valleculae into the lateral food channels. The epiglottis closes back over the laryngeal vestibule so that its ventral surfaces now slope laterally down to the right and left. This continues the shunting of the bolus down lateral chutes to one or both sides of the larynx, the way melting snow slides down the slopes of a steep gable roof with overhanging eaves. As the bolus is squeezed downward, the larynx is pulled up sharply with an ever-tightening closure of the laryngeal outlet, which gets it quickly out of the way of possible leakage from the bolus. This is the critical area of most speedy movement of the bolus.

Clearly the larynx creates an obstruction in the food channel. But since it is a construct vital to the protection of the airway, it is designed to act with alacrity and precision. When the larynx is at rest, the epiglottis stands erect against the tongue base in front. The arytenoid cartilages are also erect in lateral view, but their vertical axes lean laterally at an angle of some 40 degrees. In this position they rest on the upper, outer, posterior surfaces of the articular facets on the cricoid cartilage. In this situation their vocal processes are turned up and out, carrying the vocal folds into the laryngeal ventricles and obliterating them except for a small anterior slit. Thus at rest, in quiet breathing, the larynx is held widely open and its walls are smooth, showing no impinging folds except at the anterior end where the vocal and vestibular folds converge in the corner angle of the thyroid cartilage.

The mechanism of laryngeal closure is essentially sphincteric, but it is effected by a peculiar double valve action. As the bolus is driven down the tongue base, the larynx is brought into a distinctive alert posture in which its lumen is partially closed by a downward, inward, and forward spiraling of the arytenoid cartilages on their cricoid articular facets. This causes the vestibular and vocal folds and the arytenoid, corniculate, and cuneiform cartilages to bulge into the lumen in conjunction with the backward tilt of the epiglottis. This is the point of vallecular arrest during which the bolus collects against the epiglottis.

Immediately after this momentary pause, several activities occur simultaneously. The hyoid bone lifts toward the lower border of the jaw, pulled up principally by the geniohyoid and stylohyoid muscles and adjusted to by the digastric, mylohyoid, and infrahyoid muscles. As part of this movement the hyoid drifts forward and tilts down behind to lower its greater cornua. The thyroid cartilage follows closely to overtake and narrow the gap between hyoid and thyroid until its upper margin reaches above the level of the down-turned hyoid cornua. This provides slack in the lateral thyrohyoid ligaments, allowing the thyroid cartilage to rock back on its articulation with the cricoid cartilage. This movement helps further laryngeal closure, since it creates slack in vocal and ventricular ligaments.

The arytenoids can now complete their downward, forward, and inward screwlike twist, which swings around a center of rotation at the anchorage of the major cricoarytenoid ligament on the tiny tubercle at the upper medial margin of its cricoid facet. Close scrutiny of this articular facet reveals a groove running downward, forward, and inward, resembling a shallow thread of a screw.

The completed movement brings the tips of the vocal processes down to meet in the midline, carrying the vocal and ventricular folds into tight midline contact. Although the bases of the arytenoid cartilages must remain separated because of the space between their articulations on the cricoid cartilage (see Fig. 6-7), the triangular gap thus formed at the back of the laryngeal passage is closed from above by the forceful forward tilt of the arytenoid cartilages. In this prone position the flexible corniculate cartilages on the arytenoid tips are squeezed and fitted tightly against the epiglottic tubercle as the epiglottis swings back to the "gable roof" position described previously. Also, in this position, the interarytenoid musculature lies snugly above the posterior gap in the laryngeal lumen to close the airway completely. Thus two closely connected valvular systems are distinguishable in laryngeal closure, one formed by the vocal and vestibular folds together with the transverse arytenoid muscles, and one formed by the upper laryngeal margin pulled together by the purse string effect of the oblique arytenoids in continuity with the aryepiglottic muscles (see Figs. 6-12 and 6-13).

Speaking

Speech is the behavior that distinguishes man from even his closest relatives. It is a highly complicated phenomenon in which special brain and auditory systems are obviously major integrals, although their modes of contribution are by no means clearly understood. Even the mechanics of phonetics are yet to be satisfactorily defined. Although the act of speaking employs the same oropharyngeal system as that used for swallowing, its patterns of activity have distinct differences.

In swallowing, the pattern is essentially an unvarying sequence of movements that squeeze a closely contained mass from the front of the mouth, back, then down, into the esophageal portal beyond the larynx. The larynx must be closed tightly at a particular stage of the performance. Thus, in relation to the *total* organism, the behavior is an input function. It brings food energy in.

In speaking, on the other hand, patterns are composed of varying sequences of movements that intermittently modify pulses of humming air blown from the larynx, up, then forward, out of the front of the mouth. The vocal folds of the larynx must be slightly ajar during the performance, with the rims of the quavering gap under continuous neural control. In this case, in relation to the *total* organism, the behavior is an output function. It puts coded information out.

Basically the output is the result of energy transformed into air pulses used as signals coded to represent information, which are made audible at a distance. Hence the human system has an energy source, which is the pumping lung; a sound producer, which is the vibrating larynx; and a "filtering" resonator complex, which is the oropharyngeal tube. But since most of these parts were already present in early mammals, they were not evolved primarily for speech. All air-breathing vertebrates have some sort of larynx, and most make various sorts of sounds. The specific equipment that molds the specific sounds of speech is the highly mobile, locally elaborated, tortuous tubing extending from the rima glottis to the lips. This is called the vocal tract. Just as the foremost gill arches were fortuitously situated to become vertebrate jaws, this chain of feeding structures was fortuitously lined up to become speech structures. Then, with the drastic warping of skull and neck structures in adjustment to the vertical body posture resulting from bipedal locomotion, the oropharyngeal channel was bent sharply below the cranial base. This pulled the larynx down to separate the epiglottis widely from the soft palate, whereas they are in overlapping contact in other mammals. In this way a broad continuity became established between laryngeal orifice and posterior oral portal, on which selection could act in evolving a speaking tube (see Fig. 6-1).

Puffs of air waves are sent up the tube by vibrating the vocal folds with the breath. The folds are long, slim, ligamentous strips with rolled edges covered by closely bound stratified squamous epithelium and fitted with finely inserted special musculature. Frequency of vibration (hence pitch) is a direct function of tension of these highly effective structures. Their movements, positions, and tension are adjusted by the intrinsic laryngeal musculature.

VOCAL TRACT

Vibrations of the vocal cords alone can hardly make sounds perceptible to an outsider. The human supraglottic (vocal) tract thus acts as a compound resonator that amplifies and filters glottal pulses to produce audible sounds. It is formed by the oral and pharyngeal cavities, which are bent at their junction to follow closely the skull base and the cervical vertebral column (see Fig. 6-1). The vocal tract can then be defined as a serially coupled, instantaneously adjustable, double resonator system bent at a right angle. The nasal cavities and associated sinuses may contribute to the resonance but not to the mechanics of the tract.

Blowing soundless air across the open mouth of a jug produces an audible tone whose fundamental wave frequency depends on the volume of vibrating air. The tone is changed by adding fluid, which decreases the column of air. The air in the coupled oropharyngeal cavities is resonated much in this manner, the same as in the pipes of an organ. The different lengths and widths of the pipes are simulated by the vocal pipe when its segments are momentarily readjusted by its special musculature. In addition, the vocal resonators function as filters, since they can fortify some sound wave lengths, mask others, and add fundamental frequencies and harmonics of their own. Wave frequencies at which resonances occur are called *formant frequencies*. Given frequencies are resonated by given configurations of the vocal tract. The effect of the configuration is defined as an area function, or the relation between cross-sectional area and the distance from glottis to lips. Since resonation is the primary factor differentiating vowels, the mechanics of vowel formation exemplify these functions best.

Each vowel is a distinct, complex vibration containing a fundamental tone and a set of overtones. The two vocal resonators filter this complex to produce at least two prominent formant frequencies apparently corresponding to the conformations of the oral and pharyngeal cavities. The result is the sound we recognize as a particular vowel. Diphthongs are simply glides combining two vowels. In English there are at least ten vowellike sounds that require different contours of the vocal tract.

Three of these vowels, /i/, /a/, /u/, are recognized as "language universal." They are formed at the extremes of vocal tract posturing and thus illustrate vocal mechanics clearly in exaggerated form. In all three the palatopharyngeal sphincter is closed, raising the soft palate to form a deflecting plane shunting air out through the mouth (Fig. 6-15, *B*, *C*, and *D*).

The vowel /i/, pronounced as in t*ee*m, is produced by reducing the oral resonator area and expanding the pharyngeal resonator area. The tongue mass is raised and flattened forward to bring its dorsum close and parallel to the contours of the palate. The tongue tip is poised just below and behind the gap between slightly parted incisors. Thus a short, narrow tunnel is formed from parted lips back to a level anterior to the insertion of the tensor palati muscles above, and forward of the foramen cecum below. The vertical posterior portion of the tongue is pulled forward, away from the posterior wall of the pharynx. Thus a long, broad cavern is formed from the glottis to the raised dome of the soft palate above (Fig. 6-15, *B*).

The vowel /a/, as in t*o*p, is produced by the reverse of the above; the oral resonator is expanded and the pharyngeal resonator reduced. The tongue mass is lowered and bulged backward. The tongue tip is depressed and withdrawn to uncover the lowered anterior oral floor. Thus a long, wide, deep cavern is formed from parted lips back to the posterior limit of the soft palate. In this situation the vertical posterior third of the tongue has been brought down and back, close and parallel to the posterior pharyngeal wall as the transverse pharyngeal diameter is contracted by a third. Thus a short, narrow tunnel is formed from the level of the lowered foramen cecum to the glottis (Fig. 6-15, *C*).

The vowel /u/, as in t*oo*l, is produced by a combination of these two movements; both oral and pharyngeal resonators are expanded but separated by an abrupt constriction. The tongue mass is further lowered anteriorly so that the tongue tip is nearly obscured and the oral resonator is thus deepened. It is also lengthened by pursed protrusion of the lips. The posterior third of the tongue is bunched forward, up, and away from the posterior pharyngeal wall, thus deepening the pharyngeal resonator in sagittal dimension. As a result of this severe contraction of the tongue from front to back, a sharp, raised angle at the level of the junction of posterior and middle thirds is formed. Thus this region approaches the palate closely, at the level of the downwardly bulged insertion of the contracted tensor palati muscles. This produces a markedly narrowed isthmus between front and back resonators (Fig. 6-15, *D*). As noted previously, there are varieties of modifications within these extremes.

It is convenient to describe the roles of the muscles in these activities in groups related to the resonator formation. Closing off of the nasal space is often not as complete in phonation as in swallowing. However, certain features of the closure are significant for proper resonation. Strong contraction of the tensor palati muscles causes a downward curve of the anterior third of the soft palate, since their tendons pull from the hamular grooves which lie well below the level of the hard palate as noted previously. The levator palati muscles, on the other hand, cause a marked upward buckling of the posterior portion of the palate when strongly contracted. The result forms an undulating S-shaped curve (Fig. 6-15, A).

The tongue plays the lead in controlling the resonator complex because it alone acts in both oral and pharyngeal resonators. Although the tongue is anchored on the hyoid bone, which moves in stabilized patterns, it lacks an internal bony skeleton. It performs its innumerable gradations of movements on the principle of a hydrostatic skeleton. A system of this sort depends on two fundamental properties, the incompressibility of water and contractibility in three planes of space. Thus the tongue is actually a fluid-filled bag that can contract in three planes by the action of its intrinsic longitudinal, vertical, and transverse muscles. This exquisitely mobile mass is attached to the skull directly and indirectly by four pairs of extrinsic muscles.

The palatoglossi and styloglossi arise directly from the skull and act as synergists. The palatoglossus arises from the aponeurotic extension of the hard palate. It curves out, down, and around the isthmus between oral and pharyngeal cavities to enter the tongue at the apex of its bend between middle and posterior thirds. It courses medially to continue with its counterpart of the opposite side. The styloglossus arises from the styloid process. It runs down and forward also to enter the tongue at its bend. Here it separates into three segments. The first, proximal portion turns medially immediately, to course with the palatoglossus and join its counterpart from the opposite side. The second, longest portion runs forward along the edge of the tongue to fuse with its counterpart around the tongue tip. Thus the muscles form two continuous loops, one around the tongue bend and one around the tongue tip. These look much like check reins, pulling the tongue bend up and back, increasing its angle with the aid of the palatoglossus, and pulling the tongue tip back (Fig. 6-16). The third portion dwindles downward to interlace with bundles of the hyoglossus.

The genioglossi and hyoglossi arise indirectly from the skull since they spring from mandible and hyoid bone, both of which are slung from the skull base.

The oral resonator is expanded by the combined action of extrinsic and intrinsic muscles of the tongue and by movements of the mandible and hyoid. The hyoglossus muscles pull the body of the tongue downward, assisted by intrinsic vertical fibers and perhaps by anterior genioglossus fibers. At the same time the superior and inferior longitudinal bundles pull the tongue mass backward in conjunction with the upper fibers of the styloglossus muscles, which reach to the tip of the tongue. The floor of the oral cavity is thus exposed anteriorly, and this is lowered by depression of the jaw and hyoid bone.

The pharyngeal resonator is expanded by the integrated action of a number of muscles. The geniohyoids pull the hyoid forward and with it the entire tongue. Horizontal fibers of the genioglossus muscles pull the erect tongue base strongly forward. Slight contraction of the lower fibers of the middle and upper pharyngeal constrictors, which pull upward and forward, as well as those of the palatopharyngeus and salpingopharyngeus muscles, permit slack in the pharynx, which can thus be broadened by the outward traction of the stylopharyngeus muscles. Finally, the length of the pharynx is augmented by the lifting of the back of the soft palate in a strong upward curve due to the pull of the levator palati muscles.

Augmenting or diminishing the double resonator effect is managed by controlling the constriction between segments of the tongue and soft palate. The junction of the middle and posterior thirds of the tongue at rest forms nearly a right angle, which can be made more acute for the coupled resonator function. This is done by depressing the anterior two thirds of the tongue and bunching its mass strongly back against the vertical, forwardly thrust posterior third in the manner already described. The apex of this angle is then raised further by the styloglossus muscles, assisted by the palatoglossals. It thus approaches the soft palate closely, just at the level of its anterior curvature, which is pulled down toward the tongue by the tensor palati muscles (Fig. 6-17). The final effect forms raised lateral margins on the tongue, walling a narrow midline groove roofed above by the tensely depressed anterior segment of the soft palate. In this way the bore and length of the tunnel connecting the oral cavity and pharynx can be controlled with remarkable precision (Figs. 6-15, *D* and 6-17).

SPEECH ARTICULATORS

Certain structures along the vocal tract have been classified as "articulators." They are mostly concentrated around the oral cavity and are listed in textbooks as the lips, cheeks, teeth, alveolar process, palate, velum, tongue, posterior pharyngeal wall, mandible, hyoid, and lips of the glottis. However, when these articulators are pictured within the frame of the coupled resonator model, a vivid functional scheme can be seen. Here the articulators act simply as valves that stop, slow, or release resonating exhaled air. The tongue takes the lead, bouncing about the oral resonator in a precisely programmed dance, momentarily contacting the teeth, alveolar process, and palate (front, back, or sides), while the exact relations of the tongue to these regions are constantly readjusted by the shifting jaw. These activities are closely integrated with contributions from the lips in front and the velum and upper pharynx in back. The act of correct articulation depends on precise timing and accuracy in direction of movement and in positioning of the parts, as well as in the forces exerted in each movement. The sounds produced are broadly classified as consonants, which include the stops, or plosives, /p/, /b/, /t/, /d/, /k/, /g/, the fricatives /f/, /v/, /s/, /z/, and, in English, /θ/, and /ð/, pronounced as variations of *th*, and the liquids /l/ and /r/. All of these sounds are made with the nasal spaces closed off by the velopharyngeal sphincter. In addition there are three English speech sounds characterized by noticeable nasal resonation. Thus they are called nasals, /m/ as in *man*, /n/ as in *note*, and /ŋ/ as in si*ng*, in which the velopharyngeal sphincter is opened to allow a leak of sound into the nasal resonators.

The primary factor differentiating articulated sounds is the particular point of valvelike action. Plosives are formed at the lips, at the tongue front, and at the tongue back. Fricatives are formed at the lip and tongue tip in specific relations to front teeth. Since the positions are definitive, the anatomic configurations for making these particular sounds will be used to exemplify articulatory mechanisms. Liquids and nasals seem to be blurred variations of plosives and fricatives.

Plosives (explosive modulation) are characterized by stopping and then suddenly releasing an output breath flow, and they may be made with or without an accompanying voice sound. Fricatives (frictional modulation) are characterized by forcing an uninterrupted output breath flow through a highly restricted opening, and they also may be made with or without an accompanying voice sound.

The plosives /p/ and /b/ are made at the lips. The lips are brought together over slightly parted front teeth. The dorsum of the tongue is moderately and evenly separated from the palate along its entire length. The velopharyngeal sphincter is closed so that air pressure can be built up behind the lips. Air is released suddenly by parting the lips; /p/ is voiceless, /b/ includes a resonated glottal tone.

The plosives /t/ and /d/ are made at the tongue tip. The lips are parted, but the tongue closes the vocal tract at the front by contact between its anterior margin and the palatal alveolar process in an arch on the gingivae of the front teeth. The dorsum of the tongue is further separated from the palate posteriorly. The velopharyngeal sphincter is closed, and air pressure is built up behind the raised anterior rim of the tongue. Air is released suddenly by rapid depression of the tongue tip; /t/ is voiceless and /d/ includes a resonated glottal tone.

The fricatives /f/ and /v/ are made at lip and teeth. The lower lip is rolled back between slightly parted incisors. The dorsum of the tongue is moderately separated from the palate along its entire length, and the velopharyngeal sphincter is closed. Air is forced through the restricted slit formed between the incisal edges of the upper teeth and the edge of the approximated lower lip. It causes a frictional (rubbing) sound, which is voiceless in /f/ and includes a resonated glottal tone in /v/.

The fricatives /s/ and /z/ are formed at the tongue tip and the teeth. The tongue tip is raised close behind the lingual surface of the upper front teeth. The dorsum of the tongue is lowered from the palate posteriorly. Air is forced through a restricted central slit formed by the raised sides of the tongue and by its tip near the upper incisal edges. It causes a frictional (hissing) sound that may be accentuated by the edges of the slightly parted lower incisors. It is voiceless in /s/ and includes a resonated glottal tone in /z/.

The tongue plays a major part in both resonation and articulation. Observations on the rapidity of movement of the parts record that the tongue leads, the jaw follows, and the lips and palate move slowest. But even a crude estimate of timing points up a certain close association between parts of the tongue and the jaw: tongue tip, 8.2 movements per second; jaw, 7.3 per second; tongue base, 7.1 per second; lips and velum, 6.7 per second. Thus there is a gradient from front to back, with the tongue base and mandible moving at almost the same rate. An examination of the structural arrangement clarifies the integration of tongue and jaw function.

The tongue is, in effect, slung from the skull by hawserlike muscles that pull from moorings situated strategically about the cranial base. They control the postures and shifts of position of the tongue by acting either directly on its mass or indirectly through the mandible and hyoid bone. From the temporal bone, via the styloid process, the styloglossus muscles act directly on the tongue, pulling it upward and backward and aiding in buckling it up at the junction of the posterior and middle thirds. From the palatine bone, via the palatine aponeurosis, the palatoglossus muscles descend in the anterior pillars of the fauces to become continuous through the transverse fibers of the tongue near the junction of its middle and posterior thirds. Thus they form a sling much like the sling of the levator palati muscles and assist in the kinking up of the back of the tongue. From the temporal bone, via the styloid processes, the stylohyoid muscles act indirectly on the position of the tongue through the hyoid bone. Again from the temporal bone, but now via the craniomandibular joint and along the jaw, the geniohyoid muscles act indirectly on the tongue through the hyoid bone. Together both geniohyoids and stylohyoids shift the tongue mass forward and backward by tugging on the hyoid bone. Finally through the hyoid bone thus suspended from the skull and supported in this position by the infrahyoid strap muscles, the hyoglossus muscles plait their fibers throughout the middle tongue mass and act on its form and position.

At the front of the oral cavity, the mechanisms manipulating the oral orifice are essentially sphincteric. The encircling orbicularis oris fibers produce the pursing effect, which lengthens the oral resonator. The radiating musculature controls parting of the lips and spreading and widening of the mouth opening. The special arrangement of these radiating fibers at the angles of the lips, plaited through the "modiolus," produces an overriding lateral component of force that maintains the normally approximated horizontal lip slit at rest.

At the back of the oral cavity, mechanisms operating the oropharyngeal portal have already been considered. Behind this, the sphincteric activity closing off the nasal spaces from the pharynx has been noted. Special bands of the palatopharyngeus muscles run back lateral to the inserting levator palati muscles. These fibers meet in the raphe at the midline of the posterior wall of the pharynx, where they become difficult to distinguish from fibers of the superior constrictor. This forms an encircling band of fibers from velum to upper pharynx, which contracts in conjunction with upward pull of the levators. The shortened, thickened, raised palatal margin and uvula are thus clamped within this ring to produce a tight seal.

From this brief analysis of swallowing and speaking mechanisms it becomes evident that even the slightest impingement on the neuromuscular structures of this complexly coordinated system will have some deleterious effect on the normal performance of these vital activities. Among these disruptive influences are disturbances of relative growth, deformities such as palatal clefts, distortions of neck postures such as torticollis, infections or tumors of the tract, neurologic effects such as bulbar poliomyelitis impinging on the suspension apparatus of the pharynx and larynx, trauma, malpositioning of the jaw, reconstructive dental procedures, and prosthetic appliances.

CHAPTER 7

The blood vessels

ARTERIES

The arteries of the oral cavity and the adjacent regions are, with a few exceptions, branches of the external carotid artery. Only parts of the nasal cavity and the upper parts of the face receive branches of the internal carotid artery. The external carotid artery is sometimes termed the facial carotid, supplying superficial and deep structures of the face, whereas the name cerebral carotid applies to the internal carotid artery, which sends its blood almost exclusively to the brain.

The external and internal carotid arteries arise from the division of the common carotid artery (Fig. 7-1). The common carotid on the right side is a branch of the brachiocephalic (innominate) artery; on the left side it is a direct branch of the aortic arch. The common carotid, as a rule branchless, runs lateral to the trachea and larynx to the level of the upper border of the thyroid cartilage. In a candelabra-like division, it gives rise to the internal carotid artery situated posteromedially and the external carotid artery situated anterolaterally. At the division, the internal carotid artery is slightly widened to form the carotid sinus, which is important for the reflex regulation of blood pressure. The division of the common carotid is frequently situated somewhat above, more rarely below, the level of the superior border of the thyroid cartilages.

External carotid artery

The external carotid artery (Fig. 7-2), arising under the cover of the anterior border of the sternocleidomastoid muscle, can be followed upward and slightly anteriorly and is, shortly after its origin, superficially located. It is covered only by the investing layer of the deep cervical fascia, the platysma, the subcutaneous tissue (or superficial fascia), and the skin. The external carotid runs straight upward to reach the lower border of the posterior belly of the digastric muscle and the stylohyoid muscle. Farther cranially, it lies medial to these two muscles and at the same time bends slightly posteriorly. The artery traverses the most posterior part of the submandibular triangle to enter the retromandibular fossa behind the mandibular angle. Here the external carotid again changes its course and ascends, embedded in the substance of the parotid gland, parallel to the posterior border of the mandible through the retromandibular fossa. At the level of the mandibular neck, the artery splits into its two terminal branches, the superficial temporal artery and the maxillary artery. However,

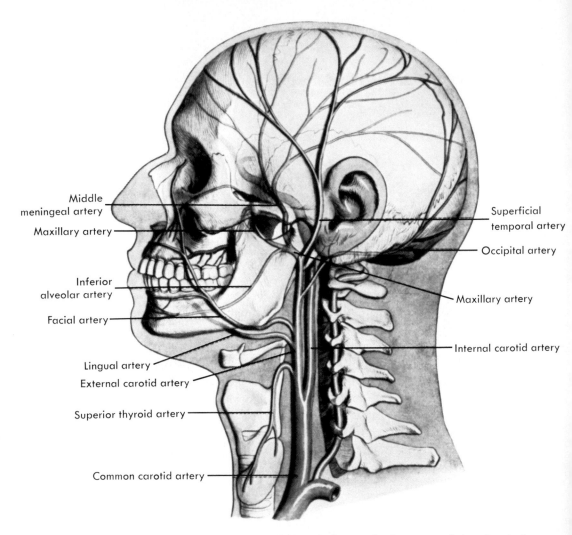

Fig. 7-1. General plan of the arteries of the head showing relations to hard structures. Only major arteries are indicated; for detail of branching see following figures. Since we are only concerned with the branches *above* the origin of the common carotid, the figure has been reversed for consistency with figures that follow. (Sicher and Tandler: Anatomie für Zahnärzte.)

it would be more correct to regard the temporal artery as the last branch of the external carotid and the maxillary artery as the continuation of the external carotid.

In its course the external carotid artery follows first the lateral wall of the pharynx. Higher up it is separated from the pharynx by the styloglossal and the stylopharyngeus muscles, which intervene between the external and internal carotid arteries. The hypoglossal nerve crosses the external carotid artery before it reaches the lower border of the digastric muscle (see Fig. 13-8). In the retromandibular fossa, the

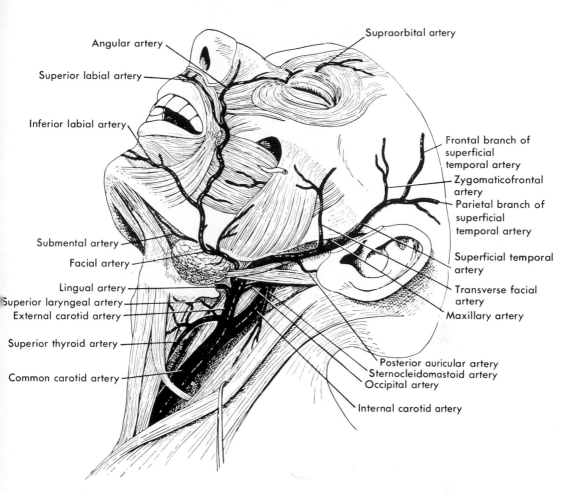

Fig. 7-2. Superficial branches of external carotid artery. (Modified and redrawn from Sicher and Tandler: Anatomie für Zahnärzte.)

retromandibular (posterior facial) vein lies on the lateral side of the artery (see Fig. 7-9); artery and vein are crossed by the superficially situated facial nerve or its two main branches. Almost at the same level at which the hypoglossal nerve crosses the external carotid artery on its lateral side, it is crossed by the superior laryngeal nerve on its medial or deep surface.

According to the location of their origin, the branches of the external artery can be divided into anterior, posterior, and medial branches, to which the terminal branches of the artery have to be added.

ANTERIOR BRANCHES OF EXTERNAL CAROTID ARTERY

Three arteries arise from the anterior wall of the external carotid artery: the superior thyroid artery, the lingual artery, and the facial artery.

Superior thyroid artery. This artery (Fig. 7-2) arises from the external carotid artery at or immediately above the bifurcation of the common carotid. Not too rarely it is a branch of the common carotid artery. The superior thyroid artery, arising at some distance above the upper pole of the thyroid gland, curves anteriorly and downward to reach this organ. This arch of the superior thyroid artery is characteristic and can serve as a diagnostic landmark in surgical exposure of the external carotid. Where the superior thyroid artery reaches the thyroid gland, it divides, as a rule, into an anterior and a posterior branch. Both send secondary branches into the substance of the thyroid gland. The anterior branch anastomoses with the corresponding branch of the other side; the posterior branch joins with branches of the inferior thyroid artery of the thyrocervical trunk of the subclavian artery.

Aside from muscular branches to neighboring muscles and a small hyoid branch that follows the hyoid bone at its inferior border, the superior thyroid artery gives off two extraglandular branches, the superior laryngeal artery and the cricothyroid artery. The main branch of the superior laryngeal artery perforates the thyrohyoid membrane and thus enters the larynx. Here it supplies the mucous membrane and the muscles of the larger upper part of the larynx and anastomoses with branches of the inferior laryngeal artery of the inferior thyroid artery. The cricothyroid branch, a seemingly insignificant small twig, gains its importance from its relation to the cricothyroid, or conic, ligament (see Fig. 15-5). It crosses this ligament in a horizontal course and, anastomosing with the same artery of the other side, forms the cricothyroid arch.

Lingual artery. This artery (Fig. 7-5) arises from the external carotid artery approximately at the level of the greater horn of the hyoid bone. Frequently it has a common origin with the facial artery, which normally arises a short distance above the origin of the lingual artery. The common origin is called the linguofacial trunk. From the place of its origin, the lingual artery courses almost horizontally forward to the posterior border of the hyoglossus muscle and continues forward and upward on the deep surface of this muscle. Normally it disappears at the posterior border of the hyoglossus muscle; sometimes, however, it crosses the most posterior bundles of the muscle on their lateral surface and then passes through a slit of the hyoglossus muscle. Covered by the muscle, the artery turns steeply upward to reach the space between the genioglossus muscle and the inferior longitudinal muscle of the tongue. Here it bends again into a horizontal plane and reaches, in a tortuous course, the tip of the tongue. The curves of the artery are situated in a vertical plane and develop as an adaptation to the great mobility of the tongue, especially to its power of elongation.

Before the lingual artery enters the substance of the tongue, it releases a hyoid branch that follows the upper border of the hyoid bone, sends branches to the muscles attached to the bone, and finally anastomoses with the hyoid branch of the other side.

One or more dorsal lingual branches leave the first part of the lingual artery where it approaches the base of the tongue. Ascending vertically, they distribute blood to the basal part of the tongue.

Before the lingual artery turns into the body of the tongue, it releases the sublingual artery (see Figs. 7-5, 13-2, and 13-3). This vessel is situated in the floor of the mouth medial to the sublingual gland and supplies the gland, the mucous membrane at the floor of the mouth, and the mylohyoid muscle. Through the substance of the latter, the sublingual artery anastomoses with muscular branches of the submental artery, a branch of the facial artery. If the sublingual artery is missing, it is replaced by a perforating branch of the submental artery. This variation, the origination of the sublingual artery from the facial instead of from the lingual artery, is clinically important (see Chapter 13).

After giving off the sublingual artery, the lingual artery itself, now situated in the body of the tongue, is called the deep lingual artery. In its anterior course, it lies near the inferior surface of the tongue, close to the covering mucous membrane. The numerous branches of the lingual artery supply the body and apex of the tongue. One of its terminal branches anastomoses with the deep lingual artery of the other side to form the arcus raninus.

Facial artery. This artery (Figs. 7-2 to 7-4) arises from the external carotid just below the posterior belly of the digastric muscle, sometimes even higher up so that the muscle covers its origin. It has been mentioned that the facial and the lingual arteries frequently have a common origin, the linguofacial trunk. From its origin, the facial artery courses obliquely upward and forward, crossing the posterior belly of the

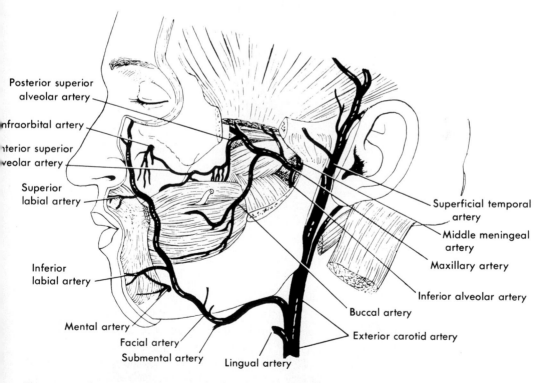

Fig. 7-3. Facial (external maxillary) and maxillary arteries. (Modified and redrawn from Sicher and Tandler: Anatomie für Zahnärzte.)

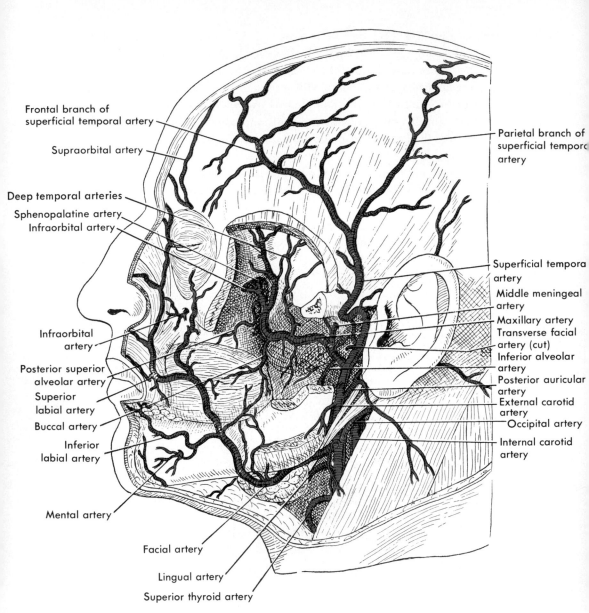

Frontal branch of superficial temporal artery

Supraorbital artery

Deep temporal arteries

Sphenopalatine artery

Infraorbital artery

Infraorbital artery

Posterior superior alveolar artery

Superior labial artery

Buccal artery

Inferior labial artery

Mental artery

Facial artery

Lingual artery

Superior thyroid artery

Parietal branch of superficial temporal artery

Superficial temporal artery

Middle meningeal artery

Maxillary artery

Transverse facial artery (cut)

Inferior alveolar artery

Posterior auricular artery

External carotid artery

Occipital artery

Internal carotid artery

Fig. 7-4. Superficial and deep arteries of the face. (Modified and redrawn from Tandler: Lehrbuch der Anatomie.)

digastric muscle and the stylohyoid muscle on their medial surface, and enters the submandibular triangle. Here the facial artery is covered by the submandibular salivary gland. After reaching the superior border of the gland, the artery turns sharply laterally, situated either in a groove of the gland or even embedded in its substance. The convexity of this sharp turn is, as a rule, covered by the angle of the mandible and reaches close to the lower pole of the palatine tonsil, from which it is separated by fibers of the superior pharyngeal constrictor. The horizontal part of the artery above the submandibular gland is directed obliquely anteriorly, laterally, and slightly downward to the lower border of the mandible, which the artery reaches just in front of the anterior border of the masseter muscle. At this point, the artery describes a second sharp turn, swinging around the mandibular border under the antegonial notch to enter the face.

The facial part of this artery, which gave to the artery the name facial artery, is characterized by the tortuous course of the vessel, an adaptation to the varying expansion of the lips and cheek. From the point where the artery crosses the lower border of the mandible, it is directed toward the corner of the mouth and then follows the lateral border of the nose to the inner corner of the eye. Here it ends as the angular artery, anastomosing with branches of the ophthalmic artery of the internal carotid artery.

The branches of the facial artery can be divided into two sets, the cervical branches and the facial branches. In the neck the artery sends small branches to adjacent muscles and larger branches into the submandibular gland. The two most important cervical branches are the ascending palatine artery and the submental artery.

The *ascending palatine artery* takes its origin from the highest point of the first bend of the facial artery, close to the lateral pharyngeal wall. The vessel courses cranially along the outer surface of the superior pharyngeal constrictor to reach the levator palati muscle, along which its terminal branch enters the soft palate. In addition to small branches to the pharyngeal muscles and the mucous membrane of the pharynx, the ascending palatine artery gives rise to a tonsillar branch, which often is the main artery for the palatine tonsil. The tonsillar artery sometimes arises independently from the facial artery.

The submental artery arises from the horizontal part of the facial artery before it turns upward into the face. The main branch of the submental artery converges with the mylohyoid nerve and, following it, reaches the inferolateral surface of the mylohyoid muscle. The submental artery supplies lymph nodes in the submandibular triangle, the anterior belly of the digastric muscle, and the mylohyoid muscle. Branches perforating the mylohyoid muscle anastomose with branches of the sublingual artery. The sublingual artery may be substituted by a branch of the submental artery, but sometimes the reverse is true; that is, the submental artery is lacking, and the blood supply to the structures in the anterior part of the submandibular triangle is taken over by a perforating branch of the sublingual artery. In the region of the chin a terminal branch of the submental artery turns upward into the face, where it anastomoses with branches of the inferior labial artery.

In the face, the facial artery lies superficially at first, covered only by the platysma muscle, superficial fascia, and skin. The pulse of the artery can easily be felt at the lower border of the mandible or slightly above it and in front of the masseter muscle. In its course upward and forward toward the corner of the mouth, the facial artery lies deep to the depressor anguli oris, risorius, and major zygomatic muscles and then between the elevator of the upper lip and levator anguli oris muscles. In this part of its course, the artery is situated closer to the mucous membrane of the cheek than to the skin, and its pulse can be felt from the oral cavity.

In the lower part of the face, the facial artery supplies a varying number of small branches to the neighboring muscles. The two most important branches are the arteries to the lips, the inferior and the superior labial arteries. These two blood vessels arise at a variable distance from the corner of the mouth to enter the lips, where they are found close to the free border of the lips and deep to the orbicularis oris muscle. In the lower as well as in the upper lip, right and left labial arteries anastomose widely in the midline to form an arterial circle surrounding the oral fissure. The inferior labial artery anastomoses with branches of the mental artery of the inferior alveolar artery of the maxillary artery. Close to the midline, anastomoses are established between the inferior labial artery and the terminal part of the submental artery. The upper labial artery sends ascending branches to the inferior border of the nasal wings and septum, where these branches anastomose with nasal branches of the ophthalmic artery of the internal carotid.

Ascending at the lateral border of the nose, the facial artery supplies the lateral parts of the nose and the adjacent part of the cheek and anastomoses with the infraorbital artery of the maxillary artery. The facial artery then ends as the angular artery, anastomosing with branches of the ophthalmic artery.

In addition to the anastomoses already mentioned, branches of the facial artery connect with the buccal artery of the maxillary artery and the transverse facial artery of the superficial temporal artery.

The upper part of the facial artery may be lacking, the artery terminating as the inferior or superior labial artery. In such cases the missing part and its branches are replaced by branches of either the ophthalmic or the infraorbital artery.

POSTERIOR BRANCHES OF EXTERNAL CAROTID ARTERY

Two branches arise from the posterior wall of the external carotid artery: the occipital artery and the posterior auricular artery.

Occipital artery. This artery (Figs. 7-2, 7-4, and 7-5) takes its origin, as a rule, at the same level as the facial artery. However, lower or higher origin of this artery is not rare. The occipital artery runs obliquely upward and backward parallel to the lower border of the posterior belly off the digastric muscle, often covered by this muscle, and reaches the space between the transverse process of the atlas and mastoid process. The occipital artery now turns into a more horizontal course, crossing the mastoid process on its medial side in the narrow and deep occipital groove of the temporal bone. In the dense connective tissue between the deep posterior muscles of the neck, the occipital artery turns upward again and perforates the aponeurotic connection between the tendons of the trapezius and sternocleidomastoid muscles. There the artery becomes superficial and divides its branches in the posterior part of the scalp.

Before the occipital artery approaches the superficial structures, it gives off a descending branch for the deep musculature of the neck. This branch anastomoses with branches of the deep cervical artery of the costocervical trunk of the subclavian artery.

Of the many smaller muscular branches of the occipital artery, only one is distinguished by a separate name. It is the sternocleidomastoid branch, which arises from the first part of the occipital artery. Characteristically it loops around the hypoglossal nerve from above and enters the sternocleidomastoid muscle at its deep surface close to the point of entrance of the accessory nerve.

Posterior auricular artery. This artery (Fig. 7-2), the second posterior branch of the external carotid artery, arises in the retromandibular fossa just above the stylo-

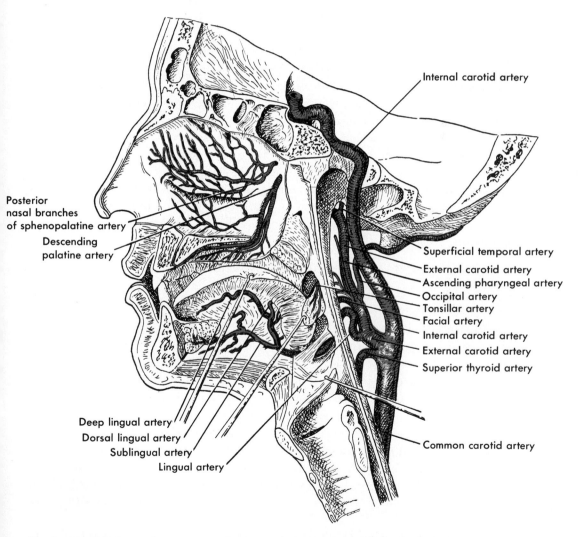

Fig. 7-5. Lingual artery, palatine artery, and posterior nasal arteries. (Modified and redrawn from Tandler: Lehrbuch der Anatomie.)

hyoid muscle. Following the upper border of this muscle and the anterior border of the styloid process, the posterior auricular artery reaches the groove between the cartilage of the outer ear and the mastoid process. It distributes its branches partly to the outer ear and partly to the adjacent area of the scalp. It anastomoses with branches of the occipital artery and with the auricular branches of the superficial temporal artery. A small branch of the posterior auricular artery, the stylomastoid artery, enters the stylomastoid foramen and runs along the facial nerve to contribute to the blood supply of the tympanic cavity.

MEDIAL BRANCH OF EXTERNAL CAROTID ARTERY

Ascending pharyngeal artery. This artery is the only medial branch of the external carotid artery. Normally it arises from the medial or posteromedial wall of the external carotid immediately above the division of the common carotid. Frequently, however, the ascending pharyngeal artery arises at a higher level, or even as a branch of the occipital artery. The vessel ascends along the lateral pharyngeal wall to the base of the skull. In its course, branches are given off to the wall of the pharynx and to adjacent muscles, for instance, to the stylopharyngeus, the tensor and levator palati muscles, and to the deep muscles in front of the vertebral column. The branches of the ascending pharyngeal artery anastomose with those of the ascending palatine artery and others contributing to the blood supply of the pharynx and, in the prevertebral fascia, with branches of the ascending cervical artery of the thyrocervical trunk of the subclavian artery. At the base of the skull, the ascending pharyngeal artery anastomoses also with the pterygoid artery of the maxillary artery and terminates in several branches that enter the cavity of the skull along the trigeminal, vagus, and hypoglossal nerves.

TERMINAL BRANCHES OF EXTERNAL CAROTID ARTERY

The terminal branches of the external carotid artery are the superficial temporal artery and the maxillary artery.

Superficial temporal artery. This artery (Figs. 7-3 and 7-4) continues the course of the external carotid artery in the retromandibular fossa and, ascending vertically, crosses the posterior root of the zygomatic arch immediately in front of the outer ear. The pulse of this artery can be felt at this place because of the superficial position of the artery, which, after emerging from the substance of the parotid gland, is covered only by superficial fascia and skin. Before the superficial temporal artery leaves the parotid gland, it releases the transverse facial artery; originating at the level of the mandibular neck, this branch turns horizontally forward between the parotid gland and masseter muscle (Fig. 7-2). The transverse facial artery is usually found between the zygomatic arch and parotid duct; it sends branches to the masseter muscle and parotid gland and terminates below the outer corner of the eye, where it may anastomose with palpebral arteries.

After sending a few small branches posteriorly to the outer ear and anteriorly to the joint capsule, the superficial temporal artery divides, at a variable distance above the zygomatic arch, into its two main branches, the parietal and the frontal. The parietal branch continues almost vertically upward and supplies a wide lateral area of the scalp. The frontal branch runs obliquely upward and forward and is, like the parietal branch, often tortuous. The winding artery is clearly seen through the skin. In the scalp, the branches of the temporal artery anastomose with branches of the posterior auricular and occipital arteries behind, with supraorbital and frontal arteries in front, and, across the midline, with the arteries of the other side.

One superficial branch, the zygomatico-orbital artery, arises either from the main stem of the superficial temporal artery above the zygomatic arch or from its anterior branch, runs almost horizontally forward toward the outer corner of the eye, sends branches to the orbicularis oculi muscle, and anastomoses with branches of the lacrimal artery.

In addition to the superficial branches, the superficial temporal artery sends one branch into the depth, the middle temporal artery. Arising slightly above the zygomatic arch, the middle temporal artery perforates the temporal fascia and the temporal muscle to continue in the periosteum of the temporal squama, lying in a vertical groove of the bone. The middle temporal artery ramifies in the periosteum of the temporal bone and anastomoses in the substance of the temporal muscle with branches of the posterior deep temporal artery of the maxillary artery.

Maxillary artery. The (internal) maxillary artery (Figs. 7-3, 7-4, and 7-5) arises from the external carotid artery just below the level of the mandibular neck in the substance of the parotid gland. Although the superficial temporal artery continues the course of the external carotid artery upward, whereas the maxillary artery arises at a right angle, the maxillary artery is embryologically and phylogenetically the continuation of the external carotid. The maxillary artery follows an anterior, slightly upward, and medial course through the infratemporal fossa. It is deeply situated on the inner surface of the mandible and in a varying relation to the lateral pterygoid muscle. In slightly more than 50% of all persons the artery is found on the outer side of this muscle after passing through the space between the mandible and the sphenomandibular ligament. In the remaining individuals the artery lies medial to the lateral pterygoid muscle. In the latter cases the artery crosses the lingual and inferior alveolar nerves between the lateral and medial pterygoid muscles. The maxillary artery is, in most persons, situated lateral to these two nerves but is sometimes at their medial side. In rare cases the artery crosses one of the two nerves on its lateral side and the other on its medial side. The artery also supplies the jaw joint (see Chapter 4).

At the anterosuperior end of the infratemporal fossa, the maxillary artery passes through the pterygopalatine gap, or pterygopalatine hiatus, into the pterygopalatine fossa, where it splits into its terminal branches. When the maxillary artery lies on the outer surface of the lateral pterygoid muscle, it reaches the pterygopalatine hiatus by passing between the two heads of the lateral pterygoid muscle.

The maxillary artery may arbitrarily be divided into four parts. The first, or mandibular, part is that short section which lies medial to the mandibular neck. The second part, the muscular, or pterygoid, part is the longest of the four and is in close relation to the lateral pterygoid muscle. The third section is the maxillary part, which is here in close relation to the posterior surface of the maxilla. The fourth and terminal part of the maxillary artery is best termed the pterygopalatine part, because the artery divides into its terminal branches in the pterygopalatine space, which it enters through the pterygopalatine gap.

The branches of the maxillary artery are numerous and, with the exception of one, are destined for the deep structures of the face, lower and upper jaws and teeth, masticatory muscles, palate, and part of the nasal cavity. In addition, the artery sends a branch into the cranial cavity as the main supply of the dura mater of the brain.

An understanding of the complicated ramification of the maxillary artery can be gained if one coordinates the different branches to the relations of the four sections of the artery. From the mandibular, or first, part of the maxillary artery arises the middle meningeal artery for the dura mater and the inferior alveolar artery, the main artery for the mandible. From the second, the muscular, or pterygoid, part of the maxillary artery arises the set of muscular branches, the temporal, pterygoid, masseteric, and buccal arteries. The third, or maxillary, part releases the branches for the upper jaw, namely, the posterior superior alveolar and the infraorbital arteries. The main terminal branches of the maxillary artery, released from its fourth, or pterygopalatine, part, are the sphenopalatine and the descending palatine arteries. In addition to these larger and more important branches, a number of smaller ones are given off by the maxillary artery.

The first, or mandibular, segment of the maxillary artery gives off two small branches to the ear. The deep auricular artery runs up through the parotid gland behind the jaw joint and pierces the cartilaginous or the bony wall of the external acoustic meatus to supply its lining and the outer surface of the tympanic membrane. Next the anterior tympanic branch enters the tympanic cavity of the middle ear through the petrotympanic fissure to supply the inner surface of the tympanic membrane and surrounding lining. Following these, the two main branches of this mandibular segment are released, the middle meningeal artery and the inferior alveolar artery.

The *middle meningeal artery* (Figs. 7-3 and 7-4) runs straight up to enter the foramen spinosum. On its way it usually passes between two roots of the auricular temporal nerve. (see Chapter 9). Below the cranial base the accessory meningeal artery originates; it supplies the auditory tube, adjacent muscles, and with one branch, which passes through the foramen ovale, the semilunar ganglion. Immediately after entering the cranial cavity, the middle meningeal artery sends several small tympanic branches into the tympanic cavity. These twigs perforate the roof of the middle ear. At a variable distance from the spinous foramen, the middle meningeal artery splits into a posterior branch and an anterior branch. The middle meningeal artery and its branches are embedded in deep and branching grooves on the inner surface of the cranial bones. They supply the dura mater and send branches into the bones over which they pass. The anterior branch of the middle meningeal artery anastomoses regularly with the lacrimal artery of the ophthalmic artery of the internal carotid.

The *inferior alveolar artery* (Figs. 7-3 and 7-4) varies in its origin according to the different relation of the maxillary artery to the lateral pterygoid muscle. If the maxillary artery lies superficial to the lateral pterygoid, the inferior alveolar artery is a direct branch of the maxillary artery. If, however, the main artery follows a deep course, the inferior alveolar artery frequently arises with the posterior deep temporal artery by a common trunk that winds around the lower border of the lateral pterygoid muscle. The posterior deep temporal artery reaches the temporal muscle by crossing the lateral surface of the lateral pterygoid, whereas the inferior alveolar artery arises at the lower border of the lateral pterygoid muscle. From its origin, the inferior alveolar artery turns almost vertically downward to reach the mandibular foramen, the entrance into the mandibular canal. The first part of the artery is, in most persons, closely applied to the inner surface of the mandible itself. Before entering the canal, the inferior alveolar artery releases the mylohyoid artery, which follows the mylohyoid nerve to the mylohyoid muscle, where it anastomoses with branches of the submental artery.

In the mandibular canal, the inferior alveolar artery sends branches into the marrow spaces of the bone and to the teeth and the alveolar process. The mental artery, the larger of the two terminal branches of the inferior alveolar artery, is released through the mental canal. The mental artery supplies the soft tissues of the chin and anastomoses with branches of the inferior labial artery. The second smaller terminal branch of the inferior alveolar artery is the incisive branch, which continues the course of the inferior alveolar artery inside the mandible to the midline, where it anastomoses with the artery of the other side.

The blood vessels that turn from the inferior alveolar artery upward into the alveolar process are of two distinct types. One set of branches enters the root canals through the apical foramina and supplies the dental pulps. They can be termed dental arteries. A second set of branches, alveolar, or perforating, branches, enter the interdental and interradicular septa. The alveolar branches ascend in narrow canals, which often are visible on radiographs, especially in the anterior part of the mandible. Many small branches, arising at right angles, enter the periodontal ligaments of adjacent teeth or adjacent roots of one tooth. The interradicular alveolar arteries end in the periodontal ligament at the bifurcation of the molars. The interdental alveolar arteries perforate the alveolar crest in the interdental spaces and end in the gingiva, supplying the interdental papilla and the adjacent areas of the buccal and lingual gingiva. In the gingiva these branches anastomose with superficial branches of arteries, which supply the oral and vestibular mucosae, for instance, with branches of the lingual, buccal, mental, and palatine arteries.

The second part, the muscular, or pterygoid, part of the maxillary artery supplies the masticatory muscles and the buccinator muscle. The temporal muscle receives two arteries arising from the superior wall of the maxillary artery, the *posterior* and *anterior deep temporal arteries.* They enter the temporal muscle from its deep surface. The posterior deep temporal artery anastomoses with the middle temporal artery. If the maxillary artery lies deep to the lateral pterygoid muscle, the posterior deep temporal artery winds around the lower border and the outer surface of the lateral pterygoid muscle to reach the temporal muscle, releasing the lower alveolar artery at the lower border of the lateral pterygoid muscle.

The *masseteric artery* leaves the maxillary artery on its lateral surface and passes through the mandibular notch following the masseteric nerve. Between the condylar process of the mandible and the posterior border of the tendon of the temporal muscle, the masseteric artery reaches the inner, or deep, surface of the masseter muscle, which it supplies. It also supplies the joint capsule (see Chapter 4).

Lateral and medial pterygoid muscles are supplied by a variable number of smaller *pterygoid branches* of the maxillary artery. The number and the location of these pterygoid branches depend on the relation of the maxillary artery to the lateral pterygoid muscle.

The last branch of the muscular part of the maxillary artery is the *buccal artery* (Figs. 7-3 and 7-4). If the maxillary artery is situated on the outer surface of the lateral pterygoid muscle, the buccal artery is given off just before the maxillary artery enters the slit between the two heads of the lateral pterygoid muscle. If the maxillary artery follows a deep course, the buccal artery passes laterally through the slit between the superior and inferior heads of the lateral pterygoid muscle. On the outer surface of this muscle the buccal artery turns downward and forward between the inferior head of the external pterygoid muscle and the temporal muscle. Crossing the temporal tendons obliquely, the buccal artery reaches the space between the masseter muscle and buccinator muscle below the buccal fat-pad, which fills this space. At the outer surface of the buccinator muscle, the buccal artery breaks up into its terminal branches. They supply the buccinator muscle and the mucous lining of the cheek and anastomose with branches of the facial artery and the transverse facial artery.

The third, or maxillary, segment of the maxillary artery runs along the posterior surface of the maxilla near its upper border. Here it gives off the posterior superior alveolar and infraorbital branches before entering the pterygomaxillary fissure.

The *posterior superior alveolar artery* (Figs. 7-3 and 7-4) is a fairly large vessel that winds down and out around the convexity of the maxillary tuberosity, where it is closely applied to the periosteum of the bone. On the way the artery gives off one or two branches that enter the posterior superior alveolar canals accompanied by the posterior superior alveolar nerves (see Chapter 9). The terminal, or gingival, extensions of the posterior superior alveolar artery continue to supply the mucosa covering the buccal surface of the alveolar process of the molars and premolars up to their gingival margins. Several branches extend into the cheeks. The posterior superior alveolar artery may sometimes be a branch of the buccal artery.

The *infraorbital artery* (Figs. 7-3 and 7-4) arises from the maxillary artery close to the posterior superior alveolar artery. Often the two arteries arise from the maxillary artery by a common trunk. The infraorbital artery enters the orbit through the inferior orbital fissure and runs anteriorly, first in the infraorbital sulcus and then in the infraorbital canal. Emerging through the infraorbital foramen, the infraorbital artery supplies the anterior part of the cheek and the root of the upper lip and anastomoses with branches of the superior labial artery of the facial artery and the angular artery, which it may replace. On its way through the orbit, the infraorbital artery sends small branches to the inferior muscles of the eyeball, the inferior rectus and the inferior oblique muscles, and participates in supplying the lower lid. Before leaving the infraorbital canal through the infraorbital foramen, the anterior superior alveolar artery is given off. It follows the anterior superior alveolar nerves through the narrow canals in the anterior wall of the maxillary sinus to the alveolar process. Here the anterior superior alveolar artery anastomoses with branches of the posterior superior alveolar artery and, in the neighborhood of the piriform aperture, with nasal arteries. The branches that the superior alveolar arteries release are, in principle, arranged like those in the mandible. The dental arteries enter the apical foramina of the roots and supply the dental pulps. These arteries send only small twigs to the periodontal membrane in the apical region of the teeth. The alveolar, or perforating, arteries descend in the septa between the sockets of adjacent teeth or roots as interdental or interradicular arteries. The former end in the gingival papillae, the latter in the periodontal membrane at the furcation of the roots. On their way through the inter-dental and interradicular septa the perforating arteries send many branches into the periodontal membrane of the adjacent roots.

The fourth, or pterygopalatine, part of the maxillary artery is short because the artery divides into its terminal branches immediately after entering the pterygopal-atine fossa through the pterygomaxillary fissure, the gap between the maxilla and the pterygoid process of the sphenoid bone.

The *descending palatine artery* (Fig. 7-5) is one of the terminal branches of the maxillary artery and arises in the pterygopalatine fossa. Descending through the pter-ygopalatine fossa and then through the pterygopalatine canal, the main branch of the descending palatine artery reaches the oral cavity through the major palatine fora-men.

In the pterygopalatine canal the descending palatine artery emits inferior poste-rior nasal branches, which enter the nasal cavity together with nasal branches of the palatine nerves. The nasal branches supply the inferior concha and the adjacent region of the lateral wall of the nasal cavity.

The main branch of the descending palatine artery emerging through the major palatine foramen is called the major palatine artery. One or two smaller branches, the minor palatine arteries, arise inside the pterygopalatine canal and reach the oral cavity through the minor palatine foramina. They supply the soft palate and the upper part of the palatine tonsil and anastomose with branches of the ascending palatine artery. The major palatine artery turns anteriorly from the major palatine foramen in the submucosa of the hard palate in a groove between the horizontal palatine process of the maxilla and the inner plate of the alveolar process. With numerous branches, the major palatine artery supplies the mucous membrane and the glands of the hard palate and the gingiva on the lingual surface of the upper alveolar process. The gingival branches of the palatine artery anastomose with gingival branches of the perfo-rating arteries of the upper aleovar arteries. The terminal part of the major palatine artery, the nasopalatine branch, reaches the incisive foramen and, ascending through the incisive canal, enters the nasal cavity where it anastomoses with septal branches of the sphenopalatine artery.

The second of the three terminal branches of the maxillary artery, the *artery of the pterygoid canal,* is a small branch that enters the pterygoid canal through its anterior opening and anastomoses in the canal with a branch of the ascending pharyngeal artery.

The *sphenopalatine artery* (Fig. 7-5) is the last of the terminal branches of the maxillary artery and supplies a large area of the nasal cavity. This artery passes from the uppermost part of the pterygopalatine fossa through the sphenopalatine foramen into the nasal cavity. Close to its roof the sphenopalatine artery divides into its lateral and septal branches. The posterior lateral nasal artery divides on the lateral wall of the nasal cavity into branches that supply the middle and upper nasal conchae and the mucous membrane in the corresponding nasal passages; smaller branches perforate the lateral nasal wall and reach the mucous membrane of the maxillary sinus. The posterior septal artery reaches the nasal septum over the roof of the nasal cavity and takes a diagonal course downward and forward along the septum. After supplying branches to the nasal septum, the septal artery passes through the incisive canal to anastomose with the nasopalatine branch of the major palatine artery.

In addition to the nasal branches, a branch to the pharynx arises from the sphe-nopalatine artery, which anastomoses with branches of the ascending pharyngeal artery.

Internal carotid artery

The internal carotid artery (Figs. 7-1, 7-2, and 7-5) ascends from its origin along the lateral wall of the pharynx to the base of the skull. It is at first situated behind and slightly medial to the external carotid artery. In its course upward the internal carotid moves away from the external carotid artery, and, where the internal carotid artery reaches the lateral wall of the pharynx, it is separated from the external carotid by the styloglossal and stylopharyngeus muscles. At the base of the skull, the internal carotid artery enters the carotid canal and passes through it into the cranial cavity. Here, the internal carotid artery is situated above the fibrocartilage, which fills and closes the foramen lacerum. The internal carotid now enters the cavernous sinus (see Fig. 14-3), through which it passes in a tight S-shaped curve. Perforating the dura mater at the roof of the cavernous sinus, the internal carotid artery reaches the intradural space and the brain.

The internal carotid artery can be divided into a cervical and a cranial part. The cervical part is branchless and slightly curved so that the artery can follow the move-ments of the neck without being stretched. The curves increase with advancing age because of the gradual loss of elasticity of the arterial wall. In elderly persons the internal carotid artery sometimes follows a strongly tortuous course, and then its normal relation to the external carotid artery may be altered; for some distance the internal carotid artery may lie in the same layer as the external carotid or even superficial to it. In the upper part of its course, a tortuous internal carotid artery may bulge toward the lateral wall of the pharynx, and the pulse of the internal carotid artery then can be seen through the wide-open mouth.

The cervical part of the internal carotid artery is closely related to the internal jugular vein. The vein is at first situated lateral and slightly anterior to the internal carotid artery, then at its lateral surface, and, still higher up, the vein moves gradually toward the posterior surface of the internal carotid artery. At the base of the skull, the jugular foramen is located posterior and slightly medial to the entrance into the carotid canal. Thus the vein describes half a spiral around the artery.

The internal carotid artery is also closely related to the vagus nerve, which lies between the internal jugular vein and the internal carotid artery and somewhat deep to the blood vessels. The cervical sympathetic trunk is separated from the vessels by the prevertebral fascia.

The internal carotid artery releases a few small and rather insignificant branches in its course through the carotid canal of the temporal bone. Of these, the caroticotympanic branches enter the tympanic cavity; others supply the dura mater around the cavernous sinus. In the cavernous sinus, the internal carotid artery supplies fine twigs to the ophthalmic nerve and to the pituitary gland. After emerging through the roof of the cavernous sinus, the internal carotid artery releases the ophthalmic artery, which follows the optic nerve into the orbit, then emits its cerebral branches.

The anterior cerebral artery turns medially and then anteriorly; where it bends it is connected with the anterior cerebral artery of the other side by the anterior communicating artery. The middle cerebral artery leaves the internal carotid at its lateral circumference to enter the deep lateral, or Sylvian, fissure between the frontal and temporal lobes of the brain. The posterior communicating artery is given off at the posterior circumference of the internal carotid artery together with the anterior choroid artery. The right and left posterior communicating arteries join the posterior cerebral arteries, which are the terminal branches of the unpaired basilar artery. Thus an irregular hexagonal chain of anastomosing arteries, the circle of Willis, is closed around the optic chiasm and the stalk of the hypophysis.

Ophthalmic artery. This branch of the internal carotid artery supplies the eyeball, its muscles, and the lacrimal gland and sends branches into the eyelids and into the upper part of the face. The central artery of the retina and the ciliary arteries are destined for the eyeball. The lacrimal gland and the muscles of the eyeball are supplied by the lacrimal artery and muscular branches. Posterior and anterior ethmoid branches enter the nasal cavity through the ethmoid foramina. Medial and lateral palpebral branches, the latter arising from the lacrimal artery, ramify in the eyelids. The supraorbital branch (Figs. 7-2 and 7-4) swings around the upper rim of the orbital entrance into the forehead, passing with the supraorbital nerve through the supraorbital notch, or supraorbital foramen. It supplies the frontal muscle and the skin of the forehead.

A frontal, or supratrochlear, branch leaves the orbit near the medial corner of the eye and sends its branches to the soft tissues of the forehead. The supraorbital and frontal branches anastomose with each other, with the anterior branch of the superficial temporal artery, and, across the midline, with the arteries of the other side.

The last facial branch of the ophthalmic artery is the nasal, or dorsal nasal, branch, which courses downward on the lateral surface of the nose and anastomoses with the angular artery, the terminal part of the facial artery. The nasal artery and angular artery are in a reciprocal relation; if one of these arteries is weak or missing, the other is proportionately stronger or may even replace the missing branch. The nasal artery anastomoses not only with the angular artery, but also with the infraorbital artery.

VEINS

The venous blood of the head and neck is drained almost entirely by the internal jugular vein (Figs. 7-6 and 7-7), which, behind the sternoclavicular articulation, joins

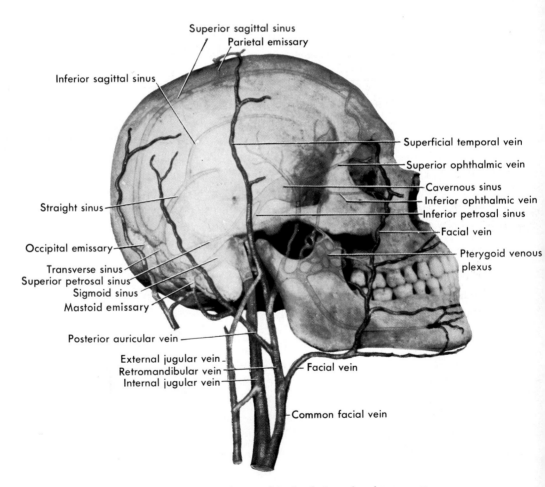

Fig. 7-6. Diagram of veins of the head. See color plate opposite.

the subclavian vein to form the brachiocephalic (innominate) vein. The two brachio-cephalic veins unite to form the superior vena cava. Along the neck itself, two super-ficial veins are added to the deep internal jugular vein, namely, the external and the anterior jugular veins (Fig. 7-8). At the root of the neck the superficial veins finally open into the deep vein.

As in other parts of the body, the superficial and deep veins are united by several anastomoses. Moreover, the superficial veins themselves are connected with each other, and the great variability of the veins in the face and neck is caused by the great

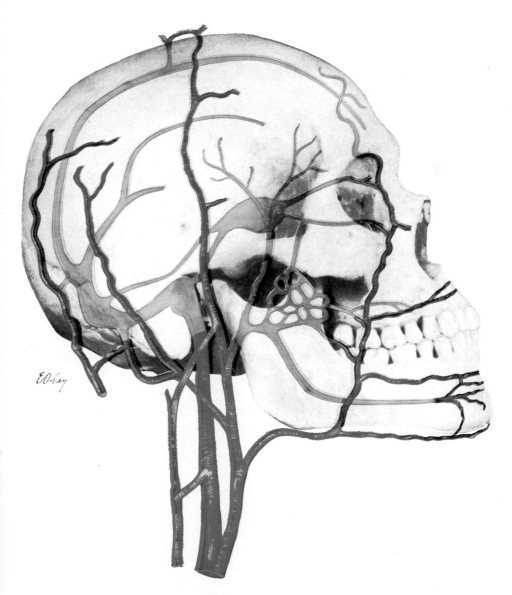

Fig. 7-6, cont'd. For legend see opposite page.

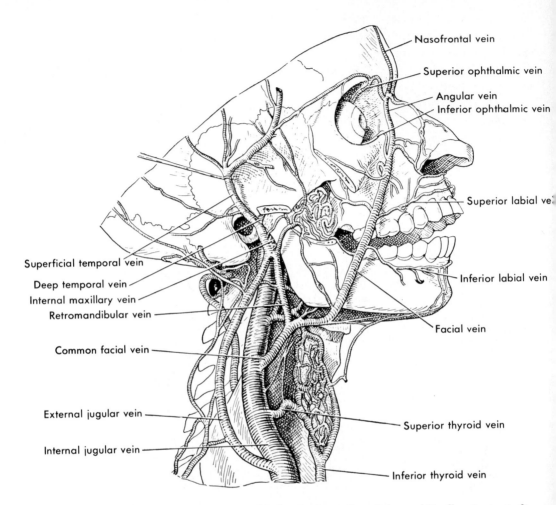

Fig. 7-7. Veins of the head and neck. (Modified and redrawn from Sicher and Tandler: Anatomie für Zahnärzte.)

number of possible outlets for the drained venous blood. In other words, anastomotic branches may assume greater proportions, whereas parts of the typical veins may diminish in caliber or even become obsolete.

The complications of the system of veins in the head and neck are further enhanced by the fact that intracranial veins, draining the blood of the brain, and extracranial veins are connected by multiple anastomoses, which permit a flow of blood in both directions. The anastomoses between the veins of the brain, enclosed in a rigid bony capsule, and the extracranial veins are safety outlets. Their existence prevents a rise of the intracranial pressure, which would occur if the internal jugular vein, the main drainage of the cerebral blood, were compressed. In this case the venous blood of the brain can escape in many directions. These communications are, however, a potential danger because an infection, involving primarily an extracranial

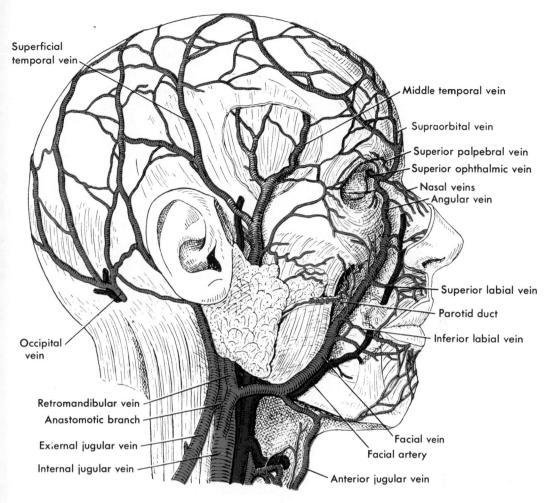

Superficial temporal vein

Middle temporal vein

Supraorbital vein

Superior palpebral vein

Superior ophthalmic vein

Nasal veins

Angular vein

Superior labial vein

Parotid duct

Inferior labial vein

Occipital vein

Retromandibular vein

Anastomotic branch

External jugular vein

Internal jugular vein

Facial vein

Facial artery

Anterior jugular vein

Fig. 7-8. Superficial veins of the face and scalp. (Modified and redrawn from Tandler: Lehrbuch der Anatomie.)

vein, for instance one of the facial veins, may spread to the intracranial veins and involve the meninges, the covering membranes of the brain. The danger of a retrograde spread of infection is the graver, because the veins of the face have few, if any, valves, which in other veins prevent a backflow of blood. In addition one has to remember that the intracranial veins, collecting the blood of the brain, are not collapsible. The sinuses of the dura mater have, in fact, no wall of their own, but are spaces or canals between layers of the dura mater. They are lined by endothelium characteristic of all blood vessels. The rigidity of the walls of the sinus prevents any change in their lumen and renders them open ways for the spread of an infection.

Internal jugular vein. This vein (Fig. 7-7) commences at the jugular foramen, the main outlet of the venous blood of the brain. Immediately below the jugular foramen the internal jugular vein is considerably widened to form the superior bulb of the internal jugular vein, contained in the jugular fossa on the inferior surface of the temporal bone. The internal jugular vein is here located posterior to the internal carotid artery, which enters the skull through the carotid canal. Descending with the internal carotid artery and, farther below, with the common carotid artery and the vagus nerve, the internal jugular vein moves first to the lateral and then to the anterolateral circumference of the artery. At its lower end, at the junction with the subclavian vein, the internal jugular vein is again widened to form the inferior bulb. At this junction or slightly above it the internal jugular vein carries its only valve. Right and left jugular veins are rarely of equal diameter, the right jugular vein as a rule being wider than the left. The difference in the caliber is caused by the asymmetry of the sinuses of the dura mater.

The tributary branches of the internal jugular vein are as follows. Into the superior bulb opens the inferior petrosal sinus, which leaves the skull through the jugular foramen or in front of it. Veins of the pharynx, of the root of the tongue, and of the sublingual area drain into the upper part of the internal jugular vein. The next branch is the (common) facial vein, which drains the blood of the superficial and deep parts of the face. In the upper corner of the carotid triangle, where these veins empty into the internal jugular vein, there is normally a wide anastomosis between the internal jugular vein and the superficial external jugular vein (Figs. 7-8 and 7-9). In the lower part of the neck, the veins of the larynx and thyroid glands are the main tributaries of the internal jugular vein. Into its terminal part empty the external and the anterior jugular veins.

The lingual veins drain the tongue and sublingual region. Corresponding to the three main branches of the lingual artery, the veins are arranged as dorsal lingual veins, deep lingual veins, and a sublingual vein. Most of these veins accompany the corresponding arteries; the smaller branches of the artery are, as a rule, flanked by two veins that anastomose with one another. The largest of these veins is the sublingual vein, which accompanies the hypoglossal nerve for some distance. The veins of the tongue may join to a single large trunk or may empty separately into the internal jugular vein. In many persons the lingual veins drain into the common facial vein; in others some of these veins may open into the internal jugular and some into the common facial vein. Some veins from the pharynx often join the lingual veins, whereas others drain directly into the internal jugular vein.

Facial (common facial) vein. This vein (Figs. 7-7 to 7-9) drains the blood of the superficial and deep parts of the face, that is, in general, the blood of the areas supplied by the facial, the maxillary, and the superficial temporal arteries. Typically the common facial vein originates below the angle of the mandible from the junction of the facial and retromandibular veins. The vein turns downward and backward, perforates the investing layer of the deep fascia, and reaches the internal jugular vein approximately at the level of the hyoid bone. In most persons an anastomosis connects the common facial vein with the external jugular vein.

Facial (anterior facial) vein. This vein (Figs. 7-7 to 7-9) corresponds in the main to the facial artery. The facial vein takes its origin from the junction of the veins of the

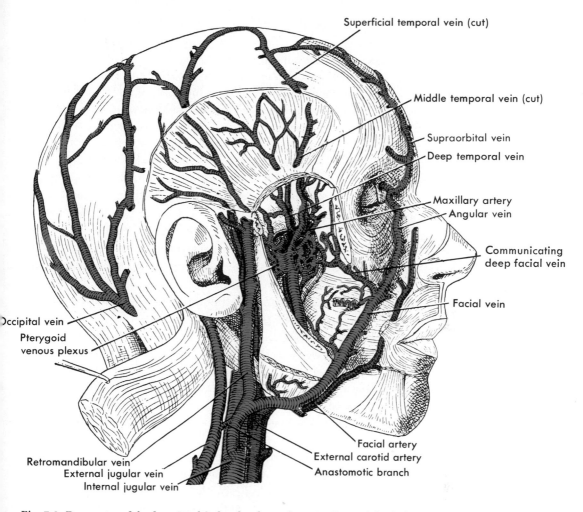

Fig. 7-9. Deep veins of the face. (Modified and redrawn from Tandler: Lehrbuch der Anatomie.)

forehead and nose. Its upper part is termed the angular vein and accompanies the angular artery, the terminal part of the facial artery. The angular vein receives the frontal vein, the supraorbital vein, and veins from the lower lid and from the bridge of the nose.

The frontal vein collects the blood from the anterior parts of the scalp and descends close to the midline in the superficial fascia toward the inner corner of the eye. Right and left frontal veins are often fused to an unpaired, slightly asymmetrically situated vein, which may empty into one of the angular veins or connect with both right and left angular veins. If the two frontal veins are fused, the unpaired vein is termed the median frontal vein. The frontal vein is often readily visible through the skin.

The supraorbital vein, draining the blood from the region of the eyebrow, empties either into the frontal vein or into the angular vein. Frontal and supraorbital veins anastomose through wide venous nets with the other veins of the scalp, the superficial temporal, posterior auricular, and occipital veins.

Where palpebral and nasal veins join at the inner corner of the eye, the angular vein is constantly in wide communication with the superior ophthalmic vein. The anastomotic branch is situated above the medial palpebral ligament. The superior ophthalmic vein, which opens into the cavernous sinus, thus forms a wide link between the facial vein and the intracranial sinuses of the dura mater (see Chapter 14).

From the inner corner of the eye the facial vein descends in a fairly straight line to the lower border of the mandible, which it reaches at the anterior border of the masseter muscle. The facial vein lies behind the facial artery. In the upper part of the face and at the mandible, the artery and the vein are in close relation. In the middle part of the cheek, however, the vein lies at some distance behind the artery and is also more superficial, the elevator of the upper lip being interposed between the vessels. In its course along the cheek, the facial vein receives the upper and lower labial veins and veins from the cheek itself.

Branches of the facial vein anastomose with the infraorbital vein and the mental vein. One anastomotic vein connects the pterygoid venous plexus, which drains into the retromandibular vein, with the facial vein and is therefore of importance. This branch, the communicating, or deep facial, vein (Fig. 7-9), courses anteriorly and inferiorly on the inner surface of the temporal and masseter muscles and appears between the masseter and buccinator muscles below the zygomatic process of the maxilla to open into the facial vein. Below the mandible the facial vein, running backward and downward, receives the submental vein and palatine veins, which also drain the tonsil.

Retromandibular (posterior facial) vein. This vein (Figs. 7-7 to 7-9) drains approximately the regions that are supplied by the maxillary and the superficial temporal arteries. The retromandibular vein is made up by the union of the superficial temporal and the maxillary veins in the substance of the parotid gland behind the neck of the mandible. The retromandibular vein descends in the gland and is superficial or lateral to the external carotid artery. The vein emerges at the lower pole of the gland to unite in typical cases with the facial vein. In most persons the retromandibular vein and the external carotid artery diverge inferiorly and are separated by a fairly thick layer of the parotid gland. The vein continues downward on the outer surface of the stylohyoid and digastric muscles, but the artery lies deep to these muscles (Fig. 7-9). In some persons, however, a deep branch of the retromandibular vein follows the external carotid artery in its deep course and empties into the internal jugular vein.

The superficial temporal artery and its branches are often accompanied by two veins. Above the root of the zygomatic arch, a middle temporal vein opens into the superficial temporal vein. The middle temporal vein drains a venous plexus that is situated underneath the temporal fascia and receives blood from the temporal muscle. The two maxillary veins are the outlet of the large and dense pterygoid venous plexus, which surrounds the maxillary artery in the infratemporal fossa. The ptery-goid plexus of veins (Figs. 7-7 and 7-9), into which the veins of the deep structures of the face open, is situated between temporal and lateral pterygoid, or between lateral and medial pterygoid muscles, depending on the variable course of the maxillary artery. Anteriorly it reaches from the tuberosity of the maxilla, superiorly to the base of the skull. Aside from the veins of the masticatory muscles, the following blood vessels empty into the pterygoid plexus: sphenopalatine veins, draining the posterior part of the nasal cavity and the greater part of the palate; middle meningeal veins, draining the dura mater, which leave the cranial cavity through the spinous foramen; articular veins from the rich plexus in and around the capsule of the mandibular joint; auricular veins from the external ear; and a transverse facial vein, draining the posterior part of the cheek and the parotid gland.

The dense venous plexus surrounding the maxillary artery serves to protect the artery from compression when the masticatory muscles contract. During their contraction the bulging muscles drive blood from the veins. During relaxation of these muscles the veins fill again. Such a "mechanical" protective function of veins is by no means rare in the human body; an example is the venous plexus surrounding the internal carotid artery in the carotid canal.

External jugular vein. This vein (Fig. 7-7) is one of the two superficial veins of the neck. It originates below the lobe of the ear by the union of the posterior auricular veins and the occipital veins, which correspond to the arteries of the same names. The external jugular vein courses almost vertically downward and therefore crosses the sternocleidomastoid muscle diagonally. This course leads the vein toward the posterior border of the muscle above its insertion to the clavicle; the vein curves around the posterior border of the sternocleidomastoid muscle and passes into the depth. From its origin to this point the vein is covered only by the platysma muscle and the skin and is, in many individuals, visible through the skin as a blue line. Above the clavicle the external jugular vein perforates the deep fascia and empties into the inferior end of the internal jugular vein. At this point, or somewhat higher up, the external jugular vein possesses a pair of valves. A second pair of valves is sometimes found at a variable height, but most frequently in the lower half of the external jugular vein. Aside from the two veins, which, by their union, constitute the external jugular vein, it receives only few tributaries. One is the variable cutaneous vein of the neck, which drains the blood from the occipital region and the neighboring area of the neck and reaches the external jugular vein about halfway down the neck. A more important vein emptying into the external jugular vein is an anastomotic branch from the common facial vein.

Anterior jugular vein. A second superficial venous drainage on the neck is provided by the anterior jugular vein (Fig. 7-8). This vein, however, is variable and often absent on one or both sides. Sometimes the two veins fuse and form a median vein of the neck. Not far above the sternoclavicular articulation, the anterior jugular vein curves around the anterior border of the sternocleidomastoid muscles and, perforating the deep fascia, turns laterally to open into the lowermost part of the internal jugular vein, or into the angle formed by the union of the internal jugular and subclavian veins, or into the terminal part of the external jugular vein. The anterior jugular vein drains the skin and superficial fascia of a narrow anterior part of the neck close to the midline.

Above the superior border of the sternum, in the suprasternal space of Burns, the two anterior jugular veins are commonly united by a transverse anastomosis, the jugular arc. If the anterior jugular veins are absent, this transverse venous vessel may connect the two external or the two internal jugular veins. If the anterior jugular veins are replaced by a median vein, the vessel divides in the interfascial space into two branches that turn laterally to reach the internal or external jugular veins (see Fig. 15-2).

VARIATIONS OF THE SUPERFICIAL CERVICAL VEINS

The variations of the superficial veins of the neck and their relations to the facial veins are of some importance from a practical point of view. These variations are explained by the fact that the superficial veins develop from a rather uniform subcutaneous venous net through a widening of some of its meshes. Moreover, superficial and deep cervical veins are, as elsewhere in the body, connected by several anastomotic branches. The most important and frequent variations are the following: (1) The common facial vein does not exist. The retromandibular vein continues into the external jugular vein; the facial vein opens into the internal jugular vein. (2) The retromandibular vein opens into the internal jugular vein, the facial vein continues into the anterior jugular vein, and a common facial vein again is absent. (3) The common facial vein loses its connection with the internal jugular vein and empties instead into the external jugular vein. (4) The retromandibular vein continues into the external jugular vein; the facial vein continues into the anterior jugular vein.

The superficial veins of the neck are more often different than symmetrical on the right and the left side.

SINUSES OF THE DURA MATER

The blood of the brain and the eye is collected by a system of specialized veins in the dura mater called sinuses (Figs. 7-6 and 7-10). These sinuses are not collapsible, and their lumen is unchangeable because their walls are formed by the dense, rigid, and inelastic tissue of the dura mater. They drain eventually into the internal jugular vein, but there are numerous communications between sinuses and the extracranial veins. A short description of these sinuses is necessary to understand the clinical implication of their communications with the veins of the face and head that are located outside the cranial cavity.

Superior sagittal sinus. This sinus commences in the region of the crista galli of the ethmoid bone and, gradually gaining in volume, curves posteriorly in the midline over the frontal, parietal, and occipital bones. On its way it receives numerous veins from the convexity of the brain.

Inferior sagittal sinus. A narrow sinus, the inferior sagittal sinus, is enclosed in the lower free border of a sickle-shaped median fold of the dura, the falx cerebri, which separates the two hemispheres of the cerebrum.

Straight sinus. Where the falx and the tentorium, a roughly horizontal fold of the dura between cerebrum and cerebellum, meet, the inferior sagittal sinus joins with a deep vein of the brain and continues backward and downward as the straight sinus. The straight sinus unites with the superior sagittal sinus at the inner occipital eminence.

Occipital sinus. This small vein begins on either side of the great occipital foramen and ascends in the midline. It ends at the inner occipital eminence.

Transverse sinuses. The point where the superior sagittal sinus, straight sinus, and occipital sinus unite is called the confluence of the sinuses. From here the blood is drained by the paired transverse sinuses. A symmetrical arrangement is, however, the exception rather than the rule; more often the division of the blood is asymmetrical. Sometimes the superior sagittal sinus and the straight sinus do not join but continue each into one transverse sinus. Even if the sinuses join, a greater amount of blood usually enters the right transverse sinus than the left. As a consequence the right internal jugular vein is often much larger than the left. In a small number of persons, the division of the blood is reversed, so that more blood is drained toward the left than toward the right jugular vein.

The transverse sinus runs almost horizontally across the occipital bone, the inferoposterior corner of the parietal bone, and then over the temporal bone to the point where the superior crest of the temporal pyramid commences. From this point the transverse sinus continues in an S-shaped curve as the sigmoid sinus; the convexity of

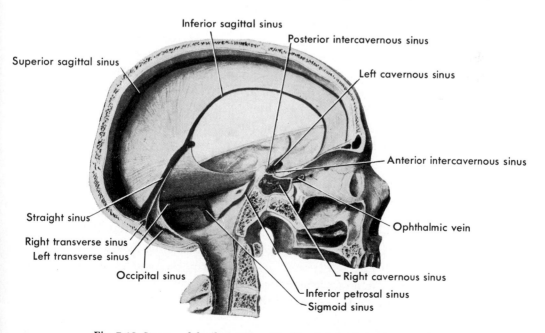

Fig. 7-10. Sinuses of the dura mater. (Tandler: Lehrbuch der Anatomie.)

the upper curve is directed anteriorly, whereas the lower convexity faces posteriorly. Descending toward the cranial base, the sigmoid sinus continues through the jugular foramen into the internal jugular vein (Fig. 7-10).

Cavernous and intercavernous sinuses. In the anterior part of the cranial base lies a second system of venous sinuses, the center of which is the paired cavernous sinus. This name was chosen because the cavernous sinus is not a uniform, wide-open space but is subdivided by thin strands and trabeculae of connective tissue into a system of communicating smaller spaces, which create a similarity with an erectile cavernous body. The cavernous sinus is situated on the lateral slope of the body of the sphenoid bone, on either side of the sella turcica, which houses the pituitary gland. In front of the gland and in back of it, right and left cavernous sinuses communicate with each other through the anterior and posterior intercavernous sinuses.

The venous channels draining into the cavernous sinus anteriorly are two on either side. Along the posterior edge of the lesser wing of the sphenoid bone runs the sphenoparietal sinus into the anterolateral corner of the cavernous sinus. At its beginning the sphenoparietal sinus communicates with a branch of the middle meningeal vein.

The most important tributary of the cavernous sinus is the ophtalmic vein. It originates from the union of a larger superior and a smaller inferior ophthalmic vein, which drain the eyeball and its auxiliary organs. The ophthalmic vein reaches the cavernous sinus through the superior orbital fissure. Sometimes superior and inferior ophthalmic veins open separately into the cavernous sinus.

Superior and inferior petrosal sinuses. The blood that has been collected in the cavernous sinus is drained posteriorly by two venous sinuses on either side, the superior and the inferior petrosal sinuses. The superior petrosal sinus originates from the posterosuperior corner of the cavernous sinus, courses posteriorly and laterally along the superior crest of the temporal pyramid, and reaches the transverse sinus, where the latter bends to continue into the sigmoid sinus. Near the apex of the pyramid, the sinus bridges the trigeminal notch.

The inferior petrosal sinus is shorter but wider than the superior. It arises from the inferoposterior corner of the cavernous sinus and follows the petro-occipital fissure backward to the anterior border of the jugular foramen. It passes through the most anterior portion of this foramen or through the petro-occipital fissure in front of the jugular foramen, crosses the glossopharyngeal, vagus, and accessory nerves, and empties into the superior bulb of the internal jugular vein.

Through the cavernous sinus runs the internal carotid artery, surrounded by the carotid plexus of sympathetic nerves. Lateral to the S-curved artery, the abducent nerve traverses the sinus in an almost sagittal direction. During their passage through the sinus, the internal carotid artery, the sympathetic plexus, and the abducent nerve are covered by endothelium. Oculomotor, trochlear, and ophthalmic nerves are situated in the roof and the lateral wall of the sinus and have, therefore, less intimate relations to the sinus (see Fig. 14-3).

The internal carotid artery enters the sinus through its posteroinferior wall and leaves through the anterior part of its roof. The abducent nerve enters the most anterior part of the inferior petrosal sinus on the clivus and then runs into the cavernous sinus. It leaves the cavernous sinus through its anterior wall, which borders the superior orbital fissure, where the abducent nerve converges with the oculomotor, trochlear, and ophthalmic nerves.

Basilar plexus. A loose network of veins, the basilar plexus, extends on the clivus from the cavernous sinus to the anterior border of the foramen magnum and drains here into the veins of the vertebral canal.

COMMUNICATIONS BETWEEN INTRACRANIAL AND EXTRACRANIAL VEINS

The connections between the sinuses and the veins outside the cranial cavity are important outlets for the blood of the brain but are also potential passages for infections into the cranium. They are mainly of four types.

Short but sometimes wide veins form a direct communication between a sinus and a vein on the outside of the brain capsule. These communicating veins are termed emissary veins, or emissaries.

Cranial nerves and the internal carotid artery are surrounded by venous plexuses where they leave or enter the skull. These veins are a second but less important connection between intracranial and extracranial veins.

A third indirect communication between the two systems of veins is provided by the diploic veins, the veins of the bones of the cranial vault.

The fourth and last indirect but highly important connection is mediated by the ophthalmic veins, which drain into the cavernous sinus but anastomose with veins of the face.

Venous emissaries (Fig. 7-6). The emissaries are characterized by thin walls that are tightly attached to the surrounding bone or fibrocartilage and are therefore not collapsible. The parietal emissary perforates the parietal bone close to the midline at the boundary between the middle and posterior thirds of the sagittal suture. It connects the superior sagittal sinus with a branch of the superficial temporal vein. The parietal emissary frequently is missing on one or both sides.

The mastoid emissary is found in the suture between the occipital bone and the mastoid plate of the temporal bone or in the mastoid plate close to the suture. It is a connection between the sigmoid sinus and a branch of the occipital veins.

The condylar emissary perforates the lateral part of the occipital bone in an almost horizontal course from the posterior part of the jugular notch to the condylar foramen behind the occipital condyle and connects the terminal part of the sigmoid sinus with one of the deep occipital or cervical veins.

The inconstant occipital emissary is unpaired. It perforates the occipital bone close to the internal occipital protuberance and forms a communication between the confluence of the sinuses and an occipital vein.

In front of and medial to the foramen ovale, the greater wing of the sphenoid bone is perforated (foramen of Vesalius) by the inconstant sphenoid emissary, linking the cavernous sinus and the pterygoid venous plexus. In other instances the sphenoid emissary perforates the fibrocartilage of the foramen lacerum.

In the child only, the anterior end of the superior sagittal sinus communicates with the nasal veins through the foramen cecum. The communicating emissary is known as Zuckerkandl's vein.

Venous plexuses. In contrast to the emissaries, the veins that connect the sinuses and the extracranial veins along the internal carotid artery and many of the cranial nerves are loosely connected with the surrounding tissues and are therefore collapsible. This is especially obvious in the carotid plexus of veins, which is, in fact, a compressible cushioning, allowing for the changes in volume of the artery during its pulsation. During systole the expanding artery empties the veins of the accompanying plexus; during diastole, when the artery narrows, blood again fills the surrounding veins.

The internal carotid plexus of veins connects the cavernous sinus with the pterygoid plexus of veins. Another, more important, plexus of veins accompanies the hypoglossal nerve through the hypoglossal canal.

Diploic veins. The diploic veins (see Fig. 2-4) are wide, valveless, and noncollapsible veins in the flat bones of the cranial roof. The diploic veins are variable. They are situated in the diploe, the spongy layer of the cranial bones, and drain partly into a neighboring sinus, partly to the outside into an adjacent vein. Thus they provide an indirect communication of the intracranial and extracranial veins.

The frontal diploic vein descends in the squama of the frontal bone close to the midline and drains into the superior sagittal sinus and one of the frontal veins.

In the temporal region an anterior and a posterior temporal diploic vein are found. The anterior temporal diploic vein is contained in the posterior part of the frontal squama and empties into the sphenoparietal sinus and the middle temporal vein. A posterior temporal diploic vein in the posterior part of the parietal bone sends its blood to the sigmoid sinus and to an occipital vein.

An occipital diploic vein situated in the occipital squama connects with the transverse sinus and a branch of the occipital vein.

Communications of the ophthalmic veins. The communications of the ophthalmic veins with the facial (Figs. 7-6 to 7-9) and retromandibular (Fig. 7-6) veins are of special importance in the pathology of facial infections. A communication is established via ophthalmic veins between the system of the facial veins and the cavernous sinus, into which the ophthalmic veins drain. The superior ophthalmic vein is, at the inner corner of the eye, in constant and wide communication with the angular vein, which continues into the facial vein. The inferior ophthalmic vein has inconstant anastomoses with the infraorbital veins or the inferior palpebral veins at the lower border of the orbital entrance and thus has indirect connections with the facial vein.

Of equal importance is an anastomosis between the veins of the orbit and the retromandibular vein that connects the posterior end of the inferior ophthalmic vein with the pterygoid plexus of veins, from which the retromandibular vein receives most of its blood. The anastomosing branch passes through the inferior orbital fissure and links the system of the retromandibular vein with the cavernous sinus behind the orbit.

CHAPTER 8

The lymphatic system

As in all other regions of the human body, lymph vessels and lymph nodes of the head and neck are of great clinical importance. Infections as well as malignant tumors may spread via lymph vessels. Despite the frequent and wide communications between smaller and larger lymph vessels, the lymph of any specific region is carried, in the great majority of persons, to certain well-localized lymph nodes. Lymph nodes that receive the lymph of a definite region before it has passed through other lymph nodes are called regional lymph nodes. They are the first site at which pathologic processes will manifest themselves if they spread from their primary location via lymph vessels.

Knowledge of the regional lymph nodes is important for two reasons: One is able to prognosticate the possible or probable involvement of certain lymph nodes if the site of a tumor or an infection is known, and, conversely, knowledge of the regional nodes permits the diagnosis of an obscure site of a pathologic process if a lymph node or a group of lymph nodes is found diseased. It is, however, necessary to remember that the lymph, after passing the regional node or nodes, is carried farther to more centrally located lymph nodes. The regional lymph nodes may also be called primary lymph nodes of a certain organ or region; the more central lymph nodes can be described as secondary, tertiary, etc., in the order in which they receive the lymph. Furthermore, it is important to realize that a group of lymph nodes that are secondary to a certain region may be primary nodes for another region. Despite these complications and despite the frequent major variations in the relations of lymph vessels and lymph nodes, knowledge of the regional coordination of lymph nodes is of paramount importance in diagnosis and therapy of infections and malignant tumors.

LYMPHATIC TISSUE OF THE ORAL CAVITY AND PHARYNX

The posterior part of the oral cavity, the fauces, and the neighboring parts of the pharynx contain an accumulation of lymphatic tissue, forming some distinct lymphatic organs. These are the pharyngeal tonsil at the roof of the pharynx, the two palatine tonsils between the anterior and posterior palatine pillars, and the less circumscribed lingual tonsil at the base of the tongue. An accumulation of lymphatic tissue at the opening of the auditory tube into the pharynx is called the tubal tonsil. In addition, the pillars and the adjacent parts of the pharyngeal mucosa contain numerous solitary lymph follicles.

The lymphatic organs, guarding, as it were, the entrance into the deeper parts of the digestive tract, are known as the pharyngeal lymphatic ring of Waldeyer. The lymphatic tissue is highly developed in the infant and child but undergoes later regressive changes and almost disappears in old age.

The pharyngeal tonsil occupies the entire breadth of the pharyngeal roof, extending between the openings of the auditory tubes. It is a rounded, variably protruding body into which are cut deep and narrow, irregularly branching furrows, the tonsillar crypts. Sometimes a much deeper groove, situated at the center of the pharyngeal tonsil, extends through the lymphatic tissue into the underlying connective tissue. This deep recessus is known as the pharyngeal bursa.

The palatine tonsils, or *the* tonsils, are ovoid of lymphatic tissue, cleft by deep crypts, as is the pharyngeal tonsil. The tonsils are situated in the tonsillar niche between the palatoglossal and palatopharyngeal arches. A triangular groove above the tonsil and below the common origin of the arches is known as the supratonsillar fossa. The anterior border of the tonsil is sometimes covered by a variably high extension of the palatoglossal arch. This duplication of the mucous membrane is called the semilunar fold where it covers the upper pole of the tonsil and triangular fold at the lower pole of the tonsil.

The palatine tonsils are bounded toward the superior pharyngeal constrictor by a well-differentiated capsule. The blood supply of the palatine tonsil is provided by several smaller arteries, branches of neighboring blood vessels. One branch, however, gains prominence in most cases, namely, the tonsillar branch of the ascending palatine artery; sometimes it is an independent branch of the facial artery (see Chapter 7).

Along the palatoglossal arch isolated lymphatic follicles sometimes form a link between the palatine and lingual tonsils. The latter consist, as previously described, of the aggregation of the lingual follicles that occupy the surface of the base of the tongue.

The solitary lymphatic follicles of the pharyngeal mucosa are especially numerous in a small area just below the pharyngeal ostium of the tube. If this aggregation of lymphatic tissue gains more than average prominence it is referred to as the tubal tonsil.

LYMPH NODES OF THE HEAD AND NECK

Although the site of lymph nodes is fairly constant, there is a great variability as to their number and size. Ordinarily it is best to speak of groups of lymph nodes rather than of a single node because one node in any one region may be subdivided into two or more smaller nodes. In the regions of the face and neck that are of practical importance for the oral surgeon, the lymph nodes are distributed in superficial and deep groups. To the many typical groups of nodes have to be added accessory nodes, which are present in a smaller or larger percentage of persons. If accessory lymph nodes are present, they are always found along larger lymph vessels, which, in turn, usually follow the veins; the potential sites of accessory lymph nodes are therefore predictable with a fair degree of accuracy.

Around the outer ear and close to it lie several groups of lymph nodes, the auricular lymph nodes (Fig. 8-3). They can be subdivided into anterior, inferior, and posterior groups. The posterior auricular, or postauricular, lymph nodes receive the lymph from a part of the ear and a wide region of the scalp above and behind the ear. The anterior auricular lymph nodes, or preauricular lymph nodes, are situated in front of the external ear. It is of importance that some of these small nodes are superficial to the capsule of the parotid gland, whereas others are found inside the capsule and even in the substance of the parotid gland. The preauricular lymph nodes are regional to the skin of the anterior temporal region, to the lateral parts of the forehead and of the eyelids, to the posterior part of the cheek, to a part of the outer ear, and, finally, to the parotid gland itself. The lymph nodes of the preauricular group that are more intimately related to the parotid gland are often described as parotid lymph nodes. Preauricular and postauricular lymph nodes send their efferent lymph vessels to the infra-auricular group below the ear lobe or to the superficial and deep cervical lymph nodes.

The anterior and lateral surfaces of the face are not infrequently the site of accessory lymph nodes. They are found along the facial vein and can be subdivided into three groups. The upper group is situated close to the inner corner of the eye or a little farther down along the lateral boundary of the nose to the level of the nasal wing. Such infraorbital nodes are fairly rare. More frequent is a node or a group of two or three smaller nodes, buccal lymph nodes, in the cheek at or about the level of the corner of the mouth. In some persons they lie close to the corner of the mouth; in others they lie closer to the anterior border of the masseter muscle. The last and most inferior group of the accessory facial lymph nodes is found at or slightly above the lower border of the mandible, where the facial vein and facial artery cross the mandible. These nodes are called mandibular, or supramandibular, lymph nodes. All of these accessory facial lymph nodes are regional to the skin on the anterior surface of the face. However, the buccal, and especially the supramandibular, lymph nodes also receive lymph from deeper parts of the face, the mucous membrane of the lips and cheek, and occasionally even from upper or lower teeth and the adjacent gingiva.

Below the mandible and close to its lower border are situated one unpaired and two paired groups of lymph nodes. The unpaired group of submental lymph nodes (Figs. 8-1 and 8-3) lies between the chin and the hyoid bone and between the anterior bellies of the digastric muscles in the submental triangle. In some persons the submental node or nodes are found close to the chin; in others they are found farther below in the neighborhood of the hyoid bone. According to their position, they are characterized as superior and inferior submental nodes. Frequently both groups are represented in the same person. The submental nodes are regional to the middle part of the lower lip, to the skin of the chin, and to the tip of the tongue. Lymph from the lower incisors and the gingiva in this region flows also, at least partly, into the submental nodes. The secondary lymph nodes of the described regions are in part the submandibular and in part the superior deep cervical lymph nodes.

The submandibular lymph nodes (Figs. 8-1 to 8-3) are located in the submandibular triangle between the two bellies of the digastric muscle and the lower border of the mandible. The submandibular lymph nodes can be subdivided into an anterior, a middle, and a posterior group, each represented by one larger or two or more smaller lymph nodes. Some of these nodes, located in the submandibular niche, the space between the mylohyoid muscle and the medial surface of the mandible, are hidden by the mandibular body and can be palpated only by passing the finger upward on the inner surface of the lower jaw. This manipulation is facilitated if the patient bends the head forward and toward the side being examined, because in this position skin and deep fascia are relaxed.

The anterior submandibular node or group of nodes is found along the submental vein close to the chin. In the majority of persons there is a single anterior submandibular lymph node. The middle group is almost always represented by two or three small nodes, situated around the facial vein and facial artery above the submandibular salivary gland. The posterior group of submandibular lymph nodes is located behind the facial vein. One of the nodes of this group often is found at the union of the facial and retromandibular veins and therefore at a greater distance from the mandible.

The submandibular lymph nodes collect the lymph of the upper and lower teeth,

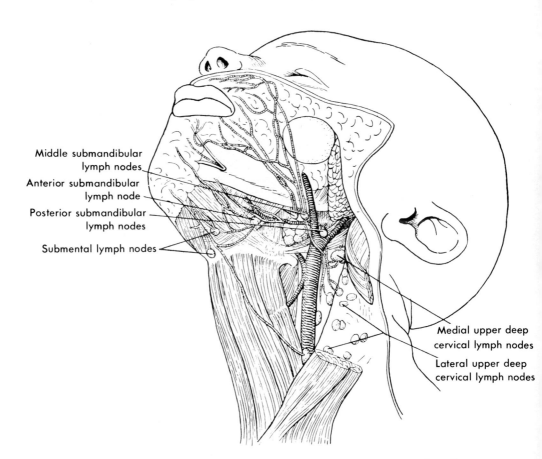

Middle submandibular lymph nodes

Anterior submandibular lymph node

Posterior submandibular lymph nodes

Submental lymph nodes

Medial upper deep cervical lymph nodes

Lateral upper deep cervical lymph nodes

Fig. 8-1. Lymph nodes in upper part of neck. (Modified and redrawn from Sicher and Tandler: Anatomie für Zahnärzte.)

with the exception of the incisors of the lower jaw; the lymph from the upper and lower lips, with the exception of the median part of the lower lip; the lymph from the anterior parts of the nasal cavity and palate; and, finally, the lymph from the body of the tongue. Because of their relation to the teeth, the submental and submandibular lymph nodes are sometimes described as dental lymph nodes. The submandibular lymph nodes drain into the deep cervical lymph nodes.

Accessory lymph nodes are frequently found associated with the submandibular lymph nodes and closely related to the submandibular salivary gland. They are situated inside the capsule of the gland or even in its interlobular connective tissue. If they are present, the accessory lymph nodes receive lymph from the tongue and possibly from the lower lip, but always, however, from the submandibular salivary gland itself. These accessory lymph nodes are called paramandibular lymph nodes. Other accessory lymph nodes sometimes are found in the deep layers of the submandibular region on the hyoglossus muscle. They receive lymph from the substance of the tongue and therefore are of special importance in tumors of the tongue.

The different groups of cervical lymph nodes are distributed along the external

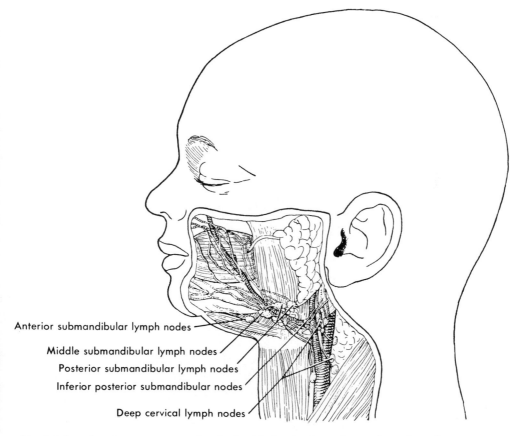

Anterior submandibular lymph nodes

Middle submandibular lymph nodes

Posterior submandibular lymph nodes

Inferior posterior submandibular nodes

Deep cervical lymph nodes

Fig. 8-2. Lymph nodes in upper part of neck. (Modified and redrawn from Sicher and Tandler: Anatomie für Zahnärzte.)

and internal jugular veins. A subdivision into superficial and deep groups is made according to the relation of the nodes to the deep fascia of the neck. The superficial cervical lymph nodes are, as a rule, restricted to the upper region of the neck and are found in the angle between the mandibular ramus and the sternocleidomastoid muscle. The superficial cervical lymph nodes are adjacent to the inferior auricular lymph nodes, and these two groups are often inseparable. The superficial cervical lymph nodes receive the lymph directly from the ear lobe and the adjacent part of the skin and are secondary to the preauricular and postauricular lymph nodes.

The deep cervical lymph nodes may be subdivided into an upper and a lower group; the latter sometimes are called supraclavicular lymph nodes. If a continuous chain of nodes accompanies the internal jugular vein, the omohyoid muscle is taken as the arbitrary boundary between the upper and lower deep cervical lymph nodes. In addition, each of these two groups again is subdivided into an anterior, or medial, and a posterior, or lateral, group according to the relation of the nodes to the sternocleidomastoid muscle. The superior and inferior deep cervical lymph nodes that are

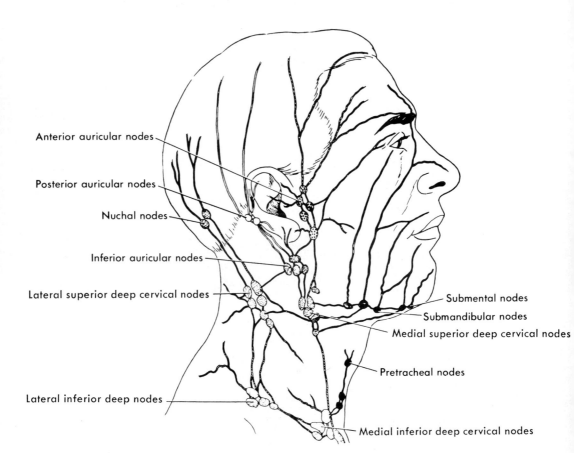

Fig. 8-3. Regional lymph nodes and lymph vessels of superficial structures of head and neck. (Modified from Tandler: Lehrbuch der Anatomie.)

situated in front of, or covered by, the sternocleidomastoid muscle are classified as anterior, or medial, deep cervical lymph nodes; those situated in the posterior triangle of the neck behind the sternocleidomastoid muscle are called posterior, or lateral, deep cervical lymph nodes. Surgical terminology often uses other names for the medial and lateral deep cervical lymph nodes. Since the medial group follows the internal jugular vein, they are referred to as the jugular chain. Since the lateral group is in close relation to the accessory nerve, it is known as the accessory chain.

The deep cervical lymph nodes are primary for the base of the tongue, the sublingual region, and the posterior part of the palate. They are secondary and tertiary nodes into which the lymph of the auricular, submental, submandibular, and accessory nodes of the face empty. They are also secondary to the nuchal nodes, which are regional to the occipital part of the scalp and to deep lymph nodes of the neck, the retropharyngeal, infrahyoid, pretracheal, and paratracheal nodes, which collect the lymph from the viscera of the neck.

Two nodes of the chain following the internal jugular vein are singled out because they receive lymph from a large part of the tongue. One, the jugulodigastric node at the level of the greater horn of the hyoid bone, is part of the superior deep cervical nodes. The other, the jugulo-omohyoid node, belongs to the inferior group of the deep cervical nodes and is found just above the intermediate tendon of the omohyoid muscle.

The superior deep cervical lymph nodes send their lymph into the inferior deep cervical, or supraclavicular, lymph nodes. The lymph on the right side is then collected by the right lymphatic trunk, on the left side by the thoracic duct. These two main lymphatic vessels empty on either side into the "venous angle," where internal jugular and subclavian veins unite; thus the lymph enters the system of the superior vena cava.

LYMPH VESSELS OF THE HEAD AND NECK

The lymph vessels take their origin from closed lymph capillaries and, as a rule, follow the veins. After a variably long course, the lymph vessels enter and pass through a lymph node, and the outgoing lymph vessels again may pass through one or more nodes until they join the larger lymph trunks, which empty into the veins.

The lymph vessels of the scalp drain the lymph in three different directions (Fig. 8-3). The lymph of the occipital region is drained into the occipital, or nuchal, lymph nodes, which are situated at the tendons of trapezius and sternocleidomastoid muscles. Fom here originate lymph vessels that reach the posterior superior deep cervical lymph nodes.

The lymph from the lateral surface of the head, including the greater part of the forehead, is drained into the auricular lymph nodes. From here the lymph is sent into the superficial cervical nodes and into the anterior superior deep cervical lymph nodes. The lymph vessels that originate in the most medial part of the forehead above the root of the nose follow the facial vein and reach the submandibular lymph nodes and then the superior deep cervical nodes. Eyelids, external nose, upper lip, and cheeks are also drained into the submandibular lymph nodes. However, the lower lip and chin send their lymph partly into the submandibular and partly into the submental nodes, and latter receiving the lymph from the middle part of the lower lip. The submental nodes drain directly or via submandibular nodes into the deep cervical lymph nodes.

Lymph from the skin and the superficial soft tissues of the entire head converges, therefore, toward the superior deep cervical lymph nodes and from here into the supraclavicular nodes, the last lymphatic station before the lymph empties into the veins.

The deep structures of the face are drained, for the most part, into the submental, submandibular, and anterior superior deep cervical lymph nodes (Fig. 8-4). The lymph of the nasal mucosa flows in two different directions that correspond to its divided blood and nerve supply. The posterior parts of the nasal cavity are drained posteriorly into retropharyngeal nodes and from here into deep cervical lymph nodes. The anterior parts of the nasal cavity are drained toward the outer surface of the face and from here into the submandibular nodes.

The soft palate and the larger part of the hard palate send their lymph posteriorly along the branches of the retromandibular vein. The lymph enters the anterior supe-

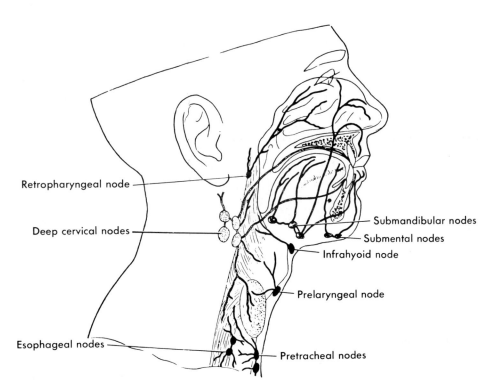

Fig. 8-4. Regional lymph nodes and lymph vessels of deep structures of head and neck. (Modified from Tandler: Lehrbuch der Anatomie.)

rior deep cervical lymph nodes. Into the same nodes flows the lymph from the base of the tongue and from the larger part of the sublingual region. The anterior part of the hard palate sends the lymph into the submandibular lymph nodes via the anterior facial lymph vessels, and into the same nodes flows the lymph from the body of the tongue. The tip of the tongue, however, drains not into the submandibular but into the submental lymph nodes.

The lymph vessels of the gingiva collect in small branches on the inner and outer surface of the alveolar process. The vessels at the labial and buccal surfaces of the upper and lower jaws unite distally and reach one of the submandibular nodes. Lymph from the incisal region of the lower jaw usually drains into one of the submental nodes. The lymph vessels of the inner, or lingual, surface of the upper jaw course backward to unite with those of the palate and finally reach the superior cervical lymph nodes. The lingual lymph vessels of the mandibular gingiva are divided; the posterior vessels follow those of the base of the tongue to the cervical lymph nodes; the anterior vessels collect toward the front, perforate the mylohyoid muscle, and reach the anterior group of the submandibular nodes.

The long controversy as to the existence of lymph vessels in the dental pulp has been decided in a positive way. The lymph vessels draining the pulp and periodontal membrane have a common outlet. It is not possible to correlate exactly a certain tooth or group of teeth with a certain lymph node, because variations of the smaller lymph vessels are too numerous. Only a general plan for the distribution of the dental and periodontal lymph vessels can be worked out. The lymph vessels draining the incisors and the canines of the upper and lower jaws run anteriorly; those draining the molars are directed posteriorly. The premolars are situated in a critical area, and their lymph may be drained anteriorly or posteriorly. The dental lymph vessels from the anterior part of the upper jaw pass through the anterior superior alveolar canals and emerge into the face through the infraorbital foramen. The posterior maxillary lymph vessels collect at the maxillary tuber after passing through the posterior superior alveolar canals. From the infraorbital foramen the anterior maxillary lymph vessels follow the facial vein. The posterior lymph vessels find their way along tributaries of the retro-mandibular vein.

The posterior superior dental lymph vessels are joined in the infratemporal fossa by those that drain the posterior part of the mandible. The latter run posteriorly in the mandibular canal and leave the mandible through the mandibular foramen. The anterior mandibular teeth send their lymph vessels through the mental foramen into the superficial region of the face where they open into lymph vessels along the facial vein. The incisors of the lower jaw usually have their own drainage system, leading into the submental nodes.

Ordinarily the lymph of all the teeth, with the exception of the lower incisors, reaches the submandibular lymph nodes. However, some dental lymph vessels, arising in the molar region of the upper and lower jaws, may reach directly one of the deep superior cervical lymph nodes, which otherwise are secondary to the submandibular and submental nodes. A specific correlation between lymph nodes and teeth is, as was previously mentioned, impossible. One can only state that submental and anterior submandibular lymph nodes receive lymph from the anterior parts of the lower jaw only. Lymph from the lower wisdom tooth and its surroundings is drained into a posterior submandibular node, which usually lies below the angle of the mandible.

The lymph vessels of the parotid gland empty into the parotid lymph nodes or anterior auricular lymph nodes; the lymph vessels of the submandibular salivary gland drain into the paramandibular or submandibular nodes; the sublingual salivary gland is drained toward the deep cervical lymph nodes.

The lymph vessels of the tonsils can be followed to the anterior superior deep cervical lymph nodes, especially to a node situated behind the mandibular angle close to the internal jugular vein.

Major variations of the lymph vessels have occasionally been observed. It is not known, however, how frequent they are. Such variations are clinically of considerable importance. It has been observed, for instance, that lymph vessels from the lower lip and tongue, which normally drain into one of the submental or submandibular lymph nodes, may pass downward directly into the deep cervical nodes (Fig. 8-1).

It is a general rule that some of the lymph vessels that take their origin close to the midline cross to the other side. The median parts of the lips, of the tongue, and of the palate are, therefore, drained to both sides. It is clear that this behavior of the lymph vessels influences the propagation of infections or malignant tumors and that surgical therapy has to take this circumstance into consideration.

CHAPTER 9

The nerves

GENERAL FEATURES

The peripheral nervous system is composed of 12 pairs of cranial nerves emerging from the brain stem and 31 pairs of spinal nerves from the spinal cord. The system is divided functionally into somatic and visceral categories. Each category is further subdivided into afferent, or sensory fibers, and efferent, or motor fibers. *Somatic* nerves are defined as those afferent fibers that transmit stimuli from the skin, special sense organs, voluntary muscles, tendons, ligaments, and joints, as well as those efferent fibers that activate the voluntary, striated, skeletal musculature. *Visceral* nerves are defined as those afferent fibers that transmit stimuli from the viscera, as well as those efferent fibers that activate the involuntary, smooth musculature of the viscera, the cardiac musculature, and the secretion of glands.

Because of the looseness of common usage, a clear distinction in the meaning of certain terms must be understood at the outset. A nerve is a gross conduit made up of many fibers. A fiber is a long process of a neuron of specific function. Therefore, by far most of the nerves one dissects are mixed nerves; they are made up of fibers of various functions.

The somatic component. Somatic nerves are concerned with the external environment. Thus somatic afferent fibers receive *exteroceptive* stimuli conveying sensations of touch, pressure, pain, and temperature. They also receive stimuli from the body proper, *proprioceptive* stimuli conveying sensations of bodily posture and position and movement in the environment, from the muscles, tendons, joints, etc. All these stimuli go to make up most of what we know as consciousness, but they may also initiate unconscious reflex motor responses. Somatic efferent fibers send voluntary stimuli to the striated skeletal musculature, but here again, the voluntary skeletal musculature can react involuntarily to visceral stimuli by reflex motor response.

The visceral component. Visceral nerves are concerned with the internal environment. Thus visceral afferent fibers receive *interoceptive* stimuli from the organs in the body cavities. These stimuli do not normally reach the level of consciousness. In abnormal or pathologic conditions, however, they may reach consciousness to be perceived as discomfort or pain. Visceral efferent fibers send involuntary stimuli to the smooth and cardiac musculature of the viscera.

The whole visceral motor outflow is placed in a separate category called the autonomic nervous system because it acts "automatically," or independently of volition. This system is itself subdivided into *sympathetic* and *parasympathetic* systems, which

391

act, more or less, as antagonists; where one excites, the other is silent or inhibits. Sympathetic fibers emerge from the thoracic and upper lumbar segments of the spinal cord and are therefore also known as the *thoracolumbar* outflow. Parasympathetic fibers emerge directly from the brain stem and from the upper sacral segments of the spinal cord and are therefore also known as the *craniosacral* outflow.

SPECIAL FEATURES

The major innervation of the head and neck is supplied by the cranial nerves, a minor portion by the upper cervical spinal nerves. A difficult problem arises in the functional classification of cranial nerves. The customary classification modifies the four categories defined above by the term *general* somatic afferents and efferents, and *general* visceral afferents and efferents. Cranial nerves add three more categories: *special* somatic afferents only, and *special* visceral afferents and efferents. Special somatic afferents include only the nerves from the special sense organs of vision and hearing. Special visceral afferents include the nerves from the special sense organs of smell and taste (which obviously makes the classification inconsistent). Special visceral efferents include the motor nerves to the facial, masticatory, pharyngeal, and laryngeal muscles (among others). But these muscles are indistinguishable from ordinary somatic muscles (which again seems inconsistent).

Perhaps some confusion is unavoidable because, at the complicated head end of the animal, the entodermal feeding channel of the visceral realm coalesces with the ectodermal face of the somatic realm. But conflict has been further compounded because two different criteria for classification have emerged during the historical course of neurologic study. One is based on the embryologic derivation of the innervated structure, the other on the function with which the innervated structure is associated. For example, the special somatic afferent fibers from eye and ear are so classified because these sense organs are ectodermically derived, but fibers from the olfactory sense organ, which is also derived from the ectoderm (nasal pit) are classified special visceral afferents because they are associated with the visceral function of feeding.

Somatic (voluntary, striated) muscles are derived from the segmental somites along the trunk of the embryo or from their homologues in the head, such as the muscles that move the eyeball and the muscles of the tongue. On the other hand, facial muscles, masticatory muscles, pharyngeal and laryngeal muscles, and even certain massive neck muscles (sternocleidomastoid and trapezius), are derived from the mesoderm of the branchial, or visceral, arches. The situation is unique in that these muscles are not in any way comparable to other visceral musculature. They are voluntary, striated muscles indistinguishable in their microscopic structure and neural arrangement from all ordinary somatic musculature.

But while the motor side of the fifth cranial nerve to the masticatory muscles is classified *special visceral efferent* because it serves a visceral function, the sensory side comes under the category of *general somatic afferent* because its fibers come from ectodermal structures—the same cranial nerve in two categories! It is possible that the muscles of mastication were once truly visceral in their structure and nerve supply in earlier vertebrate forms. If this is so it seems reasonable to assume that the present structure and behavior is a phylogenetic somatization of muscle and nerve from the primitive state. (It is also possible that they were derived from migrant somites.)

Additional conflicts in classification can be readily pointed out, but prolonged discussion is not useful in the present context. As long as the *nature* of the problem is grasped no troublesome misconceptions need arise.

All of the sensory nerves, whether somatic or visceral, consist of fibers that are the peripheral processes of nerve cells situated in ganglia outside of, but close to, the central nervous system. These ganglia are called sensory, or root, ganglia. They are found as dorsal ganglia or spinal ganglia in the dorsal or sensory roots of the spinal nerves. In the cranial nerves they occupy a comparable position in the sensory roots of these nerves. There is one noteworthy exception to this rule: the sensory proprioceptive fibers of the trigeminal nerve do not arise from cells of the trigeminal, or semilunar, ganglion, but from cells that compose the mesencephalic nucleus of the trigeminal nerve situated within the midbrain. Apart from the nerves of special sense, the olfactory, optic, and statoacoustic (auditory) nerves, the following cranial nerves contain somatic or visceral sensory fibers and therefore possess root ganglia: trigeminal, facial, glossopharyngeal, and vagus nerves.

The somatic motor, or efferent, nerves are composed of axons that are processes of nerve cells situated inside the central nervous system. The axon of such a motor nerve cell continues uninterruptedly from its origin in the central nervous system to its end on a group of voluntary, striated muscle fibers. In other words, the connection between the central nervous system and the effector organ is established by *one* neuron.

The visceral motor or secretory efferent stimuli are transmitted from the central nervous system to the effector organ (smooth muscle, cardiac muscle, or glandular cells) by *two* neurons. The first, or central, of these two neurons arises from a nerve cell inside the central nervous system (brain or spinal cord) whose axon emerges in one of the cranial or spinal nerves. At a variable distance the fiber of this neuron ends in synaptic contact with cell bodies of several second, or peripheral, neurons; these cells are usually clustered together in one of the many visceral ganglia. The axons of the second neuron then can be followed to the effector organ. Because of their relation to this intercalated ganglion, the central neuron of the visceral efferent system is called preganglionic; the peripheral neuron is called postganglionic. The preganglionic nerve fiber is, as a rule, myelinated; the postganglionic is nonmyelinated. Therefore the preganglionic nerves are white like the somatic nerves, whereas the postganglionic visceral nerves appear gray. Ordinarily one preganglionic neuron synapses with a group of postganglionic neurons, spreading, as it were, the central impulse to a wider peripheral area.

The visceral ganglia, which serve as relay stations in the course of the parasympathetic nerves for the head, are topographically adjacent to branches of the trigeminal nerve. They are the ciliary, pterygopalatine (sphenopalatine), otic, and submandibular ganglia. The sympathetic fibers, which are destined for the head and neck, arise, as mentioned before, in the upper thoracic segments of the spinal cord. The synapsis of the preganglionic fibers with the cells of the postganglionic neurons occurs almost exclusively in the superior cervical ganglion of the sympathetic chain (see section on the autonomic nervous system, this chapter).

CRANIAL NERVES

Traditionally 12 pairs of cranial nerves are counted, although this enumeration no longer fits the present-day knowledge. The 12 pairs are the following.

The *first pair*, the *olfactory nerve*, transmits the sense of smell. Its branches, arising from the sensory cells of the nasal mucosa, enter the cranial cavity as olfactory fila through the openings of the cribriform plate of the ethmoid bone. They enter the olfactory bulb singly. The bulb is the vestige of the olfactory lobe of macrosmatic mammals, those animals with a highly developed olfactory sense.

The *second pair*, the *optic nerve*, the nerve of visual sense, arises in the ganglion cells of the retina and enters the cranial cavity through the optic foramen.

The *third pair*, the *oculomotor nerve*, contains somatic and parasympathetic visceral efferent fibers. The somatic fibers are destined for most of the extrinsic muscles of the eye—the superior, medial, and inferior rectus muscles, the inferior oblique muscle, and the levator of the upper eyelid. The parasympathetic fibers of the oculomotor nerve are relayed in the ciliary ganglion. The postganglionic fibers, arising from the cells of the ciliary ganglion, enter the eyeball and supply the muscle of accommodation, or ciliary muscle, and the sphincter of the pupil. The oculomotor nerve reaches the orbit through the superior orbital fissure.

The *fourth pair*, the *trochlear nerve*, carries somatic motor fibers that supply the superior oblique muscle of the eyeball. The trochlear nerve passes through the superior orbital fissure.

The *fifth pair*, the *trigeminal nerve*, consists of a greater somatic sensory and a small somatic (somatized visceral) motor portion. Its motor fibers supply the masticatory muscles, that is, masseter, temporal, lateral, and medial pterygoid muscles. The motor fibers of this nerve also supply the tensor palati muscle, the mylohyoid muscle, the anterior belly of the digastric muscle, and, in the middle ear, the tensor tympani muscle. The sensory fibers of the trigeminal nerve, with the exception of proprioceptive fibers, arise in the large semilunar, or Gasserian, ganglion and supply the skin of the entire face and the mucous membrane of the cranial viscera, with the exception of the pharynx and the base of the tongue. The first of its three divisions passes through the superior orbital fissure, the second through the foramen rotundum, and the third, which is joined by the entire somatized visceral motor portion, through the foramen ovale.

The *sixth pair*, the *abducent nerve*, supplies, with its somatic motor fibers, the lateral rectus muscle of the eyeball after passing through the superior orbital fissure.

The *seventh pair*, the *facial nerve*, is a composite of two nerves, the facial nerve proper and the intermediate nerve (of Wrisberg). The facial nerve proper consists of somatized efferent fibers for the muscles of facial expression, including the platysma, the muscles of the outer ear, and the epicranius, or occipitofrontal, muscles; the facial nerve also supplies the stapedius muscle, the posterior belly of the digastric muscle, and the stylohyoid muscle. The intermediate nerve consists of general and special somatic afferent fibers and visceral parasympathetic efferent fibers. The general somatic sensory fibers serve the deep sensibility of the face; the special sensory fibers mediate the taste sensation from the anterior two thirds of the tongue. The sensory fibers originate from the cells of the geniculate ganglion of the facial nerve, located at the bend, or knee, of the facial canal. The visceral efferent fibers of the intermediate nerve supply the lacrimal gland, the submandibular and sublingual glands, and other smaller glands in the nasal and the oral cavity. The fibers for the lacrimal gland are relayed in the pterygopalatine ganglion; the fibers supplying the two lower salivary glands are relayed in the submandibular ganglion. The facial nerve enters the internal acoustic meatus and emerges after a lengthy course through the temporal bone at the stylomastoid foramen.

The *eighth pair*, the *statoacoustic (auditory) nerve*, consists of two functionally different nerves, the cochlear and the vestibular nerves. The first, arising in the cochlea of the labyrinth, transmits the sensation of hearing. The second, arising from the semicircular canals, utriculus, and sacculus of the labyrinth, transmits sensations of position and movement. The two parts of the statoacoustic nerve reach the labyrinth through the inner acoustic meatus.

The *ninth pair*, the *glossopharyngeal nerve*, contains general and special somatic afferent, somatized efferent, and visceral efferent fibers. The somatic afferent fibers from the base of the tongue and the pharynx serve partly general sense and partly the special sense of taste in the posterior third of the tongue. They arise from cells of the two ganglia of the glossopharyngeal nerve, the superior and the inferior (petrous) ganglion. The somatized motor fibers of the glossopharyngeal nerve supply, with fibers of the vagus nerve, the striated voluntary muscles of the pharynx, including the stylopharyngeus muscle. Visceral efferent fibers, relayed in the otic ganglion, supply the parotid gland.

The *tenth pair*, the *vagus nerve*, is the largest of the parasympathetic visceral nerves. It contains, however, not only visceral, but also somatic fibers. The sensory fibers of the vagus arise from cells of two ganglia, the superior (jugular) ganglion and the inferior (nodose) ganglion. The vagus nerve sends its somatized motor fibers to the musculature of the pharynx and larynx. Somatic sensory fibers supply the skin behind the ear and the lining of a part of the external acoustic meatus. Special sensory fibers serve the sense of taste in the region of the epiglottis. Visceral afferent fibers come from a large part of the digestive tract, the lungs, the bronchi, the heart, and the mucous membrane of the lower part of the pharynx and larynx. Since fibers from the last-named regions transmit conscious sensations, it can be argued whether they should be called visceral or somatic afferent nerves. The visceral efferent fibers pass through visceral ganglia of the chest and the upper abdominal cavity to the thoracic and abdominal viscera, with the exception of the lower parts of the large intestine, the bladder, and the sex organs, all of which receive parasympathetic fibers from the sacral segments of the spinal cord. The parasympathetic vagus fibers are relayed in ganglia that are situated in or near the respective organs.

The *eleventh pair*, the *accessory nerve*, consists of a cranial and a spinal portion. The former is functionally a part of the vagus nerve, and in the periphery its fibers are indistinguishable from those of the vagus. The spinal part of the accessory nerve arises from the upper five or six cervical segments of the spinal cord, enters the cranial cavity through the foramen magnum, joins the cranial accessory, and, together with the glossopharyngeal and vagus nerves, leaves the skull through the jugular foramen. The spinal fibers continue as the external branch of the accessory nerve and supply parts of sternocleidomastoid and trapezius muscles. The somatized motor fibers of the eleventh nerve are said to reach the muscles of pharynx and larynx as branches of the vagus nerve.

The *twelfth pair*, the *hypoglossal nerve*, is the motor nerve of the tongue, and therefore contains only somatic efferent fibers. It leaves the skull through the hypoglossal canal.

Trigeminal nerve

The trigeminal nerve arises with a larger sensory and a smaller motor root from the ventral surface of the cerebral pons at the boundary between its body and arm (middle cerebellar peduncle). The origin is closer to the anterior or superior than to the posterior or inferior border of the pons. At the emergence from the substance of the brain, the motor portion is located anteromedial to the sensory portion. The root of the trigeminal nerve travels from its point of origin anteriorly and slightly laterally to cross the upper edge of the temporal pyramid close to its apex. At this point the motor root has already slipped to the inferior surface of the sensory root.

At the edge of the pyramid, between bone and the superior petrosal sinus, the trigeminal root enters a space that extends anteriorly and inferiorly between the layers of the dura mater. The dural compartment widens considerably anteriorly to accommodate the sensory root ganglion of the trigeminal nerve, the semilunar, or Gasserian, ganglion. The space in which the ganglion is contained, Meckel's cavity, is situated partly in the lateral wall of the cavernous sinus, partly on the anterior slope of the temporal pyramid, and partly above the fibrocartilage that fills the lacerated foramen. The semilunar ganglion (Fig. 9-1) is crescent-shaped, its convexity facing forward and downward. The sensory root fibers enter fanwise into the concave margin. From the convexity arise the three sensory divisions of the trigeminal nerve. The motor root of the trigeminal nerve lies, at the pyramidal edge, at the inferomedial surface of the sensory root and then crosses the deep surface of the semilunar ganglion in a lateral direction to become part of the mandibular nerve.

The first trigeminal division, the ophthalmic nerve, courses anteriorly in the lateral wall of the cavernous sinus to the medial part of the superior orbital fissure, through which it enters the orbit. The second division, the maxillary nerve, is directed downward and forward. It enters the uppermost part of the pterygopalatine fossa through the foramen rotundum. The third division, the mandibular nerve, runs steeply downward to the foramen ovale, where motor and sensory fibers intermingle. It then passes through the foramen into the infratemporal fossa.

Each of the three divisions sends a small recurrent branch to the dura mater. These branches are given off by the first and second divisions inside the skull. The recurrent branch of the third division arises in the infratemporal fossa and re-enters the skull, together with the middle meningeal artery, through the foramen spinosum.

The cutaneous areas that are supplied by the three trigeminal divisions comprise

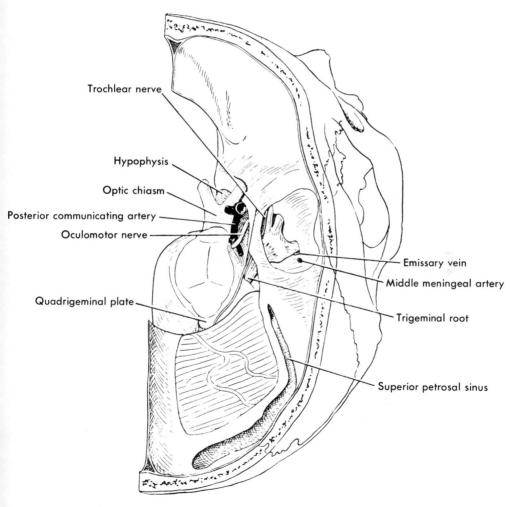

Fig. 9-1. Semilunar ganglion and its relation to the cavernous sinus. (Modified and redrawn from Tandler and Ranzi: Chirurgische Anatomie des Zentral Nervensystems.)

the entire face, with the exception of a variably large area at the mandibular angle (Fig. 9-2). The line that separates the trigeminal area from that supplied by the posterior and anterior branches of the upper cervical nerves is called the vertex-ear-chin line. It starts at the top of the head, runs down on its lateral surface to the anterior edge of the outer ear, encircles a small area of the auricle, and then reaches the posterior border of the mandible. The line turns forward above and in front of the mandibular angle, reaches, in an anteriorly convex curve, the lower border of the mandible in front of the mandibular angle, and follows the inferior margin of the lower jaw to the chin.

The areas supplied by the three divisions are roughly separated by two lines, the upper passing through the palpebral fissure between the lids and the lower passing through the oral fissure between the lips. However, several branches of the three divisions cross these diagrammatic boundaries. The external nasal branch of the oph-

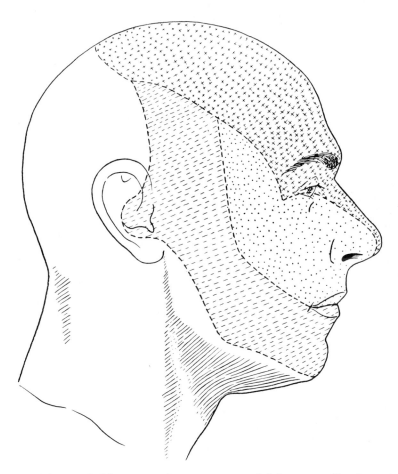

Fig. 9-2. Areas of skin supplied by trigeminal nerve. *Crosses,* ophthalmic nerve (first division); *stippled,* maxillary nerve (second division); *broken lines,* mandibular nerve (third division); *blank areas,* upper cervical nerves.

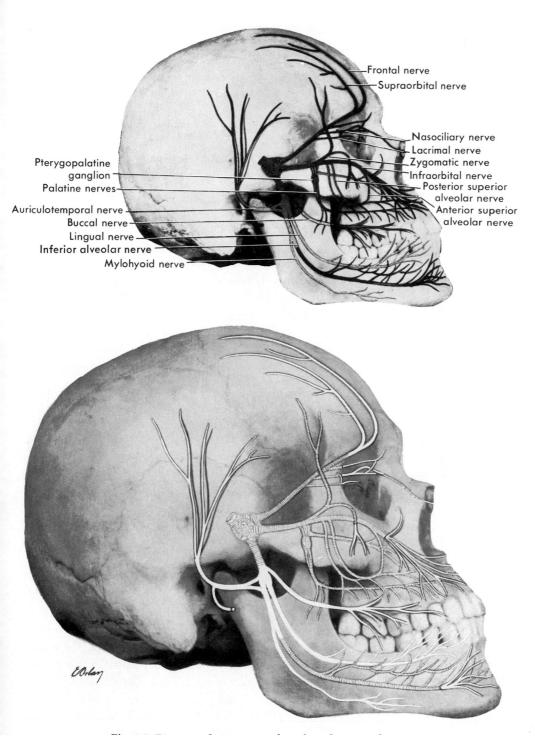

Frontal nerve
Supraorbital nerve
Nasociliary nerve
Lacrimal nerve
Zygomatic nerve
Infraorbital nerve
Posterior superior alveolar nerve
Anterior superior alveolar nerve

Pterygopalatine ganglion
Palatine nerves
Auriculotemporal nerve
Buccal nerve
Lingual nerve
Inferior alveolar nerve
Mylohyoid nerve

Fig. 9-3. Diagrams of main sensory branches of trigeminal nerve.

Table 2. Main sensory branches of the trigeminal nerve

Division	Internal branches	Intermediate branches	External branches
I. Ophthalmic nerve	Nasociliary nerve	Frontal nerve	Lacrimal nerve
II. Maxillary nerve	Pterygopalatine nerve	Infraorbital nerve	Zygomatic nerve
III. Mandibular nerve	Buccal nerve and lingual nerve	Inferior alveolar nerve	Auriculotemporal nerve

thalmic nerve supplies the skin of the nasal bridge down to the tip of the nose and thus seems to trespass into the area of the maxillary nerve. Maxillary and mandibular nerves, on the other hand, send branches upward on the lateral surface of the face into the temporal region. The zygomaticotemporal branch of the second division supplies a small anterior area of the temple; the auriculotemporal branch of the third division supplies the larger posterior part of the temporal area.

A study of the complicated ramification of the sensory branches of the trigeminal nerve (Fig. 9-3) can be facilitated by subdividing each division into three sets of branches. Each division sends fibers to the mucous membrane of the nasal or oral cavity; these branches may be designated as internal rami. The skin on the anterior surface of the face is supplied by the intermediate rami of each division. External rami finally supply the skin on the lateral surface of the face. Table 2 contains a synopsis of the most important sensory branches of the trigeminal nerve. The motor fibers of the third division are not considered at this time.

Ophthalmic nerve

The ophthalmic nerve, the first division of the trigeminal nerve (Fig. 9-4) splits, immediately after reaching the orbit, into its three main branches. The internal branch, the nasociliary nerve, follows the medial border of the orbital roof, releases branches to the nasal cavity, and ends in the skin at the root of the nose. The intermediate branch, the frontal nerve, courses straight anteriorly to reach the skin of the forehead. Finally, the external branch, the lacrimal nerve, runs anteriorly and laterally along the lateral border of the roof of the orbit toward the lacrimal gland and to the skin at the outer corner of the eye.

Nasociliary nerve. This nerve is the internal branch of the ophthalmic nerve. It sends a communicating branch to and through the ciliary ganglion, which may be wrongly called the sensory root of the ciliary ganglion. As will be discussed in the section on the parasympathetic nerve supply of the head, this branch of the nasociliary nerve has no relation to the cells of the ciliary ganglion; its fibers continue through the ganglion into the eyeball. The next branches of the nasociliary nerve are two or three long ciliary nerves that run directly to the eyeball. The nasociliary nerve now turns medially between the optic nerve and the superior rectus muscle of the eyeball and follows the upper border of the medial rectus muscle of the eye. Here arises the ethmoid nerve, which passes through the anterior ethmoid foramen into the cranial cavity, crosses the anterior end of the cribriform plate, and passes into the nasal cavity through an anteromedial slit of this plate. In its short passage through the cranial cavity the nerve is situated extradurally.

In the nasal cavity the ethmoid nerve divides into medial and lateral anterior nasal branches. They supply a small anterior area of the mucous membrane on the lateral nasal wall and on the nasal septum. One of the branches, the external nasal branch, runs downward along the inner surface of the nasal bone and turns into the skin of the nasal bridge below the lower border of the nasal bone or through a small opening in the bone. In the skin of the nasal bridge the external nasal branch can be followed to the tip of the nose.

The terminal branch of the nasociliary nerve is the small infratrochlear nerve, which runs anteriorly, passes below the pulley, or trochlea, of the superior oblique muscle, and emerges from the orbit into the skin at the inner corner of the eye. The infratrochlear nerve exchanges fibers with the supratrochlear nerve, a branch of the frontal nerve, and supplies the inner part of the upper eyelid and the adjacent skin at the root of the nose.

Frontal nerve. This nerve, the intermediate branch, is the largest branch of the ophthalmic nerve. Curving around the lateral border of the superior rectus eye muscle, it reaches its superior surface and then reaches the upper surface of the levator of the upper eyelid. Continuing its forward course between the roof of the orbit and the levator of the upper eyelid as the supraorbital nerve, it divides into three branches: the medial and lateral branches of the supraorbital nerve, and the supratrochlear nerve. The largest of these, the lateral branch, continues anteriorly as the supraorbital nerve and emerges into the skin of the forehead through the supraorbital notch,

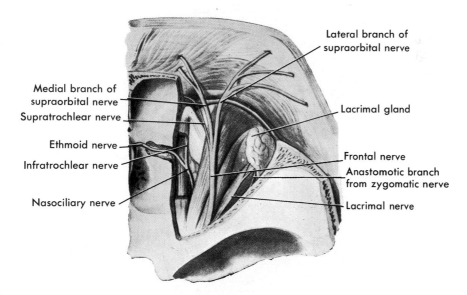

Fig. 9-4. Main branches of ophthalmic nerve, exposed after removal of orbital roof. (Sicher and Tandler: Anatomie für Zahnärzte.)

or the supraorbital foramen. The lateral branch of the supraorbital nerve supplies the greater lateral part of the forehead and the skin of the scalp upward and backward to the vertex, the highest point of the head. The medial branch of the supraorbital nerve, which is sometimes wrongly called the supratrochlear nerve, turns from its origin slightly medially. Reaching the forehead through the frontal notch of the superior orbital rim, the frontal branch supplies a smaller medial area of the skin of the forehead. The last and smallest branch of the frontal nerve, the supratrochlear nerve, is its most medial branch and arises from the frontal nerve itself or from its medial branch. It crosses above the pulley (trochlea) of the superior oblique muscle of the eye and reaches the upper eyelid near the inner corner of the eye. There it exchanges fibers with the infratrochlear nerve and participates in supplying the skin of the upper lid and nasal root.

Lacrimal nerve. This is the external branch of the ophthalmic nerve. In its course toward the lacrimal gland, it receives a branch from the zygomatic nerve of the second division. The connecting branch contains postganglionic parasympathetic fibers from the pterygopalatine ganglion, which reach the lacrimal gland via the lacrimal nerve (see Fig. 9-14). After passing through or along the lacrimal gland, the lacrimal nerve

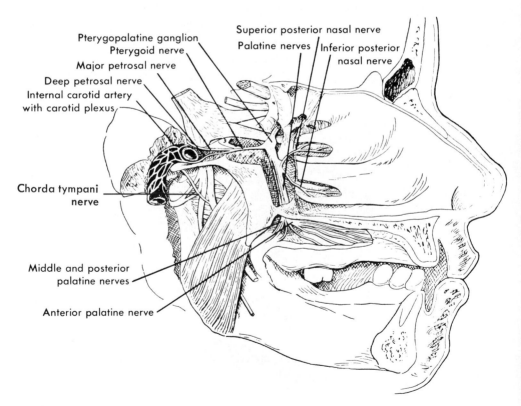

Fig. 9-5. Pterygopalatine ganglion with nasal and palatine nerves. (Modified and redrawn from Sicher and Tandler: Anatomie für Zahnärzte.)

reaches the upper eyelid near the outer corner of the eye and supplies the lateral part of the upper eyelid and a small adjacent area of the skin.

Maxillary nerve

The maxillary nerve, the second division of the trigeminal nerve, leaves the skull through a short, almost horizontal canal, the foramen rotundum. The anterior opening of the canal leads the second division into the pterygopalatine fossa. Immediately after entering the fossa, the maxillary nerve splits into its three major branches. The internal ramus is represented by the pterygopalatine nerve; the intermediate ramus is the infraorbital nerve; the external ramus, the smallest of the three, is the zygomatic nerve.

Pterygopalatine nerve. This nerve, which is sometimes simple but sometimes divided into two or three roots, turns straight downward after it has left the trunk of the second division. The pterygopalatine ganglion is attached to the medial side of the nerve (Figs. 9-5 and 9-7). The pterygopalatine nerve or nerves seem to enter the ganglion after a course of only 2 or 3 mm. The fibers of the pterygopalatine nerve have, however, only a topographic connection with the pterygopalatine ganglion and do not enter into a synapse with its cells. Instead, they pass through the ganglion or

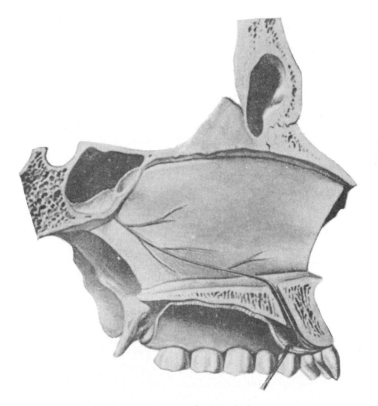

Fig. 9-6. Nasopalatine nerve. (Sicher: Anatomie und Technik der Leitungsanästhesie im Bereiche der Mundhöhle.)

along its lateral surface, to which they are tightly bound. The superior posterior nasal branches are given off at the level of the ganglion. They enter the nasal cavity through the sphenopalatine foramen behind the posterior end of the middle nasal concha and below the body of the sphenoid bone. Lateral branches of the superior posterior nasal nerves supply the larger posterior parts of the upper and middle conchae. Medial branches pass over the roof of the nasal cavity to the nasal septum. One of the medial branches of the posterior superior nasal nerves is distinguished by its great length and by its diagonal course downward and forward along the nasal septum; it is the nasopalatine nerve (of Scarpa) (Fig. 9-6). The nasopalatine nerve supplies branches to the septal mucosa and then passes through the incisive canal into the oral cavity. Immediately after entering the incisive, or nasopalatine, canal, the nasopalatine nerve exchanges fibers with the anterior superior alveolar nerves and consequently may participate in the innervation of the upper central incisor. In the nasopalatine canal, the right and left palatine nerves approach each other and enter the oral cavity through the unpaired incisive foramen. They supply a small anterior area of the palatine mucosa behind the incisor teeth, which, diagrammatically, is bounded posteriorly by a line from one canine to the other.

The main part of the pterygopalatine nerve continues below the pterygopalatine ganglion in a straight downward course through the entire height of the pterygopalatine fossa and then through the pterygopalatine canal. These descending nerves are called palatine nerves (Fig. 9-5). Two or three branches leave the palatine nerve in the pterygopalatine canal to enter the nasal cavity. They are the inferior posterior nasal nerves, which supply mainly the inferior nasal concha and the middle and inferior nasal meatus.

Before reaching the lower, oral end of the pterygopalatine canal, the palatine nerve divides into one larger and one or two smaller terminal branches. The larger branch, the anterior palatine nerve, enters the oral cavity through the major palatine foramen and turns immediately anteriorly. It soon splits into numerous branches that spread fanwise anteriorly, laterally, and medially and supply the mucosa of the hard palate to the canine line, where they exchange fibers with the nasopalatine nerve.

The smaller middle and posterior palatine nerves emerge into the oral cavity through the lesser palatine foramina and supply the tonsil and soft palate with sensory twigs.

Infraorbital nerve. This nerve (Fig. 9-7), the intermediate branch of the maxillary nerve, the second trigeminal division, continues the course of the main trunk anteriorly and slightly laterally. This course takes the infraorbital nerve through the pterygomaxillary fissure into the anteromedial corner of the infratemporal fossa only to leave it immediately through the inferior orbital fissure, through which it enters the orbit; here it runs in the infraorbital groove at the orbital floor almost straight forward. Farther anteriorly, at a variable distance from the posterior border of the orbit, the infraorbital groove is roofed to form the infraorbital canal, which leads the infraorbital nerve through the infraorbital foramen to the superficial structures of the face. The infraorbital nerve splits into its terminal branches immediately after leaving the infraorbital canal.

The infraorbital nerve releases three branches or, sometimes, three sets of branches before it emerges at the infraorbital foramen. These branches are the superior alveolar nerves, which supply the upper teeth, their periodontal membranes, and the gingivae on the outer surface of the upper jaw (Fig. 9-7).

The posterior superior alveolar nerve arises from the infraorbital nerve in the infratemporal fossa before it reaches the maxillary tuberosity. The posterior superior alveolar nerve runs downward, anteriorly, and laterally to reach the convex posterior surface of the maxilla at about the center of this surface. At a variable distance from its origin the posterior superior alveolar nerve splits into two or three branches. The division sometimes occurs before the nerve arrives at the maxillary tuberosity, sometimes on the posterior surface of the maxilla, and sometimes after the nerve has entered the posterior superior alveolar foramen. The second type of division is by far the most frequent. If the division takes place at the surface of the maxilla, the alveolar nerves enter two or three small openings that lead into the narrow posterior superior alveolar canals in the posterolateral wall of the maxillary sinus. In these canals the posterior superior alveolar nerves finally reach the base of the alveolar process. A gingival branch may run downward and forward along the outer surface of the maxillary tuberosity.

The middle superior alveolar nerve leaves the infraorbital nerve somewhere in the infraorbital sulcus. Enclosed in a narrow canal, the middle superior alveolar nerve

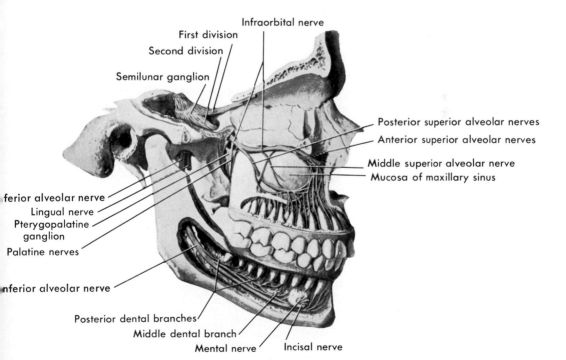

Fig. 9-7. Alveolar nerves. (From Sicher: Anatomie und Technik der Leitungsanästhesie im Bereiche der Mundhöhle.)

travels first in the roof of the maxillary sinus and then in its lateral walls to converge with the posterior superior alveolar nerves toward the base of the alveolar process. The middle superior alveolar nerve is frequently absent, probably in about 60% of persons, and its fibers are then incorporated into the posterior or, more often, into the anterior superior alveolar nerves.

The anterior superior alveolar nerve or nerves leave the infraorbital nerve in the infraorbital canal either as one common branch or as two or three smaller branches. The canals that contain the anterior superior alveolar nerves are situated in the anterior wall of the maxillary sinus. The nerves run at first downward and laterally and then curve medially and divide into two sets of branches below the infraorbital foramen. An anterior set continues the inferior and medial course to the inferomedial circumference of the piriform, or anterior nasal, aperture. At this point a small nasal branch is given off; the alveolar branches continue into the most medial part of the alveolar process. A posterior set of branches of the anterior superior alveolar nerve turns from the point of divergence downward and backward and reaches the alveolar process in the region of the canine.

In the base of the alveolar process the superior alveolar nerves exchange fibers and form a loose plexus, the superior alveolar, or superior dental, plexus. The terminal branches of the superior alveolar nerves emerge from this plexus in two sets that accompany the corresponding arteries. The first group of nerves are the dental nerves. Their number corresponds to the number of the roots of the superior teeth. Each dental nerve enters the apical foramen of one of the roots and branches in the dental pulp. The second group of the terminal branches of the superior alveolar nerves are the perforating, or interdental and interradicular, nerves. Each interdental branch runs through the entire height of an interalveolar septum between two adjacent teeth and supplies, during this part of its course, numerous branches to the periodontal ligaments of the adjacent teeth through the alveolar bone proper. At the crest of the interalveolar septum, the interdental nerves emerge into the gingiva and supply the interdental papilla and the labial or buccal gingiva. The interradicular nerves traverse the entire height of an interradicular or intra-alveolar septum and send branches to the periodontal membranes of two adjacent roots. The interradicular nerves end in the periodontal ligament at the furcation of the roots.

The terminal branches of the infraorbital nerve itself spread fanwise from the infraorbital foramen toward the lower eyelid, nose, and upper lip. The palpebral branches turn upward into the eyelid; the nasal branches supply the lateral slope of the nose and the nasal wing. The three or four superior labial branches enter the lip between its muscles and the mucous membrane. They supply not only the mucous membrane of the upper lip, but also its skin, which they reach by perforating the orbicularis oris muscle.

Zygomatic nerve. This nerve, the small external ramus of the maxillary nerve, often appears to be a branch of the infraorbital nerve. The division occurs either before or while the infraorbital nerve passes through the inferior orbital fissure. In the orbit the zygomatic nerve follows the lateral edge of the orbital floor anteriorly and laterally. The zygomatic nerve sends a branch upward to the lacrimal nerve; this communicating branch consists of postganglionic parasympathetic fibers, which arise from the cells of the pterygopalatine ganglion (see Fig. 9-14). At first incorporated into the zygomatic nerve, these visceral efferent fibers are shunted to the lacrimal nerve and thus reach the lacrimal gland.

After having released the communicating branch, the zygomatic nerve enters the zygomatic-orbital foramen in the orbital surface of the zygomatic bone. In the zygomatic bone, the zygomatic nerve divides into two branches. One branch, the zygomaticofacial nerve, emerges at the anterior, or malar, surface of the zygomatic bone and supplies the skin over the height of the cheek. The second branch of the zygomatic nerve, the zygomaticotemporal nerve, emerges at the posterior, or temporal, surface of the frontal process into the temporal fossa. After perforating the temporal fascia, the zygomaticotemporal nerve supplies a small anterior area of the skin in the temporal region. The zygomatic nerve may split into zygomaticofacial and zygomaticotemporal branches before entering the zygomatic bone.

Mandibular nerve

The mandibular nerve, the third trigeminal division, is a mixed nerve and contains the entire motor portion. The mandibular nerve, the largest of the three divisions of the trigeminal nerve, leaves the skull through the foramen ovale and enters

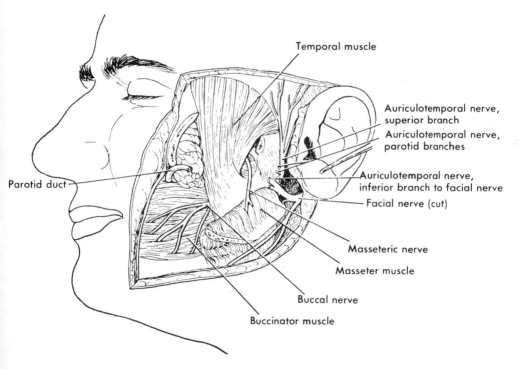

Fig. 9-8. Mandibular nerve, superficial layer. Zygomatic arch and masseter muscle are reflected downward. (Modified and redrawn from Sicher and Tandler: Anatomie für Zahnärzte.)

the infratemporal fossa. Below the foramen ovale the mandibular nerve is in close relation to the anterolateral, membranous wall of the auditory tube. The otic ganglion is attached to the medial surface of the third division (see Fig. 9-16).

At their origin, motor and sensory branches of the mandibular nerve cannot be entirely separated. However, the motor fibers mass for the greater part on the anterior and anterolateral circumference of the sensory fibers.

The *motor* nerves for the four muscles of mastication are given off in the following way (Figs. 9-8 to 9-10).

Masseteric nerve. This nerve leaves the trunk of the mandibular nerve at its lateral circumference close to the cranial base. It runs laterally between the infratemporal surface of the greater sphenoid wing and the lateral pterygoid muscle, passes behind the tendon of the temporal muscle through the mandibular notch, and enters the masseter muscle from its deep surface. The masseteric nerve is accompanied by the masseteric artery and vein.

Posterior and anterior deep temporal nerves. The posterior temporal nerve arises from the mandibular nerve close to, or together with, the masseteric nerve. The anterior temporal nerve is at its origin, as a rule, united with the buccal nerve. The

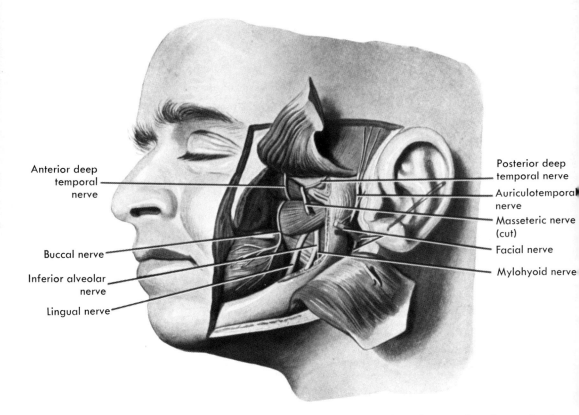

Fig. 9-9. Mandibular nerve, middle layer. Temporalis with coronoid attachment reflected upward and masseter reflected downward. (Sicher and Tandler: Anatomie für Zahnärzte.)

common trunk turns anteriorly and slightly laterally in a groove on the anterolateral circumference of the oval foramen. The sulcus is bridged by a ligament. If it ossifies, an abnormal foramen is found between the base of skull and the ossified ligament. This foramen was named temporobuccal foramen after the old term for the common trunk of the anterior temporal and buccal nerves (see Fig. 2-14). Posterior and anterior temporal nerves wind around the infratemporal crest, and, proceeding superiorly, enter the temporal muscle from its deep or medial surface.

Medial pterygoid nerve. This branch, the nerve for the medial pterygoid muscle, arises from the anteromedial circumference of the mandibular nerve. In most persons the nerve is connected closely with the otic ganglion or passes through it (see Fig. 9-16). Descending anteriorly, the medial pterygoid nerve reaches the medial pterygoid muscle close to its posterior border and not far below its origin from the pterygoid process.

The nerve for the tensor palati muscle is often a branch of the medial pterygoid nerve, or it arises from the mandibular nerve close to the origin of the medial pterygoid nerve.

The nerve for the tensor tympani muscle usually arises together with the medial

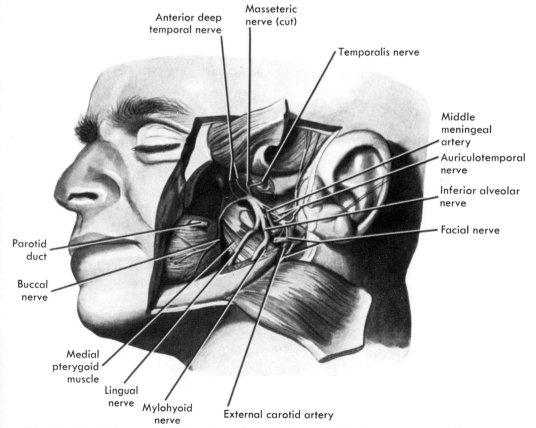

Fig. 9-10. Mandibular nerve, deep layer. Lateral pterygoid muscle and entire ramus removed. (Sicher and Tandler: Anatomie für Zahnärzte.)

pterygoid nerve and passes posteriorly along or through the otic ganglion into the canal for the tensor tympani muscle, which is situated above the bony auditory tube.

Lateral pterygoid nerve. This nerve to the lateral pterygoid muscle is usually incorporated with the buccal nerve. It branches off as the buccal nerve passes between the two heads of the lateral pterygoid, and it sends twigs into both heads immediately.

The motor fibers for the anterior belly of the digastric muscle and for the mylohyoid muscle are part of the mylohyoid nerve, a branch of the inferior alveolar nerve.

The four *sensory* branches of the mandibular nerve (Figs. 9-8 to 9-10) separate from each other usually 5 to 10 mm. below the base of the skull. Buccal and lingual nerves, destined to supply large areas of the oral mucosa, represent the internal branch. The inferior alveolar nerve, the intermediate branch, supplies the mandibular teeth, the skin and mucous membrane of the lower lip, and the skin of the chin. The external surface of the face, that is, the posterior part of the cheek and posterior area of the temporal region, including parts of the outer ear, is supplied by the auriculotemporal nerve, which represents the external branch of the mandibular nerve.

Buccal nerve. This nerve leaves the trunk of the mandibular nerve at its anterolateral circumference. In its first part it is combined with motor fibers, which will constitute the anterior temporal and the lateral pterygoid nerves. The buccal nerve runs at first anterolaterally, close to the inferior surface of the greater wing of the sphenoid bone. After releasing the anterior deep temporal nerve, the buccal nerve descends behind the superior head of the lateral pterygoid muscle, then turns laterally between the two heads of this muscle. At this point the nerve releases the fibers that enter the lateral pterygoid muscle. The buccal nerve turns sharply downward to descend on the outer surface of the inferior head of the lateral pterygoid muscle, between the lateral pterygoid and temporal muscles and often closely attached to the fascia of the temporalis. The nerve may even pass through the substance of the temporal muscle near its anterior border. At the anterior border of the tendons of the temporal muscle, the buccal nerve emerges and follows the outer surface of the buccinator muscle in a forward and downward course, splits into several branches in or underneath the outer fascia of the buccinator muscle, and here exchanges fibers with branches of the facial nerve. Singly, the branches of the buccal nerve perforate the buccinator muscle and reach the mucous membrane of the cheek. Almost the entire mucosa of the cheek is supplied by the buccal nerve, with the exception of a posterosuperior area, which may receive sensory fibers from the gingival branch of the posterior superior alveolar nerves. The buccal branches of the superior alveolar nerve and the buccal nerve itself are in a reciprocal relation. Often the buccal nerve participates in the nerve supply of a small area of the buccal gingiva in the distal part of the upper jaw. Branches of the posterior superior alveolar nerves, on the other hand, may supply a larger area of the cheek and may, in rare cases, even replace the buccal nerve.

The area supplied by the buccal nerve may extend for a short distance into the mucous membrane of the upper and lower lips close to the corner of the mouth. Only the cutaneous branches of the buccinator nerve supply the skin around the commissure of the lips. Of importance are branches of the buccal nerve that supply the gingiva on the outer surface of the lower alveolar process in an area varying considerably in its mesiodistal extent. In the majority of persons the nerve serves a field of the gingiva buccal to the second premolar and the first molar of the lower jaw. However, the area may extend mesially into the region of the canine and distally into that of the third molar. In other extreme cases the buccal nerve may be entirely excluded from supplying any part of the gingiva.

Lingual nerve. Below the foramen ovale, this nerve is united closely with the inferior alveolar nerve (Fig. 9-10). Separating from the alveolar nerve, usually 5 to 10 mm. below the cranial base, the lingual nerve lies anterior and slightly medial to the inferior alveolar nerve. The lingual nerve descends between the lateral and medial pterygoid muscles and may be separated from the inferior alveolar nerve by the pterygospinous ligament. This ligament connects the posterior border of the lateral pterygoid plate with the angular spine of the sphenoid bone and may partly or entirely ossify. If the ligament intervenes between the two nerves, the lingual nerve is found on the medial, the alveolar nerve on the lateral, side of the ligament. At the lower border of the lateral pterygoid muscle, the lingual nerve receives the chorda tympani, which runs medially in the depth of the petrotympanic fissure to the angular spine of the sphenid, where it swings anteriorly, running in a groove on the medial surface of the spine. It then turns down to join the lingual nerve at an acute angle after crossing the inferior alveolar nerve on its medial side (see Figs. 9-5, 9-16, and 16-2). The chorda tympani carries visceral efferent and taste fibers from the facial (intermediary) nerve.

Below the lateral pterygoid muscle the lingual nerve, coursing downward and slightly laterally, follows the lateral surface of the medial pterygoid muscle. At the level of the upper end of the mylohyoid line the nerve turns in a sharp curve anteriorly to continue horizontally on the superior surface of the mylohyoid muscle into the oral cavity. The lingual nerve is, at this point, in close relation to the upper pole of the submandibular gland and here releases the fibers to the submandibular ganglion. In the most posterior part of the oral cavity the nerve is superficial and can even be seen through the mucous membrane above the mylohyoid line at the level of the third and second lower molars. At the same point gingival branches are given off that supply the mucous membrane on the inner surface of the mandible and the gingiva on the lingual surface of the lower teeth.

Farther anteriorly the lingual nerve is in close relation to the posterior part of the sublingual gland, which receives several fine branches, whereas other branches supply the mucous membrane of the sublingual region. The nerve then turns medially, spirals under the submandibular duct, and divided into a variable number of branches, enters the substance of the tongue. After exchanging fibers with the hypoglossal nerve, the branches of the lingual nerve perforate the muscles of the tongue lateral to the genioglossus muscle and end in the mucous membrane on the lower and upper surface of the body of the tongue. Posteriorly the area of the nerve extends to the line of the circumvallate papillae. At its origin the lingual nerve carries only fibers of general sense, that is, fibers for the perception of touch, pressure, pain, and temperature. The taste fibers for the anterior two thirds of the tongue, derived from the facial nerve, are carried to the lingual nerve by the chorda tympani nerve and are distributed to the taste buds in branches of the lingual nerve.

Inferior alveolar nerve. This nerve, the intermediate branch of the mandibular nerve (the third trigeminal division), descends behind and slightly lateral to the lingual nerve between the two pterygoid muscles. It winds around the lower border of the lateral pterygoid muscle, which separates the alveolar nerve from the mandibular ramus, and then turns sharply outward and downward to reach the inner surface of the mandible at the mandibular foramen, which it enters. It is important to stress the fact that the inferior alveolar nerve has no contact with the mandible above the entrance into the mandibular canal (see Fig. 12-1).

Before the nerve disappears into the canal of the mandible, it releases the mylohyoid nerve. This small nerve turns downward and anteriorly in the mylohyoid groove of the mandible, which is bridged by the sphenomandibular ligament, partial ossification of which is not rare. Leaving the mylohyoid groove, the mylohyoid nerve converges with the submental artery and vein in the submandibular fosa and approaches the inferolateral surface of the mylohyoid muscle near its posterior border. Here the mylohyoid nerve releases several branches for the mylohyoid muscle and one or two branches for the anterior belly of the digastric muscle.

The mylohyoid nerve has, however, not exhausted its fibers after supplying these two muscles, but sensory fibers contained in it continue in most persons as a thin sensory nerve toward the chin, where it supplies the skin on the inferior and sometimes on the anterior surface of the mental prominence. The cutaneous branch of the mylohyoid nerve is frequently asymmetrical and sometimes even is missing on one side. In about 10% of the examined cadavers, a twig of the terminal sensory branch of the mylohyoid nerve enters the mandible in the mental region and may participate in the nerve supply to the lower incisors, which is important in local anesthesia.

The inferior alveolar nerve passes through the length of the mandibular canal and divides in the premolar region into its two unequal terminal branches, the incisive and mental nerves. The mental nerve leaves the body of the mandible through the mental canal; emerging at the mental foramen, the nerve usually divides into three branches. One branch turns forward and downward to the skin of the chin. The other two branches course anteriorly and upward into the lower lip, where they supply the skin and mucous membrane of the lip and mucosa on the labial alveolar surface. The incisive branch is one of the dental branches of the inferior alveolar nerve.

The dental branches of the inferior alveolar nerve (Fig. 9-7) vary in number and are arbitrarily divided into posterior, middle, and anterior sets. The posterior dental branch leaves the alveolar nerve in the most posterior part of the mandibular canal; the middle branches separate from the nerve trunk below the first molar or the second premolar; the anterior dental nerve is the incisive nerve. Before the lower dental nerves send out their terminal branches, they exchange fibers, thus forming the loose inferior alveolar, or inferior dental, plexus. The terminal branches of this plexus are arranged in the same way as in the upper jaw and can be divided into dental nerves proper and interdental and interradicular nerves. The dental nerves enter the roots of the lower teeth and supply their pulps. The interdental nerves perforate the interalveolar septa, supply the periodontal ligaments of the adjacent teeth, and end in the gingival papilla. Where the buccal gingiva is not supplied by the buccal nerve, it receives fibers from the perforating interdental nerves. The interradicular nerves pass through the intraalveolar or interradicular septa and are distributed to the periodontal ligamets of two adjacent roots. They end in the periodontal ligament at the bifurcation.

Auriculotemporal nerve. This is the external branch of the mandibular nerve, the third trigeminal division. The nerve separates from the trunk of the third division immediately below the base of the skull, turns almost directly backward, and encircles the middle meningeal artery with two branches (Fig. 9-10). These two branches unite behind the artery, and the nerve continues posteriorly and slightly downward and outward to the posterior surface of the mandibular neck. Then the auriculotemporal nerve crosses the neck of the mandible and enters the parotid gland, where it divides into two almost equal branches. One branch bends sharply upward and continues its course in front of the cartilage of the outer ear between the superficial temporal artery and vein. This superior branch crosses the root of the zygoma to reach up across the temporal region. On its way it sends auricular branches back to the anterosuperior area of the outer ear and the external auditory meatus, articular

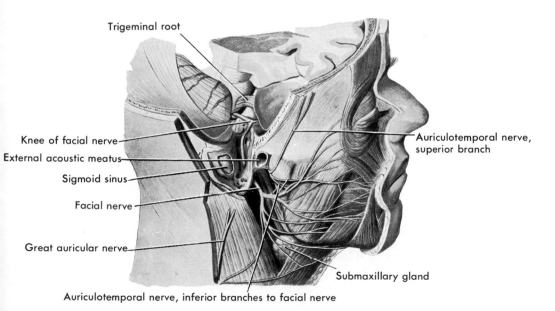

Fig. 9-11. Facial nerve. (Sicher and Tandler: Anatomie für Zahnärzte.)

branches forward to the jaw joint, and other branches inward, into the parotid gland. The terminal, or superficial temporal, branches of the auriculotemporal nerve supply the skin over the posterior part of the temple. The second, inferior, branch of the auriculotemporal nerve is sometimes split into two or three twigs. It turns in the substance of the parotid gland downward and laterally and joins the superior division of the facial nerve. In the sheath of the facial nerve, the fibers of the buccal branch of the auriculotemporal nerve continue anteriorly and are distributed to the skin of the greater posterior part of the cheek. The inferior branch of the auriculotemporal nerve is usually described as the "anastomotic branch to the facial nerve" (Fig. 9-11).

Facial nerve

The facial nerve (Figs. 9-11 and 9-12) in reality consists of two nerves, the facial nerve proper and the intermediate nerve. The facial nerve proper contains the somatized motor fibers, which are destined for the muscles of facial expression, including the occipital and auricular muscles and the platysma, and for the stapedius muscle, the posterior belly of the digastric, and the stylohyoid muscle. The intermediate nerve contains proprioceptive sensory fibers, which serve the deep sensitivity of the face, and special sensory fibers mediating the taste sensation in the anterior two thirds of the tongue and on the palate. The sensory fibers arise from the cells of the genic-

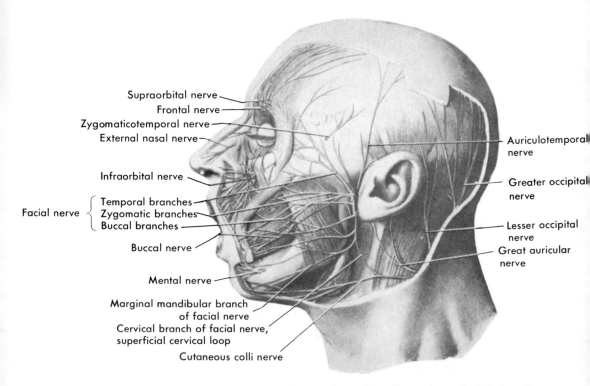

Fig. 9-12. Superficial nerves of the face. (Sicher and Tandler: Anatomie für Zahnärzte.)

ulate ganglion. The intermediate nerve also contains preganglionic visceral efferent fibers which supply the lacrimal gland, the sublingual and submandibular salivary glands, and smaller glands of the oral cavity. The visceral fibers end around the cells of the pterygopalatine and submandibular ganglia, respectively.

Facial and intermediate nerves emerge from the brain at the pontocerebellar angle in front of and medial to the statoacoustic nerve. Facial and intermediate nerves unite, as a rule, a short distance from their emergence and enter, with the statoacoustic nerve, the inner auditory meatus. At the outer blind end of the meatus the facial nerve continues its lateral course in a separate canal. Where the facial canal reaches the sagittal plane of the medial wall of the tympanic cavity, it bends sharply posteriorly. At this bend, the knee, or genu, of the facial nerve, lies the small sensory geniculate ganglion (Figs. 9-11 and 9-16). From the knee, the facial canal and nerve run backward, to pass above the oval window; then, below the lateral semicircular canal, the nerve turns in a smooth curve downward and continues in the posterior wall of the tympanic cavity. The facial canal opens finally at the stylomastoid foramen (Fig. 9-16).

The first important branch of the facial nerve leaves at the knee of the facial nerve. It is the major (greater superficial) petrosal nerve. This nerve contains some taste fibers for the palate, but mainly it contains the preganglionic parasympathetic fibers, which carry impulses to the pterygopalatine ganglion, whence they are relayed to the lacrimal gland and some nasal and palatine glands. The major petrosal nerve leaves the facial canal through the hiatus, or slit, of the facial canal and runs forward, downward, and inward in a furrow on the anterior surface of the pyramid of the temporal bone. The major petrosal nerve leaves the cranial cavity, perforating the fibrocartilage that fills the lacerated foramen, after joining the deep petrosal nerve from the sympathetic plexus of the internal carotid artery (see Fig. 9-5). Superficial and deep petrosal nerves form the pterygoid, or Vidian, nerve, which passes through the pterygoid canal into the pterygopalatine fossa to the pterygopalatine ganglion.

After emitting the major petrosal nerve, the facial nerve releases a small contribution to the minor petrosal nerve. The next branch of the facial nerve is given off in the descending part of the facial canal. It is a small motor nerve for the stapedius muscle, which is attached to the stapes or stirrup, the innermost of the three auditory ossicles.

One more branch leaves the facial nerve in its canal above the stylomastoid foramen, that is, the chorda tympani, which contains taste fibers and preganglionic parasympathetic secretory fibers. From the facial nerve the chorda tympani turns upward and forward and enters the tympanic cavity through a small opening in its posterior wall. In an upward convex arch it runs forward in a fold of the mucous membrane that lines the tympanic cavity. After passing between hammer and anvil, the chorda tympani leaves the tympanic cavity through an opening in its anterior wall and enters the petrotympanic fissure between the petrosal and tympanic bones. In the depth of the petrotympanic fissure (see Fig. 16-2), the chorda tympani runs medially and reaches the angular spine of the sphenoid bone on its posterior edge. Then it turns downward and forward in a shallow groove on the medial surface of the angular spine, crosses the inferior alveolar nerve on its medial side, and joins the lingual nerve. The fibers of the chorda tympani continue now in the sheath of the lingual nerve. The secretory fibers leave the lingual nerve where it lies close to the upper pole of the submandibular gland and enter the submandibular ganglion. The taste fibers of the chorda tympani follow the lingual nerve into the substance of the tongue and are distributed to the taste buds, which are most numerous on the vallate papillae and less so on the fungiform papillae in the body and tip of the tongue. Taste buds signal sweet and salt from the tongue tip, sour (acid) from the sides, and bitter from base. The dorsum is silent.

Immediately after emerging through the stylomastoid foramen, the facial nerve gives off two small branches. One of these, the posterior auricular branch, turns backward and upward between the mastoid process and the auricle and supplies the posterior auricular and the occipital muscles. The second of the two branches turns downward as a long twig to the stylohyoid muscle and then enters the posterior belly of the digastric muscle, which it suplies. Some fibers perforate the digastric muscle and join the glossopharyngeal nerve.

At the stylomastoid foramen the main trunk of the facial nerve enters the substance of the parotid gland, in which its ramification takes place. The first separation of the facial nerve into an upper and lower division usually occurs behind the mandible (Fig. 9-11). These two branches swing around the posterior border of the mandible, surround the isthmus of the gland that connects superficial and deep lobes, and divide further between the two lobes and between the parotid gland and the masseter muscle. Exchanging fibers, they form the parotid plexus. The terminal branches of the facial nerve diverge, the uppermost running almost vertically upward, the lowermost running downward and slightly anteriorly. All of these branches emerge at the borders of the parotid gland. However, they leave the parotid gland on its deep surface and course for a variable distance between the gland and the masseter muscle. From above downward these branches are the temporal, zygomatic, buccal, mandibular, and cervical branches. The upper, or temporal, division releases the temporal, zygomatic, and upper buccal branches. The lower, or cervical, division gives off lower buccal, mandibular, and cervical branches. Variations in the distribution of the facial nerve are rather frequent, but do not ordinarily influence the final, or terminal, ramification.

The temporal branch or branches emerge from the parotid gland at its upper pole slightly in front of the superficial temporal artery. Posterior branches are given off to the anterior and superior auricular muscles; the anterior temporal branches supply the frontal muscle, the superior part of the orbicularis oculi muscle, the corrugator of the eyebrows, and the slender muscle of the nose.

The zygomatic branches leave the parotid gland on its anterosuperior border and run upward and forward. Crossing the body of the zygomatic bone, the zygomatic branches of the facial nerve supply the inferior part of the orbicularis oculi muscle.

The buccal branches of the facial nerve emerge at the anterior border of the parotid gland and are often divided into an upper and a lower group according to their relation to the parotid duct. The upper buccal branches supply the muscles of the upper lip and the muscles of the nose. The lower buccal branches supply the buccinator muscle and the risorius muscle. The orbicularis oris muscle also receives its nerve supply from the buccal branches of the facial nerve.

The mandibular branches run parallel with the lower border of the mandible, sometimes above but more often below this border. One of them, the marginal mandibular branch, follows almost exactly the lower border of the lower jaw. In their course anteriorly the mandibular branches cross the facial vein and the facial artery lying superficial to the vessels. If there is only one mandibular branch, it usually follows the course of the marginal mandibular branch. The mandibular branches of the facial nerve supply the muscles of the lower lip and the mental muscle.

The cervical branch of the facial nerve leaves the parotid gland at or slightly above its inferior pole. The cervical branch runs downward and anteriorly underneath the platysma muscle, which it supplies.

The branches of the facial nerve exchange fibers with almost all of the sensory cutaneous branches of the trigeminal nerve. The connections between the facial and trigeminal branches result in the formation of small mixed terminal nerves, which carry motor and sensory fibers to a limited area of the face. The most important of these connections are the following: a branch of the auriculotemporal nerve joins the upper branch of the facial nerve; the upper buccal branches of the facial nerve join branches of the infraorbital nerve in the canine fossa; the cervical branch of the facial nerve exchanges fibers with the transverse colli (cutaneous colli) nerve of the cervical plexus. The loop-shaped connection between the facial and cutaneous colli nerve is known as the superficial cervical ansa.

Glossopharyngeal nerve

The glossopharyngeal nerve (Fig. 9-13) emerges from the brain on the lateral surface of the medulla oblongata behind the olive and passes in front of the vagus nerve through the jugular foramen. The glossopharyngeal nerve contains motor fibers for the stylopharyngeus muscle and participates with the vagus in supplying the constrictors of the pharynx and the palatopharyngeus muscle. Parasympathetic secretory fibers are sent to the otic ganglion, from which the impulses are relayed to the parotid gland. General sensory fibers supply the region of the tonsil, the adjacent parts of the pharyngeal mucosa, and the entire base of the tongue. The taste sensation originating in the vallate and foliate papillae at the base of the tongue is also transmitted by the glossopharyngeal nerve.

The sensory fibers of the glossopharyngeal nerve arise from ganglion cells of two small ganglia, the superior ganglion and the inferior (petrosal) ganglion. The superior ganglion lies in the jugular foramen; the inferior ganglion, the larger of the two, is found in a small fovea on the inferior surface of the petrous temporal bone in front of the jugular foramen.

At the inferior ganglion a small branch, the tympanic nerve, leaves the glosso-pharyngeal nerve. The tympanic nerve perforates the floor of the tympanic cavity in the narrow tympanic canal. Then the tympanic nerve and branches from the sympathetic carotid plexus form a loose network in the mucous membrane on the medial wall of the tympanic cavity, the tympanic plexus of Jacobson. The tympanic nerve contains sensory and secretory fibers. The secretory fibers pass through the tympanic plexus, perforate the roof of the tympanic cavity, and form, with a small contributory branch of the facial nerve, the minor petrosal nerve. The minor petrosal nerve runs parallel and close to the major petrosal nerve and on its lateral side, downward and forward on the anterosuperior surface of the pyramid, and leaves the skull through the sphenopetrosal fissure. Below the base of the skull, the minor petrosal nerve enters the otic ganglion.

After emerging from the skull, the glossopharyngeal nerve exchanges fibers with the vagus nerve and the sympathetic chain. Running downward and forward on the medial side of the styloid process, the glossopharyngeal nerve winds around the posterior border of the stylopharyngeus muscle to its lateral surface. The glossopharyngeal nerve supplies the stylopharyngeus muscle and sends through it a perforating branch to exchange fibers with the facial nerve. On the lateral wall of the pharynx and

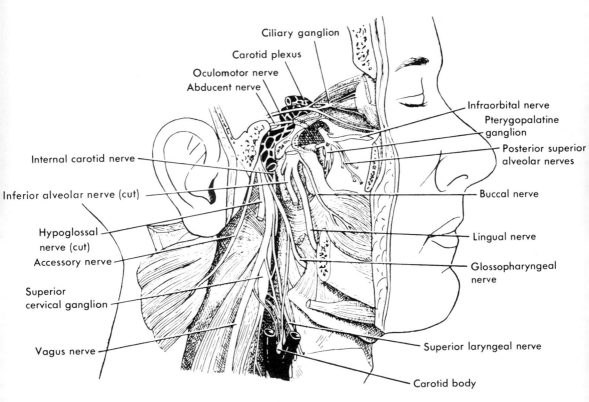

Fig. 9-13. Sympathetic nerves of the head. (Modified and redrawn from Sicher and Tandler: Anatomie für Zahnärzte.)

above the stylopharyngeus muscle the pharyngeal branches are released, some of which join branches of the vagus nerve to form the pharyngeal plexus and others of which perforate the middle constrictor of the pharynx to supply its mucous membrane.

The glossopharyngeal nerve itself enters the base of the tongue below the styloglossus muscle and deep to the hyoglossus muscle. Its terminal branches supply the base of the tongue, including the vallate and foliate papillae, with fibers of general sense and with taste fibers. Branches also are sent to the palatine tonsil and the palatine arches.

At a variable level the glossopharyngeal nerve releases a fine carotid branch, usually where the nerve crosses the internal carotid artery on its lateral side. The carotid branch joins with fibers of the vagus nerve and can be followed along the internal carotid artery to the carotid body (Fig. 9-13), which it supplies; other fibers reach the carotid sinus. The carotid nerve plays an important role in the reflex regulation of respiration, heart action, and blood pressure.

Hypoglossal nerve

The hypoglossal nerve arises from the anterior surface of the medulla oblongata between the olive and the pyramid. The root fibers of the nerve are collected in two bundles that pass through two separate openings of the dura mater. The bony hypoglossal canal also may be divided by a horizontal bar of bone. The hypoglossal nerve is a somatic motor nerve, supplying all extrinsic and intrinsic muscles of the tongue.

After emerging through the hypoglossal canal, the nerve spirals around the posterior and lateral surface of the vagus nerve. The two nerves are tightly bound to each other by connective tissue. The hypoglossal nerve descends steeply and crosses the stylohyoid and digastric muscles on their medial surfaces. Below the lower border of the digastric muscle the hypoglossal nerve turns in a flat curve anteriorly and slightly upward. It crosses the internal and external carotid arteries and the occipital and lingual arteries on their lateral sides and reaches the hyoglossus muscle. Running forward and upward on the outer surface of this muscle, the hypoglossal nerve, accompanied by the sublingual vein, crosses a second time the tendon of the digastric and the stylohyoid muscle on their deep surfaces. Slightly above the digastric tendon the hypoglossal nerve enters the oral cavity at the posterior border of the mylohyoid muscle and continues on its superomedial surface. After exchanging fibers with the lingual nerve, the hypoglossal nerve splits into several branches that continue into the substance of the tongue on the lateral surface of the genioglossus muscle. The lingual branches of the hypoglossal nerve diverge fanwise and supply all of the muscles of the tongue, except the palatoglossus.

The ramification of the hypoglossal nerve is complicated by its connection with the upper cervical nerves. Not far below the base of the skull the hypoglossal nerve is joined by a nerve that arises from the loop between the first and second cervical nerves. Most of these cervical fibers again detach themselves from the hypoglossal nerve where it crosses the internal carotid artery, and these fibers constitute the superior branch of cervical ansa (descending hypoglossal nerve). Descending superficially along the internal carotid artery, this nerve joins at a variable level with a branch of the second and third cervical nerves, the inferior branch of cervical ansa, in the deep cervical loop or hypoglossal ansa. From the loop arise branches for the omohyoid, sternothyroid, and sternohyoid muscles. Not all cervical fibers leave the hypoglossal nerve in its descending branch. Those that continue in the sheath of the hypoglossal nerve are released as two more branches. The nerve for the thyrohyoid muscle is given off at the posterior end of the greater hyoid horn; the nerve for the geniohyoid muscle arises above the mylohyoid muscle in the oral cavity.

AUTONOMIC NERVOUS SYSTEM

The visceral efferent component of the nervous system is a distinct entity, structurally and functionally. It is therefore assigned a separate category called the autonomic nervous system. As previously pointed out, it is composed of a sympathetic system and a parasympathetic system. Visceral efferent nerves supply the smooth muscles of the eye and orbit, the lacrimal gland, major and minor salivary glands, and perhaps nasal glands. Sympathetic fibers innervate the dilator of the pupil and the superior and inferior palpebral (tarsal) muscles. Parasympathetic fibers innervate the sphincter of the pupil, the ciliary muscle of lens accommodation, and the lacrimal gland. The salivary, and perhaps nasal, glands receive both sympathetic and parasympathetic innervation.

All sympathetic fibers in the head are postganglionic. The preganglionic cell bodies lie in the upper segments of the thoracic spinal cord; their axons end on the cells of the superior cervical ganglion. The sympathetic fibers in the head therefore have no synaptic relation to cells of the ciliary, pterygopalatine, otic, or submandibular ganglia. Sympathetic fibers pass through these ganglia, as do sensory fibers of the adjacent branches of the trigeminal nerves. Branches emanating from the ganglia are thus mixed nerves. The eyeball, for instance, receives parasympathetic fibers for the pupillary sphincter and the muscles of accommodation, sympathetic fibers for the pupillary dilator, and somatic sensory fibers for sensitive coats of the eye, all contained in the short ciliary nerves.

Parasympathetic fibers incorporated in the oculomotor, facial, glossopharyngeal, and vagus nerves are preganglionic. The vagus fibers, however, do not involve areas of concern here. Parasympathetic fibers of the oculomotor, facial, and glossopharyngeal nerves enter the ganglia related to branches of the trigeminal nerve, namely, the ciliary, pterygopalatine, otic, and submandibular ganglia. Each single preganglionic fiber ends in synaptic connection with a group of cells forming the ganglion. These multiple cells give rise to the postganglionic axons, which carry the impulse on to smooth muscle fibers or secretory cells called effector organs. The parasympathetic ganglia of the head, therefore, are the relay stations for parasympathetic neurons, but they are also meeting places for fibers of other functions, which pass directly through and make up the "mixed" nerves.

Traditionally all of the nerves that enter one of the ganglia of the head are called roots of the ganglion. The ciliary ganglion for instance is said to have a parasympa-thetic "short," or "motor," root, a sensory "long" root, and a sympathetic root. It should be understood that only the "root" that carries parasympathetic fibers is a root in the true sense, because only its fibers will synapse on the cells of the ganglion, whereas the fibers of the other "roots" merely pass through it. Since it is known that only oculomotor, facial, and glossopharyngeal nerves contain preganglionic parasym-pathetic fibers that are connected with the ganglia under consideration, it is a simple matter to recognize the true root of the ganglion; it is that branch entering the gan-glion that arises from one of these three nerves: oculomotor, facial, or glossopharyn-geal.

Sympathetic nerve supply of the head

The preganglionic fibers of the sympathetic nerves that are destined for the head and neck arise in the upper segments of the thoracic part of the spinal cord. They reach the sympathetic trunk through white rami communicantes at the level of the stellate, or the inferior cervical, ganglion and run upward in the cervical part of the sympathetic chain. They finally reach the superior cervical ganglion, on the cells of which they end to establish synaptic contact with the postganglionic neurons.

The postganglionic fibers that leave the superior cervical ganglion (Fig. 9-13) are in part destined for the heart and the great vessels. Those that end in the organs of the head and neck follow either the external carotid artery and its branches or the internal carotid artery. The fibers that follow the internal carotid leave the upper pole of the superior cervical ganglion and accompany the internal carotid artery as the internal carotid nerve, which soon splits to form a loose plexus around the artery and its branches. The internal carotid nerve and plexus and its branches consist of postgan-glionic nonmyelinated fibers and are therefore "gray" nerves.

The internal carotid plexus sends communicating branches to a great number of cranial nerves. In the carotid canal arise the two caroticotympanic nerves, which enter the tympanic cavity and participate in forming the tympanic plexus. Where the internal carotid artery enters the cavernous sinus, the deep petrosal nerve is given off. It joins the parasympathetic major petrosal nerve to form the pterygoid nerve, which penetrates the fibrocartilage of the lacerated foramen and continues through the pterygoid canal to the pterygopalatine ganglion. The fibers of the sympathetic part of the pterygoid nerve pass through the ganglion and are destined for glands and blood vessels of the nasal cavity, palate, and pharynx.

The internal carotid plexus finally releases the so-called sympathetic root of the ciliary ganglion. The sympathetic fibers reach the ciliary ganglion through the supe-rior orbital fissure either independently or incorporated in a branch of the nasociliary nerve. These fibers merely pass through the ganglion and then become part of the short ciliary nerves, enter the eyeball, and end in the dilator of the pupil.

The postganglionic sympathetic fibers arising in the superior cervical ganglion, which follow the external carotid artery and its branches, supply the muscles of the blood vessels and smooth muscles and glands of the skin. They also send branches to

Table 3. Parasympathetic ganglia associated with trigeminal nerve

Division	Ganglion	Source of preganglionic fibers	Main effector organs
I. Ophthalmic nerve	Ciliary	Oculomotor	Muscle of accommodation (ciliary muscle) Sphincter of pupil
II. Maxillary nerve	Pterygopalatine	Facial: greater petrosal	Lacrimal gland
III. Mandibular nerve	Submandibular	Facial: chorda tympani	Submandibular gland Sublingual gland
	Otic	Glossopharyngeal: lesser petrosal	Parotid gland

the large salivary glands. The fibers for the submandibular and sublingual glands are derived from the plexus surrounding the facial artery. They reach the glands by passing through the submandibular ganglion. The sympathetic branches for the parotid gland come from the plexus surrounding the middle meningeal artery and pass through the otic ganglion.

Parasympathetic nerve supply of the head

The parasympathetic nerves of the head can best be described if the parasympathetic ganglia are taken as the means of classification. It then becomes clear that the ciliary ganglion relays the parasympathetic fibers that are contained in the oculomotor nerve. Pterygopalatine (sphenopalatine) and submandibular ganglia are relay stations for the parasympathetic fibers of the facial (intermediate) nerve. The otic ganglion, finally, receives and relays the glossopharyngeal parasympathetic outflow. Table 3 summarizes briefly the salient facts of the distribution of parasympathetic nerves in the head.

Ciliary ganglion. The ciliary ganglion (Fig. 9-13) is situated in the posterior part of the orbit between the optic nerve and the lateral rectus muscle of the eye. It is an oval body 2 by 1 mm. in size and of a reddish gray color. The parasympathetic fibers of the oculomotor nerve, arising in the Edinger-Westphal nucleus, are carried in the inferior branch of the oculomotor nerve, which passes below the ganglion on its way forward and downward to the inferior rectus and inferior oblique muscles of the eye. The parasympathetic fibers reach the ganglion as a short and relatively thick nerve, the short, or motor, root of the ciliary ganglion. The short root is, in a functional sense, the true root of the ciliary ganglion. The postganglionic parasympathetic fibers, which arise from the cells of the ciliary ganglion, leave it at its anterior pole as six to ten fine nerves, the short ciliary nerves. Divided into 20 or more branches, they enter the eyeball at its posterior surface in a circular area around the optic nerve.

The short ciliary nerves also contain sensory and postganglionic sympathetic fibers. The sensory fibers are derived from the nasociliary nerve of the first division of the trigeminal nerve. These fibers pass through the ganglion and reach the eyeball in the short ciliary nerves. The branch of the nasociliary nerve that goes to and through the ciliary ganglion is often described as its sensory, or long, root.

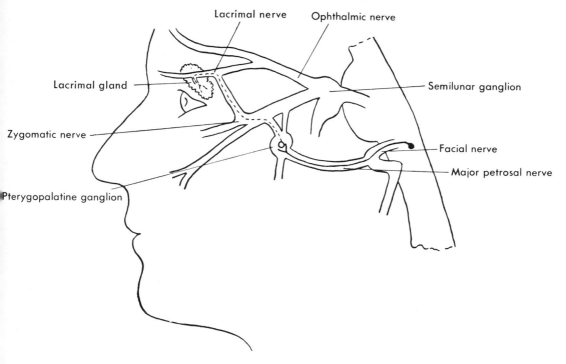

Fig. 9-14. Diagram of parasympathetic innervation of lacrimal gland. *Solid line*, preganglionic neuron; *broken line*, postganglionic neuron.

The postganglionic sympathetic fibers contained in the short ciliary nerves are derived from the plexus of the internal carotid artery and enter the orbit through the superior orbital fissure either as a separate filament or joined with the nasociliary nerve. If the sympathetic fibers form a separate nerve, it is called the sympathetic root of the ciliary ganglion. The sympathetic fibers merely pass through the ganglion and are then incorporated into the ciliary nerves.

The parasympathetic fibers derived from the cells of the ciliary ganglion supply the muscle of accommodation, or ciliary muscle, and the sphincter of the pupil. The sympathetic fibers derived from cells of the superior cervical ganglion end in the dilator of the pupil. The sensory fibers are destined for the coats of the eyeball.

Pterygopalatine ganglion. The pterygopalatine (sphenopalatine, or Meckel's ganglion) (Figs. 9-5 and 9-14) is a triangular flat body situated in the pterygopalatine fossa below the trunk of the maxillary nerve and medial to the pterygopalatine nerve. The ganglion is accessible from the nasal cavity through the sphenopalatine foramen at the posterior end of the middle nasal concha.

The parasympathetic fibers, which enter the ganglion to end in synaptic contact with its cells, are derived from the superior salivary nucleus and emerge from the brain in the facial nerve. They leave the facial nerve at its outer knee as the major petrosal nerve. This nerve joins with the deep petrosal nerve, which consists of postganglionic sympathetic fibers from the internal carotid plexus. Major petrosal and deep petrosal nerves form the pterygoid, or Vidian, nerve, which reaches the pterygopalatine fossa through the pterygoid canal. The pterygoid nerve shows its composition of preganglionic and postganglionic fibers clearly by the white and gray colors of its two components. The white bundle contains the preganglionic parasympathetic myelinated fibers; the gray bundle contains the postganglionic sympathetic nonmyelinated fibers. The former are the continuation of the major petrosal nerve; the latter represent the deep petrosal nerve.

The sympathetic fibers that enter the pterygopalatine ganglion have no relation to its cell and pass through the ganglion into its efferent nerves. Through the pterygopalatine ganglion, or closely attached to its outer surface, pass sensory fibers of the second division of the trigeminal nerve, the pterygopalatine nerve. The postganglionic parasympathetic and sympathetic fibers are incorporated in the trigeminal branches, which, emerging from the pterygopalatine ganglion, reach the nasal cavity and the palate to supply the nasal and palatine glands and blood vessels. A small pharyngeal branch of the pterygopalatine ganglion also contains visceral fibers. Through the pterygopalatine ganglion also pass the taste fibers, which are carried in the major petrosal nerve. They reach the few taste buds of the palate in the palatine nerves.

Some of the parasympathetic fibers derived from the cells of the pterygopalatine

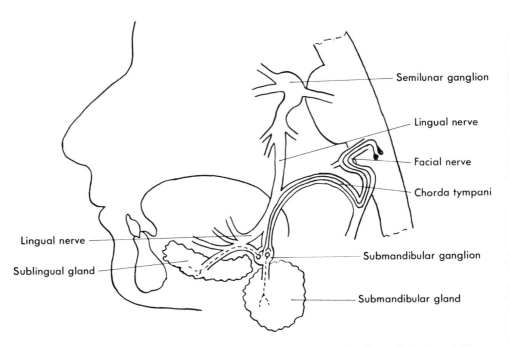

Fig. 9-15. Diagram of parasympathetic innervation of submandibular and sublingual glands. *Solid lines,* preganglionic neurons; *broken lines,* postganglionic neurons.

ganglion turn laterally and are incorporated in the zygomatic nerve. These fibers are led from the zygomatic nerve by a connecting branch to the lacrimal nerve and finally reach the lacrimal gland, which they supply. A sympathetic supply of the lacrimal gland has not been established.

Submandibular ganglion. The submandibular ganglion (Figs. 9-15 and 13-5) lies above the submandibular gland in the plexus of nerves connecting the lingual nerve with the gland. The parasympathetic preganglionic fibers, which are relayed in the submandibular ganglion, originate in the superior salivary nucleus and become part of the facial (intermediate) nerve. They leave the facial nerve, together with most of its taste fibers, as the chorda tympani. After passing through the tympanic cavity, the chorda tympani joins the lingual nerve. Where the lingual nerve turns anteriorly above the submandibular glands, the parasympathetic fibers leave the lingual nerve and enter the submandibular ganglion. Some of the postganglionic fibers enter the submandibular gland as fine filaments; the others return upward and forward to the lingual nerve and are carried in its branches to the sublingual and lingual glands. Sensory trigeminal fibers of the lingual nerve pass through the ganglion and, with its efferent branches, into the submandibular gland. Sympathetic postganglionic fibers also enter and pass through the ganglion to the salivary glands. The sympathetic fibers reach the ganglion from the sympathetic plexus around the facial artery.

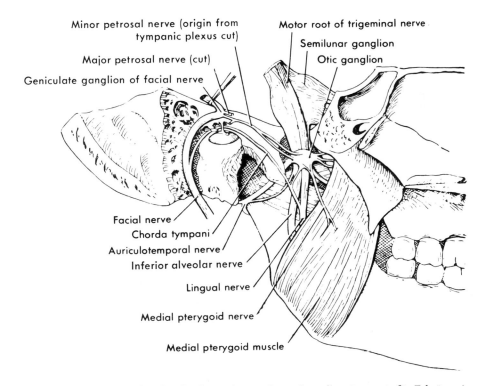

Fig. 9-16. Otic ganglion. (Modified and redrawn from Sicher and Tandler: Anatomie für Zahnärzte.)

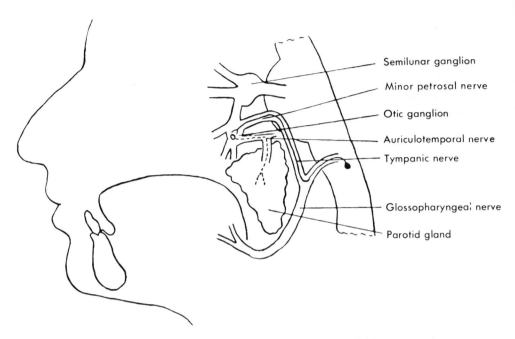

Fig. 9-17. Diagram of parasympathetic innervation of parotid gland. *Solid line,* preganglionic neuron; *broken line,* postganglionic neuron.

Otic ganglion. The otic ganglion (Figs. 9-16 and 9-17) is attached to the medial surface of the mandibular nerve immediately below the oval foramen. The parasympathetic preganglionic fibers, which end in synaptic relation on the cells of the otic ganglion, originate in the inferior salivary nucleus and are incorporated in the glossopharyngeal nerve. They leave this nerve as the tympanic nerve, enter the tympanic cavity, pass through the tympanic plexus, and emerge through the roof of the tympanic cavity as the lesser petrosal nerve, which, after receiving fibers from the facial nerve, reaches the otic ganglion through the sphenopetrosal fissure. The postganglionic parasympathetic fibers, which arise from the cells of the otic ganglion, join the auriculotemporal nerve and reach, through its parotid branches, the parotid gland, which they supply.

The sympathetic fibers that are destined for the parotid gland make their way through the otic ganglion to join its efferent nerves. They reach the otic ganglion from the sympathetic plexus of the middle meningeal artery.

Motor fibers of the mandibular nerve pass through the otic ganglion. The nerve to the medial pterygoid muscle passes through the ganglion or along its surface, and the nerves of the tensor tympani and the tensor palati muscles, branching off the medial pterygoid nerve, ordinarily also pass through the otic ganglion.

PART II

Regional and applied anatomy

In many textbooks, references to applied anatomy are made after the description of an organ or a region of the human body. By necessity these practical notes are too general because they are addressed at the same time to the general practitioner in medicine and to the different specialists, including the dentist and the oral surgeon.

Applied anatomy should be the link between theory and practice. It should provide the solid basis for any medical or dental techniques. Therefore there is not *one* applied anatomy but as many as there are specialties of the healing arts. The following chapters, selected and arranged from the clinical point of view, are presented not as an applied anatomy of the head and neck, but rather as the anatomic basis for the practice of general dentistry and all associated specialties, particularly oral, maxillofacial, and plastic surgery.

CHAPTER 10

Palpability of the facial skeleton

The bones of the facial skeleton and of the adjacent parts of the skull can be felt partly through the skin and partly through the mucosa of the oral vestibule or the oral cavity. How much of the bony surface can be felt is dependent on the thickness and firmness of the covering soft tissues. Thus the extent of the palpable areas not only is restricted by the relation of soft to hard parts in general, but also differs widely individually, according to the varying amount of subcutaneous fat and the volume of the overlying musculature.

Through the skin of the forehead the squama of the frontal bone can be felt in its entire extent from one temporal line to the other. Although it is covered by the temporal muscle and the temporal fascia, the temporal surface of the frontal squama behind the temporal line can be palpated in most persons since, in this region, the muscle is almost always thin enough to allow an examination of the underlying bone by the palpating finger. During this examination, the patient should relax the masticatory muscles, with the mouth slightly open. The more peripheral areas of the temporal fossa can be felt easily just below the temporal lines of the parietal and temporal bones because of the thinness of the temporal muscle in this region. The central part of the temporal fossa, however, is overlaid by the more voluminous portion of the temporal muscle and is made still less accessible by the firm and tightly stretched temporal fascia. The closer the palpating finger is brought to the zygomatic arch, the less it can feel of the bones at the floor of the temporal fossa; the tension of the temporal fascia can be so great that it gives the impression of bony resistance. Skull fractures in this region may, therefore, be obscured and should never be excluded without proper radiographic examination.

In the lower part of the forehead the superciliary arches are visible and clearly palpable through the skin and the frontal muscle. Above the root of the nose, between the superciliary arches, the prominence of the glabella can be found. The bony skeleton of the external nose is covered by a relatively thin skin and, therefore, is palpable in its entirety.

The borders of the orbital entrance can be felt in all their parts through the extremely thin skin of the eyelids. On the upper orbital rim, the shallow frontal notch can be felt close to the root of the nose, and lateral to this notch, the deeper supra-orbital notch can be felt. The latter is often transformed into a foramen by ossification of the normally thin ligament bridging the notch. In such cases there is no supraor-

429

bital notch. The supraorbital rim is continuous from the shallow depression for the frontal nerve laterally to the end of the zygomatic process of the frontal bone. However, the location of the emerging supraorbital nerve can still be palpated. The upper orbital border is shaped in two parts. The medial third is thick and rounded, the lateral two thirds is thin and sharp. It is at the juncture of these two parts that the supraorbital notch or foramen is found. The formation of the superior orbital rim is often asymmetrical, a notch being present on one side, a foramen on the other. This variation is of practical importance for the examination of the sensitivity of the supraorbital nerve to pressure. The pressure should not be exerted from below against the superior orbital rim but against the frontal bone just above the supraorbital notch or foramen, so that the pressure is independent of the variations of the skeleton at this point.

The lateral orbital rim, composed of the zygomatic process of the frontal bones and the frontal process of the zygomatic bone, is easily accessible, and the suture between these two bones can be felt as a rough prominence. On the medial boundary of the orbital entrance the frontal process of the maxilla can be palpated posterior to and including the anterior lacrimal crest. The inferior orbital rim is also easily felt through the thin skin of the lower eyelid. In most persons the suture between the maxilla and the zygomatic bones, at about the middle of the inferior orbital rim, is marked by a slight prominence of the otherwise smooth bony edge. This point is important as a landmark for the location of the infraorbital foramen, which is situated directly below the point where the maxillozygomatic suture crosses the inferior orbital rim.

The anterior surface of the maxillary body and the adjacent parts of the upper alveolar process are palpable through the skin, but in obese persons the upper part of the canine fossa is not easily felt. The lateral border of the piriform aperture can be recognized, whereas its lower border and the anterior nasal spine are usually obscured. As a rule the shape and depth of the canine fossa can be examined as well as its posterior boundary, the prominent zygomaticoalveolar crest. Easily felt are the alveolar eminences of the incisors, canine, and premolars. Of the maxillary body behind the zygomaticoalveolar crest, only a rather small part can be felt through the skin because the masseter muscle intervenes between the skin and bone.

The zygomatic bone and the entire zygomatic arch are accessible to the examining finger. At its lower border, the outline of the articular tubercle and the articular notch can be established if the subcutaneous fat is of not more than moderate volume. The localization of the articular tubercle and the notch is facilitated if the mandible is moved, since during opening of the mouth the mandibular head is level with the height of the tubercle, and during closing it glides back toward the mandibular fossa. Parts of the head of the mandible can be palpated through the skin and from the external auditory meatus. Especially during movements, the lateral pole of the condyle is easily felt and is sometimes seen through the skin, and restrictions or aberrations of its movements can be diagnosed. This is considerably aided by simultaneous examination of the posterior surface of the condyle from the ear passage.

How much of the posterior border of the mandible can be felt through the skin is dependent not only on the development of the subcutaneous fat, but also on the thickness of the parotid gland. In most persons the entire posterior border of the mandibular ramus can be examined from the condyle to the mandibular angle. Immediately below the condyle, part of the outer surface of the mandibular ramus itself can be palpated; most of it, however, is made inaccessible by the overlying masseter muscle. This muscle extends anteriorly farther than the anterior border of the mandibular ramus, which can be felt only in its inferior parts and then only if the masseter muscle is relaxed. The oblique line that continues the anterior border of the ramus downward and forward is always easily felt through the skin. The entire body of the mandible, its outer surface as well as its lower border, and the alveolar process and the alveolar eminences, with the exception of the region of the third molar, can be palpated through the skin. The posterior region is covered by the masseter muscle and is often made inaccessible.

At the mandibular angle and in front of it a variable area of the inner surface of the mandibular body can be felt through the skin. The palpation of this bony surface is facilitated by bending the head toward the chest and toward the examined side to relax the skin and the fascia below the mandible. The inner surface of the chin itself is inaccessible because the digastric and mylohyoid muscles, inserting at the lower border of the mandible, restrict the examining finger.

The digital examination from the oral vestibule reveals clearly the entire outer plate of the upper and lower alveolar processes. On the mandible the oblique line can be felt in the region of the second molar; following this ridge backward and upward, the finger is led to the anterior border of the mandibular ramus and higher up to the root of the coronoid process. The zygomaticoalveolar crest, marking the boundary between the anterior and posterior surfaces of the maxilla, can be located in all persons. The crest starts in the region of the first molar and can be followed upward and outward to the zygomatic process of the maxilla.

The line of the vestibular fornix is generally found at the level of the apical one third of the roots of the upper and lower teeth. If the jaws are closed and the lips and cheeks relaxed, the palpating finger can examine the entire height of the alveolar process and even the adjacent parts of the maxillary and mandibular bodies; the loose fixation of the vestibular mucosa permits the necessary extension of the fornix. The expansion of the fornix is somewhat restricted in the anterior part, especially in the mandibular region, because the mental and lower incisive muscles arise high on the alveolar process. The mobility of the vestibular mucosa is also restricted in the posterior parts of the vestibule in consequence of the restricted mobility of the posterior part of the cheek. This is especially true for the upper fornix in the molar region, whereas the mobility of the lower jaw itself necessitates a certain mobility of the mucosa in the mandibular molar area.

The accessibility of the posterior part of the upper fornix is also restricted by the temporal and masseter muscles and by the coronoid process of the mandible, which protrude strongly toward the upper alveolar process. It is, however, easy to widen this narrow space by moving the mandible toward the side that is being examined. In this movement the anterior border of the mandibular ramus and the adjacent muscles are shifted laterally, away from the maxilla. The widening of the posterior end of the upper fornix is still further enhanced if the jaws are kept almost closed so that the soft tissues of the cheek are relaxed.

From the oral cavity wide parts of the mandible can be palpated. The inner surface of the alveolar process is accessible in its entire extent. Of the body of the mandible, the area above the mylohyoid line and the insertion of the mylohyoid muscle can be felt. In the region of the lower third molar the finger can glide below the posterior end of the mylohyoid line and approach the region of the mandibular angle. In all persons the attachment of the deep temporal tendon to the temporal crest can be located medial and posterior to the anterior border of the mandibular ramus. The tendinous attachment, however, makes it impossible to feel the bony crest itself, although the great resistance of the tendon is often taken for the bony elevation. Between the anterior border of the ramus and the prominent deep temporal tendon the retromolar fossa can be palpated. The temporal crest is most easily found at its lower end immediately behind the lower third molar because it is bulkiest at this level. The inner surface of the mandibular ramus behind the temporal crest cannot be reached by the examining finger because it is covered by the medial pterygoid muscle.

In the upper jaw the inner plate of the alveolar process and the central area of the hard palate can be palpated from the oral cavity. The lateral area of the roof of the oral cavity and the root of the alveolar process in the molar region cannot be felt. Here the mucous membrane forms an arch between the roof and lateral wall of the oral cavity and hides the skeleton from the examining finger. The claim that one can localize the major palatine foramen by palpation is erroneous. One can, however, feel the soft connective tissue pad covering the foramen and its neighborhood. Behind the distal end of the upper alveolar process and slightly medial to it, in the root of the soft palate, the tip of the pterygoid hamulus can be felt as a bony prominence the size of a large pinhead.

CHAPTER 11

Structure and relations of the alveolar processes

Differential diagnosis of the source, or the course, of pathology in the facial area may, in many instances, depend on an understanding in depth of the structure and relations of the alveolar processes. The extraction of teeth, surgical exposure of root tips, surgical access to the maxillary sinus, surgical preparation for oral prosthesis, etc., must obviously proceed from a familiarity with the detail and variation found in alveolar structures and their relations. Planning local anesthesia where the anesthetic fluid must penetrate the cortical plates to reach the nerves within the medullary bone clearly depends on knowing the structural minutiae of these parts. Finally, familiarity with the relations, immediate and distant, of these processes is indispensable for an appreciation of the modes of spread of inflammatory reactions arising from the teeth. All of these concerns are preliminary to the study of more serious, penetrating extensions of infections of dental origin (see Chapter 14).

ALVEOLAR PROCESS OF THE MAXILLA

The alveolar process of the maxilla is in relation with the floor of the nasal cavity and the floor of the maxillary sinus. Its relation to these cavities is determined by the functional structure of the maxilla (see Figs. 2-60 and 2-61). The canine pillar of the maxilla, arising from the socket of the canine and extending upward along the lateral border of the piriform aperture into the frontal process of the maxilla, is the most constant bony structure in the base of the alveolar process. The canine pillar is situated lateral to the entrance into the nasal cavity. Being a functional reinforcement of the bone, it determines the medial and anterior expansion of the maxillary sinus, which replaces nonfunctional bone. It is, therefore, a general rule that the incisors are below the floor of the nasal cavity, the premolars and molars are below the floor of the maxillary sinus, and the canine occupies a neutral position between the two cavities. This is true even if the nasal cavity is abnormally wide, because the widening does not markedly involve the area in front of the incisive canal.

The relations of the apices of the incisors to the nasal floor are dependent on two factors: height of the face, especially height of the upper alveolar process, and length of the incisor roots. Since these two measurements are not correlated, it is necessary to examine each case individually and to ascertain the relations between the incisor sockets and the nasal floor by radiographic examination. It is a general rule that the root of the lateral incisor does not show as close a relation to the nasal floor as does the root of the central incisor, because the root of the lateral incisor tends to curve toward the outer rim of the nasal aperture. In addition, it has to be remembered that the floor of the nasal cavity ascends slightly laterally, which also increases the distance between the fundus of the socket of the lateral incisor and the nasal floor.

In persons with a relatively short alveolar process and long roots, the central incisor may actually reach the thin compact bony plate that forms the floor of the nasal cavity (Fig. 11-1, *A*). The apex of the tooth is then separated from the nasal cavity by only a thin plate of bone. In the other extreme a rather thick layer of spongy bone may be interposed between the nasal floor and the socket of the central incisor (Fig. 11-1, *B*). The distance between these two structures may reach 10 mm. and even more. The apex of the lateral incisor shows, in principle, the same variations in its relation to the nasal floor, but it rarely actually comes into contact with the nasal floor (Fig. 11-2, *A* and *B*).

The configuration of the alveolar process in the incisal region is, to a high degree, dependent on the formation of the palate. The inner palate of the alveolar process ascends at a moderate angle if the palate is low and then curves without a break into the horizontal roof of the oral cavity (Fig. 11-2, *A*). If the palate is high, the inner plate of the alveolar process is steep in its anterior part, and there is a fairly sharp angle between the alveolar process and the roof of the mouth (Fig. 11-2, *B*). These variations decisively influence the amount and the configuration of the spongy bone, the retroalveolar spongiosa, between the outer and inner plates of the alveolar process and the nasal floor. In a flat or low palate this space is roughly triangular and rather wide. In a high palate the retroalveolar spongiosa is restricted and occupies, in sagittal section, a more rectangular area.

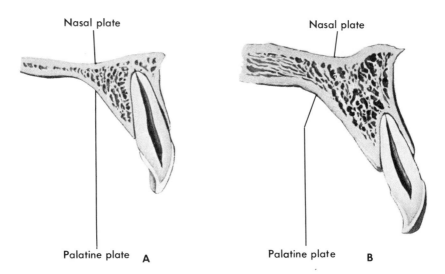

Nasal plate   Nasal plate

Palatine plate   **A**   Palatine plate   **B**

Fig. 11-1. Labiolingual sections through upper first incisor. (Sicher and Tandler: Anatomie für Zahnärzte.)

It has to be remembered that the difference between a low and a high palate is expressed not only in quantitative measurements but also in the changed configuration of the palate. In the incisor region the differences in shape and in the molar region the differences in relative size are more prominent, whereas the premolar area is a zone of transition. In the anterior region of the maxilla the inclination of the inner alveolar plate, or palatine plate, is slight in the low palate and steep in the high palate. In the molar region of the maxilla the angle between the oral roof and the inner surface of the alveolar process is always nearly a right angle, so that here the high palate is characterized mainly by an increase in the length of the alveolar process.

The sockets of the incisors are eccentrically placed into the alveolar process, the axis of the root and socket being more nearly vertical than the axis of the alveolar process as a whole (Figs. 11-1 and 11-2). Thus the alveolar bone proper on the labial surface of the root fuses with the external plate of the alveolar bone, whereas lingually a wedge-shaped area of spongy bone is found between the alveolar bone proper and the palatine, or inner, plate of the alveolar process. This is why abscesses originating in the incisor teeth in most instances perforate the labial plate of the alveolar process and open into the vestibule of the oral cavity. There is, however, one important exception to this rule. In a rather high percentage of incisors the apical part of the root of the lateral incisor is sharply curved lingually, and its apical foramen is placed in or near the center of the retroalveolar spongiosa and rather distant from the outer alveolar plate (Fig. 11-2, C). Periapical abscesses that take their origin from a lateral incisor of this type tend to expand lingually and may perforate the palatine plate of bone and cause a palatine abscess.

The relations of the incisors to the nasal floor explain the fact that an abscess

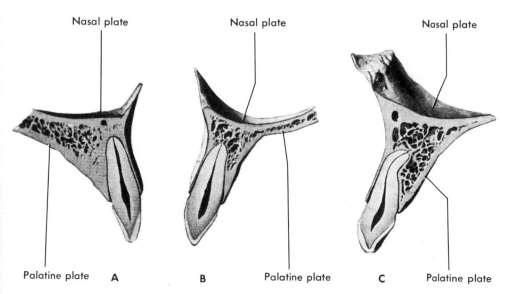

Nasal plate   Nasal plate   Nasal plate

Palatine plate   A   B   Palatine plate   C   Palatine plate

Fig. 11-2. Labiolingual sections through upper second incisor. (Sicher and Tandler: Anatomie für Zahnärzte.)

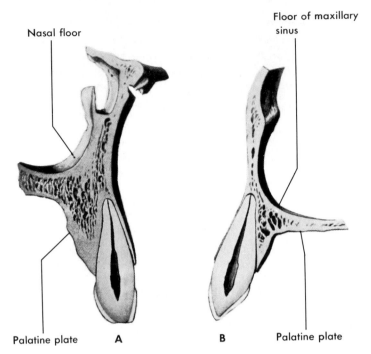

Fig. 11-3. Labiolingual sections through upper canine. (Sicher and Tandler: Anatomie für Zahnärzte.)

arising from the central incisor may open into the nasal cavity or that a radicular cyst of an incisor may bulge into the inferior nasal meatus, even causing an occlusion of the nostril.

The canine is embedded in the lower part of the canine pillar of the maxilla (Fig. 11-3, *A*). If this pillar contains a great amount of spongy bone, it is continuous with the retroalveolar spongiosa in the incisal region. Because of the position of the canine tooth in the canine pillar, neither nasal cavity nor maxillary sinus has intimate relations to the socket and the root of the canine. In extreme cases, however, the maxillary sinus may extend forward so far that it approaches the distolingual circumference of the socket of the canine in a rather broad front (Fig. 11-3, *B*). The same is sometimes true for the nasal cavity, which approaches the mesiolingual surface of the canine. The relation of the canine to the plates of the alveolar process is, in principle, the same as that of the incisors, its root being eccentrically embedded in the alveolar process. The compactness and the size of the canine roots cause an even greater bulging of the socket toward the labial surface of the alveolar process, and the alveolar eminence of the canine tooth is the most prominent in the upper jaw.

The premolars and molars are, as a rule, situated below the floor of the maxillary sinus. Whether the relations between the tooth and the sinus are intimate or not depends most of all on the development of the inferior, or alveolar, recess of the maxillary sinus (Figs. 11-4 to 11-6). But even in cases in which the base of the alveolar process is deeply excavated by the maxillary sinus, the first premolar is almost always

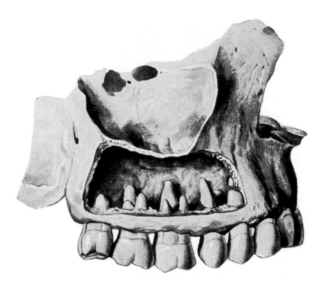

Fig. 11-4. Relations between maxillary sinus and teeth. Spongy trabeculae removed to show relation of sinus floor to roots. Alveolar recess of the sinus is lacking. (Sicher and Tandler: Anatomie für Zahnärzte.)

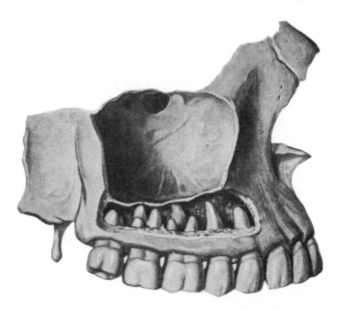

Fig. 11-5. Relations between maxillary sinus and teeth. There is a deep alveolar recess of the sinus. (Sicher and Tandler: Anatomie für Zahnärzte.)

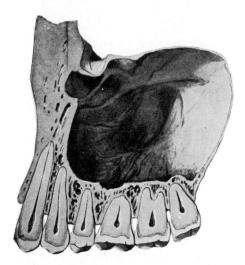

Fig. 11-6. Extreme expansion of maxillary sinus. (Sicher and Tandler: Anatomie für Zahnärzte.)

farther removed from the floor of the sinus than are the second premolar and the molars, because in the premolar area the floor of the sinus rises before continuing into the anterior wall. This, in turn, is correlated to the widening of the canine pillar at its base. Thus, with exception of extreme expansion of the maxillary sinus, the alveolar fundus of the first premolar is separated from the sinus floor by a layer of spongy bone.

The transition of the inner plate of the alveolar process into the horizontal part of the hard palate occurs in the region of the first premolar in a more pronounced angle (Fig. 11-7), and differences between a low and a high palate are here of a more quantitative character than they are in the anterior region of the maxilla. The relation of the first premolar socket to the alveolar process as a whole and to the retroalveolar spongiosa varies according to the formation of the root. If the first premolar has a single root, the socket is in close relation to the outer alveolar plate and is separated from the inner plate by spongy bone. As in the incisor-canine area, the outer alveolar plate is, in reality, a fusion between the alveolar bone proper and the alveolar plate and often is extremely thin. In many persons the outer plate may even be defective, or fenestrated, especially in the apical third of the alveolar eminence. If the first premolar possesses two roots, the buccal one is closely applied to the outer alveolar plate, whereas the socket of the lingual root is placed almost in the center of the retroalveolar spongiosa (Fig. 11-7).

The relations of the second premolar to the maxillary sinus are, as a rule, closer than those of the first premolar. Only if the alveolar recess of the maxillary sinus is absent or poorly developed does a layer of spongy bone intervene between the socket of the second premolar and the floor of the sinus (Fig. 11-8). In the majority of persons the floor of the sinus dips down into the immediate neighborhood of the second premolar (Fig. 11-9). Its socket is then separated from the sinus only by a thin layer of

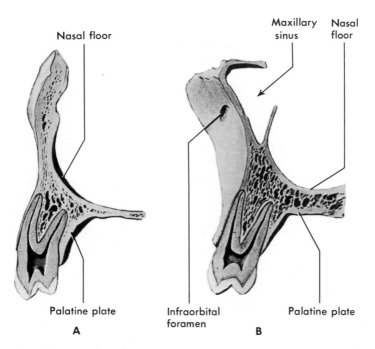

Fig. 11-7. Buccolingual sections through upper first premolar. (Sicher and Tandler: Anatomie für Zahnärzte.)

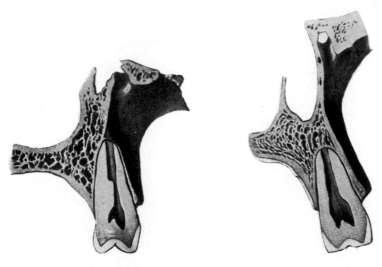

Fig. 11-8. Buccolingual sections through upper second premolar. (Sicher and Tandler: Anatomie für Zahnärzte.)

compact bone. The sinus may even extend below the level of the alveolar fundus of the second premolar, and the socket causes a slight prominence at the floor of the sinus (Fig. 11-9, *A*). If the expansion of the sinus goes further, the thin bony plate between the sinus and the socket of the second premolar may even disappear, so that only soft tissues separate the apex of the root from the cavity of the sinus; in other words, the periodontal tissue is then in direct contact with the mucoperiosteal lining of the sinus.

In the region of the second premolar the inner alveolar plate is more nearly vertical, except in cases of extremely low palate. The retroalveolar spongiosa is reduced, and it almost disappears in the region of the molars.

Intimate relations between the tooth and the maxillary sinus are the rule in the region of the molars. The intervention of a substantial layer of bone between the alveolar fundus and the maxillary sinus is here an exception (Figs. 11-10, *A*, and 11-11, *B*). The sockets of the molars almost always reach the floor of the sinus, and frequently the alveolar fundi of some or all of the molar roots protrude into the sinus, where small rounded prominences at the floor of the sinus mark the position of the root apices. Bony defects at the height of these prominences are not at all rare and sometimes are of fairly large extent (Fig. 11-13). The divergence of the molar roots, especially in the first molar, frequently permits an extension of the sinus downward toward the furcation of the roots (Figs. 11-11, *A*, and 11-12). Often sickle-shaped buttresses of bone traverse the floor of the sinus in a frontal plane between the molars whose roots protrude into the sinus. Sometimes these ridges connect the prominence of one of the buccal roots with that of the lingual root (Fig. 11-13). Branches of the alveolar nerves, destined for the lingual roots of the molars, use these sickle-shaped

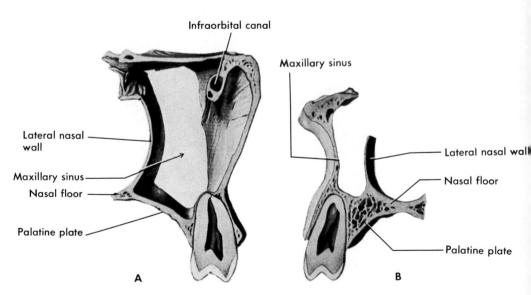

Fig. 11-9. Buccolingual sections through upper second premolar. (Sicher and Tandler: Anatomie für Zahnärzte.)

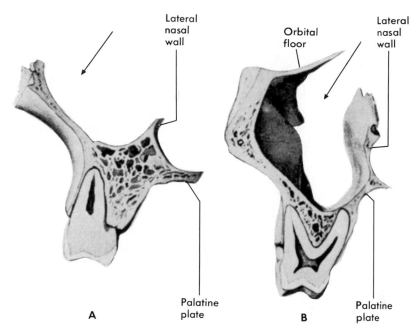

Fig. 11-10. Two buccolingual sections through upper first molar. Arrows point into maxillary sinus. **A,** Through mesiobuccal root. **B,** Through distobuccal and lingual roots. (Sicher and Tandler: Anatomie für Zahnärzte.)

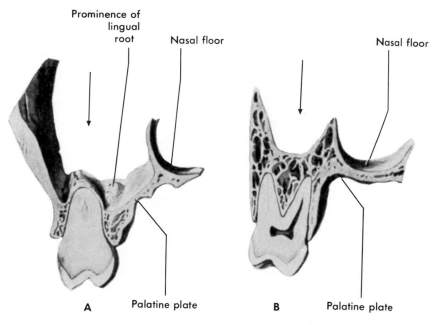

Fig. 11-11. Two sections through upper second molar. Arrows point into maxillary sinus. **A,** Through mesiobuccal root. **B,** Through distobuccal and lingual roots. (Sicher and Tandler: Anatomie für Zahnärzte.)

folds as bridges; they run in narrow canals that often are open toward the sinus for a variable length. The bony crests divide the alveolar recess into several chambers, a peculiarity that should be kept in mind in the search for a root fragment that has been displaced into the sinus.

Differences in the relation between the first and the second molars to the sinus are caused mainly by the greater divergence of the lingual and the buccal roots in the first molar. The lingual root of the first molar frequently extends toward the base of the bony partition between the nasal cavity and the maxillary sinus (Fig. 11-10, *B*) and may, in extreme cases, even extend toward the lateral area of the nasal floor.

Behind the socket of the upper third molar the posterior end of the alveolar process forms a variably large knob-shaped bony prominence, the alveolar tubercle. The junction of the maxilla and the pterygoid process of the sphenoid bone, mediated usually by the palatine bone, occurs at a variable level above the free margin of the alveolar process behind the last molar. If this junction is high and if the alveolar tubercle is hollowed out by the maxillary sinus, the bone behind the maxillary third molar is weak (see Fig. 11-6). If the extraction of a third molar is attempted by applying an instrument that exerts pressure distally, the entire corner of the maxilla may be broken off and the wisdom tooth is not removed from its socket, but the tooth and socket are severed from the maxilla. As a consequence of this fracture, the oral cavity and the maxillary sinus communicate through a wide opening. The possibility of this alveolar fracture should caution against attempts to extract or to loosen the upper third molar by introducing an elevator between the second and third molars and exerting pressure distally.

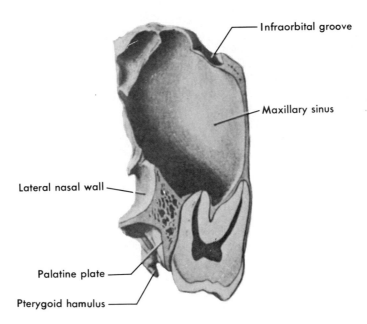

Infraorbital groove

Maxillary sinus

Lateral nasal wall

Palatine plate

Pterygoid hamulus

Fig. 11-12. Buccolingual section through upper third molar. (Sicher and Tandler: Anatomie für Zahnärzte.)

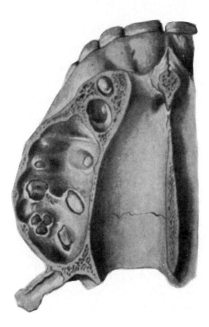

Fig. 11-13. Horizontal section through upper jaw above nasal floor. Defects of bone at floor of maxillary sinus correspond to root apices of molars. (Sicher and Tandler: Anatomie für Zahnärzte.)

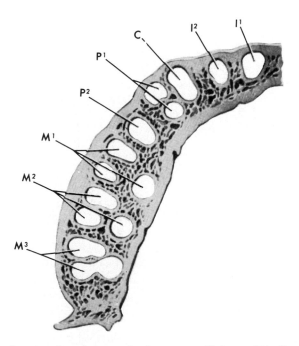

Fig. 11-14. Horizontal section through upper alveolar process. (Sicher and Tandler: Anatomie für Zahnärzte.)

The vertical position of the inner plate of the alveolar process in the molar region restricts the retroalveolar spongiosa to small areas lingual to the mesiobuccal root because the lingual root is situated alongside the distobuccal root (Fig. 11-14). The socket of the lingual root fuses with the inner plate of the alveolar process or is at least close to it. Mesial to the lingual root, however, a block of spongy bone intervenes between the socket of the mesiobuccal root and the lingual plate of the alveolar process (Figs. 11-10, A, 11-11, A, and 11-14). This arrangement of the spongy bone is the rule in the region of the first and the second molars; it is, however, often obscured around the third molar because of the great variability of third molar roots.

ALVEOLAR PROCESS OF THE MANDIBLE

Conforming to the great strength and more uniform solidity of the mandible, the lower alveolar process is in most areas far stronger than that of the upper jaw. Only in the incisor and canine areas are the outer and inner plates of the alveolar process thin; distally, however, they increase rapidly in thickness.

It is of clinical importance that the relation of the alveolar bone proper to the compact plates and the spongiosa of the alveolar process varies widely. In the anterior part of the mandible, in the region of the incisors and the canine, the alveolar process is narrow in the labiolingual direction, and in most jaws the alveolar bone proper fuses for the entire length of the root, or at least for most of its length, with the outer and the inner alveolar plates (Figs. 11-15 and 11-16). Only rarely is there a restricted zone of spongiosa lingual to the apical part of the socket.

The position of the sockets of the premolars and molars in the spongy bone of the

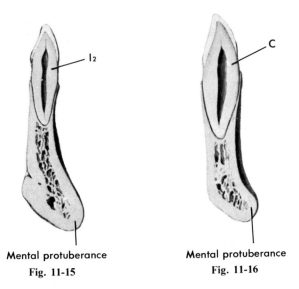

Mental protuberance

Fig. 11-15

Mental protuberance

Fig. 11-16

Fig. 11-15. Labiolingual section through lower second incisor. (Sicher and Tandler: Anatomie für Zahnärzte.)

Fig. 11-16. Labiolingual section through lower canine. (Sicher and Tandler: Anatomie für Zahnärzte.)

mandible varies. Only infrequently is the socket symmetrically placed between the outer and inner plates. In most cases the position of the socket is asymmetrical; that is, the axis of the root and the socket is inclined against the axis of the alveolar process. The alveolar bone proper is then fused for a variable length with one of the alveolar plates. The premolars and the first molar are mostly in close relation to the outer alveolar plate (Figs. 11-17 and 11-18). The second and third molars, however, often show a reversed relation, which is almost a rule for the third molar (Figs. 11-19 and 11-20). This is not so much the consequence of a different inclination of the last mandibular teeth but of a medial shift of the alveolar process itself in relation to the bulk of the mandibular body. The oblique line juts considerably on the outer surface of the mandible in the region of the second and third molars, and a fairly thick layer of spongy bone is interposed between the socket and the outer compact layer of the bone (Figs. 11-20 and 11-21), but this bone cannot be regarded as part of the alveolar process in a strict sense. The described relations are of clinical importance because an inflammation originating in the second and especially in the third molar will often perforate the inner compacta of the mandible. The variable relations of the socket and root can best be evaluated in buccolingual sections through the mandible at the level of the third molar. In such sections the socket of the wisdom tooth projects on the inner, or medial, surface of the mandible somewhat like a balcony (Fig. 11-21), and in

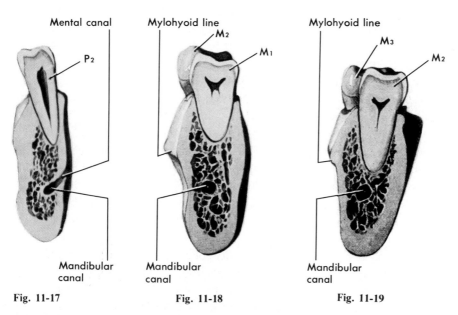

Fig. 11-17   Fig. 11-18   Fig. 11-19

Fig. 11-17. Buccolingual section through lower second premolar and through mental canal and foramen. (Sicher and Tandler: Anatomie für Zahnärzte.)
Fig. 11-18. Buccolingual section through distal root of lower first molar. (Sicher and Tandler: Anatomie für Zahnärzte.)
Fig. 11-19. Buccolingual section through distal root of lower second molar. (Sicher and Tandler: Anatomie für Zahnärzte.)

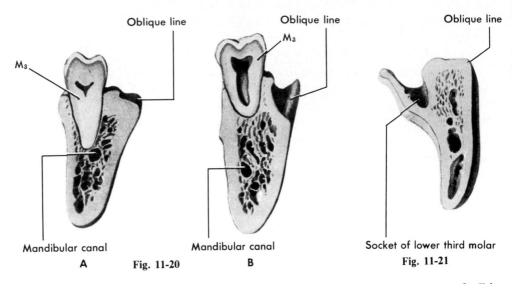

Oblique line   Oblique line   Oblique line

M₃

M₃

M₃

Mandibular canal   Mandibular canal   Socket of lower third molar

A   **Fig. 11-20**   B   **Fig. 11-21**

Fig. 11-20. Buccolingual sections through lower third molar. (Sicher and Tandler: Anatomie für Zahnärzte.)

Fig. 11-21. Buccolingual section through lower jaw in third molar region. (Sicher and Tandler: Anatomie für Zahnärzte.)

some persons it is shifted so far medially that it is in its entirety inside the arch of the mandibular body. The farther the socket projects inward, the thinner is its lingual wall and the closer is the apex of the root to the inner surface of the bone.

At or above the level of the fundus of the socket the mylohyoid line can be seen on the medial surface of the jaw. The variations in the relation of this line to the third molar are of great importance because the mylohyoid muscle, which forms the floor of the oral cavity, is attached to this line. The relations of the mylohyoid line to the apex of the third molar depend on three factors: the height of the mandibular body, the anteroposterior length of the mandibular alveolar process, and the length of the roots of the third molar. The level of the apex of the third molar roots is found, as a rule, below the level of the mylohyoid ridge, especially if the roots of the wisdom tooth are long, if the alveolar process is relatively short, and if the mandibular body is of below-average height. It is clear that in such cases a perforating abscess of the wisdom tooth will not appear in the oral cavity but below its floor in the connective tissue of the submandibular region. The consequence of such an occurrence will be discussed in the chapter on propagation of dental infections (Chapter 14).

Lateral, or buccal, to the alveolus of the lower third molar, the massive bone forms either a variably wide horizontal ledge (Figs. 11-20, A and 11-21) or a variably wide and variably deep groove (Fig. 11-20, B). The outer edge of this bony field is the oblique line where it turns anteriorly and inferiorly in continuation of the anterior border of the mandibular ramus. According to the relative length of the alveolar process, the wisdom tooth is either entirely in front of the ascending ramus or its distal part is flanked by the most anterior part of the ramus. In the latter case the

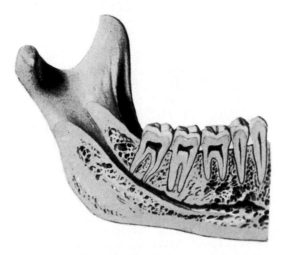

Fig. 11-22. Sagittal section through lower jaw. Note close relation of apices of third molar to mandibular canal. (Sicher and Tandler: Anatomie für Zahnärzte.)

accessibility of the lower wisdom tooth is restricted, especially if the superficial tendon of the temporal muscle is well developed and accentuates the anteriorly projecting border of the ramus.

Distal to the socket of the lower third molar is a rough bony triangle that can be regarded as the posterior end of the lower alveolar process; it is comparable to the alveolar tuberosity of the upper jaw. The posterior corner of the retromolar triangle continues into the temporal crest of the mandible. The deep tendon of the temporal muscle reaches downward along the entire length of the temporal crest to the level of the retromolar triangle, in other words, to the level of the alveolar process behind the lower wisdom tooth (see Figs. 3-6 and 3-9). The deep tendon is generally longer and more prominent than the superficial tendon.

Of special importance are the relations of the lower teeth to the mandibular canal and to its contents, the lower alveolar nerve and the accompanying blood vessels. The second premolar and the molars may be in rather close relation to the mandibular canal itself, whereas the first premolar shows relation to the mental canal. Canines and incisors are placed in the region of the narrow incisive canal, the anterior continuation of the mandibular canal.

In the relation of the root apices to the mandibular canal three types can be established. The most frequent type is that in which the canal is in contact with the alveolar fundus of the third molar, and the distance between the canal and the roots increases anteriorly (Fig. 11-22). When the canal is in proximity to the third molar root, the thin lamella of bone that bounds the mandibular canal may even show a fairly large defect, and the periapical connective tissue of the third molar is in direct contact with the contents of the mandibular canal. Severe pain of a neuralgic character after the extraction of a lower wisdom tooth or during inflammations of its periodontal ligament is easily explained by these relations.

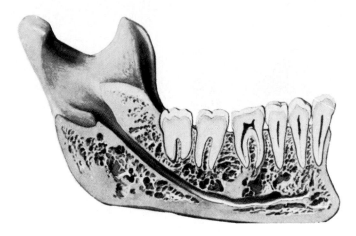

Fig. 11-23. Sagittal section through lower jaw. Note presence of spongy bone between roots of all teeth and mandibular canal. (Sicher and Tandler: Anatomie für Zahnärzte.)

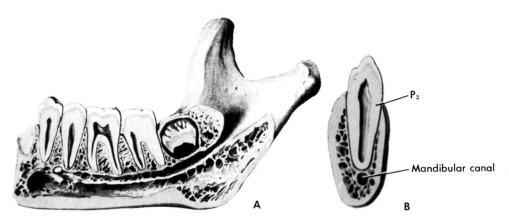

Fig. 11-24. A, Sagittal section through lower jaw of a young individual. Note close relation of all posterior teeth to mandibular canal. **B,** Buccolingual section through lower second premolar. Mandible is abnormally low. Note proximity of root apex and mandibular canal (Sicher and Tandler: Anatomie für Zahnärzte.)

The other two types of topography of the mandibular canal occur only in a small number of persons. In cases of a relatively high mandibular body combined with roots of moderate length, the mandibular canal has no intimate relations to any one of the posterior teeth (Fig. 11-23). The reverse is true in those who have a low mandible and relatively long roots. In these cases the mandibular canal may be in close contact with the roots of all the three molars and the second premolar.

The last-described type is normal for children and most young persons in whom the definite height of the mandible has not yet been attained (Fig. 11-24). During further growth, the mandibular body increases in height by apposition at the free border of the alveolar process, and the teeth, by their correlated vertical eruption, move away from the mandibular canal.

The frequent impaction of the lower third molar may bring about a still closer and more complicated relation of its roots to the mandibular canal and its contents. In impaction of the wisdom tooth the developing roots grow into the bone. If the tooth is in an oblique or nearly vertical position, and if the growing roots are not stunted or bent, they frequently extend beyond the level of the mandibular canal. However, an actual meeting between roots and canal is rare, although a routine radiograph may give this illusion. Since the impacted lower third molar is usually lingually inclined (Fig. 11-20, *B*), its roots pass the mandibular canal on its buccal side. Only in a minority of cases are the roots located lingual to the canal (Fig. 11-20, *A*) if the wisdom tooth is abnormally inclined and especially if there is a considerable lingual shift of the posterior end of the alveolar process.

In rare instances the roots of an impacted third molar grow straight toward the mandibular canal and then, continuing to grow, envelop its contents. The wisdom tooth then has a root that is, to a variable extent, divided into a buccal and a lingual part. The mandibular canal may lie in this abnormal bifurcation, or, if the apices of the roots fuse below the canal, the alveolar nerve and blood vessels may pass through a canal in the roots of the wisdom tooth. The complications caused by this fortunately rare anomaly during extraction of such a wisdom tooth are self-evident. It is as though the loosened wisdom tooth were held in its socket by an elastic band. Cutting of this "band" means cutting the alveolar nerve and blood vessels. In view of these complications, the routine radiographs should be supplemented by one taken in vertical projection with the film in the occlusal plane. If by such a picture the diagnosis of the described anomaly can be made, division of the wisdom tooth into a buccal and a lingual part should be attempted to liberate the contents of the mandibular canal.

The relations of the first premolar to the mental canal and foramen deserve special attention. Ordinarily the mental canal arises from the mandibular canal in the plane of the first premolar; sometimes its origin is slightly distal to this plane. From its origin inside the mandible, the short mental canal runs outward, upward, and backward to open at the mental foramen, situated between the two premolars or in the plane of the second premolar. The oblique course of the mental canal (see Fig. 11-17) makes it understandable that its outer end is at a higher and more posterior plane than its inner end. This explains the fact that in radiographs the mental foramen often is projected on the apex of the second premolar but rarely on the apex of the first premolar. Since at this point the mandibular canal is seldom in the immediate neighborhood of the apices of these teeth, the mental foramen appears to have no connection with the mandibular canal and often is diagnosed wrongly as a pathologic defect of the bone, for instance as a periapical granuloma.

It was mentioned that in the premolar and molar region the outer and inner plates of the lower alveolar process consist of a fairly thick layer of compact bone. Attempts to anesthetize the inferior dental nerves by subperiosteal or supraperiosteal injections in this region are doomed to failure. In the region of the canine and incisors this method of injection is successful if the anesthetic is injected into the mental fossa above the mental tuberosity. Two facts make it advisable to inject fairly close to the lower border of the mandible and rather far below the level of the apices of the anterior teeth. The first is the fact that the incisal canal is situated at a lower level than the mandibular canal itself; the second is that the outer compacta of the mandible in the mental fossa is always perforated by a few small openings that allow an entrance of the injected fluid into the spongy core of the bone and thus to the incisive nerve.

CHAPTER 12

Anatomy of local anesthesia

The technique of local anesthesia can be sound only if it is built on exact anatomic knowledge. Although the topographic anatomy of the nerves that are the objects of local anesthesia in oral and maxillofacial surgery will be the primary topic of discussion in this chapter, it is unavoidable that certain technical conclusions drawn from the anatomic point of view will have to be included.

Some general principles are valid for all types of local anesthesia. The first and most important is that the technique has to integrate individual variations. This cannot be done by using average linear or angular measurements. It has to be done by selecting landmarks for the injection that are correlated to each other, so that their recognition makes the operator independent of individual variations. Most landmarks are points of the skeleton, but not all of these are accessible to the eye or to the palpating finger. One has to project the examination into the depth, and this can be done by extending, as it were, the palpating finger into the tissues by using the point of the needle as a probe. If such a procedure is to be successful, an inflexible, rigid needle must be used.

Anesthesia induced by injection of an anesthetic drug can attempt either to paralyze the nerve endings in the tissues or to reach the more centrally located nerves and block conduction in these nerves. The first type of local anesthesia is infiltration, or field, anesthesia; the second type is conduction anesthesia, or nerve blocking. The anatomic basis of infiltration, or field, anesthesia is simple enough. Here the primary consideration is the density of the tissues into which the anesthetic fluid is to be injected. The denser the tissue, the less fluid can be injected without using a pressure that would cause injury to the injected area. In oral and maxillofacial surgery, infiltration anesthesia has limited usefulness; it is used primarily to anesthetize small areas of the mucous membrane of the oral cavity or of the skin.

Conduction, or block, anesthesia, as applied in oral surgery, can be subdivided into two types. The attempt can be made to anesthetize the dental and periodontal nerves as close to the tooth as possible. The anatomic point at which these nerves can be reached is the dental plexus, or alveolar plexus, in the upper and lower jaws. It is the network of nerves in the spongy bone immediately above or below the root apices, respectively. This type of oral anesthesia can be called plexus anesthesia. It is ordinarily restricted to smaller areas of the jaws or to a small group of teeth. If the alveolar nerves or the trigeminal branches that give origin to the alveolar nerves are blocked, the term trunk anesthesia seems to be appropriate.

APPLIED ANATOMY OF THE DENTAL PLEXUS

The accessibility of the dental plexus (see Fig. 9-7) depends entirely on the thickness and density of the alveolar plates because the injection has to be made at the base of the alveolar process on its outer or inner surface. Therefore, the premolar and molar region of the lower jaw, which is characterized by the great thickness of the compact alveolar plates, cannot be anesthetized by plexus anesthesia. In the region of the lower canine and incisors, the outer plate of the bone is thin enough to permit the diffusion of the injected fluid into the spongy core of the mandible. The incisive nerve, which is the source for the loose and rather simple dental plexus in this region, is situated between the lower border of the mandible and the roots of the incisors. Thus the incisive nerve is found at the level of the mental fossa, a depression above and lateral to the mental prominence, and the injection should be made into the depth of the mental fossa; this technique is made still more advisable by the fact that the outer compacta of the mandible in the region of the mental fossa is always perforated by a few small openings. The plexus anesthesia for the lower incisors aims, therefore, for a point beyond and below the level of the apices of these teeth.

The outer alveolar plate of the upper jaw is almost always thin enough and porous enough to make plexus anesthesia successful. Only in the region of the upper first molar, where one encounters the lower end of the zygomaticoalveolar crest, the middle (or zygomatic) pillar of the maxillary skeleton, is the bone on the outer surface sometimes relatively thick.

It is generally believed that plexus anesthesia in the upper jaw should be attempted by injection at or above the level of the root apices. Two considerations, however, speak against this method and for an injection at the level of the apical third of the root length. One reason for the advisability of this technique is the formation of the skeleton itself, especially in the regions of the incisors and the first molar (see Figs. 11-1, 11-2, and 11-10). In these areas the outer surface of the maxilla is buccally concave; in other words, the outer surface of the bone is farther away from the plane of the root the farther upward one goes. This is caused in the incisor region by the often pronounced anterior projection of the lower border of the piriform aperture, especially above the central incisor at the base of the anterior nasal spine. In the area of the first molar, it is the zygomaticoalveolar crest that turns in a more or less sharp arch upward and lateral to the zygomatic process of the maxilla. It is also important that in the regions of the incisors and the first molar the outer alveolar plate gains in thickness and density at the base of the alveolar process.

A second reason for injecting somewhat below the level of the root apices of the upper teeth is the structure of the submucous connective tissue into which the injection is made (see Fig. 5-2). The injection for a maxillary plexus anesthesia is made in the area of the loosely attached vestibular mucosa above the mucogingival junction, the border line of the dense and immovably fixed gingiva. In injecting at or above the level of the root apices, the fluid enters the connective tissue at or above the vestibular fornix. Here the submucous connective tissue is loose and voluminous, and the injected fluid tends to expand away from the bone and spread over a rather large area.

If the operator follows the instinctive feeling that the injection will be more successful the deeper the needle is introduced, the chances of a rapid penetration of the anesthetic fluid into the spongy bone are decreased. If, however, the injection is made at or slightly below the line of the fornix, one injects into a more restricted and not so loosely textured submucous tissue. The injected fluid is retained in a smaller area and in closer contact with the bone, and the penetration of an adequate amount of sufficiently concentrated anesthetic solution is assured.

A subperiosteal injection is everywhere contraindicated because the detachment of the periosteum from the bone entails the rupture of blood vessels entering the bone and causes subperiosteal hematomas and postoperative pain. Any advantages a subperiosteal injection might have are negligible in the face of these complications. If the injected fluid can penetrate the compact bone of the alveolar plate, the delicate periosteum of the maxilla cannot possibly be a serious obstacle.

In the spongy bone the fluid diffuses rather uniformly, and the direction of its diffusion is determined by the extent of the marrow spaces. After the anesthetic solution has reached the spongy bone below the root tip, its spread is automatically directed upward into the base of the alveolar process because the outer alveolar plate is fused to the alveolar bone proper in the cervical parts of the socket.

The opinion is widely held that a palatine injection adds to the efficiency of a buccal injection, if the latter is not wholly satisfactory. Such a procedure is successful only in exceptional cases. Normally the lingual plate of the alveolar bone in the incisor, canine, and premolar regions is arched and bends away from the apices of these teeth. In the molar region, where the inner alveolar plate ascends steeply, the most that can be expected from a palatine injection is an influence on the nerves that enter the lingual root of the molars. These nerves, however, are but branches of the buccally located dental plexus and reach their destination by running through the spongy bone above the molars or sometimes in one of the bony ridges on the floor of the maxillary sinus. If a buccal injection in the molar region is not successful, the palatine injection will at best achieve a partial anesthesia of the tooth.

The exceptions in which a lingual anesthesia may be helpful concern individuals with an extremely high palate and a long, narrow alveolar process. In such persons the inner alveolar plate in the premolar and canine regions and sometimes even in the incisor region ascends so steeply that the distance from the inner alveolar plate to the apices of the teeth is greatly reduced.

After a successful plexus anesthesia, the anesthesia area comprises the tooth itself, its periodontal ligaments, the gingiva on the buccal surface of the alveolar process, and the interdental papillae. The soft tissues on the lingual surface of the alveolar process are not anesthetized. The lingual mucosa of the lower jaw is supplied by branches of the lingual nerve in its entire extent, whereas the palatine and nasopalatine nerves supply the lingual gingiva and mucosa of the upper jaw. The lingual mucosa of the mandible can be anesthetized easily by the injection of a small quantity of the anesthetic solution below the inferior border of the lingual gingiva. In the upper jaw a palatine anesthesia should be made only in distinct areas because of the peculiar structure and density of the palatine mucosa. The anatomic basis for the technique of these injections is discussed later.

APPLIED ANATOMY OF THE NERVES OF THE UPPER AND LOWER JAWS

The alveolar nerves of the upper jaw are branches of the infraorbital nerves; those of the lower jaw are branches of the inferior alveolar nerve. Although the latter is easily accessible for local anesthesia just before entering the mandibular canal, the postorbital part of the infraorbital nerve cannot be reached by as simple a technique. One injection to the lower alveolar nerve can anesthetize all of the inferior dental branches, but in the upper jaw the superior alveolar nerves must be approached separately. The posterior superior alveolar nerves can be reached at the posterior convex surface of the maxilla; the anterior superior alveolar nerves can be reached in the anterior part of the infraorbital canal; the middle superior alveolar nerve, if it is present, is almost inaccessible.

In addition to the anesthesia of the alveolar nerves that supply the teeth, their periodontal ligaments, and certain areas of the gingiva, the palatine nerve and the nasopalatine nerve must be blocked if a complete anesthesia of the upper jaw is intended. For full anesthesia of the lower jaw not only the inferior alveolar nerve but also the lingual nerve and, in most persons, branches of the buccal nerve, which supplies a variably large area of the buccal gingiva, must be blocked.

Topography of the posterior superior alveolar nerves

The posterior superior alveolar nerves can best be reached where they enter the bony canals in the posterolateral wall of the maxillary sinus (see Figs. 2-28 and 9-7). This area can be located by drawing a vertical line immediately behind the last molar and bisecting it between the alveolar border and the orbital surface of the maxilla. Since the anterior and posterior heights of the maxilla are almost equal, a usable estimate of the level of the superior posterior alveolar foramina can be gained by bisecting the distance between the inferior orbital rim and the gingival border at the level of the first premolar. In using half of this distance as a measure, the operator automatically eliminates most individual variations.

The statement that the posterior superior alveolar foramina are situated in a plane erected behind the last molar needs some clarification. Since the eruption of the molars is correlated to the anteroposterior growth of the jaws, the second molar must be used as a landmark in young persons between 10 and 16 years of age. The same is true in adults if the upper third molar is absent and if the end of the alveolar process, the alveolar tubercle, is immediately behind the second molar. However, since growth of the jaws is not dependent on the presence of teeth, the space behind the second molar is sometimes of considerable length even if the wisdom tooth is missing. In such individuals the determination of the anteroposterior plane of the foramina must be done as if the upper third molar were present or had been lost by extraction.

To reach the target area, the needle has to glide along the surface of the maxilla in an oblique direction; a vertical insertion of the needle is impossible because of the interference of the lower lip and lower jaw. If a third molar is present, the puncture of the oral mucosa should be done at the height of the vestibular fornix and at the level of the distal half of the second molar. This rule is also valid if the third molar has been lost, or if there is a fairly wide space distal to the second molar. In the case of absence of the third molar and shortness of the alveolar process, and in persons under 16 years of age whose wisdom tooth has not yet started to erupt, the injection starts at the level of the distal half of the first molar; one then operates in the region of the prominent zygomaticoalveolar crest. In such cases the puncture always must be made distal to this crest, which otherwise would be a formidable obstacle in the path of the needle.

From the moment the needle comes into contact with the bone until the target area is reached, the needle should never for a moment lose contact with the bone. This is necessary not only because the bone is the only reliable landmark in this region, but also because of the danger of inserting the needle into the rich and dense network of veins, the pterygoid venous plexus, which lies immediately behind the convex posterior surface of the maxilla. To eliminate difficulties sometimes encountered in this procedure, it is well to perform the anesthesia while the patient's mouth is almost closed so that the cheek is fully relaxed. Moreover, if the patient moves the chin toward the side of operation, the narrow space between the mandibular ramus and posterior part of the maxilla is greatly widened and the maneuverability of the needle is greatly enhanced.

The depth to which the needle is introduced is equal to half the maxillary height. The distance between the point of puncture and the target area is practically the same as that between the alveolar border and the target area because the triangle described between these three points is an isosceles triangle. The needle should not be inserted any deeper. The posterior superior alveolar nerves arises from the infraorbital nerve at some distance behind the posterior surface of the maxilla and reaches the bone at the point of the posterior superior alveolar foramen.

During anesthesia of the posterior superior alveolar nerves, often called "tuber" or "zygomatic" anesthesia, rather large, deep-seated hematomas may occur, which cause considerable swelling of the cheek. It is characteristic for this hemorrhage to spread in a surprisingly short time. The belief has often been expressed that an injury to the pterygoid venous plexus gives rise to the described internal bleeding. The rapid development, however, disproves this contention unequivocally. Only an artery bleeding under relatively high pressure can gain so great an extent in so short a time. It is an injury of the posterior superior alveolar artery or its external, gingival branch that causes the accident. This artery (see Fig. 7-4) runs in a more or less tortuous course downward and forward along the posterolateral surface of the maxilla and is here closely applied to the thin periosteum. The artery, which is sometimes fairly large, is situated directly in the path of the needle, which is guided upward and backward along the bone. Piercing of one of the coils of the artery, therefore, cannot always be avoided. The artery bleeds into the loose fat-containing connective tissue that fills the spaces between the masticatory muscles and the skeleton, and the bleeding finally reaches the subcutaneous tissue of the cheek just in front of the masseter muscle. The only possible way to restrict this hematoma is to exert digital pressure upward, inward, and slightly forward against the bone below the zygomatic arch and in front of the masseter muscle. During a tuber injection the possibility of a fast-spreading arterial hematoma has to be kept in mind, so that the first sign of this accident finds the operator fully prepared.

After a successful anesthesia of the posterior superior alveolar nerves, the anesthetic zone comprises the three molars and the buccal gingiva in this region. The anesthetic zone is sometimes smaller; it may, although more rarely, reach farther anteriorly into the area of the second premolar or even into that of the first premolar. This can be observed in persons who lack a middle superior alveolar nerve and in whom some or all of the fibers normally constituting this nerve are incorporated into the superior posterior alveolar nerve.

Topography of the anterior superior alveolar nerves

The anterior superior alveolar nerves arise in the infraorbital canal at a distance varying from 6 to 10 mm. behind the infraorbital foramen. To secure a full anesthesia of the anterior superior alveolar nerves, the injection has to be made into the infraorbital canal. Therefore it is necessary to describe in detail the position of the infraorbital foramen and the course of the most anterior part of the infraorbital canal.

The infraorbital foramen is situated 5 to 8 mm. below the middle part of the inferior orbital rim. The point of the orbital border just above the infraorbital foramen is marked by a slight roughness where the zygomaticomaxillary suture crosses the inferior orbital rim (see Fig. 2-3). The suture can be easily located through the thin skin of the lower eyelid and the projection of the infraorbital foramen to the skin can, in the majority of persons, be determined with a fair degree of accuracy. In a minority of individuals, especially in women, the slight roughness at the zygomaticomaxillary suture is missing. In these cases the pupillary distance can be taken as a landmark. If the patient looks straight forward into space, the distance between the centers of the pupils is 8 to 10 mm. greater than the distance between the two infraorbital foramina. If a vertical line is dropped through the center of the pupil, the infraorbital foramen lies 4 to 5 mm. medial to this line and 5 to 8 mm. below the lower border of the orbit.

The anterior, terminal part of the infraorbital canal follows an oblique course. If traced anteriorly, it deviates medially and inferiorly. If the axes of the two infraorbital canals are extended, they cross each other 1 to 2 cm. anterior to the crowns of the maxillary first incisors. If a needle is to be introduced into the infraorbital canal through the infraorbital foramen, the needle must be placed into the direction of the axis of the canal. In any other direction the needle would soon come into contact with one of the walls of the canal and could not enter the canal for a sufficient distance. Therefore the needle must point backward, upward, and outward.

If the projection of the infraorbital foramen to the skin is determined and if this point is marked, for instance, with iodine, the skin has to be punctured medial and inferior to this point so that the obliquely inserted needle can reach the bone at or in the immediate neighborhood of the infraorbital foramen. The thickness of the soft tissue in the region of the infraorbital foramen determines how far medially and inferiorly from the projection of the infraorbital foramen the skin should be punctured. The thickness of the soft tissues at this point varies considerably, depending on the amount of fat in the subcutaneous tissue and on the depth of the canine fossa of the maxilla. The dimensions can, however, easily be estimated by palpating the soft tissues between the thumb and index finger; while the jaws are closed and the lips relaxed, the thumb is inserted into the upper fornix and the index finger is placed on the skin.

The needle should penetrate the infraorbital canal to a maximum depth of 2 to 4 mm. to reach the superior anterior alveolar nerves. Since the injected anesthetic fluid is propelled deeper into the canal, the origin of these nerves will also be reached in individuals in whom they arise somewhat farther posteriorly. In inserting the needle into the canal, caution is necessary because the bony plate separating the canal from the orbit thins out posteriorly to disappear where the infraorbital canal continues into the roofless infraorbital sulcus. If the needle penetrates the entire length of the canal itself, the point of the needle may then pierce the connective tissue that separates the sulcus from the orbit, and the anesthetic fluid may be injected into the orbital fat. The inferior branch of the oculomotor nerve, which supplies the inferior rectus and oblique muscles of the eye, may then be paralyzed. Double vision is the consequence of this accident, and, although temporary, it is disturbing to the patient. There is even the possibility that the injected fluid may reach the optic nerve and cause temporary blindness or blurring of vision.

After successful infraorbital anesthesia the incisors and the canine are anesthetized, as well as the periodontal ligaments of these teeth, the labial mucosa, and the gingiva in the anterior region of the jaw. The anesthesia extends further to the upper lip, to the anterior area of the cheek, to the medial part of the lower eyelid, and to the wing of the nose. Fairly often the first premolar is also anesthetized, more rarely the second premolar. The enlargement of the anesthetic area is explained by the inclusion of fibers of the middle superior alveolar nerve into the anterior group of nerves.

The anesthetic zone frequently does not reach to the midline, and pulp and periodontal ligament of the first incisor are not anesthetized or are only partly anesthetized. It has been claimed that this is caused by a crossing of the alveolar nerves over the midline of the face from one side to the other. Although such an overlapping nerve supply is true for the skin, it has been proved that the anterior superior alveolar nerves are entirely restricted to one side of the upper jaw. The paramedian defect of the infraorbital anesthesia is, in fact, caused by the participation of fibers of the nasopalatine nerve in supplying this area. The nasopalatine nerve and the superior alveolar plexus exchange nerve fibers by a connection just below the nasal floor. The connecting nerve leaves the nasopalatine nerve in the most superior part of the incisive canal and reaches the alveolar plexus in its most medial extension.

To anesthetize the remaining sensitive zone after an otherwise successful blocking of the infraorbital nerve, one of two methods is applicable. If the region of the central incisor is free of inflammation, an additional plexus anesthesia in the region of the central upper incisor will block all the nerve fibers to the first incisor regardless of their origin. However, if an inflammatory infiltration in the incisor region contraindicates a local injection, the nasopalatine fibers can be anesthetized by inserting the needle into the nasopalatine canal through the incisive foramen. The direction of the nasal part of the incisive canal is oblique; the canal starts lateral to the base of the nasal septum and converges downward with the canal of the other side. To introduce the needle into the right incisive canal, the palatine mucosa is punctured on the left side of the palatine papilla. The needle is directed upward, slightly backward, and toward the midline. The distance to which the needle can be introduced into the incisive canal without entering the nasal cavity can be judged by the level of a horizontal plane through the junction of the nasal septum and the upper lip, which marks rather accurately the level of the nasal floor.

Topography of the palatine nerves

The soft tissues covering the hard palate and the lingual gingiva of the upper jaw are supplied by the branches of the anterior palatine nerves and by the oral branch of nasopalatine nerves of Scarpa. The boundary between the two areas corresponds roughly to a line that connects the canine of one side with that of the other. The border zone between the anterior and posterior areas of the palate is supplied by both the palatine and nasopalatine nerves so that the two areas are not sharply limited from each other.

The anterior palatine nerve enters the oral cavity through the major palatine foramen. Accompanied by the palatine artery and veins, the nerve courses anteriorly in a groove between the alveolar process and the roof of the oral cavity. This furrow loses depth rather rapidly, because nerve and blood vessels send numerous larger branches toward the midline and smaller branches laterally into the gingiva. In the molar region the nerve and the blood vessels are embedded in loose connective tissue, which is most voluminous around and immediately in front of the major palatine foramen. This loose connective tissue fills the space between the alveolar process and the palatine process of the maxilla, which join almost at a right angle, and the mucous membrane of the palate, which bridges the corner in a sweeping arch (see Fig. 5-4, *B*). On frontal sections the space is triangular or wedge-shaped.

The posterior area of the palatine mucosa and submucosa, with the exception of the loose connective tissue in the described location, is densely textured, and an injection into this tissue needs a fairly high pressure. If more than a few drops of fluid are injected into the dense areas of the palatine mucosa, small blood vessels are almost unavoidably torn. The patient experiences, as a consequence, sometimes long-lasting postoperative pain. Even ulceration and necrosis of the injected palatine mucosa have been observed.

All of these complications can be avoided if one does not attempt a strictly local anesthesia in the premolar and first molar region of the palate. Trunk anesthesia of the anterior palatine nerve at or immediately in front of the major palatine foramen should be the method of choice. The injection is made into the loose connective tissue surrounding the nerve and blood vessels, which can take up a fair amount of fluid; up to 0.5 ml. of anesthetic solution can be injected without any undue pressure. In fact, the lack of resistance during this injection is a sign that the needle has been introduced at the right place.

To reach the anterior palatine nerve as close as possible to the major palatine foramen, the location of this opening must be known. The foramen, which cannot be palpated in the living, is situated in the sagittal part of the suture between the horizontal plate of the palatine bone and the maxilla in the groove between the alveolar process and the roof of the oral cavity (see Figs. 2-30 and 2-62, B). The foramen lies at the level of the distal half of the last molar, 3 to 4 mm. in front of the posterior border of the hard palate. If the molars are missing, the border between the hard and soft palates can be taken as a landmark. This border is marked in the living by the sudden change in color between the soft and hard palates (see Fig. 5-4, A). The soft palate is dark red with a yellowish hue; the hard palate is pale with a grayish blue tinge.

Since syringe and needle cannot be introduced vertically, the puncture of the mucous membrane should be made at the level of the distal half of the molar in front of the last molar. The puncture is made at the height of the curving arch of the mucous membrane between the roof of the mouth and the alveolar process, and the needle is directed upward, backward, and outward.

The anesthesia of the oral branches of the nasopalatine nerve is best done at the oral opening of the incisive canal, the incisive fossa. This opening is covered by the palatine, or incisive, papilla, immediately behind the central incisors. An injection through the highly sensitive papilla should be avoided. Instead, it is advisable to insert the needle immediately lateral to the papilla and to direct the needle upward and slightly medially and backward. The needle then reaches the loose connective tissue in the wide oral part of the incisive canals, and a few drops of the anesthetic fluid, injected without great pressure, suffice to anesthetize both the right and left nasopalatine nerves, which enter the palatine mucosa close to the midline. Since the right and left nasopalatine nerves are closely applied to each other, it is also possible to reach these nerves in patients in whom a palatine inflammation or abscess exists on one side. It is then possible to puncture the mucous membrane on the unaffected side close to the palatine papilla and to avoid any injection into the inflamed area.

Topography of the inferior alveolar nerve

The inferior alveolar nerve releases all of the lower dental nerves in the mandibular canal and also participates in supplying the interdental papillae and the most distal and mesial areas of the buccal gingiva. Its cutaneous branch, the mental nerve, supplies the mucous membrane, the skin of the lower lip, and a variable area of the skin of the chin. The buccal gingiva in the middle part of the lower jaw is supplied by the buccal nerve; the entire lingual gingiva is supplied by branches of the lingual nerve.

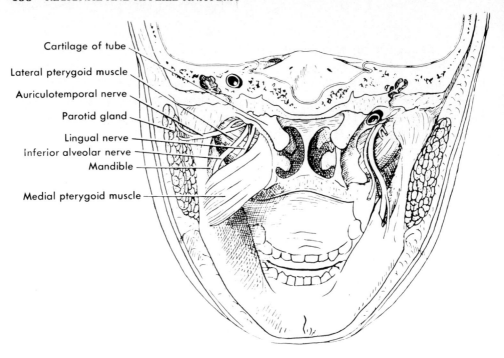

Fig. 12-1. Pterygomandibular space and inferior alveolar nerve dissected from behind.

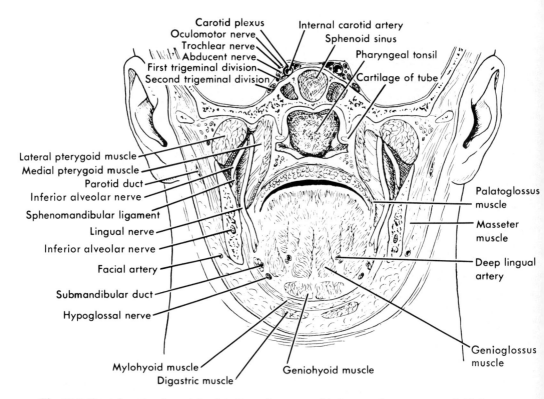

Fig. 12-2. Frontal section through head, in front of craniomandibular articulation; posterior half of section. (Modified and redrawn from Sicher and Tandler: Anatomie für Zahnärzte.)

The inferior alveolar nerve can be reached in the pterygomandibular space just before the nerve enters the mandibular foramen. The anterior branches of the alveolar nerve can also be anesthetized by injecting into the mental canal. The pterygomandibular space (Figs. 12-1 and 12-2) is a well-defined space between the mandibular ramus and the pterygoid muscles. Its lateral wall is formed by the inner surface of the ramus of the mandible, its medial wall is formed by the medial pterygoid muscle, and its roof is formed by the lateral pterygoid muscle. In frontal section (Fig. 12-2) the pterygomandibular space is triangular, narrowing downward where the medial pterygoid muscle converges with the mandible to which it is attached. The pterygomandibular space communicates posteriorly with the retromandibular space, containing the parotid gland. Lingual and inferior alveolar nerves enter the pterygomandibular space from the roof of the infratemporal fossa (see Fig. 9-10).

Anteriorly the pterygomandibular space is accessible between the deep tendon of the temporal muscle, where it is attached to the temporal crest of the mandibular ramus, and the anterior border of the medial pterygoid muscle (Figs. 12-3 and 12-5). The entrance into the pterygomandibular space is separated from the oral cavity by the thin plate of the buccinator muscle and the oral mucosa of the most posterior part of the cheek. Anteriorly, at its narrow inferior corner, the pterygomandibular space communicates with the niche containing the submandibular gland. This passageway is used by the lingual nerve to enter the submandibular region, through which it curves forward to cross above the mylohyoid muscle and proceed on to the floor of the oral cavity (Figs. 12-2 and 12-5).

The pterygomandibular space is filled with loose connective tissue, which contains a variable amount of fat. The contents of the space are the lingual nerve in front and the inferior alveolar nerve behind. Posterior and lateral to the alveolar nerve are found the inferior alveolar artery and veins, which converge with the nerve toward the mandibular foramen.

The inferior alveolar nerve passes through the pterygomandibular space obliquely from above and medially downward and laterally. It separates from the lingual nerve a few millimeters below the foramen ovale and is here situated on the medial side of the lateral pterygoid muscle. Farther downward it crosses the posterosuperior border of the medial pterygoid muscle and enters the pterygomandibular space through the narrow cleft between the two pterygoid muscles. Only a short distance in front of the inferior alveolar nerve lies the lingual nerve. The latter receives the chorda tympani just where it enters the pterygomandibular space. Where the alveolar nerve reaches the pterygomandibular space, it is separated from the mandible by the lateral pterygoid muscle and then below this muscle it converges with the mandibular ramus, which it reaches at the mandibular foramen (Fig. 12-1).

Since the inner surface of the mandibular ramus must be used as a landmark for the injection to the inferior alveolar nerve, it becomes clear that this injection has to be done as close to the mandibular foramen as possible. The higher up the bone one injects, the farther away the injected fluid will be from the alveolar nerve. Since the mandibular foramen is situated in the posterior extension of the occlusal plane of the

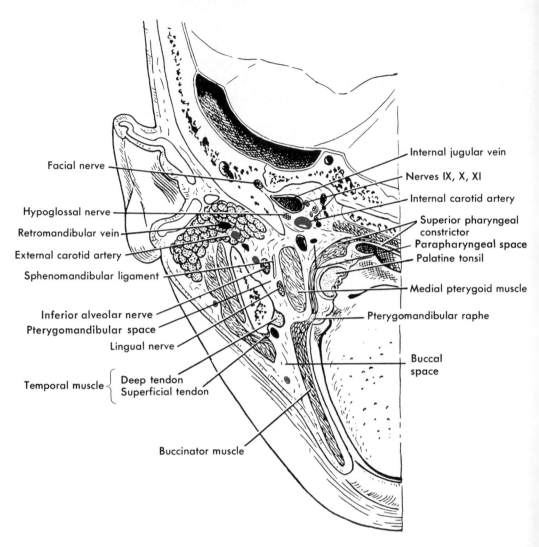

Fig. 12-3. Oblique section through head that had been fixed with the mouth wide open. Plane of section is plane of mandibular injection. (Modified and redrawn from Sicher: Leitungsanästhesie.)

lower molars, the injection should be made not more than 3 to 4 mm. above this plane. If molars are absent, the plane of the foramen can be found by bisecting the posterior border of the ramus and placing an imaginary line through this point and parallel to the lower border of the mandible or by locating the level of the narrowest part of the mandibular ramus.

A shallow groove extends from the mandibular foramen upward and backward to the neck of the mandible, the groove of the mandibular neck (see Fig. 2-41). Formerly this groove was called the groove of the mandibular nerve because the inferior alveolar nerve (mandibular nerve) was believed to lie in this depression of the bone. However, the alveolar nerve has no relation to the inner surface of the mandibular

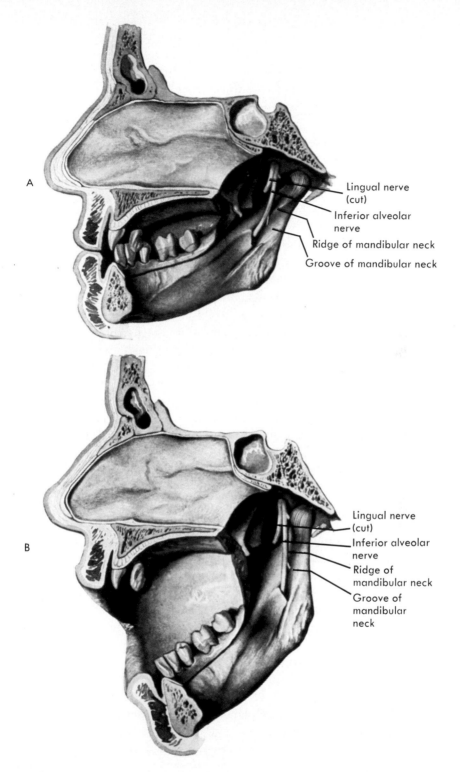

Lingual nerve
(cut)

Inferior alveolar
nerve

Ridge of mandibular neck

Groove of mandibular neck

Lingual nerve
(cut)

Inferior alveolar
nerve

Ridge of
mandibular neck

Groove of
mandibular
neck

Fig. 12-4. A, Relation of relaxed inferior alveolar nerve to ridge and groove of mandibular neck, mouth closed. **B,** Relation of stretched inferior alveolar nerve to ridge and groove of mandibular neck, mouth wide open. (Sicher: Leitungsanästhesie.)

ramus above the mandibular foramen. Traced back from this point, the inferior alveolar nerve can be followed upward and inward to the foramen ovale when the plane of the ramus is vertical. In addition, the groove of the mandibular neck runs from the mandibular foramen upward and backward (Fig. 12-4, A), so that this groove and the alveolar nerve diverge in two dimensions of space.

The suggestion to use the groove of the mandibular neck as a landmark for the anesthesia of the lower alveolar nerve was originally made because of the supposedly close relation of the nerve to the inner surface of the mandibular ramus. Despite the fallacy of this reasoning, the injection into this sulcus is entirely justified. This paradoxical statement can be made because of the peculiar and radical change in the relation between the alveolar nerve and the groove of the mandibular neck that occurs during the movements of the lower jaw (Fig. 12-4). As long as the mouth is closed, there is a double divergence between groove and nerve. If the mouth is opened as wide as possible, the mandibular head glides from its position in the articular fossa forward and downward to the height of the articular eminence and often even somewhat farther forward. At the same time the mandible rotates around a horizontal transverse axis, which, passing through the condyles, moves forward and downward with the condyles. During the opening movement the mandibular foramen, the point of entrance of the inferior alveolar nerve into the mandibular canal, drops a few millimeters without deviating anteriorly or posteriorly. This behavior of the mandibular foramen can also be expressed by stating that the entrance of the nerve and blood vessels into the bone is at the point of least relative movement.

The inferior alveolar nerve thus does not alter its course during the opening movement of the jaw and is only straightened. The flat S-shaped curve described by the nerve in the rest, or occlusal, position of the mandible (Fig. 12-1) provides the necessary slack for the straightening of the nerve at the end of the opening movement. While the nerve remains in its position, the groove of the mandibular neck changes from the oblique course upward and backward, which it had assumed in occlusal position of the mandible, into an almost vertical position at the end of the opening movement (Fig. 12-4, B). At this moment the inferior alveolar nerve and the groove of the mandibular neck are almost in the same frontal plane, although the nerve never comes to lie in the groove. The nerve always runs from the mandibular foramen upward and inward, away from the inner surface of the mandibular ramus.

The target site for depositing the anesthetic is, therefore, the lowest part of the groove of the mandibular neck, just above the entrance of the nerve into the mandibular foramen. The nerve is still accessible here, the nerve-bone relations are closest here, and bony landmarks are palpable. Thus two important rules for block anesthesia of the inferior alveolar nerve emerge from these anatomic relations. First, the injection must be done with the patient's mouth open to the maximum; second, the injection must be made into the lowest part of the groove of the mandibular neck. It is obvious that the higher the anesthetic is deposited, the farther away it will be from the nerve.

To locate the target site, the index finger is laid on the occlusal plane of the lower molars. The finger is pressed straight back for its tip to palpate the concavity of the anterior border of the ramus. Medial to the concavity, the palpating finger can locate the inner bulge of the deep tendon of the temporal muscle (see Figs. 3-6 and 12-3). The needle is laid along the midline of the finger parallel to, and thus slightly above, the occlusal plane.

Entrance into the pterygomandibular space is between the anterior border of the medial pterygoid muscle and the deep tendon of the temporal muscle (Figs. 12-3 and 12-5). The deep tendon attached to the temporal crest of the mandible juts considerably medially and thus narrows the entrance to the space. It is inadvisable to try to contact bone with the needle in front of the tendon. If this is done, the syringe must be swung around to skirt the bony crest to reach the groove of the neck behind. It is obvious that fracture of the needle, stuck in this tough tendon, is a serious hazard.

To reach bone behind the crest by the most direct route, the injection site is approached from the opposite side of the mouth; the syringe is positioned in as nearly a transverse plane as the cheek of the opposite side will permit. The puncture site between the temporal tendon and the medial pterygoid passes through the posterior portion of the buccinator muscle until the needle touches bone behind the temporal tendon. The needle can then be rotated toward the injected side through loose, fatty connective tissue and directed posteriorly. The needle slides along the smooth surface of bone between the temporal crest and the crest of the mandibular neck. Its passage over the crest of the neck into the groove behind is clearly felt, and the needle acts as a direct extension of a palpating finger.

In inserting the needle into the pterygomandibular space, one should avoid an injury to the medial pterygoid muscle. The pterygomandibular fold (see Fig. 5-5) may serve as a landmark for the anterior border of this muscle. This fold arises from the pterygoid hamulus, medial and posterior to the posterior end of the upper alveolar process, and extends downward and outward to end behind the lower last molar. The fold is elevated by the pterygomandibular raphe, which gives rise to fibers of the buccinator muscle anteriorly and fibers of the superior constrictor of the pharynx posteriorly. The tendinous band is stretched while the mouth is opened, and thus the fold of the mucous membrane becomes clearly visible. If the needle pierces the mucous membrane lateral to the pterygomandibular fold, an injury to the medial pterygoid muscle can be avoided easily.

It is interesting to note that the injected fluid does not, as is commonly believed, spread concentrically in the loose connective tissue but, according to Max Sadove, has a tendency to spread upward, as seen in radiographs after injection of a radiopaque substance. This peculiar spread is, in all probability, caused by the guiding influence of the sphenomandibular ligament, lateral to which the fluid is deposited.

From the foregoing description it is clear that a secure intraoral technique for anesthesia of the inferior alveolar nerve is impossible if the patient cannot freely open the mouth. In such cases an extraoral approach is indicated. Two ways of getting close to the alveolar nerve are feasible, one from the lower border of the mandible along its inner surface to the mandibular foramen, the other through the mandibular notch into the pterygomandibular space.

For the first method the following landmarks can be used. The mandibular foramen is situated halfway between the anterior and posterior borders of the mandibular ramus. It is found in a plane that is laid parallel to the lower border of the mandible through the midpoint of the posterior border of the ramus.

The needle is inserted in front of the geometric mandibular angle (that is, the intersection of the extended posterior and inferior borders) at a distance corresponding to half of the width of the ramus (Fig. 12-6). The needle should reach the bone just above the lower border. From here the needle travels along the bone, always in contact with the bone, upward and backward parallel to the posterior border of the ramus until its point is 3 to 4 mm. above the plane of the midpoint of the posterior

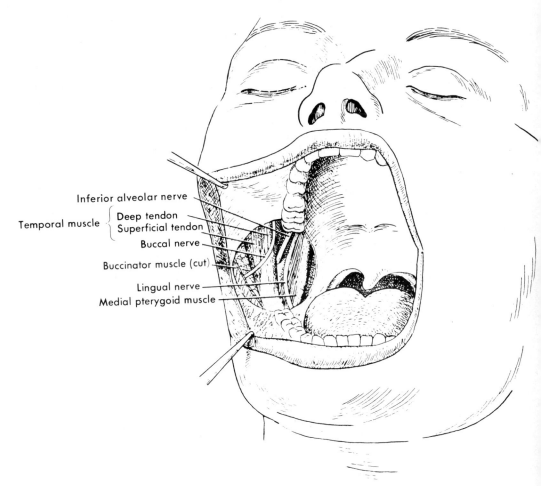

Inferior alveolar nerve

Temporal muscle { Deep tendon
Superficial tendon

Buccal nerve

Buccinator muscle (cut)

Lingual nerve
Medial pterygoid muscle

Fig. 12-5. Pterygomandibular space dissected from oral cavity.

border. The point of the needle is then just lateral to the inferior alveolar nerve above its entrance into the mandibular foramen. The fluid is injected into the loose connective tissue of the pterygomandibular space. The needle enters this space by passing through the most posterior part of the submandibular niche in front of the attachment of the medial pterygoid muscle. Anterosuperior fibers of this muscle may be perforated by the needle not far below the level of the mandibular foramen.

The approach to the inferior alveolar nerve through the mandibular notch is less reliable, and therefore the injection of a larger quantity of anesthetic fluid is necessary. If one tries to inject the anesthetic solution as close to the nerve as possible, it should be remembered that at the level of the lowest point of the mandibular notch the alveolar nerve is at a considerable distance from the medial surface of the ramus, which it approaches in a lateral and inferior course (Fig. 12-2). It is therefore advisable to direct the needle slightly downward while it passes over the bony edge of the mandibular notch. The needle should be inserted through the skin just below the zygomatic arch. Passing through the skin and masseter muscle, the needle may pierce the posterior fibers of the temporal muscle or may enter the pterygomandibular space behind this muscle. Traveling downward and inward, the needle should not be inserted deeper than about 8 to 12 mm. beyond the plane of the coronoid process. The fluid will then infiltrate the connective tissue of the pterygomandibular space and thus reach the nerve, provided that 4 to 6 ml. are injected.

Assuming that by using one of the described methods the inferior alveolar nerve

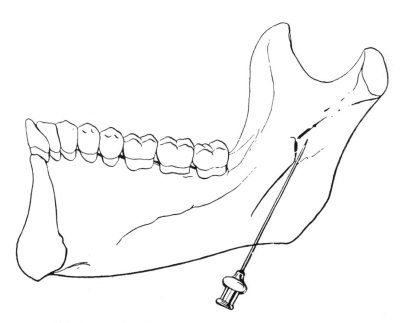

Fig. 12-6. Position of needle in percutaneous injection to inferior alveolar nerve. (Sicher: Leitungsanästhesie.)

has been blocked, the anesthetic zone comprises the teeth of half of the mandible, the buccal gingiva in the posterior and anterior regions of the mandible, separated by the area supplied by the buccal nerve, the skin and mucous membrane of the lower lip, and the skin of the chin. However, the anesthesia in the region close to the midline is often not complete. The cause for this incomplete anesthesia is generally believed to be a crossing of nerves over the midline, so that the first incisor or the area of both incisors receives fibers from the right and left inferior alveolar nerves. This behavior of the nerves has not been proved and is somewhat improbable, since the two mandibular halves are separated by the symphyseal cartilage until the end of the first year of life. Nerves are not known to cross a median cartilage.

A second explanation of the near median defect of a mandibular block anesthesia postulates the participation of a branch of the transversus (cutaneous) colli nerve of the cervical plexus in supplying sensory fibers to the mandibular incisor region. This legendary branch is supposed to enter the mandible on its inner surface close to the lower border in the premolar area. Careful investigations have shown that such a branch of the cervical nerves does not exist, as could have been expected from developmental facts. However, an injection to the area of the entrance of this imaginary nerve into the bone is sometimes helpful. The additional injection is, in fact, an injection to the anterior branch of the mylohyoid nerve, situated between the lower border of the mandible and the mylohyoid muscle. The mylohyoid nerve is known regularly to contain sensory fibers to the chin and, in one out of ten of the examined cadavers, it sends a branch into the mandible. It enters the bone in the mental region not far from the midline and just above the lower border of the mandible.

To assume that dental fibers may occasionally travel in the mylohyoid branch of the inferior alveolar nerve is in full accord with known facts of the anatomy and of the variations of peripheral nerves. In individuals in whom the mylohyoid nerve separates from the inferior alveolar nerve at some distance above the mandibular foramen, the anesthetic fluid, injected between the alveolar nerve and bone, may not reach the mylohyoid nerve, which, at this point, is situated posteromedial to the alveolar nerve. If the mylohyoid nerve contains dental fibers, they can then be reached just before they enter the mandible.

In some rare cases an otherwise successful mandibular block anesthesia will leave the third molar sensitive. The reason for this anomalous behavior is a variation in the branching of the inferior alveolar nerve. The branch to the third molar, the posterior dental branch, is normally given off shortly after the alveolar nerve has entered the mandibular canal. Sometimes, however, the posterior dental branch arises from the anterior surface of the alveolar nerve above the mandibular foramen and, descending anteriorly, enters a small foramen in front of and above the mandibular foramen. This abnormal branch in front of the main nerve may escape the influence of an anesthetic, since the fluid is injected lateral to and slightly behind the alveolar nerve. An injection of a few drops of anesthetic fluid just in front of the typical site of injection will block an abnormal posterior dental branch.

A typical, although not too frequent, accident during mandibular block is a temporary paralysis of the facial nerve or of one of its two main branches. The motor paralysis is caused by a direct influence of the injected "anesthetic"* on the facial nerve. The explanation of this accident is based on the fact that almost invariably in such cases the sensory auriculotemporal nerve is also blocked. This nerve crosses the posterior border of the mandible at the level of its neck and supplies part of the outer ear and the skin of the temporal region and posterior part of the cheek. The involvement of the auriculotemporal nerve indicates that the injection was made too high above the mandibular foramen. If this is done, the needle is automatically guided toward the posterior border of the mandibular neck because of the obliquity of the ridge and the groove of the mandibular neck, which reach the posterior border close to the mandibular neck. The facial nerve crosses almost at the same level from the retromandibular fossa into the face. In the majority of persons the facial nerve is here embedded in the substance of the parotid gland and is protected from being reached by an injected fluid, placed close to the posterior border of the mandible. However, in some persons the parotid gland fails to envelop the facial nerve or one of its two main branches in the retromandibular fossa. Then the nerve or its superior or inferior branch may be infiltrated if a mandibular injection is placed too high and too close to the posterior border of the ramus. The ensuing paralysis is temporary and disappears with the absorption of the injected fluid.

A more frequent complication of the mandibular block is the accidental intravenous injection of all or a part of the anesthetic drug. It is surprising how often the needle is found to have entered a vein. The fact can easily be ascertained by routinely aspirating before the syringe is emptied, to check whether blood will enter the syringe. The frequency of positive tests and the obvious danger of intravenous injection make it imperative that only a syringe which permits aspiration be used. The reason for the high percentage of venous injuries seems to be the course of the inferior alveolar artery and veins. The course of these vessels and their relation to the alveolar nerve and mandible do not depend on the position of the maxillary artery and veins in the region of the mandibular neck; the alveolar vessels are, in all individuals, much closer to the bone than to the inferior alveolar nerve. If the maxillary artery lies superficially on the lateral surface of the lateral pterygoid muscle, the inferior alveolar artery arises directly from the maxillary artery and runs downward to the mandibular foramen between the nerve and bone. If the maxillary artery follows a deep course on the medial surface of the lateral pterygoid muscle, the alveolar artery arises in a common trunk with the posterior deep temporal artery, which swings around the lower border of the lateral pterygoid muscle to its lateral surface. The inferior alveolar artery and veins, therefore, are always closely related to the bone, and thus one of the veins is frequently punctured.

---

*The term "anesthetic" drug is misleading in many ways. The term "nerve-blocking" drug seems to be more adequate.

Topography of the mental nerve

In some instances anesthesia of the anterior region of the mandible, involving the area from the left to the right premolars, is desirable. If a bilateral mandibular block is not indicated, for instance, after extensive injuries to the cheeks and the ascending ramus, an approach to the anterior branches of the alveolar nerve through the mental foramen is helpful. This foramen is situated in a vertical plane between the two premolars or distal to this plane below the second premolar. The mental foramen lies midway between the free alveolar border and the lower border of the mandible, or closer to the latter. If teeth are missing, the location of the foramen sometimes is possible by careful palpation. After loss of premolars and the disappearance of the alveolar process, the opening of the foramen usually can be felt by the finger.

The mental foramen is the opening of a short canal, the mental canal, which is a branch of the mandibular canal. The mental canal is directed outward, backward, and upward toward the surface of the mandible. The mandibular canal itself continues toward the midline as a narrow canal containing the anterior dental branch, or incisive nerve.

The premolar, canine, and incisor areas of the mandible can be fully anesthetized only if the anesthetic solution is injected into the mental canal. The needle has to be placed into the direction of the axis of the canal. Entering the foramen, the needle and syringe must point inward, downward, and forward (Fig. 12-7). This position can be achieved easily if the jaws are closed and the lips and cheek are fully relaxed so that they can be readily retracted. As in other regions, the first attempt to enter a small foramen is often not successful. If the needle has reached the bone close to the foramen, a careful and systematic palpation of the bony surface with the needle will soon locate the opening. Injecting while the needle is slowly inserted into the mental

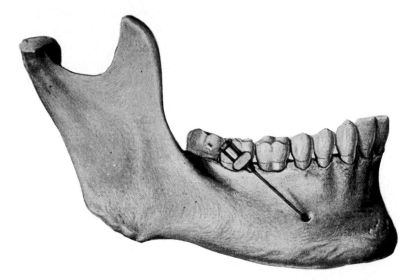

Fig. 12-7. Position of needle in injection into mental canal. (Sicher: Leitungsanästhesie.)

canal does not only render the injection almost painless, but also prevents injury to the nerve and blood vessels, which are pushed aside by the injected fluid. The injection has to be made as slowly as possible and under the least possible pressure. Only a few drops of the solution should be injected.

Topography of the lingual nerve

Branches of the lingual nerve supply the lingual gingiva and the adjacent mucosa of the lower jaw. Anesthesia of the lingual nerve is necessary for any operation on the lower jaw that is not restricted to the teeth themselves. It can easily be reached in the pterygomandibular space, which it enters in front of the inferior alveolar nerve. The two nerves, at first closely related, diverge as they descend. The lingual nerve deviates anteriorly to lie between the medial pterygoid muscle and mandibular ramus a short distance behind the temporal crest and attached deep temporal tendon (Figs. 12-3 and 12-5). In the intraoral approach to the inferior alveolar nerve the needle, reaching the bone just behind the deep temporal tendon and temporal crest, passes between the bone and the lingual nerve while it slides toward the groove of the mandibular neck. Injection of 0.25 ml. of the anesthetic solution just posterior to the point where the needle touches the bone suffices to anesthetize the lingual nerve.

Turning anteriorly toward the floor of the mouth, the lingual nerve becomes superficially located. It can often be seen on oral examination through the translucent mucous membrane in the sublingual sulcus, close to the alveolus of the last molar. Here it can be pressed against the bone with the finger. Although this point seems to be especially well suited for isolated anesthesia of the lingual nerve, care must be exercised in this area. A submucous injection at this site is in danger of introducing an infection directly into the submandibular space. The posterior border of the mylohyoid muscle, which forms the floor of the mouth, attaches to the end of the mylohyoid ridge at this point. Fluid forced behind this border passes into the fascial spaces of the neck; limited injection anterior to this border tends to be confined to the oral floor (see section on interfascial spaces of the neck, Chapter 14).

Topography of the buccal nerve

In the majority of persons a small area of the buccal gingiva and mucosa of the lower jaw is supplied by the buccal nerve. As a rule this area extends along the second premolar and first molar; however, it varies greatly. It may be reduced in size and may even be missing, or it may be larger and may, in extreme cases, extend from the canine to the third molar.

In most instances anesthesia of the buccal nerve fibers can be achieved by local infiltration of the buccal mucosa near the fornix of the vestibule. There are, however, cases in which an infection in this area precludes a local injection and the trunk of the buccal nerve has to be blocked.

The buccal nerve passes through the infratemporal fossa in a downward and forward direction. After crossing the deep surface of the temporal muscle (Fig. 12-5), the nerve is situated between the most anterior part of the masseter muscle and the posterior part of the buccinator muscle. Turning more sharply forward, the buccal nerve divides into several branches on the outer surface of the buccinator muscle. The single branches perforate the muscle to end in the mucous membrane of the cheek and in the described area of the mandibular gingiva (see Figs. 9-8 to 9-10).

The anterior border of the mandibular ramus is crossed by the buccal nerve at, or slightly below, the level of the occlusal plane. If the mouth is wide open, this plane corresponds to the occlusal surface of the upper molars. The nerve crosses the upper part of the retromolar fossa, and it is at this point that it can be reached for a block anesthesia. The anterior border of the ramus and the temporal crest with the tendons of the temporal muscle attached to these two bony ridges can easily be palpated, and the needle is then inserted between the ridges at the level of the upper occlusal plane. If the needle has entered tendinous tissue, it can be diagnosed by the greater pressure necessary to empty the syringe. The needle should then be retracted just enough so that the injection does not encounter tissue resistance. Since the exact depth of the buccal nerve cannot be ascertained, it is advisable to infiltrate a thicker layer of tissues by continuing to inject slowly while the needle is withdrawn. In reaching the buccal nerve the needle perforates the mucous membrane, the submucosa, and the thin plate of the buccinator muscle.

It should be recognized that the plane of injection to the buccal nerve, suggested here, is some distance above the plane for the mandibular block anesthesia. This is why it is inadvisable to try a simultaneous block of the inferior alveolar, lingual, and buccal nerves.

Topography of the maxillary nerve

For major operations in the upper jaw, the blocking of the entire maxillary nerve (second division of the trigeminal nerve) is desirable. Since this nerve splits into its branches in the upper part of the pterygopalatine fossa, the injection has to be made into this deeply situated space of the skull.

The pterygopalatine fossa is accessible by two routes: from the cheek through the pterygomaxillary fissure and from the oral cavity through the greater palatine canal. The extraoral approach seems to be safer and easier.

The buccal approach (Fig. 12-8) begins below the zygomatic arch and in front of the coronoid process and leads along the posterior surface of the maxilla through the pterygomaxillary fissure into the pterygopalatine fossa. The point at which the needle should be inserted is easily determined. The angle between the ascending frontal and the horizontal temporal processes of the zygomatic bone is readily felt at the anterior end of the superior border of the zygomatic arch. If a vertical line is dropped from this angle, the point of intersection of this line with the lower border of the zygomatic arch is the point of puncture. The needle is placed into a horizontal and frontal plane. The needle perforates the skin, the superficial fascia, the deep (or parotideomasseteric) fascia, and the masseter muscle, and will in most cases pass in front of the temporal muscle through the zygomaticotemporal, or retrozygomatic, extension of the buccal fat pad.

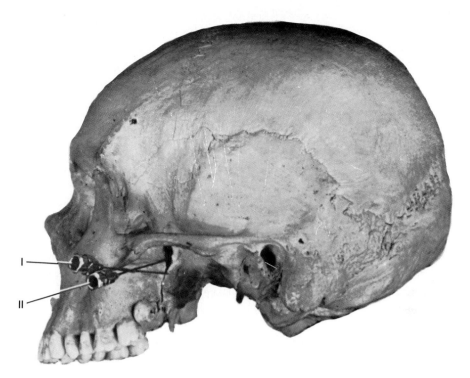

Fig. 12-8. The positions of needle in injection to maxillary nerve of trigeminal nerve in pterygopalatine fossa.

At a variable depth, depending on the degree of convexity of the maxillary tuberosity, the needle will touch the posterior surface of the maxilla. Along this surface the needle is introduced deeper until it meets with full bony resistance. The needle is now in contact with the outer plate of the pterygoid process close to its junction with the palatine and maxillary bones. If the needle is somewhat retracted and then again introduced in a slightly ascending direction, the needle passes through the pterygomaxillary fissure into the lower part of the pterygopalatine fossa. If, during the second introduction, the needle still meets the resistance of the pterygoid plate, this procedure must be repeated, and the angle must be increased.

The advisability of first contacting the pterygoid process below the entrance into the pterygopalatine fossa is twofold. The depth of the entrance, that is, its distance from the skin, can thus be measured, and by adding 2 to 3 mm. to this distance the maximum depth to which the needle can be introduced without danger is determined. The possibility of passing through the pterygopalatine fossa and the sphenopalatine foramen into the nasal cavity is thus avoided. This danger is decreased still more by the second advantage of the suggested method; the lower part of the fossa is entered and the needle is directed against the palatine bone, the medial wall of the pterygopalatine fossa, below the level of the sphenopalatine foramen, thus preventing too deep a penetration.

By placing the needle at a relatively low level it is also possible to avoid an injury to the maxillary artery, which enters the pterygopalatine fossa through the upper part of the pterygomaxillary fissure just below the point where the infraorbital nerve emerges from the fossa to reach the inferior orbital fissure.

It has been shown that an injection of 3 to 4 ml. of anesthetic solution into the inferior part of the pterygopalatine fossa suffices to anesthetize the entire ramification of the maxillary nerve, the second trigeminal division.

While the needle passes along the posterior surface of the maxilla into the pterygopalatine fossa, smaller arteries may be injured. The arteries that may be encountered are the posterior superior alveolar artery at the maxilla and the descending palatine artery in the pterygopalatine fossa. Since the injection to the maxillary nerve is reserved for major surgery, the risk of injuring one of these smaller arteries should not be a contraindication.

The intraoral route into the pterygopalatine fossa uses the greater palatine canal, which, starting at the lower end of the pterygopalatine fossa, runs downward and slightly inward and opens at the major palatine foramen. It contains, embedded in fatty tissue, the palatine nerves and the descending palatine vessels. The topography of the palatine foramen through which the canal may be entered was discussed previously. It is the exception rather than the rule that the needle reaches the foramen at the first attempt. If the needle comes into contact with the bone close to the foramen, careful and systematic palpation with the needle will soon locate the opening. The thin needle has to enter the canal in a posterior and slightly lateral direction. If some fluid is injected while the needle is pushed deeper into the canal, an injury to the contained structures can be minimized but never entirely excluded.

The needle should not pass too far into the pterygopalatine fossa and should not reach its upper part, which contains the terminal ramification of the maxillary artery. A maximum depth for the introduction of the needle can be established by measuring the height of the maxillary body between the inferior border of the orbit and the free alveolar border in the canine or premolar area. The needle should not pass above the horizontal plane of the alveolar border in the molar region for more than this distance. If the needle is introduced farther, it not only can come into conflict with the maxillary artery, but it also may enter the orbit through the most medial part of the inferior orbital fissure and even reach the optic nerve. Temporary blindness would be the mildest consequence of this incident.

Topography of the mandibular nerve

The mandibular nerve, the third trigeminal division, emerging through the foramen ovale, splits into its many branches immediately below the base of the skull. If an injection is planned to anesthetize the entire third division, the nerve must be approached at the cranial base. The landmark for this operation is the root of the pterygoid process. The foramen ovale is situated immediately behind the posterior end of the root of the lateral pterygoid plate. The long axis of the foramen extends from this point backward and outward so that the center of the foramen is closer to the cheek than is its anterior border. In other words, the center of the foramen ovale is just lateral to the plane of the lateral surface of the pterygoid process.

The relations of the nerve below the foramen ovale are of great importance. Lateral to the nerve is the upper head of the lateral pterygoid muscle, which arises from the infratemporal surface of the greater sphenoid wing. The muscle must be perforated in the lateral approach to the third trigeminal division. Medial to the nerve runs the auditory tube. Relations between the nerve and tube are close, the nerve almost touching the anterolateral, membranous wall of the tube. In front of the nerve is the pterygoid process; behind it is the middle meningeal artery ascending to the spinous foramen.

The maxillary artery and the rich venous plexus surrounding the artery and its branches lie some distance from the cranial base, either on the inner or on the outer surface of the lateral pterygoid muscle.

A variation of the skeleton is the occurrence of a temporobuccal foramen (see Fig. 2-14). It develops by ossification of a ligament that bridges a shallow sulcus lateral and

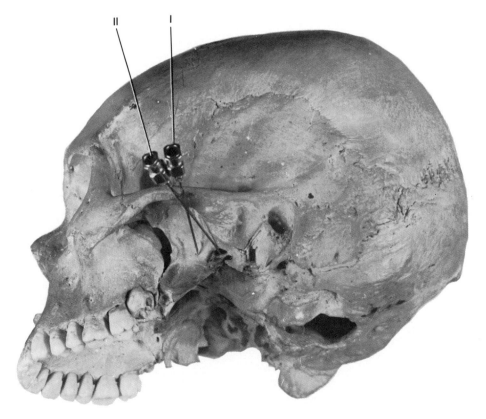

Fig. 12-9. The two positions of needle in injection to mandibular nerve of trigeminal nerve at foramen ovale.

anterior to the foramen ovale. In the sulcus, and held in place by the ligament, lies the common trunk for the buccal and anterior deep temporal nerves, sometimes called the anterior ramus of the mandibular nerve. If the ligament ossifies, it gives rise to a variably thick bony bridge that can block a lateral approach to the foramen ovale and thus to the third division of the trigeminal nerve (see Fig. 2-14).

The injection to the foramen ovale (Fig. 12-9) starts below the zygomatic arch in front of the articular tubercle. The lower border of the zygomatic arch is smooth and concave anterior to the articular tubercle, and this concavity is easily located if one follows the zygomatic arch posteriorly. It contrasts sharply with the rough and convex anterior part of the lower zygomatic margin. The movements of the mandibular condyle can also be used to fix the point of insertion for the needle. If the mouth is opened wide, this point can be found in front of the most forward position of the condyle.

After passing through the skin and subcutaneous tissue, the needle penetrates the masseter muscle and the posterior fibers of the temporal muscle and then enters the infratemporal fossa through the notch between the condylar and coronoid processes of the mandible. The needle is directed slightly upward but is kept in a frontal plane. If this is done, the needle will come in contact with bone at the horizontal roof of the infratemporal fossa, the posterolateral part of which is formed by the temporal bone; the greater wing of the sphenoid bone forms the larger anteromedial part of this surface. If the needle is introduced too steeply, it may reach the lowest part of the temporal fossa and is then stopped from further progress medially. In such a case the direction of the needle has to be gradually changed to a more horizontal position until it can pass medially below the infratemporal crest.

In gliding medially along the infratemporal plane, the needle should be kept in contact with the bone not only to control the position of the needle, but also to avoid injuries to blood vessels. The needle finally will come into contact with the outer surface of the pterygoid process at its root immediately below the cranial base. Feeling with the needle posteriorly along this bony surface, one can easily determine the moment when contact with the bone is lost, in other words, when the posterior border of the pterygoid process has been reached. At this moment the point of the needle is already at the foramen ovale and in contact with the mandibular nerve. It is most important not to let the needle penetrate deeper medially than 2 to 3 mm. beyond the plane of the pterygoid process. Otherwise the needle may perforate the thin membranous wall of the auditory tube and enter its lumen. This accident not only jeopardizes the success of the injection, but also is dangerous because the needle may become infected in the tube and may inoculate bacteria into the deep tissues while it is being retracted.

CHAPTER 13

Arterial hemorrhages and ligation of arteries

Severe arterial hemorrhages during major operations can often be prevented by a preparatory ligation of the respective artery. The numerous and wide anastomoses of all facial arteries with one another and with the contralateral arteries often make bilateral ligations necessary. Hemorrhages do sometimes occur during the lancing of abscesses if not enough consideration is given to the topographic relation of the incision to neighboring blood vessels. Accidents, too, during routine operations on the teeth or injuries sustained by external force may make the ligation of an artery necessary. Therefore one has to consider, first, the areas in which an accidental severing of an artery is possible and the means to avoid such an occurrence, and, second, the anatomic basis for ligating the afferent arteries of the facial region.

ARTERIES ENDANGERED DURING MINOR SURGICAL PROCEDURES OR DURING DENTAL TREATMENT

Three arteries are endangered during minor surgical procedures or in accidents occurring during treatment: the anterior palatine artery, the sublingual artery, and the facial artery.

Anterior palatine artery. The anterior palatine artery enters the oral cavity through the major palatine foramen (Fig. 13-1), which is situated lingual to the last molar of the upper jaw and at the border between the inner plate of the alveolar process and the roof of the oral cavity. Running forward, the artery sends its branches medially and laterally. The incision of a palatine abscess, arising, for instance, from the lingual root of the first molar, must never be made in a transverse direction but in an anteroposterior line. The incision should also be made as near to the free margin of the gingiva as possible without missing the abscess. Furthermore, the edge of the knife should be directed outward and upward and not straight upward. If these rules are kept in mind, an accidental injury to the anterior palatine artery will be avoided. If the artery is cut, it is almost impossible to stop the hemorrhage by local clamping of the artery or by tamponade, and sometimes recourse has to be taken to ligation of the external carotid artery.

Sublingual artery. Injury to the sublingual artery has been observed when sharp instruments or rotating disks slip off a lower tooth and injure the floor of the mouth. If

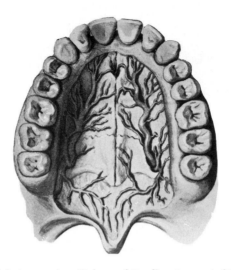

Fig. 13-1. Palatine arteries. (Sicher and Tandler: Anatomie für Zahnärzte.)

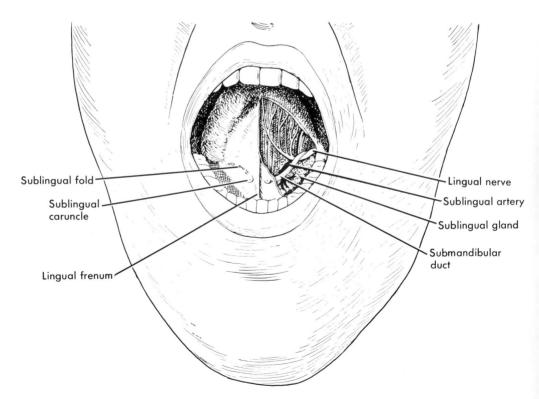

Sublingual fold

Sublingual caruncle

Lingual frenum

Lingual nerve

Sublingual artery

Sublingual gland

Submandibular duct

Fig. 13-2. Sublingual region. (Modified and redrawn from Sicher and Tandler: Anatomie für Zahnärzte.)

this injury is in the region of the premolars or the first molar, the sublingual artery may be severed where it is of considerable volume. The hemorrhage from this artery may then be a serious incident. Local clamping of the artery can be attempted, although it is rather difficult. If attempts to stop the bleeding at the place of injury fail, the lingual artery must be ligated. Mention must be made, however, of a variation in the blood supply of the sublingual region because this variation may frustrate an attempt to stop bleeding of the sublingual region by ligating the lingual artery. The sublingual artery is sometimes a small and insignificant branch of the lingual artery and may even be missing altogether. It is then replaced by branches of the submental artery, a branch of the facial artery.

The topographic relations of the sublingual regions (Figs. 7-5, 13-2, and 13-3) explain the difficulty in isolating the sublingual artery after an injury in this region. The sublingual region, or sublingual groove, extends as a horseshoe-shaped area under the lateral edges and below the tip of the tongue (see Fig. 5-6). The thin mucous membrane covering the sublingual sulcus is elevated in the anterior part of the groove by the underlying sublingual gland to an irregularly granulated fold, the sublingual (salivary) fold. Along the crest of this fold open the minor sublingual ducts. At the anteromedial end of the salivary or sublingual fold and close to the lingual frenulum the sublingual caruncula, or sublingual papilla, marks the common opening for the submandibular and major sublingual ducts.

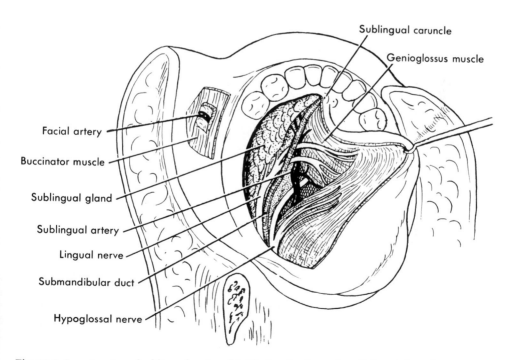

Fig. 13-3. Superior view of sublingual region. (Modified and redrawn from Sicher and Tandler: Anatomie für Zahnärzte.)

The sublingual groove extends into the depth between the mylohyoid muscle laterally and the muscles of the tongue and the geniohyoid muscle medially. In transverse section the groove is triangular with an almost vertical inner wall, whereas the outer wall, the mylohyoid muscle, is inclined downward and medially. The groove is filled with loose and fatty connective tissue surrounding the structures that are contained in the sublingual space. These structures are the sublingual gland, the submandibular duct (often accompanied in its posterior part by a flat extension of the submandibular gland itself), the lingual and hypoglossal nerves, and the sublingual artery with the accompanying veins.

The sublingual gland is closely applied to the medial surface of mandible and mylohyoid muscle. The submandibular duct runs along the medial surface of the sublingual gland. If an extension of the submandibular gland is present, it is often in contact with the posterior pole of the sublingual gland. Of the two nerves, the lingual nerve is found closer to the oral mucosa than is the hypoglossal nerve. In the region of the lower last molar the lingual nerve often can be seen through the thin mucous membrane of the sublingual groove. Farther anteriorly the nerve, at first situated lateral to the submandibular duct, crosses the duct on its inferior surface and divides into a number of branches that enter the substance of the tongue (Fig. 13-2). The hypoglossal nerve occupies the most inferior part of the sublingual space.

The sublingual artery (Figs. 5-15, 13-2, and 13-3) is situated medial and slightly inferior to the submandibular duct and lingual nerve and sends its branches to the sublingual gland and the mylohyoid, geniohyoid, and genioglossus muscles. In its course the artery is fairly close to the inner and upper surface of the mylohyoid muscle. On the outer and inferior surface of the mylohyoid muscle runs the submental artery, which arises from the facial artery where the latter passes over the submandibular gland. The submental artery supplies mainly the mylohyoid muscles, the anterior belly of the digastric muscle, and the lymph nodes of the submandibular region. The sublingual and submental arteries, almost parallel in their course, are normally linked by their branches to the mylohyoid muscle. The anastomoses of these muscular branches are the basis for the replacement of one of these arteries by a branch of the other, which perforates the mylohyoid muscle. Thus the submental artery may be replaced by a branch of the sublingual artery, just as the sublingual artery may be replaced by a branch of the submental artery.

Facial artery. Where the facial artery crosses the level of the inferior vestibular fornix in the region of the first mandibular molar (Fig. 13-3), the artery can be severed accidentally during operative procedures on the lower premolars or molars if an instrument enters the cheek in this region. It has been reported that the facial artery was severed during attempts to open a buccal abscess of the first molar. In the formation of a buccal abscess the artery is often dislocated, and instead of running an almost vertical course it circles the abscess on its inferior and lateral surfaces. Deep incisions in such a case may endanger the facial artery. If the change in relation of the artery to the vestibule during the development of an abscess is kept in mind, the rule follows that the incision should be made downward and inward instead of straight downward. At any rate the knife should not be allowed to penetrate the lateral or the inferior wall of the abscess.

LIGATION OF ARTERIES
Ligation of the facial artery

The facial artery can be easily exposed at the point where it crosses the lower border of the mandible to pass from the submandibular region into the face. This point is situated anterior to the attachment of the masseter muscle to the mandible (Fig. 13-4). Here, the pulse of the facial artery can be felt, especially if the contracted masseter muscle is used as a landmark. The artery is accompanied by the facial vein, which lies posterior to the artery. The artery and vein are crossed superficially by the marginal mandibular branch of the facial nerve. This rather small nerve runs approximately parallel to the lower border of the mandible, sometimes slightly above this border, sometimes slightly below. The nerve and vessels are covered by the platysma muscle, the subcutaneous tissue, and the skin.

Since the mandibular branch of the facial nerve supplies the muscles of the lower lip, it is necessary to plan the operation in such a way that this nerve is not in danger of being cut. To achieve this end, the incision is made at least ½ inch below the border of the mandible and parallel to it. The skin, platysma muscle, and deep fascia are cut,

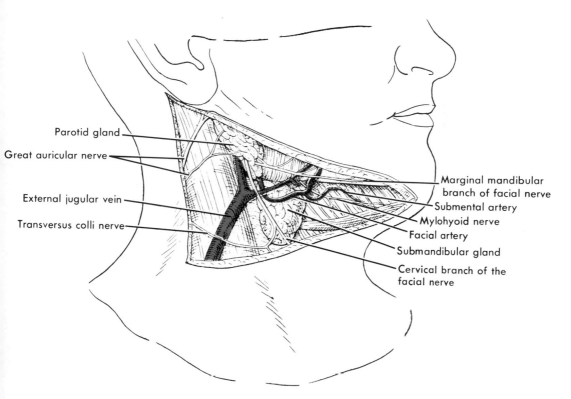

Fig. 13-4. Submandibular triangle, superficial layer.

and then the soft tissues are bluntly retracted upward until the palpating finger can feel the pulse of the facial artery. The artery then can be isolated, tied, and cut.

Ligation of the lingual artery

The exposure of the lingual artery is done in the submandibular (digastric) triangle. This region of the neck is bounded by the lower border of the mandible and the two bellies of the digastric muscle (Figs. 13-4 to 13-6). The posterior corner of this triangle behind the angle of the mandible is in open communication with the retromandibular fossa (see Basic Plan of the Neck, in Chapter 14).

EXPOSURE OF THE LINGUAL ARTERY IN THE SUBMANDIBULAR TRIANGLE

Superficially the submandibular region is covered by the superficial fascia containing the platysma muscle. After removal of these layers, the deep fascia, which extends from the hyoid bone to the lower border of the mandible, is exposed. Farther

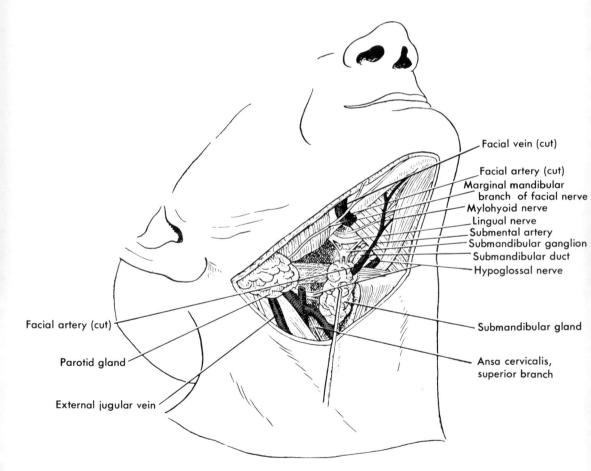

Fig. 13-5. Submandibular triangle, deep layer. (Modified and redrawn from Sicher and Tandler: Anatomie für Zahnärzte.)

posteriorly the deep fascia continues as the outer covering of the cervical lobe of the parotid gland. In the submandibular region the deep fascia is divided into several layers, the most important of which are the layer between the hyoid bone and mandible and a deeper layer that follows the mylohyoid and digastric muscles. The anterior part of the deep layer forms the wall of the submandibular niche; its posterior part takes part in forming the medial wall of the parotid niche. Between the spaces occupied by the submandibular gland and the parotid gland, the deep fascia is attached to the styloid process and its muscles and to the angle of the mandible where it continues into the fascia on the medial surface of the medial pterygoid muscle. The deep part of this fascia is known as the stylomandibular ligament, whereas the superficial part is sometimes referred to as the angular tract of the investing cervical fascia. The angular tract is a reinforcement of the deep fascia and runs from the region of the mandibular angle downward and forward to disappear gradually at the level of the hyoid bone.

The submandibular gland and its capsular space usually reach below the level of the digastric muscle (Fig. 13-4) to the level of the hyoid bone or even farther downward. If the superficial layer of the deep fascia is incised along the lower convex border of the submandibular gland, the gland itself can easily be mobilized by blunt dissection. On its superoposterior pole the gland is fixed by its connection with the facial artery. On its anterior deep pole the gland is fixed by the emerging subman-

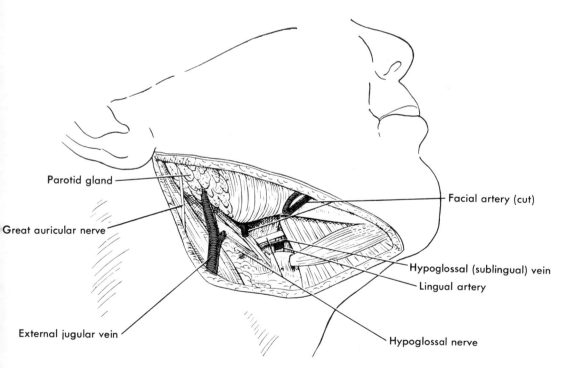

Fig. 13-6. Submandibular triangle after removal of submandibular gland. Lingual artery exposed in a slit of hyoglossus muscle.

dibular duct. The upper pole of the gland finally is connected to the lingual nerve by the afferent and efferent branches of the submandibular ganglion (Fig. 13-5).

The floor of the submandibular triangle is formed by the mylohyoid muscle in front and by the hyoglossus and styloglossus muscles posteriorly. The mylohyoid muscle itself is attached to the inner surface of the mandible; the line of attachment, the mylohyoid line, begins near the lower border of the mandible at the midline and then ascends posteriorly to the socket of the third molar. Thus a wedge-shaped space is formed between the inner surface of the mandible and the outer surface of the mylohyoid muscle; this space is shallow anteriorly and deepens considerably toward the posterior border of the mylohyoid muscle. It is the submandibular, or mylohyoid, niche and is an upward extension of the submandibular triangle on the inner surface of the mandible.

The mylohyoid muscle ends posteriorly with a sharp, well-marked free border (Figs. 13-5 and 13-6), which is directed from above and behind downward and forward. The line of the posterior border connects the region of the third molar socket with the body of the hyoid bone. This border is one of the most important landmarks in the submandibular region. Behind and below the mylohyoid muscle the hyoglossus muscle forms the floor of the submandibular region. It arises from the entire length of the greater horn of the hyoid bone. The fibers of the thin muscle plate run an almost vertical course in contrast to the oblique course of the bundles of the mylohyoid muscle. The two muscles can also readily be distinguished by the fact that the bundles of the mylohyoid muscle are thick and coarse, whereas those of the hyoglossus muscle are thin and fine.

Ascending, the vertical fibers of the hyoglossus muscle meet the horizontal fibers of the styloglossus muscle, with which they interlace. The styloglossus muscle arises from the stylohyoid process, and gradually fans out running downward and forward. Behind and below and slightly deep to the styloglossus muscle the stylopharyngeus muscle can be exposed with the glossopharyngeal nerve at its lower border (see Fig. 6-4).

The anterior end of the posterior belly and the tendon of the digastric muscle cross the hyoglossus muscle superficially and lie close to the hyoid bone. The anterior belly of the digastric muscle covers a large area of the inferior and outer surface of the mylohyoid muscle. The tendon of the digastric muscle is fastened to the hyoid bone by a pulleylike arrangement of the deep fascia. The distance of the tendon to the hyoid bone varies considerably. The posterior belly of the digastric muscle is accompanied by the stylohyoid muscle, which runs along its superior border. Near its attachment to the hyoid bone, the stylohyoid muscle often forms a slit for the passage of the digastric tendon.

Among the structures that form the content of the submandibular triangle, the submandibular gland is the largest. Its upper part, hidden in the mylohyoid niche, is here in close contact with the inner surface of the mandible. Its anterior part lies on the outer surface of the mylohyoid muscle, and the duct and a variable oral extension of the gland are found on the inner surface of the mylohyoid muscle. Thus the posterior part of the mylohyoid muscle is situated between the superficial and deep parts of the gland, or between the gland and its duct. The lower pole of the gland reaches into the upper part of the carotid triangle below the digastric tendon.

The rest of the submandibular triangle is occupied by loose connective tissue, in which the submandibular lymph nodes are embedded. The nodes are in part hidden in the mylohyoid niche on the inner side of the mandible.

The blood vessels of the submandibular region are the facial vein and sometimes the retromandibular vein and their branches, the facial artery and its branches, and, finally, in the deepest layer, the lingual artery. The facial vein reaches the submandibular region by crossing the lower border of the mandible at the anterior attachment of the masseter muscle and behind the facial artery. The vein remains fairly superficial and crosses the posterior part of the submandibular gland. It may unite with the retromandibular vein, which emerges from the lower corner of the parotid gland to form the common facial vein. However, variations of the venous vessels in this region are frequent. Where the anterior facial vein crosses the upper border of the submandibular gland, it receives the submental vein or veins.

Out of the depth, sublingual and lingual veins may communicate with the inferior end of the facial vein, the common facial vein, or the internal jugular vein.

The facial artery enters the submandibular triangle in its posterior part after crossing the posterior belly of the digastric muscle and the stylohyoid muscle on their deep surfaces. The artery is then situated on the outer surface of the hyoglossus muscle. The facial artery now runs upward and slightly forward deep to the posterior pole of the submandibular gland. In close contact with the gland, embedded in a groove of the gland, or sometimes even surrounded by lobules of the gland, the artery, turning laterally, circles the upper and posterior border of the submandibular gland. Finally, in a second turn, the artery swings around the lower border of the mandible into the face. At the height of its first turn the facial artery gives off the ascending palatine artery whose branches supply the soft palate and the palatine tonsil. Where the facial artery is closely applied to the submandibular gland, branches to the gland and the submental artery are given off. The close relation of the facial artery to the submandibular gland makes it understandable that the removal of the gland is hardly possible without ligation of the artery below and above the gland and an excision of the part of the artery between the ligatures. Converging with the submental artery and vein, the mylohyoid nerve crosses the posterior part of the mylohyoid niche. The nerve sends most of its branches to the mylohyoid muscle and the anterior belly of the digastric. The mylohyoid nerve almost always contains sensory fibers that are destined for the skin underneath the chin.

The lingual artery, arising from the external carotid artery below the facial artery or in a common trunk with the facial artery, runs in its first part almost parallel to the facial artery upward and forward. It then assumes a fairly horizontal course above the posterior end of the greater horn of the hyoid bone. At the posterior border of the hyoglossus muscle the artery turns to the deep surface of this muscle and continues forward and then forward and upward, to split into its terminal branches. Under cover of the hyoglossus muscle the artery enters the submandibular region above the digastric tendon.

If the submandibular gland is mobilized as far as possible, and if it is pulled downward and backward, the lingual nerve, connected with the upper pole of the gland (Fig. 13-5), becomes visible. Entering the submandibular triangle through the slit between the lower end of the medial pterygoid muscle and the mandible, the lingual nerve describes a sharp curve, first descending anteriorly, and then turning forward and slightly upward. Approaching the gland, the lingual nerve sends branches to the submandibular ganglion, which in turn sends some branches to the submandibular gland, whereas others return to the anterior part of the lingual nerve. Thus the lingual nerve and gland are firmly connected with each other. At the point of this connection the lingual nerve turns into An almost horizontal course and soon disappears at the posterior border of the mylohyoid muscle, where it enters the sublingual space of the oral cavity. Below the lingual nerve a tonguelike flat lobe of the submandibular gland extends, in many persons, onto the upper and inner surface of the mylohyoid muscle. The submandibular duct accompanies this oral extension or, if the latter is absent, courses upward and forward parallel to and below the lingual nerve (Fig. 13-5). The submandibular (Wharton's) duct also leaves the submandibular region at the posterior border of the mylohyoid muscle to enter the oral cavity. A third structure, in its course parallel to the lingual nerve and submandibular duct, is the hypoglossal nerve (Figs. 13-5 and 13-6). It enters the submandibular region from the carotid triangle by crossing the tendon of the digastric muscle on its deep surface

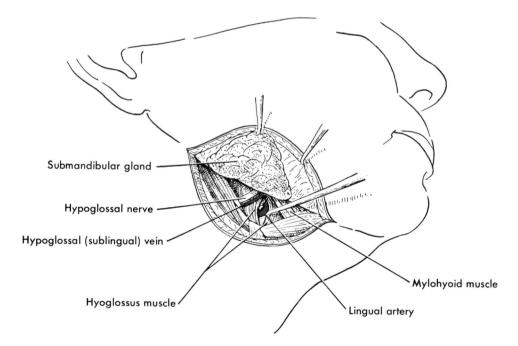

Fig. 13-7. Surgical exposure of lingual artery.

and then runs forward and slightly upward on the outer surface of the hyoglossus muscle. The nerve is here always accompanied by a small vein, which, in the living, is a characteristic mark for the recognition of the hypoglossal nerve; this vein joins the sublingual vein.

The hypoglossal nerve, the posterior border of the mylohyoid muscle, and the tendon of the digastric muscle outline a small triangle, the floor of which is formed by the hyoglossus muscle (Fig. 13-6). The triangle is sometimes referred to as the lingual triangle. The lingual artery, running upward and forward, lies on the inner surface of the hyoglossus muscle deep to the floor of the triangle. It can easily be exposed by dividing the hyoglossus muscle between its vertical bundles (Fig. 13-6). The sharp definition of the lingual triangle and the ease with which the artery can be exposed make the triangle a location of choice for the ligation of the lingual artery.

Surgical procedure. Surgically, the procedure for exposing the lingual artery is as follows (Fig. 13-7). The submandibular gland is palpated through the skin, and an incision is made that circles the lower pole of this gland. The posterior part of the incision should point toward the tip of the mastoid process; the anterior part of the incision should point toward the chin. If the skin, platysma, and deep fascia are incised, the lower pole of the submandibular gland is exposed. If the gland is lifted from its bed by blunt dissection and the entire flap is retracted upward, the tendon of the digastric muscle becomes visible. Following the tendon anteriorly, the free border of the mylohyoid muscle is easily ascertained where it is crossed by the tendon not far above the hyoid bone. If one now follows the free border of the mylohyoid muscle upward and backward, the hypoglossal nerve can be identified by the accompanying vein and by the fact that nerve and vein disappear at the posterior border of the mylohyoid muscle. Thus the lingual triangle between the digastric tendon, the posterior mylohyoid border, and the hypoglossal nerve has been circumscribed. Pulling the digastric tendon downward helps to enlarge this triangle, at the floor of which the finely bundled hyoglossus muscle with its vertical fibers becomes visible. This muscle is divided bluntly, and, in the gap between its vertical fibers, the lingual artery is found.

Ligation of the external carotid artery

Injuries of the upper part of the neck or of the superficial and deep structures of the face may make ligation of the external carotid artery or arteries necessary. There are two points at which the external carotid artery can be exposed and tied. One method exposes the artery at its origin from the common carotid artery, the ligature being placed above the origin of the superior thyroid artery from the external carotid. All of the branches of the external carotid artery with the exception of the superior thyroid—the lingual, facial, and maxillary arteries and the occipital, posterior auricular, and superficial temporal arteries—are eliminated by this method. Although ligation of the external carotid artery in the carotid triangle can be used in bleeding from any one or some of these arteries or in injuries of the external carotid artery itself, ligation higher up, behind the angle of the lower jaw, can be recommended if one deals with a hemorrhage from one of the branches of the maxillary artery. Since these branches supply the upper and lower jaws, this method should be the method of choice in injuries of the jaws and preparatory to operations on the jaws. Furthermore, the high ligation of the external carotid artery is also effective in hemorrhages from the middle meningeal artery incurred during injuries to the skull.

It must be repeated that the anastomoses of all the branches of the external carotid artery and the anastomoses of right and left arteries, across the midline, are so numerous and in summation so wide that unilateral ligation of these vessels will not stop hemorrhage or allow "dry," bloodless surgery.

EXPOSURE OF THE EXTERNAL CAROTID ARTERY IN THE CAROTID TRIANGLE

The ligation of the external carotid artery close to its origin in the carotid triangle (see Fig. 14-1) is best understood if the relations of this region are first discussed (Fig. 13-8). The carotid triangle is bounded by the posterior belly of the digastric muscle above, by the superior belly of the omohyoid muscle in front and below, and by the sternocleidomastoid muscle behind and below. However, the structures that are covered by the sternocleidomastoid muscle at this level are generally considered as part of the carotid triangle.

Superficially this region of the neck is covered by the subcutaneous platysma muscle. Underneath this muscle and between it and the investing layer of the cervical fascia are found the superficial veins and nerves of the neck. The external jugular vein originates in a variable way, in part from branches that drain the region behind the ear and in part from branches that emerge at the lower pole of the parotid gland. The latter contribution is either a branch of the retromandibular vein or, in many individuals, the retromandibular vein itself. The external jugular vein runs almost vertically downward, crossing the oblique fibers of the sternocleidomastoid muscle.

The superficial nerves in this region are mainly sensory branches of the cervical plexus. Of these only two, the great auricular nerve and the transverse cervical nerve, can be considered here (Fig. 13-4). Both nerves emerge through the deep fascia at the middle of the posterior border of the sternocleidomastoid muscle. From here the great auricular nerve, sometimes split into two branches, runs upward toward the lobe of the ear. Some of its branches pass through the parotid gland and supply the skin of a part of the outer ear and a variably wide area of the cheek in the region of the mandibular angle. The nerve lies behind the external jugular vein.

The transverse cervical nerve runs almost horizontally forward across the sternocleidomastoid muscle. One of its superior branches joins the descending, or cervical, branch of the facial nerve, which emerges at the lower pole of the parotid gland. The arching junction of these nerves is known as the superficial cervical loop, or cervical ansa (Fig. 13-4). Branches of the superficial cervical loop are mixed nerves, containing sensory fibers from the cervical plexus and motor fibers from the facial nerve. The latter supply the platysma muscle; the former perforate the muscle and supply the skin that covers it.

The carotid triangle is covered by the investing layer of the deep cervical fascia, which varies considerably in thickness. In the posterosuperior corner of the triangle, that is, below the mastoid process, it is thick and almost inseparably connected with the superficial fascia. Farther down where it covers the sternocleidomastoid muscle it is thin, but much stronger again in front of this muscle. Removal of the superficial layer of the deep cervical fascia exposes the cervical lobe of the parotid gland in the upper corner of the carotid triangle. The capsule of the gland is here closely and tightly attached to the anterior tendinous border of the sternocleidomastoid muscle. If muscle and gland are separated, and if the cervical lobe of the parotid gland is reflected upward, the posterior belly of the digastric muscle and, above it, the stylohyoid muscle can be seen running forward and downward. Retraction of the ster-

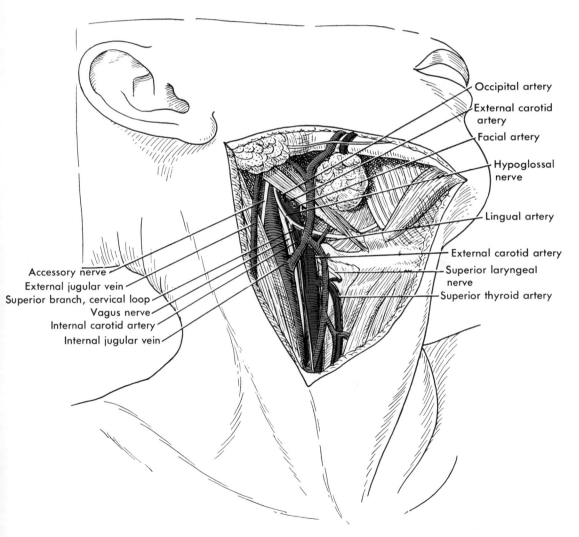

Fig. 13-8. Carotid triangle. (Redrawn from Tandler: Lehrbuch der Anatomie.)

nocleidomastoid muscle reveals that its deep surface is covered by a fascial layer that is derived from the investing fascia.

The superoposterior corner of the carotid triangle contains some of the superior deep cervical lymph nodes, packed in a variable, but generally moderate, amount of fatty tissue. Through the package of lymph nodes the spinal accessory nerve courses downward and backward (Fig. 13-8) to enter the upper part of the sternocleidomastoid muscle from its deep surface. If the lymph nodes in this region and those continuing the chain downward are removed, the great vessels and nerves in the carotid triangle can be exposed.

A carotid sheath, as a separate layer enveloping the common carotid artery, the internal jugular vein, and the vagus nerve, does not exist. However, the deep layer of the sternocleidomastoid sheath is tightly connected with the internal jugular vein. Connections of a vein with a neighboring fascia are the rule in many regions of the human body, and they seem to function as an auxiliary means of venous circulation, keeping the veins open, or even widening the veins, while the fascia is tensed under the influence of muscle action.

The common carotid artery is almost entirely covered by the superficially located internal jugular vein, and when the neck is in normal position it is just seen protruding at the anterior border of the vein. The common carotid artery and its branches are covered by an arterial sheath that may be thick and firm. This sheath is only loosely connected with the wall of the artery itself. The arterial sheath develops from the surrounding connective tissue in response to the tension generated by the pulsation of the arteries, and its loose connection to the artery permits the change in volume of the vessel during pulsation.

Superficially the internal jugular vein and the branches of the common carotid artery are crossed by the hypoglossal nerve. It enters the carotid triangle in front of the mastoid process, emerging at the lower border of the posterior belly of the digastric muscle, and describes an inferiorly convex arch, to disappear again at the inferior border of the digastric muscle just behind the hyoid bone (Fig. 13-8). Where the hypoglossal nerve enters the carotid triangle, it releases a descending branch, consisting of fibers from the first and second cervical nerves, which descends vertically in front of the internal jugular vein and superficially to the carotid artery. This branch is now considered part of the cervical plexus and is called the superior branch of the deep cervical loop, or cervical ansa. At a variable level, in most persons at the level of the lower border of the thyroid cartilage, this nerve joins the descending cervical nerve to form the deep cervical loop. The descending cervical nerve, the inferior branch of the deep cervical loop, arises from contributions of the second and third cervical nerves and crosses at an acute angle the internal jugular vein on its lateral surface. The branches of the deep cervical loop supply the omohyoid, sternohyoid, and sternothyroid muscles.

If the internal jugular vein and the common carotid artery are separated, the vagus nerve is exposed (Fig. 13-8) lying between these two vessels and deep to them. Inside the carotid triangle the vagus nerve does not usually give off any branches;

however, cardiac branches of the nerve, arising higher up in the neck, are found superficial or deep to the carotid artery on their way to the heart.

Many tributary branches of the internal jugular vein enter the vein in the upper parts of the carotid triangle. The first vein, counting from above downward, is the common facial vein (Fig. 13-8). This vein, originating from the union of the facial and retromandibular veins, runs downward and backward to perforate the deep fascia in front of the sternocleidomastoid muscle. Variations of this vein are frequent. The common facial vein may, for instance, continue into the external jugular vein, in which case it is then connected with the internal jugular vein by an anastomosing branch; in other instances only the retromandibular vein continues into the external jugular vein, and the facial vein empties into the internal jugular vein. Sometimes neither the facial nor the retromandibular vein connects with the internal jugular vein, the former continuing into the anterior, the latter into the external jugular vein.

Immediately below the common facial vein the superior thyroid vein empties into the internal jugular vein. The superior thyroid vein may receive tributaries from the tongue and pharynx; the latter may, however, join the common facial vein. In other persons the superior thyroid opens into the common facial vein (Fig. 13-8) and thus indirectly into the internal jugular vein.

The common carotid artery divides into the internal and external carotid arteries at the level of the superior border of the thyroid cartilage. However, a higher division, at the level of the hyoid bone or even slightly above this level, is by no means rare. At the point of bifurcation the external artery lies in front of the internal carotid artery. Higher up, the internal carotid artery tends toward the depth so that the external carotid artery lies anterior and lateral to the internal carotid.

The internal carotid remains branchless in its almost vertical course through the carotid triangle, but the external carotid artery is characterized and can be identified by its branching. Especially the superior thyroid artery is a landmark for the identification of the external carotid artery (Figs. 13-8 and 13-9).

The superior thyroid artery arises from the external carotid artery, sometimes at its very origin from the common carotid artery or just slightly above this point (Fig. 13-8). It curves rather sharply downward and forward toward the upper pole of the thyroid gland. From the first part of the superior thyroid artery arises the superior laryngeal artery, which enters the larynx through an opening in the hyothyroid membrane. The superior laryngeal artery is joined at this point by the internal branch of the superior laryngeal nerve, a branch of the vagus nerve. The superior laryngeal nerve, arising as a rule from the vagus nerve above the carotid triangle, crosses in its downward and forward course the branches of the carotid artery on their medial side. Behind the hyoid bone the superior laryngeal nerve sends the thin external branch downward to the cricothyroid muscle and continues as the internal branch.

At a variable distance above the origin of the superior thyroid artery the lingual artery arises from the anterior wall of the external carotid artery, and immediately above the origin of the lingual artery the facial artery is given off (Fig. 13-8). In many individuals these two arteries arise in a common trunk, the linguofacial trunk. The lingual artery, running upward and forward, disappears above the greater horn of the hyoid bone at the posterior border of the hyoglossus muscle. The facial artery, also ascending forward, disappears at the inferior border of the digastric muscle.

At about the level of the origin of the lingual artery, the external carotid emits the occipital artery from its posterior wall. The occipital artery runs upward and backward, to leave the carotid triangle close to its posterosuperior corner, where it continues medially to the posterior belly of the digastric muscle.

The ascending pharyngeal artery, the last branch of the external carotid in the carotid triangle, has a highly variable origin. It may arise at the bifurcation of the common carotid artery or from the external carotid artery at any point to the level of the origin of the occipital artery or from the occipital artery itself. The ascending

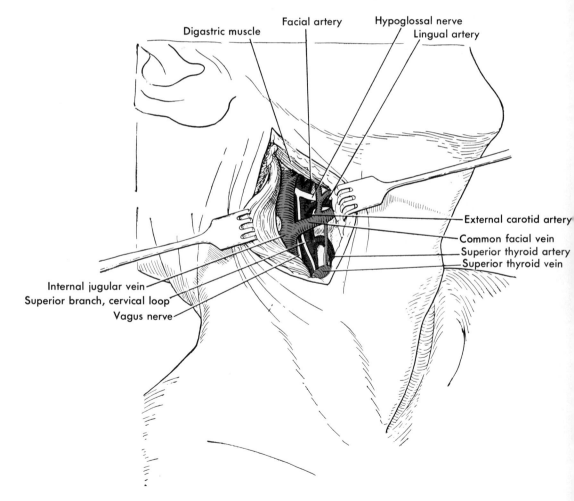

Fig. 13-9. Surgical exposure of external carotid artery in carotid triangle. (Redrawn from Tandler: Lehrbuch der Anatomie.)

pharyngeal artery turns upward and medially and continues its almost vertical course on the lateral wall of the pharynx.

If the common carotid artery and its branches are dislocated anteriorly and the vagus nerve and the internal jugular vein are dislocated posteriorly, the cervical vertebrae and the muscles attached to this part of the vertical column are exposed. These muscles, the longus colli, longus capitis, and scaleni muscles, are covered by the strong and firm prevertebral fascia. Underneath this fascia or in its substance the cervical part of the sympathetic trunk can be seen continuing upward into the large spindle-shaped superior cervical ganglion. The relation of this nerve to the prevertebral fascia immobilizes the nerve during movements of the neck and head, whereas blood vessels and the vagus nerve change their position during such movements.

Surgical procedure. Surgically the exposure and ligation of the external carotid artery in the carotid triangle can best be done in the following way (Fig. 13-9). The incision of the skin starts at the level of the angle of the mandible just behind the anterior border of the sternocleidomastoid muscle and is continued downward, parallel to the border of the muscle, to the level of cricoid cartilage. After penetrating through the skin and the platysma muscle, the superficial sheath of the sternocleidomastoid muscle is incised. Bluntly, the anterior border of the muscle is exposed and the muscle retracted; thus the deep layer of the sternocleidomastoid sheath becomes visible and through it the internal jugular vein. In front of this vein the fascia is cut to expose the arteries. The external carotid artery is identified by its first anterior branch, the superior thyroid artery, and then isolated and tied a few millimeters above the origin of the superior thyroid artery.

While the incision through the deep layer of the sternocleidomastoid sheath is made, care has to be taken not to injure the hypoglossal nerve. It is suggested that the incision through the fascia be started at the lowest point of the wound.

EXPOSURE OF THE EXTERNAL CAROTID ARTERY IN THE RETROMANDIBULAR FOSSA

The second point where the external carotid artery may be ligated lies in the retromandibular fossa behind the angle of the mandible. Here the artery crosses the stylomandibular ligament on its lateral side, and this method has also been called "ligation of the external carotid artery at the stylomandibular ligament." This approach is preferable if the hemorrhage occurs or is anticipated from a branch of the maxillary artery. The latter artery is surgically inaccessible because of its deep course.

The retromandibular space contains the bulk of the parotid gland, which extends behind the mandible, below the external auditory meatus, and in front of the mastoid process and sternocleidomastoid muscle (Fig. 13-10) into the depth to the styloid process and the muscles that arise from it. The lower pole of the gland reaches downward below the level of the inferior border of the mandible into the carotid triangle. At this point branches of the great auricular nerve, the retromandibular vein (posterior facial vein) (Fig. 13-10), and the cervical branch of the facial nerve emerge from the substance of the gland.

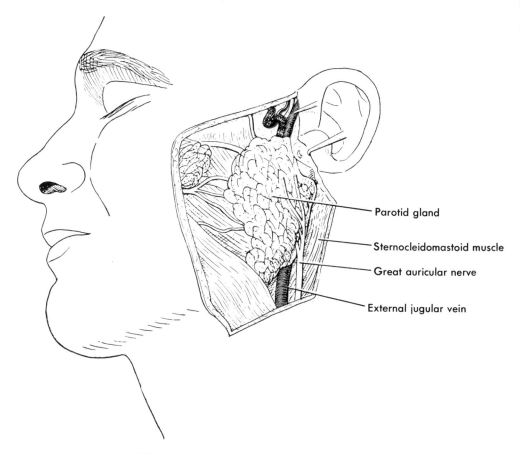

Fig. 13-10. Retromandibular fossa, superficial layer.

The parotid gland covers and partly surrounds the external carotid artery. This artery leaves the carotid triangle by passing deep to the posterior belly of the digastric and stylohyoid muscles and turns upward and slightly backward. It crosses the stylomandibular ligament on its superficial side (Fig. 13-11), and sometimes it crosses the styloid process if the latter is longer than usual. At this point the external carotid artery gives off the posterior auricular artery, which turns upward and backward, to continue between the mastoid process and outer ear. After crossing the stylomandibular ligament the external carotid artery enters the parotid gland from its deep surface and continues in the gland to the level of the mandibular neck to split into its two terminal branches, the maxillary and the superficial temporal arteries.

Superficial and parallel to the external carotid artery runs the retromandibular vein, also surrounded by tissue of the parotid gland. This vein usually continues in the parotid gland to its lower pole and is separated from the carotid artery at the stylomandibular ligament by a layer of the parotid gland itself. Below the ligament, the stylohyoid muscle and the posterior belly of the digastric muscle intervene between the external carotid artery and the retromandibular vein.

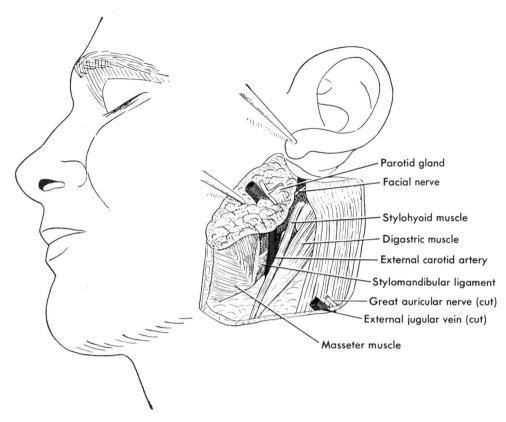

Fig. 13-11. Retromandibular fossa, deep layer. Parotid gland has been reflected upward with stumps of external jugular vein and great auricular nerve.

In some persons, however, the retromandibular vein or a deep branch of it leaves the deep surface of the parotid gland at a higher level and then follows the external carotid artery over the stylomandibular ligament and on the medial side of the digastric and stylohyoid muscles.

The retromandibular vein may turn forward and downward to join the facial vein, or downward and slightly backward to continue as the external jugular vein (Fig. 13-10). Sometimes two veins, the retromandibular vein and a branch connecting the retromandibular and external jugular veins, appear at the lower pole of the parotid gland.

The facial nerve traverses the retromandibular space in a horizontal course (Fig. 13-11). Where the nerve leaves the stylomastoid foramen its main trunk enters the parotid gland and runs downward and forward. Ordinarily it is situated superficial to both the retromandibular vein and the external carotid artery and considerably above the level of the stylomandibular ligament.

The auriculotemporal nerve is also among the contents of the retromandibular space. This nerve enters the space by crossing the posterior surface of the mandibular

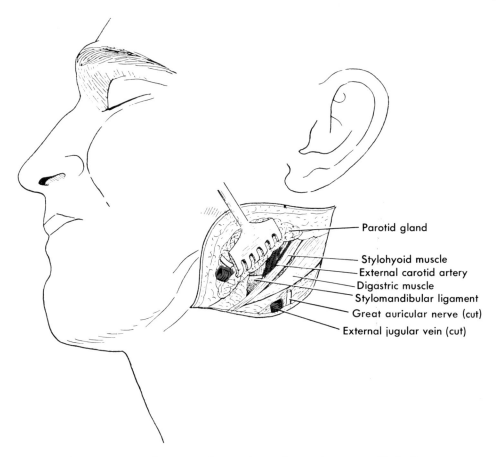

Fig. 13-12. Surgical exposure of external carotid artery in retromandibular fossa.

neck and divides here into an inferior and a superior branch. The inferior branch joins the facial nerve, and the superior branch converges with the superficial temporal artery.

Surgical procedure. The surgical exposure of the external carotid artery at the stylomandibular ligament (Fig. 13-12) is a simpler and less dangerous procedure than the exposure of the artery in the neck. The skin is incised in a line starting at the tip of the mastoid process and circling the mandibular angle, continuing forward below the mandible for about one inch. The incision is kept at an equal distance from the posterior and inferior borders of the mandible. After the scalpel has passed through the skin and some of the posterior fibers of the platysma muscle, the retromandibular vein or the external jugular vein is located, tied, and cut. Branches of the great auricular nerve must also be cut to permit the mobilization of the cervical lobe of the parotid gland. To this end, the attachment of the parotid capsule to the anterior border of the sternocleidomastoid muscle must be severed with the scalpel. If this is done, the flap of soft tissues, consisting of skin and parotid gland, is retracted anteriorly and upward. Immediately underneath the parotid gland, the posterior belly of the digastric muscle, and, slightly above it, the thin round flesh of the stylohyoid muscle become visible. Above these muscles the styloid process and the upper border of the stylomandibular ligament can be palpated, especially if at this moment the lower jaw of the patient is pulled forward. This movement of the mandible not only widens the entrance into the retromandibular fossa, but also tenses the stylomandibular ligament. At the stylomandibular ligament the pulse of the external carotid artery can be felt, and it is easy to isolate the artery and to tie it, even if it is accompanied by a larger vein.

CHAPTER 14

Propagation of dental infections

Infections originating in a tooth or its supporting structures or in the jaws can spread to far-removed parts of the body. To a high degree the path of an infection can be understood from a study of the anatomy of the head and neck. If one excludes from consideration the hematogenous spread, that is, the spread of bacteria flowing through blood vessels, there are three possibilities for the propagation of dental infections. Such infections may, as in any other part of the body, spread by the invasion of bacteria into lymph vessels and then lead to the metastatic inflammation of the regional and more remote lymph nodes (see Chapter 8). The second possibility, more frequently realized, is the spread of an infection by continuity. As far as the propagation of an infection within the jawbones and as far as the possibility of involvement of neighboring cavities and structures are concerned, the necessary data have been given in the discussion on the topographic anatomy of the alveolar processes in Chapter 11. Once outside the bones, further spread of an infection, if it is not fulminating, is dictated to a high degree by the distribution of loose connective tissue. The path of least resistance, which is the path of infections, is through the loose connective tissue. For an understanding of the configuration of the loose connective tissue, the layers of the dense connective tissue between which the loose tissue is found must be studied. This, of course, entails a study of the fasciae. The third and last possibility for the spread of an infection is by involvement of the veins, which thrombose and then form, by continued clotting of the contained blood, an open roadway for the invasion by bacteria. For an understanding of the consequences of a thrombophlebitis, the anastomoses of the facial veins with the deeper veins of the head must be studied.

DISTRIBUTION OF LOOSE CONNECTIVE TISSUE IN THE FACE

The loose, fat-containing tissue of the lips and cheeks is continuous. However, it is partially partitioned by the muscles of facial expression, which arise from the bones of the face and which, as variably wide plates, traverse the subcutaneous tissue, to end in the skin. In infections that are not caused by extremely virulent bacteria, the muscles with their thin perimysia play a role in directing the spread of the infection. In this respect it has to be remembered that dental absesses that erode and perforate the outer compact lamella of the upper or lower jaw sometimes do not progress toward the oral vestibule but find their way through the subcutaneous tissue to the skin. The formation of a cutaneous dental abscess is usually restricted to certain groups of teeth. Almost all of these abscesses take their origin from the molars of the upper and lower jaws, from the lower incisors, sometimes from a lower canine, and, more rarely, from an upper canine. Upper incisors and upper and lower premolars almost never cause a cutaneous abscess. Furthermore, cutaneous abscesses originating from the molars are much more frequent in children and in adolescents than in adults. The key to this behavior of dental abscesses can be found in the arrangement of the muscles of the lips and cheeks.

If the relation of the lines of origin of these muscles to the alveolar process is studied (Fig. 3-18), it becomes immediately clear that in the region of the upper and lower premolars muscles originate at a great distance from the base of the alveolar process. In the lower jaw the depressor anguli oris and the depressor of the lower lip (triangular and quadrate muscles of the lower lip) arise near the lower border of the mandible; the connective tissue between the mandible and these muscles that is primarily invaded after a buccal perforation of a periapical abscess is continuous with the submucous connective tissue, and an abscess in this tissue will become visible and accessible in the vestibule of this region. The path to the subcutaneous tissue, on the other hand, is effectively barred by these two muscles of the lower lip and their epimysia. In the upper jaw the relations between the premolars and the levator of the corner of the mouth (canine muscle) and the levators of the upper lip are entirely comparable. The muscles arising in the region of the upper incisors are so small that they hardly influence the spread of an infection, which will advance toward the fornix of the vestibule, where the connective tissue is always more loose in character than the subcutaneous tissue in the root of the lips. This is why the premolars and the upper incisors almost never give rise to a cutaneous abscess.

In the anterior region of the lower jaw the conditions are different. Here not only the weak inferior incisive muscle, which is the counterpart of the superior incisive muscle, but also the strong mental muscle arise from the base of the alveolar process. If the roots of the lower incisors are long, the perforation of the labial plate of the alveolar process may lead into the connective tissue below the origin of the mental muscle, that is, into the subcutaneous tissue of the chin. The path of infection then is toward the skin in front of or below the bony chin because the way toward the submucous connective tissue is barred by the mental muscle and its connective tissue sheath. The same is true for the lower canine if the mental muscle is strongly developed and its origin is widened into the region of the canine socket.

The upper canine may occasionally cause the development of a cutaneous abscess. It is characteristic for such an abscess to become visible and possibly to perforate the skin close to the inner corner of the eye. The reason for this peculiar path of infection is again to be sought in the anatomy of the muscles of the upper lip. Here the muscles are arranged in two layers. The superficial layer is formed by two muscles: the levator of the upper lip, arising just below the infraorbital rim, or infraorbital margin, and the levator of the upper lip and nasal wing, arising from the upper part of the frontal process of the maxilla. Between these two muscles, formerly known as the infraorbital and angular heads of the quadrate muscle of the upper lip, there is usually a variably wide gap that is widest at the inferior orbital border and that narrows downward where the two muscles fuse. The levator anguli oris (canine muscle) arises from the canine fossa below the infraorbital foramen in a variably long, almost horizontal line at the canine eminence. As a rule, a periapical abscess of the canine breaks through the external alveolar plate below the origin of the levator anguli oris at the corner of the mouth and then spreads into the submucous connective tissue of the vestibular fornix. However, if the root of a canine is long or if, in young patients, the canine has not moved sufficiently downward, its apex may be situated above the level of the origin of the levator of the corner of the mouth. In such cases a periapical abscess may reach the loose connective tissue containing the ramification of the infraorbital nerve and blood vessels in the space between the deep and the superficial muscles of the upper lip. If this connective tissue is involved, the infection may finally escape through the gap between the infraorbital head of the levator of the upper lip and the nasal wing of the levator of the upper lip and thus emerge under the skin just below the inner corner of the eye. Abscesses in this region imitate abscesses originating in the lacrimal sac, and the incorrect diagnosis "dacryocystitis" has often been made in cases of this type.

In the region of the molars the attachment of the buccinator muscle to the base of the alveolar process plays a decisive role for the path of a dental abscess after it has perforated the outer compact layer of the bone. Ordinarily, the line of origin of the buccinator muscle is, in the adult, beyond the level of the root apices of the molars, so that a molar abscess involves the submucous connective tissue, and its spread to the skin is blocked by the buccinator muscle and its fasciae. In persons with relatively long roots, or in young persons in whom the height of the jaws has not yet been attained and in whom the teeth have not yet sufficiently erupted from the body of the maxilla or mandibule, the apices of the molars may reach beyond the line of origin of the buccinator muscle. An abscess perforating the outer plate of the alveolar process is then barred from the submucous connective tissue by the buccinator muscle and spreads in the subcutaneous tissue toward the skin.

The buccinator muscle also plays a role in the spread of pericoronal abscesses of the lower third molar. These abscesses frequently involve the submucous connective tissue at the buccal side of the tooth. Here, at the root of the cheek where its mobility is restricted, the vestibule is shallow, and the amount of loose connective tissue at the fornix is small. The abscess, therefore, is not conspicuous before it involves more voluminous layers of loose connective tissue. The origin of the buccinator muscle near the oblique line directs the spreading abscess forward and downard, and it becomes more and more voluminous and pronounced when it reaches the level of the second or first molar. Such infections may seem to originate from a second or first molar, and only the knowledge of the peculiar anatomic relations can prevent a faulty diagnosis.

FLOOR OF THE ORAL CAVITY

The floor of the oral cavity is formed by the mylohyoid muscle. The connective tissue above this muscle is situated in the oral cavity; the connective tissue below this muscle is part of the connective tissue of the neck. However, the mylohyoid muscle is, in anteroposterior direction, shorter than the oral cavity, so that a muscular floor of the oral cavity is lacking in its most posterior part (see Fig. 3-12). The importance of these peculiarities of the mylohyoid muscle can best be evaluated if it is assumed that a fluid is injected into the submucous tissue of the sublingual sulcus. If such an injection is made in the anterior regions of this sulcus, back to about the level of the second molar, the fluid will be confined to the oral cavity. However, if such an injection is made at or slightly behind the level of the third molar, the fluid is injected into the connective tissue of the neck, that is, into the submandibular space, and may even tend to spread downward. The relation of an infection to the mylohyoid muscle will therefore be of primary importance to the path of its propagation and for the prognosis of its outcome.

In this respect it must also be remembered that the line of origin of the mylohyoid muscle begins at the midline, close to the lower border of the mandible, and ascends posteriorly diagonally across the inner surface of the mandible to the socket of the last molar (see Fig. 2-41). The obliquity of the origin of the mylohyoid muscle makes it understandable that the apical level of the roots of incisors, canines, and premolars is always above, that is, oral to, the mylohyoid line. The third molar's root tips always reach below, that is, cervical to, the mylohyoid line; the second molar shows not rarely the same relation as the third molar. The first molar usually behaves like the premolars and only rarely like the third molar. If a periapical abscess originates in the five anterior teeth and perforates the lingual plate of the lower jaw, it will involve the oral sublingual connective tissue. However, if it originates in the first or second molar, in a certain percentage of cases it may involve the connective tissue below the mylohyoid muscle, that is, the connective tissue of the submandibular space. The latter behavior is the rule for an abscess of the third molar. The infection may even spread from the submandibular niche backward into the parapharyngeal space, and its downward extension into the fascial spaces of the neck is not barred by any obstacle. Fortunately, most infections of the submandibular space remain confined in this region.

Lingual spread of a dental abscess in the mandible will therefore cause an entirely different clinical picture in the molar region from that observed in the region anterior to the molars. If a submandibular abscess spreads downward through the neck, it should be designated as descending cervical cellulitis, or Ludwig's angina; an abscess above the mylohyoid muscle should be called sublingual cellulitis.

A sublingual cellulitis involves primarily the connective tissue that surrounds the sublingual gland, submandibular (Wharton's) duct, and the neighboring structures (see Fig. 12-2). It occupies a space bounded above by the mucous membrane, medially by the geniohyoid and genioglossus muscles, and laterally and below by the mylohyoid muscle. Such an infection may, however, invade the loose connective tissue that separates the individual muscles from each other. Because of the possibility of such an invasion, the terms *intermuscular spaces* and *interfascial spaces* have been introduced. The term *spaces* should, however, be strictly reserved for those regions that are filled with loose, sometimes fat-containing, connective tissue.

The intermuscular connective tissue in the sublingual region is characterized by continuing across the midline from one side to the other (see Fig. 12-2). The connective tissue between the mylohyoid and geniohyoid muscles, as well as that separating the geniohyoid and genioglossus muscles, is not interrupted at the midline. Right and left muscles are separated in the midsagittal plane by a thin layer of loose connective tissue. A sublingual cellulitis may therefore spread across the midline and involve two distinct levels of connective tissue, the lower below and the upper above the geniohyoid muscles. In the midline itself the cellulitis will involve the tissue between the right and left geniohyoid and the right and left genioglossus muscles and will therefore cause a swelling of the body and base of the tongue itself.

A sublingual cellulitis is confined anteriorly and laterally by the mandible and posteriorly at the midline by the body of the hyoid bone. Lateral to the hyoid bone, however, the infection may spread distally and then pass the posterior border of the mylohyoid muscle. If this happens, the sublingual cellulitis passes the boundary between the submandibular niche and parapharyngeal space and may spread in the latter downward along the neck. The sublingual cellulitis then ends as a descending cervical cellulitis, or Ludwig's angina.

Usually a sublingual cellulitis is not confined to one side, and the best way of clearing the infected spaces is by draining in the midline from the chin to the hyoid bone. The incision of the skin should be made transversely so that the subsequent scar falls in the neck folds. After reflecting skin and subcutaneous tissue, the mylohyoid muscle is incised along the midline, and then the entire complicated stock of intermuscular connective tissue is accessible. It is especially important to remember that the connective tissues and thus the cellulitis extends laterally below and above the geniohyoid muscles.

MASTICATORY FAT PAD AND FASCIAE OF THE MASTICATORY MUSCLES

The masticatory muscles, masseter, temporal, and lateral and medial pterygoid, are covered by their epimysium, which is strengthened to a fascia only on the outer surface of the masseter muscle and the inner surface of the medial pterygoid muscle.

The temporal fascia is a plate of dense connective tissue enclosing the temporal fossa from temporal lines to zygomatic arch. Its structure and disposition express the biomechanical response to a complex interplay of forces. This tough fascia is, therefore, not merely a muscle sheath, it is also an essential suspensory sling upholding the zygomatic arch. At the same time, it is the aponeurotic origin for the outer fibers of the temporal muscle, which spring from the inner surface of the upper part of the fascia. These fibers slant medially to attach to the inner tendon of insertion of the temporalis, which rises from the coronoid process of the mandible (see Fig. 3-5). At about the same level as the margin of the tendon, the fascia deviates outward from the muscle to anchor on the zygomatic arch. The space between the inner tendon and outer fascia is partly occupied by loose, fat-filled connective tissue. Slightly below the deviation the temporal fascia itself splits into two well-defined layers, an inner and an outer layer. The outer layer of the temporal fascia is thicker, and it attaches to the outer surface of the zygomatic arch. The inner layer is somewhat thinner, and it attaches to the inner surface of the zygomatic arch. Both layers fuse with the periosteum of the arch, which is continuous all around the bone. Thus the zygomatic arch is literally suspended in a sling opposing the downward pull of the powerful masseter muscle. The space between the two fascial layers is filled with fat held in compartments of loose connective tissue, which connect the inner and outer layers.

The outer surface of the masseter is covered by a fairly thick fascia that is tightly attached to the superficial tendon of the masseter below the zygomatic arch. Behind the anterior border of the masseter muscle the fascia splits into a thin deep layer, which continues to the posterior border of the masseter muscle, and a thicker superficial layer, which covers the parotid gland and is firmly connected with the interlobular tissue of the gland. In the retromandibular fossa this layer ends at the external auditory meatus and the mastoid process behind, and at the root of the zygomatic arch above, continuing downward into the cervical fascia. The complex fascia of the masseter and parotid gland has been called the parotideomasseteric fascia.

A stronger fascial layer is also found on the medial, deep side of the medial pterygoid muscle. This fascia is strongest where it covers the most inferior part of the muscle near the mandibular angle. Here fibers of the stylomandibular "ligament" continue into the deep fascia of the medial pterygoid muscle, whereas others are attached to the angle of the mandible (see Fig. 4-8).

Masseter and temporal muscles in reality form an anatomic unit. The boundary between the deepest fibers of the masseter and the superficial fibers of the temporal muscle is artificial and arbitrary. Thus no space exists between these two muscles. The temporal muscle and the two pterygoid muscles, on the other hand, are separated from each other by fairly wide spaces that communicate with each other and are filled with a pad of fatty tissue. This fat is peculiarly loose in texture and is bounded by a thin connective tissue capsule of its own. The fat pad also fills the space between the masseter muscle and the buccinator muscle. At the anterior border of the masseter the fat pad protrudes as a flat, biconvex, rounded body. This part of the masticatory fat pad, which is especially well developed in the newborn and young infant, has been called the "suckling pad" because of its alleged function. The name "buccal fat pad of Bichat" is more widely used, but it would be better to speak of the *buccal part of the masticatory fat pad.*

At the anterior border of the temporal muscle the fat pad extends upward into the temporal fossa between the anterior border of the temporal muscle and the temporal surface of the zygomatic bone, the zygomaticotemporal space, and extends variably far posteriorly as a flat process between the temporal muscle and the temporal fascia.

Around the tendons of the temporal muscle, attached to the anterior border of the mandibular ramus, another extension of the masticatory fat pad reaches backward into the pterygomandibular space. This space is bounded laterally by the medial surface of the mandibular ramus, medially by the medial pterygoid muscle, and above by the lateral pterygoid muscle. The pterygomandibular extension of the fat pad, surrounding the lingual and inferior alveolar nerves and the inferior alveolar blood vessels, reaches backward to the anterior surface of the deep part of the parotid gland, which is contained in the retromandibular fossa. The masticatory fat pad also sends a rather thin process upward between the lateral and medial pterygoid muscles and finally connects, through the pterygomaxillary fissure at the anterior border of the pterygoid process, with the fat in the pterygopalatine fossa.

Corresponding to the more voluminous parts of the masticatory fat pad, three "spaces" can be differentiated. They communicate with each other and with the parapharyngeal space but are at least partly separated from each other, so that infections may, for a time, be confined to any one of the compartments. These three spaces are the buccal space, the pterygomandibular space, and the zygomaticotemporal space.

The buccal space is situated between the buccinator muscle and the masseter muscle. It communicates posteriorly with the pterygomandibular space and upward with the zygomaticotemporal space. The latter has also been called the retrozygomatic space because it is partly situated behind the zygomatic bone. The term zygomaticotemporal space seems to be preferable because it indicates the relation to the zygomatic bone and the temporal muscle.

The parapharyngeal space extends upward between the lateral wall of the pharynx and the medial surface of the medial pterygoid muscle (see Fig. 6-5). Behind the medial pterygoid muscle the parapharyngeal space widens considerably and extends laterally as far as the styloid process with its muscles and to the deep surface of the parotid gland (see Fig. 12-3). The pterygomandibular space therefore communicates with the parapharyngeal space around the anterior and posterior borders of the medial pterygoid muscle.

Infections may involve one or all of these compartments. They can be opened and explored from one key point (see Figs. 12-3 and 12-5). If a vertical incision is made in the most posterior part of the oral vestibule between the posterior ends of the upper and lower alveolar processes, lateral and parallel to the pterygomandibular fold, and if the mucous membrane and the buccinator muscle are split, the posterior part of the buccal space is opened and the tendons of the temporal muscle are exposed. A curved hemostat can be introduced in various directions through the incision. Anteriorly and laterally it enters the buccal space; posteriorly it passes into the pterygomandibular space medial to the temporal tendon. If the hemostat is guided upward along the exposed tendon of the temporal muscle, one can explore the zygomaticotemporal space. The parapharyngeal space is finally accessible from the same incision if the instrument is introduced along the inner surface of the medial pterygoid muscle, whose easily recognized anterior border serves as landmark.

Under the guidance of the introduced instrument, counterincisions can be made in the temporal region, in the cheek, and below the mandibular angle to se-

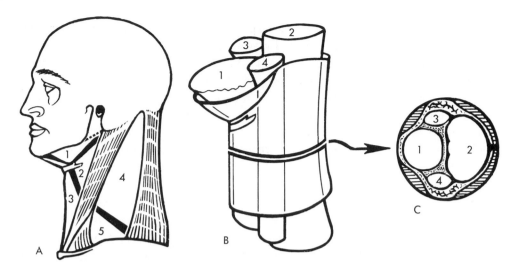

Fig. 14-1. Model of neck construction; superficial topography, fascia, and fascial clefts. **A,** Triangles of the neck (diminutive submental triangle, anterior to digastric triangle): *1,* submandibular (digastric) triangle; *2,* carotid triangle; *3,* muscular triangle; *4,* occipital triangle; *5,* supraclavicular triangle. **B,** Compartments of the neck: *1,* visceral column; *2,* supporting column; *3* and *4,* vascular columns. Note level of transverse section diagramed in C *(arrow).* **C,** Cross section of the neck (anterior at left). Note outer layer of continuous deep fascia enclosing trapezius and sternocleidomastoid muscles *(cross hatched);* deep layer of continuous fascia enclosing: *1,* visceral column; *2,* supporting column; *3* and *4,* vascular columns. Dotted central area indicates retropharyngeal and parapharyngeal fascial clefts ("surgical spaces").

cure adequate drainage of zygomaticotemporal, buccal, and parapharyngeal abscesses.

BASIC PLAN OF THE NECK

For convenience of description and clarity of conception, the neck is presented here in the form of a pitcher. It has a broad pouring spout projecting its upper front contour from the hyoid bone to the chin. The neck connects the jaw and cranial base above with the thoracic inlet below. It contains four columns extending its whole length: an anterior visceral column, two lateral vascular columns, and a posterior supporting column. Each column is wrapped separately in a fascial covering textured according to its function, and the wrappings are continuous with one another around the neck (Fig. 14-1).

Superficially, each side of the neck is divided into large anterior and posterior triangles by the oblique course of the sternocleidomastoid muscle and its relation to the midline of the neck anteriorly, and the margin of the trapezius posteriorly. These two major triangles are subdivided by easily located anatomic boundaries into lesser triangles, slightly more deeply seated. Such topographic mapping is highly valuable for locating important structures and providing landmarks in the surgical approach to deep structures in the neck (see especially the section on ligation of arteries in Chapter 13). It will be seen later that the model herein proposed is also useful in making fascial distinctions simpler.

Anterior triangle

The anterior triangle is bounded in front by the midline of the neck from the chin to the sternum. It is bounded behind by the anterior margin of the sternocleidomastoid muscle. Its base above is the body of the mandible and an imaginary line extended backward from the mandibular angle to the mastoid process. Its apex below is at the center of the jugular notch of the manubrium sterni.

The triangle is covered by skin, superficial fascia, the platysma muscle, and an underlying plate of fascia. The anterior triangle encloses the four following lesser triangles (Fig. 14-1, A).

Submental triangle. The miniature triangle of each side can be described as one midline triangle. It is bounded on each side by the anterior digastric bellies that meet in an apex at the chin. The base of the triangle is the body of the hyoid bone. Its floor is the hyoid muscle with its fascia; it is covered by skin, superficial fascia, and the platysma with its underlying fascia. This narrow space houses a few small vessels and the submental lymph nodes (see Fig. 8-1).

Submandibular (digastric) triangle. This triangle is bounded above by the body of the mandible and the line from mandibular angle to mastoid process. It is bounded behind by the posterior belly of the digastic muscle and the stylohyoid muscle; it is bounded in front by the anterior digastric belly. Its floor is the mylohyoid muscle anteriorly and the hyoglossus muscle posteriorly (see Fig. 3-12). It is covered by skin, superficial fascia, and platysma with an underlying fascia. This triangle houses the submandibular gland, the inferior extension of the parotid gland, the facial artery and vein, and, high above at the mylohyoid muscle, the mylohyoid nerve and artery and the submental artery.

Muscular triangle. This area is bounded in front by the midline of the neck. It is bounded behind and above by the superior belly of the omohyoid muscle, behind and below by the lower part of the anterior margin of the sternocleidomastoid muscle. Its floor is formed by the flat "ribbon" muscles of the neck, sternohyoid and sternothyroid (see Fig. 3-14), and the pretrachial fascia extending forward to the midline. It is covered by skin and superficial fascia and partly by platysma with an underlying fascial plate. The muscular triangle houses the highly variable anterior jugular veins and their anastomoses, with opposite sides (jugular arch) running through the "suprasternal space of Burns" (see Chapters 7 and 15).

Carotid triangle. This important triangle is bounded behind by the upper part of the anterior border of the sternocleidomastoid muscle. It is bounded in front by the posterior digastric belly and stylohyoid muscle above and the superior belly of the omohyoid below. Its floor is formed by thyrohyoid, hyoglossus, and inferior and middle pharyngeal constrictor muscles. It is covered by skin, superficial fascia, platysma muscle, and a sheet of fascia underlying it. The carotid triangle marks the position of the division of the common carotid artery into external and internal carotid arteries hidden under the anterior border of the sternocleidomastoid muscle. It contains the superior thyroid, lingual, facial, occipital, and ascending pharyngeal branches of the external carotid artery, and the corresponding veins (see Figs. 13-8).

Here the hypoglossal nerve swings down and out around the internal and external carotids to leave the triangle anteriorly and enter the tongue. The ansa hypoglossi can also be reached in this region.

Posterior triangle

The posterior triangle is bounded in front by the posterior margin of the sternocleidomastoid muscle and behind by the anterior margin of the trapezius muscle. Its blunt apex above is formed by the converging anterior and posterior muscular margins. Its base below is the middle third of the clavicle. It is covered by skin, superficial fascia, a deeper fascial plate, and the platysma muscle in its lower part. The posterior triangle encloses the two following triangles set at a slightly deeper level (Fig. 14-1, A).

Occipital triangle. This large upper triangle is bounded in front by most of the posterior margin of the sternocleidomastoid muscle, behind by the anterior margin of the trapezius, and below by the inferior belly of the omohyoid muscle. Its floor, from above downward, is composed of the splenius capitus, levator scapulae, and middle and posterior scalene muscles. It is covered by skin, superficial fascia, and platysma muscle in its lower part, and by a continuous fascial layer underlying the platysma. It contains the spinal accessory nerve and branches of the cervical plexus, that is, lesser occipital, great auricular, and transverse cervical cutaneous nerves, which curl forward around the posterior margin of the sternocleidomastoid, and the supraclavicular nerves, which run down over the clavicle.

Supraclavicular triangle. This small lower triangle varies in size with the angulation of the omohyoid and with lowering and raising of the arm. It is bounded above by the inferior belly of the omohyoid muscle, below by the middle third of the clavicle, and in front by a short segment of the posterior border of the sternocleidomastoid muscle. Its floor is formed by the first rib and the insertions on it of the scalenus medius and serratus anterior muscles. It is covered by skin, superficial fascia, and the platysma, with the layer of fascia underlying the muscle. It contains the curving subclavian artery, transverse cervical artery and vein, part of the brachial plexus, and the supraclavicular nerves.

The connective tissue underlying the skin and embedding all the deeper structures of the body varies considerably in regional distribution and texture. The variety ranges from loose, fatty, and lubricant to dense, fibrous, and tensilely supportive. In the neck, the connective tissue parcels out into compartments, the columns that run throughout its length. The connective tissue wraps the columns in blankets woven to the degrees of tissue density demanded by their separate functions.

FASCIAE OF THE NECK

Prevalent descriptions of the cervical fasciae are extraordinarily confusing. This may be due partly to the continuous splitting and fusing encountered in the numerous layers of connective tissue in the neck and partly to differences in the terminologies used, but perhaps mostly because of the lack of clarity in the usage of the term "fascia." Since dissections are usually carried out on cadavers hardened to various degrees by tissue fixatives, layers of congealed loose connective tissue may be mistakenly called fascia, or thick collections of tissue may be split artificially into several layers.

Fascia is a localized concentration of the general connective tissue permeating the body. It is broadly defined as "a sheet or layer of more or less condensed connective tissue." True fascia is found in planes where the connective tissue is regularly subjected to specific tensions. The tension can be the result of a direct pull of muscle on adjacent tissue; it can also be the result of pull on distant tissues when body parts are vigorously moved. Furthermore, tension can be the pull caused by the expansion of tissues wrapping a muscle bulging in action. It is clear that the differences in the structural orientations of fascial wrappings are to be explained on the basis of different forces arising from the various biomechanical functions of the invested parts. Fascia is commonly described under two major headings, superficial fascia (which fits the definition imperfectly) and deep fascia.

Superficial cervical fascia. Superficial fascia is a connective tissue blanket underlying the dermis. It is not a distinct membrane, but an uneven layer between skin and deep fascia. It contains a variable amount of fat and usually becomes thicker as well as more distinct over the lower anterior abdominal wall. Superficial fascia carries the subcutaneous vessels, nerves, and lymphatics, and it acts as a thermal insulator.

In the neck the superficial fascia has two distinguishing features. First, it contains the platysma muscle, which covers the anterior and lateral surfaces of the neck. Second, this layer, which is rather loose in most areas, is bound firmly to the deeper structures around the upper posterior margin of the neck. Here it is tied, by strong straps of fibrous tissue enclosing fat lobules, to the continuous aponeurotic attachments of the sternocleidomastoid and trapezius muscles along the mastoid margin and superior nuchal line.

Deep cervical fascia. Deep fascia is composed mostly of collagen fibers more or less compacted and oriented along lines of tension. The deep fascia itself is descriptively divided into superficial and deep layers. The picture becomes increasingly complicated when intermuscular septa, extending from fascial sheaths to underlying bones, are included in the description. But since the muscles within these compartments often arise from the septa, the picture is clarified when it is understood that septa are actually aponeurotic origins or insertions.

The neck is literally an isthmus that connects the head with the rest of the body. It is an adaptation that allows the sense organs in the head to scan the surrounding environment quickly, without having to turn the entire body. The neck thus balances, rotates, raises, and lowers the head independently of the torso. The great vessels that supply the head and brain must course through this twisting mass, pulsing at their own rates, without constricting impingements from turning and nodding. At the same time the visceral segments of tongue-larynx-pharynx must move independently of the rest of the neck in breathing, swallowing, and speaking. It is evident that the different functional columns, modeled in Fig. 14-1, must slip and slide, twist and bend, relative to each other in smooth, unhampered movements.

The deep cervical fascia is variably condensed, but distinct, fibroareolar tissue surrounding muscles, vessels, and viscera. It can be traced completely around the neck in a surprisingly simple general pattern of layers on two levels.

The great flat muscles immediately beneath the superficial fascia mark the outer level of the deep fascia (Fig. 14-1, C). Thus the trapezius muscle is completely ensheathed by laminae on its inner and outer surfaces, which stem from the nuchal ligament along the posterior midline of the neck. The laminae fuse to a single layer along the anterior border of the trapezius muscle. This layer extends as a fascial plate across the posterior triangle of the neck to the posterior margin of the sternocleidomastoid muscle. Here it splits again to ensheath that muscle completely in strong inner and outer laminae. At the anterior margin of the sternocleidomastoid muscle the laminae again fuse to continue across the anterior triangle of the neck as a firm single layer until it becomes continuous with its fascial counterpart from the opposite side. Posterosuperiorly the fascia ends on the superior nuchal lines and mastoid processes; inferiorly it continues into the deep fascia of the back. Anterosuperiorly it is attached to the lower border of the jaw and to the body of the hyoid bone below. It continues upward behind the mandible into the tough parotid fascia, extending to the fascia of the masseter muscle. Anteroinferiorly the fascia is attached to the sternum, clavicle, and acromion.

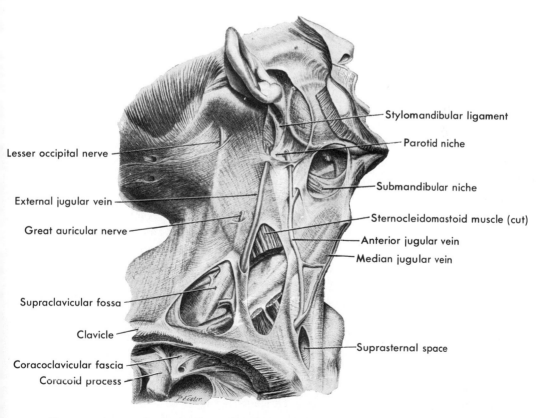

Fig. 14-2. Fasciae of neck. (Eisler: In Bardeleben: Handbuch der Anatomie des Menschen.)

Fascia at this outer level has been variously labeled "investing fascia," "superficial laminae of deep fascia," etc. Although the general plan is simple as outlined above, the tissue is unevenly textured and the details of the structures it envelopes and the structures passing through it complicate the picture locally. Where the fascia covers the trapezius, it is strong. Where it covers the supraclavicular triangle just anterior to the trapezius, it is punctured by so many holes that it has been called cribriform (sievelike) fascia. The plate of fascia below the hyoid bone is roughly triangular. Its lateral boundaries are formed by the omohyoid muscles; its base is its attachment to clavicles, the posterior surface of the sternum, and sternoclavicular and interclavic-ular ligaments. Below the thyroid gland this fascial plate splits into inner and outer layers to form the suprasternal space of Burns (Fig. 14-2). The space extends laterally on each side behind the sternocleidomastoid muscles and the omoclavicular fascia extending from the muscle to the clavicle. This continuous outer mantle of muscle and fascia is wrapped closely around the inner four columns of structures running down through the neck (Fig. 14-1, *B* and *C*).

The fascia enclosing these columns marks the inner level of the deep cervical fascia. Each column is sheathed in its own fascia, which is tailored to meet its par-ticular function. The anterior, visceral, column is supported in a fascial sleeve woven for flexibility to accommodate the brisk lifting and lowering, swelling and contracting movements of the tongue, pharynx, and larynx. The lateral vascular columns show a gradation in fibrous density. Their sheaths are continuous with the adjacent column through moderately fibrous areolar tissue. Fibrous condensation increases around veins to become heaviest around the arteries. The posterior column is fitted with the toughest fascial casing, especially anteriorly, befitting its heavy supportive func-tion.

It is informative to trace the fascial stratification at this deepest level diagramati-cally as a continuum of splitting and fusing comparable to that of the investing layer. This device points up most clearly the fascial clefts that are clinically critical (Fig. 14-1, *C*). Thus, again stemming from the ligamentum nuchae posteriorly, a fascial layer can be traced around the side of the supporting column to meet, at its antero-lateral corner, the dense fascial covering of its anterior surface. At this point the fascia extends as a loose fusion to become continuous with the fascia of the vascular column. Anteromedially, the outer and inner layers of the vascular column meet to extend and fuse with the fascia of the visceral column. Again the fascia can be considered to separate into posterior and anterior layers, which meet counterparts from opposite sides to complete the sheathing of the visceral column (Fig. 14-1, *C*). In such a model one sees immediately the interfascial cleft (or "space") between the prevertebral fascia of the supporting column and the pharyngeal fascia of the visceral column. This so-called surgical space is roughly H shaped. The crossbar represents the retropha-ryngeal cleft. The vertical arms represent the parapharyngeal spaces, limited laterally by the fascia of the vascular columns. These spaces extend upward between the pharynx and the medial pterygoid muscles and have there been called mandibulo-pharyngeal spaces. (see Figs. 12-3 and 14-1,*C*).

The visceral fascia is best developed in the region of the pharynx as pharyngobasilar fascia. It continues at the level of the cheek from the buccopharyngeal part of the upper pharyngeal constrictor forward on the outer surface of the buccinator muscle. At the level of the tongue it continues over the styloglossus and hyoglossus muscles, and below this level it covers not only the pharynx but also the larynx in a common sheath, which, however, is relatively thin in the region of the larynx itself. The visceral fascia provides the capsular covering of the thyroid gland and then continues around the trachea and esophagus. At the upper level of the esophagus and the trachea, the visceral fascia divides into two separate tubes, whose loose connection assures independent mobility of the digestive and respiratory canals. The layer that covers the trachea finds its end by fusing with the connective tissue around the great vessels in the thorax, and the esophagus carries its covering down to the diaphragm.

The investing fascia of the neck contributes to the formation of the capsule of both the submandibular and parotid glands. The niches for these glands are separated from one another by a complicated arrangement of connective tissue structures (Fig. 14-2). In the depth the boundary is formed by the stylomandibular ligament and, closer to the surface, by a reinforced part of the investing fascia, the angular tract. The fibers of this tract arise in front of the parotid gland from the angle of the mandible, where they are connected to the stylomandibular ligament and the fascia covering the deep surface of the medial pterygoid muscle. The angular tract continues downward along the anterior border of the sternocleidomastoid muscle and gains attachment to the hyoid bone.

The deep wall of the submandibular niche (Fig. 14-2) is formed in front by the fascia of the mylohyoid muscle, and behind the mylohyoid muscle by the fascia covering the hyoglossus and styloglossus muscles. The deep layer of the parotid niche is formed by the stylomandibular ligament and the fascia covering the stylohyoid muscle and the posterior belly of the digastric muscle. Above the stylomandibular ligament the deep capsule of the parotid gland is thin.

INTERFASCIAL SPACES OF THE NECK

There are actually only two locally enclosed spaces in the head and neck: the space between the split layers of the temporal fascia in the head, and the split layers forming the suprasternal space of Burns in the neck. Practically all the other fascial clefts, or "spaces," of the neck communicate with each other to a greater or lesser extent. The communications are sometimes wide, sometimes constricted. Layers or strands of connective tissue that partially separate one space from another may act as relative obstructions to the spread of infections. The spread progresses as these weak intervening layers become necrotic. At the same time it must be appreciated that all fasciae are perforated by vessels and nerves and these openings also permit the passage of infections.

On the other hand, the loose connective tissue that fills these spaces is often condensed to plates or strands of denser connective tissue. Such condensations then may incompletely subdivide otherwise uniform "spaces," but they cannot be considered to be of the same order as the typical fascial layers; they are not only variable from individual to individual in their exact location and their connections, but they also vary widely in their texture. They may be hardly recognizable and poorly differentiated from the surrounding loose areolar tissue, or they may form thick and firm bands. Such condensations, if they are present, may play the clinically important role of diverting an infection that is spreading in the common space, so that the infection is deflected in different individuals toward different walls of the space in which it is contained. This seems, at least in part, to explain the variations in the ultimate outcome of a deep cervical cellulitis.

Such condensations of loose connective tissue frequently develop where blood vessels run through loose connective tissue; then these condensations do not only envelop the vessels but also tie them to one of the neighboring fasciae. Roughly such condensations could be compared with a mesentery. Such a plate of dense connective tissue frequently extends from the prevertebral fascia forward to and around the vertebral artery and vein. This dense connective tissue is a sagittal plate, projecting into the paravisceral space from its posterior wall, but it is not broad enough to separate this space into two compartments, and it ends at the level of the sixth cervical vertebra, where the vertebral artery and vein normally enter the transverse foramina.

Other plates of the same kind are found around the inferior thyroid artery as an incomplete frontal extension of the visceral fascia, and another such plate is found at the base of the neck, extending from the prevertebral fascia to the pleura at the apex of the lung. Often such variable condensations of loose connective tissue have erroneously been described as separate and constant layers of the cervical fascia.

Clinical observations make it desirable to differentiate the paired lateral parapharyngeal and paravisceral spaces from the unpaired retropharyngeal and retroesophageal spaces behind and the pretracheal space in front. This subdivision, however, is entirely artificial, and an infection can spread fairly easily from one of these spaces into the other. The parapharyngeal space continues downward into the space on either side of the trachea and esophagus. Since this latter space is almost entirely bounded by the great blood vessels and the vagus nerve laterally, it is referred to as the vascular, or neurovascular, space.

The parapharyngeal space begins at the base of the skull. As has been mentioned before, in the region of the head the parapharyngeal space is in communication with the spaces between the muscles of mastication—the pterygomandibular space, the zygomaticotemporal space, and the buccal space. Above the styloglossus muscle the parapharyngeal space communicates also with the submandibular space in front.

The retropharyngeal space is not separated from the parapharyngeal space by an attachment of the pharyngeal fascia to the prevertebral fascia as described by some authors. That a retropharyngeal abscess develops as a clinically well-circumscribed entity is merely due to the fact that the posterior wall of the pharynx is wide and in broad contact with the vertebral column and its muscles. An infection in this region spreads downward so easily that, at least in the level of the pharynx, a horizontal expansion to either side is rare. In addition, there is an incomplete separation between the retropharyngeal and parapharyngeal spaces at the level where the stylopharyngeus and the styloglossus muscles cross the posterolateral edge of the pharynx (see Fig. 3-12).

In the lower neck the parapharyngeal space continues without any separation into the paravisceral (vascular) space. The retroesophageal space and paravisceral spaces are in wide communication. Anteriorly the vascular spaces also communicate with the pretracheal space. This communication, however, is sometimes narrowed by the presence of a frontal layer of denser connective tissue around the inferior thyroid artery.

The pretracheal space owes its existence to the divergence between the infrahyoid fascia and the trachea itself. The infrahyoid fascia is attached to the upper border of the sternum and clavicle, whereas the trachea and its fascial covering deviate posteriorly and are separated from the upper end of the sternum by the brachiocephalic artery. The pretracheal space (see Fig. 15-3) ends above the region of the isthmus of the thyroid gland or at the lower border of the larynx, where the fascial layers fuse. Contained in the pretracheal space are the inferior thyroid veins, forming a loose plexus, embedded in loose, fatty tissue.

The visceral spaces of the neck, retroesophageal, paravisceral or vascular, and the pretracheal spaces are in open communication with the mediastinal spaces of the thorax. This connection explains the danger associated with a descending cervical cellulitis. However, many cases have been reported in which the infection, descending along the neck, made its way into the supraclavicular fossa and could be opened and drained above the clavicle, between the sternocleidomastoid muscle and the trapezius muscle. In other instances the infection found its way into the axilla. In rare instances, the infection spread between the clavicle and the first rib to the anterior chest wall and could be reached in the deltoideopectoral triangle below the clavicle, between the deltoid and the greater pectoral muscle. The explanation for this variable behavior is in all probability to be sought in the existence and in the extent and density of the variable condensations of the loose connective tissue in the lower part of the neck. By such condensations the descending cellulitis may be deflected laterally above the omohyoid muscle into the fatty loose connective tissue that fills the supraclavicular fossa. If the infection reaches this region, it will pass into the subcutaneous tissue without encountering much resistance because the investing cervical fascia in this region, often described as a cribriform fascia, is not only thin, but also is perforated by a great number of irregular openings (see Fig. 12-2).

Below the level of the omohyoid muscle the omoclavicular fascia (the lateral part of the infrahyoid fascia) prevents lateral spread of a descending cervical cellulitis. But here again condensations of the loose connective tissue may cause a deviation of the infection laterally and anteriorly. Such condensations here are found not only around the vertebral artery, but also as connections of the prevertebral fascia with the fascia of the pleural covering of the apex of the lung. These condensations, described as pleurovertebral and costopleural ligaments, are extremely variable. If they are strong, they may prevent an extension of a descending cervical cellulitis into the mediastinum and may direct it along the subclavian vessels. Following the subclavian artery and the brachial plexus, the infection may then enter the axilla. If it is in a more anterior relation, it may involve the connective tissue around and in front of the subclavian vein and then become superficial below the coracoclavicular fascia in the deltoideopectoral region.

The perivisceral spaces are accessible through the investing fascia of the neck. In the upper region of the neck the spaces are reached in front of the sternocleidomastoid muscle, and in the lower regions the spaces are reached behind the same muscle. Incisions to open the vascular space should be made just behind the anterior border or just in front of the posterior border of the sternocleidomastoid muscle, which is easily exposed after the skin, the superficial fascia with the platysma muscle, and the outer lamella of the muscle sheath have been incised. The border of the muscle is then secured and retracted in the upper half of the neck or pulled forward if one operates on the lower half of the neck. Through the deep layer of the muscle sheath the vascular space can be opened. This procedure is safer than an incision passing through the different layers anteriorly or posteriorly to the sternocleidomastoid muscle because the layers are more clearly defined after the sternocleidomastoid muscle has been exposed.

The accessibility of the parapharyngeal space has already been mentioned. It is accessible from the most posterior part of the oral vestibule by a vertical incision just lateral to the pterygomandibular fold. After cutting through the buccinator muscle near its origin from the pterygomandibular raphe, the anterior border of the medial pterygoid muscle is easily exposed, and an instrument can be introduced along the medial surface of the muscle into the parapharyngeal space. If the instrument is guided downward and laterally, it can be felt below the mandibular angle through the skin, and a counterincision can be made in this location.

The communication of the submandibular niche with the parapharyngeal space above the styloglossal muscle explains the spread of an infection from the niche to the spaces of the neck; in other words, it explains the typical progress of Ludwig's angina (see the section on the floor of the oral cavity, in this chapter).

THROMBOPHLEBITIS OF THE FACE

An inflammatory involvement of any vein may be dangerous because of the possible detachment of all or part of an infected thrombus and a consecutive embolism in the pulmonary artery or one of its branches. In the face and jaws there is an added danger because of the communications between the extracranial and intracranial veins. If the thrombosis and infection extend into the veins of the dura mater, a meningitis will ensue, which may end fatally. Therefore the pathways of propagation of an infection in the veins must be studied carefully.

Extracranial and intracranial veins communicate directly by short veins that pass at typical points through the bones of the cranium (see Fig. 7-6). These veins are called emissary veins, or emissaries. The most constant of these are the parietal, the mastoid, and the condylar emissaries (see Figs. 2-7 and 2-8). The parietal emissary is a communication between the superior sagittal sinus and branches of the superficial temporal or occipital veins. It is situated between the middle and posterior thirds of the sagittal suture and close to the midline. Its size is variable, and it may be missing on one or both sides. The mastoid emissary is situated in the occipitomastoid suture, or it may perforate the posterior part of the mastoid plate of the temporal bone (see Fig. 2-21). It is a communication between the transverse sinus and tributary veins of the external jugular vein. The condylar emissary perforates the base of the skull behind the occipital condyle and provides a communication between the end of the sigmoid sinus and deep cervical veins. The mastoid and condylar emissaries also are variable and may be lacking. Sometimes an unpaired occipital emissary is found just below the occipital prominence. A more variable emissary vein connects the cavernous sinus with the pterygoid plexus of veins. It passes through an opening at the base of the greater sphenoid wing, the foramen of Vesalius, or through the fibrocartilage filling the lacerated foramen.

The emissary veins function as added drainage channels for the venous blood of the brain if the intracranial pressure is temporarily increased. Whether a reversal of the blood flow can occur by drainage from the superficial structures into the cranium is questionable. The emissaries, however, are not the only overflow channels of the cerebral veins. A plexus of veins along the clivus offers a drainage of the cavernous sinus into the veins of the vertebral canal. Functionally of less importance, but important as potential paths of a thrombophlebitis, are the plexuses of small veins that surround some nerves in the canals or foramina through which they leave the skull and a similar plexus around the internal carotid artery in the carotid canal.

Of greatest importance are the communications of the facial veins with the ophthalmic veins, which in turn enter the cranial cavity to empty into the cavernous sinus (see Figs. 7-6 to 7-9). The most constant, and usually the widest, communication between the veins of the face and the orbit is that between the superior ophthalmic vein and the facial vein at the inner corner of the eye, above the medial palpebral ligament. The communications of the inferior ophthalmic vein with the facial vein or its branches at the inferior border of the orbit above the infraorbital foramen are of secondary importance.

There is, however, one other fairly constant venous communication between the inferior ophthalmic vein and the pterygoid plexus of veins through the inferior orbital fissure (see Fig. 7-6). This communication between the roots of the retromandibular vein and the terminal part of the inferior ophthalmic vein occurs near the posterior end of the orbit.

At last an indirect communication of extracranial and intracranial veins is mediated by the diploic veins. These veins drain primarily the marrow or diploe of the flat bones of the cranium and open into the extracranial veins by perforating the outer compact plate of the bones. In their course, however, they receive small venous contributions from the dura mater, which in turn is drained by the meningeal veins.

Communications between the diploic veins and nearby sinuses of the dura mater also have been described.

Of all the communications between the extracranial and intracranial veins, those established by the ophthalmic veins are of greatest clinical importance. To understand the clinical picture and the sequence of clinical symptoms it has to be kept in mind that there are two types of propagation of a facial thrombophlebitis to the cavernous sinus. One path leads from the facial vein into the superior ophthalmic vein or sometimes, although rarely, into the inferior ophthalmic vein. The infection therefore leads into and through the orbit, and the thrombophlebitis is finally transmitted to the cavernous sinus through the superior orbital fissure.

The second path leads from the retromandibular vein into the pterygoid venous plexus, from here through the inferior orbital fissure into the terminal part of the inferior ophthalmic vein, and then immediately through the superior orbital fissure into the cavernous sinus.

In the first type of ascending fascial thrombophlebitis the involvement of the orbit, under the clinical picture of an orbital or retrobulbar cellulitis, precedes the symptoms indicating the involvement of the cavernous sinus. In the second type the intracranial of meningeal symptoms may occur without a previous orbital involvement. In the first type of ascending thrombophlebitis a danger signal occurs before the ultimate complications arise, whereas such a warning symptom is lacking in the second type.

Before discussing the relations of the cavernous sinus, it is necessary to point to the many direct or indirect communications between the anterior and posterior facial veins (see Figs. 7-7 to 7-9). These communications make it understandable that wherever an infection originates in the jaws, and whichever branches of the facial or retromandibular vein are primarily involved, the thrombophlebitis may eventually extend to either the facial or retromandibular vein or to both. This in turn means that there is no rule to determine whether the first, transorbital, or the second, retro-orbital, type of propagation is to be expected in a given case.

Facial and retromandibular veins communicate by deep, as well as by superficial, anastomoses. The anterior region of the upper jaw drains into the infraorbital veins, which anastomose freely with tributaries of the facial vein at the infraorbital foramen, whereas the infraorbital vein itself enters into the pterygoid plexus drained by the retromandibular vein. The posterior part of the upper jaws drains mainly into the posterior superior alveolar veins, which also are tributaries of the pterygoid plexus. In the jaw itself, however, there are many anastomoses between the smaller veins.

Although the venous blood of the lower jaw is primarily drained into the retromandibular vein by the inferior alveolar vein, a branch of the maxillary vein, there are wide anastomoses between the inferior alveolar vein and tributaries of the facial vein through the mental foramen. Facial and retromandibular veins are also in direct communication by the veins of the cheek, which drain forward to the facial vein and backward to the retromandibular vein. In addition, the transverse facial vein is a constant and direct anastomosis between the facial and retromandibular veins; it is in

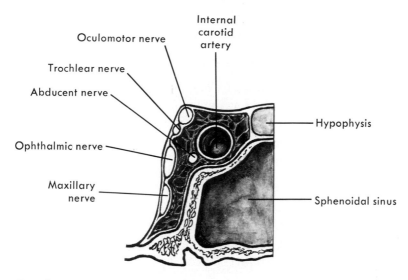

Fig. 14-3. Frontal section through the cavernous sinuses, showing relations of the structures passing through.

most instances situated deep to the masseter muscles on the outer surface of the buccinator muscle.

The structure of the cavernous sinus is identical in principle to that of the other sinuses of the dura mater. These are spaces between two lamellae of the dura mater and are lined by endothelium. The sinuses are therefore noncollapsible veins without walls of their own; they receive the veins of the brain and the eye and its accessory organs and drain into the internal jugular veins. The cavernous sinus (Fig. 14-3) is a wide venous space situated on the lateral slopes of the sphenoid body above the root of the greater sphenoid wing. Medially its upper part borders the hypophysis, and its lower part borders the sphenoid sinus; posteriorly it reaches to the tip of the temporal pyramid, and anteriorly it reaches the superior orbital fissure. The cavernous sinus is traversed by an irregular network of connective tissue trabeculae that divide its space into a system of communicating smaller compartments. This arrangement was responsible for the term "cavernous" sinus.

The cavernous sinus receives the ophthalmic veins through the superior orbital fissure. Some small tributary veins originate in the hypophysis. Along the posterior edge of the lesser sphenoid wing the sphenoparietal sinus reaches the cavernous sinus. The right and left cavernous sinuses communicate through the anterior and posterior intercavernous sinuses, which are situated in front and in back of the pituitary gland, respectively. The cavernous sinus itself is drained by the superior and inferior petrosal sinuses and in part by the plexus of veins in the dura mater of the clivus. The superior petrosal sinus empties into the first part of the sigmoid sinus; the inferior petrosal sinus reaches the superior bulb of the internal jugular vein by passing through the petro-occipital fissure or through an anterior compartment of the jugular foramen.

The cavernous sinus is furthermore distinguished by its relation to the internal carotid artery and several cranial nerves (Fig. 14-3). The internal carotid artery, accompanied by the sympathetic internal carotid plexus, enters the sinus at the tip of the temporal pyramid, forms a sharp S-shaped curve in the sinus itself, and finally emerges through the anterior part of its roof.

The sixth, or abducent, nerve runs through the cavernous sinus. The sixth nerve enters the upper part of the inferior petrosal sinus, and, through it, the nerve enters the cavernous sinus; on the lateral side of the carotid artery the abducent nerve passes through the cavernous sinus in an almost horizontal posteroanterior course, and, perforating the anterior wall of the sinus, it reaches the orbit through the superior orbital fissure.

Contained in a sleeve of the dura mater the third, or oculomotor, nerve enters the roof of the cavernous sinus, runs forward, slightly outward, and downward and passes through the superior orbital fissure into the orbit. Almost parallel to the oculomotor nerve courses the fourth, or trochlear, nerve in the roof and, farther anteriorly, in the lateral wall of the sinus.

The semilunar ganglion of the trigeminal nerve is housed in a pocket of the dura mater (see Fig. 9-1), which the trigeminal root enters from the posterior cranial fossa between the trigeminal notch and the superior petrosal sinus. The pocket for the ganglion, the trigeminal (or Meckel's) cave, is in part situated in the lateral wall of the cavernous sinus. The ophthalmic nerve (first trigeminal division) reaches the superior orbital fissure running horizontally forward in the lateral wall of the cavernous sinus. The maxillary nerve (second trigeminal division), on its way to the foramen rotundum, is also situated in the sinus wall, but there is no relation between the mandibular nerve (third trigeminal division) and the cavernous sinus.

The relation of the abducent nerve to the sinus is more intimate than that of the other nerves. In the cavernous sinus the abducent nerve and the blood contained in the sinus are separated only by a layer of endothelium, which covers not only the nerve, but also the internal carotid artery with the carotid plexus and the trabeculae of connective tissue, which traverse the sinus.

The oculomotor nerve, the trochlear nerve, the semilunar ganglion, and ophthalmic and maxillary nerves are situated not in the sinus, but in its wall. A thrombophlebitis of the sinus will therefore first involve the abducent nerve and only later the other nerves. Paresis or paralysis of the abducent nerve, diagnosed by the weakness or paralysis of the lateral rectus muscle of the eye, is therefore the first symptom of an involvement of the cavernous sinus.

CHAPTER 15

Tracheotomy and laryngotomy

Obstruction of the air passages is so serious an emergency that it demands surgical opening of the larynx or trachea below the point of obstruction. In dentistry and oral surgery the obstacle is almost without exception located at the level of the glottis between the vocal cords or above the glottis. The causes of an obstruction of the larynx are mainly three: (1) the introduction of a foreign body into the larynx, (2) laryngospasm, that is, spastic contraction of the closing muscles of the glottis, and (3) glottis edema.

If a small foreign body enters the larynx, it may pass the glottis, the narrowest point of the air passages, and lodge in a bronchus without causing immediate danger. If a foreign body is large, it will be found above the vocal folds in the laryngeal vestibule. The presence of a foreign body in this location acts not merely as a physical block of the larynx, but also as a powerful irritant, causing a reflex laryngospasm.

Laryngospasm, endangering the life of a patient, can be observed during intravenous anesthesia (for instance, with thiopental sodium) or as a reflex response if a foreign body is lodged in the immediate neighborhood of the entrance to the larynx. This may happen either in the epiglottic valleculae between the base of the tongue and the epiglottis or in the piriform sinus between the thyroid cartilage and aryepiglottic fold on either side of the laryngeal entrance. These two localities must be explored in all cases in which the entry of a foreign body into the air passages is suspected before the diagnosis of "foreign body *in* the larynx" is made.

Glottis edema is in reality a submucous edema in the region above the glottis. Its extent is determined by the extent of loose submucous tissue. The mucosa is tightly attached to the posterior surface of the epiglottis and to its anterior surface near the free superior border. A dense submucosa, firmly attaching the mucous membrane, is also characteristic of the edge of the vocal fold and the entire extent of the air passages below this level. In these areas an edema can never reach any large proportions.

The submucosa is loosely structured in the area of the epiglottic valleculae, the aryepiglottic folds, the ventricular (false vocal) folds, in the piriform sinus, and at the posterior surface of the cricoid plate with its muscles. An inflammatory or vasoneurotic edema will gain considerable volume in all of these regions (Fig. 15-1).

The aryepiglottic folds may swell for a considerable time without dangerously narrowing the laryngeal entrance. Then, however, a critical moment is reached when the swollen and flabby folds are sucked into the larynx during inspiration. At this

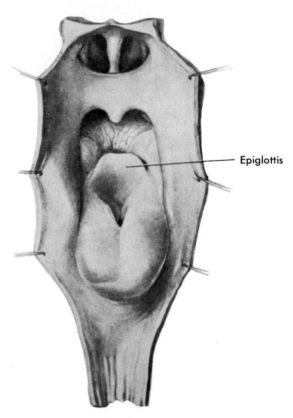

Epiglottis

Fig. 15-1. Glottis edema, artificially produced by injection of water into loose submucosa. (Sicher and Tandler: Anatomie für Zahnärzte.)

moment the folds close the laryngeal entrance as if the two wings of a door were slammed shut. The attempt of the patient to get air into his lungs by forced inspiration can only aggravate his predicament. Therefore the dangerous symptoms of glottis edema arise suddenly, in many cases without previous warning.

When suffocation threatens the life of a patient, he can be saved only by quick surgical action. Whenever it is possible (that is, if instruments and assistance are at hand) the operation of choice is the tracheotomy. However, when this opportunity is not realized, the coniotomy, a type of laryngotomy, must be considered as a lifesaving emergency operation.

INFERIOR TRACHEOTOMY

Of the two possible types of tracheotomy, the inferior tracheotomy is the preferable method. In this operation the trachea is exposed between the isthmus of the thyroid gland and the sternum. The trachea in this region lies at some distance from the skin, and this distance increases downward. The layers through which one has to pass to expose the trachea are as follows: (1) skin and subcutaneous tissue, (2) the

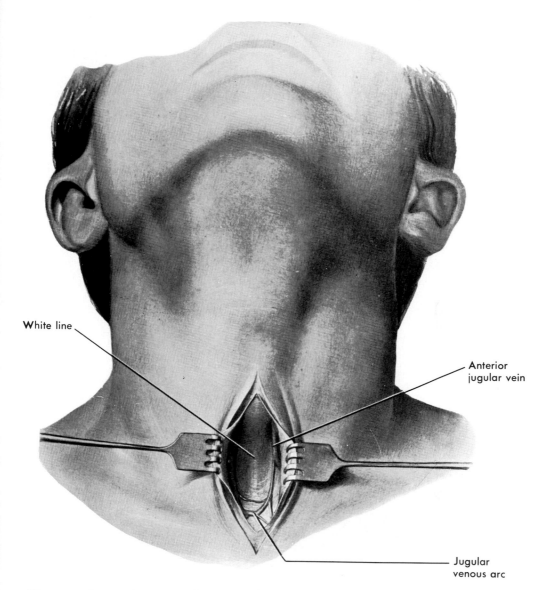

Fig. 15-2. Inferior tracheotomy. In this anatomic dissection the incision through skin was made vertically in midline; surgical incision is horizontal. Suprasternal space has been opened. (Tandler: Topographische Anatomie dringlicher Operationen.)

investing fascia of the neck, (3) the connective tissue contained in the suprasternal space of Burns, (4) the infrahyoid fascia, and (5) the tracheal fascia.

The incision in the skin is made transversely in the line of its folding. After freeing and reflecting the skin, one makes the approach to the trachea in the midline. After incising the investing fascia, the scalpel enters the space of Burns (Fig. 15-2). This space is filled with loose connective tissue that usually contains some fat. Embedded in this tissue, in a horizontal course and not far above the upper border of the sternum, runs the anastomosis between the two anterior jugular veins. This transverse vein, the jugular venous arc, has to be secured, ligated, and cut if it is situated high enough to restrict progress into the depth.

In some persons the two anterior jugular veins are replaced by a median vein that, in Burns's space, divides into a right and a left branch running horizontally to join the external jugular veins. Contrary to the remarks in some textbooks that no important structure is encountered in the midline, this median jugular vein can give rise to considerable hemorrhage.

In the posterior wall of the space of Burns the infrahyoid muscles are visible through the infrahyoid fascia. The muscles never are in contact in the midline, so that in a narrow area the fascia alone forms the posterior wall of the suprasternal space. This area, white between the red muscles, has sometimes been referred to as the

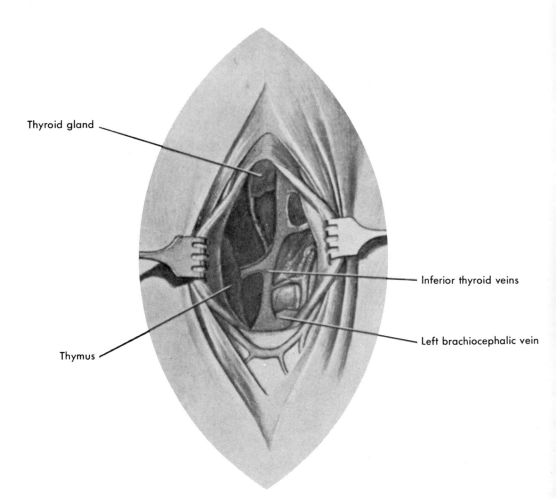

Fig. 15-3. Trachetomy; inferior thyroid veins in pretracheal space. (Tandler: Topographische Anatomie dringlicher Operationen.)

"white line," or "linea alba," of the neck (Fig. 15-2). After the infrahyoid fascia has been incised in the midline, the isthmus of the thyroid gland becomes visible in the upper corner of the wound. From the isthmus and the adjacent parts of the thyroid gland the inferior thyroid veins run downward surrounded by the loose connective tissue between the infrahyoid and tracheal fasciae (Fig. 15-3). These veins form an irregular plexus and usually empty into the left brachiocephalic vein. The inferior thyroid veins may reach considerable dimensions and are greatly extended if the patient suffers severe dyspnea. Again, these veins are not all situated lateral to the midline, but some of the principal veins and many anastomotic branches cross from right to left. Partly surrounded by the inferior thyroid veins, a lowest thyroid artery may run in front of the trachea to the middle region of the thyroid gland. This supernumerary artery originates in most instances from the arch of the aorta, but it may also

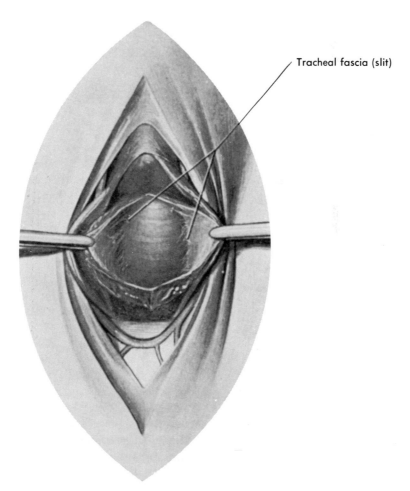

Tracheal fascia (slit)

Fig. 15-4. Tracheotomy; exposure of trachea. (Tandler: Topographische Anatomie dringlicher Operationen.)

be a branch of the brachiocephalic artery or, rarely, a branch of one of the other arteries in the base of the neck.

The brachiocephalic artery and the left common carotid artery are contained in the same layer as the inferior thyroid veins, that is, in front of the tracheal fascia. Although in adults these arteries are infrequently exposed or endangered during an inferior tracheotomy, this is not true in children, in whom the heart and its great vessels are situated at a higher level. It should be a rule, therefore, to pass the pretracheal space by blunt dissection.

Before opening the tracheal tube itself, one must sometimes dislocate the isthmus of the thyroid gland superiorly or even tie and cut it in the midline if it is so wide that the freely accessible part of the trachea below the isthmus is too short. This relation is found especially in persons with a barrel-shaped chest, a more nearly horizontal position of the first ribs, and a high position of the superior border of the sternum. In contrast to the relations in these stockily built individuals, patients with a flat chest and a long neck present a slanting position of the first ribs and a low position of the upper border of the sternum. The infrathyroid or suprasternal part of the trachea is therefore much shorter in persons of the first type than in those of the second type.

After localizing and, if necessary, disposing of the thyroid isthmus, one should split the visceral tracheal fascia in the midline and strip it from the trachea for some distance (Fig. 15-4). Then the trachea can be securely held and incised, and the cannula can be inserted into its lumen.

To avoid injury to the brachiocephalic artery that may, especially in flat-chested persons, lie dangerously close to the lower end of the surgical wound, the incision into the tracheal wall should always begin at the lowest visible point. The edge of the scalpel is directed upward, and the incision also is made in a cranial direction.

CONIOTOMY

The coniotomy was first performed by the French surgeon and anatomist Vicq d'Azyr and later described and recommended by Tandler. This emergency laryngotomy is done by opening the larynx through the cricothyroid ligament between the thyroid and cricoid cartilages. This operation has been named coniotomy from the old anatomic term "conic ligament" for the cricothyroid ligament. The short term "coniotomy" seems to be preferable to the newer term, "intercricothyroid laryngotomy."

The indications for the performance of a coniotomy are restricted. It should be employed only in case of emergency and utmost urgency if conditions for a tracheotomy are not favorable. It has to be stressed especially that the coniotomy can be done without assistance, without anesthesia, and without a tracheal cannula, the only necessary instrument being a knife.

The aim of the operation is to incise the anterior wall of the larynx between the thyroid and cricoid cartilages, where it is formed by a yellow, elastic ligament composed of vertical fibers. The mucous membrane of the larynx is tightly attached to the inner surface of this ligament. The ligament is situated in the lower space of the larynx; that is, below the level of the vocal ligaments that are attached to the inner surface of the thyroid cartilage (see Fig. 6-11).

The middle part of the cricothyroid, or conic, ligament is exposed between the two cricothyroid muscles (Fig. 15-5). It is covered by the deep cervical fascia, the subcutaneous tissue, and the skin. The cricothyroid ligament is easily located by palpation in the midline between the thyroid cartilage and the narrow anterior part of the cricoid cartilage. The palpating finger encounters here a well-circumscribed depression.

The cricothyroid ligament is sometimes crossed close to its upper border by a horizontal anastomosis between the right and left cricothyroid arteries, which are rather small branches of the superior thyroid artery. If a pyramidal lobe of the thyroid gland is present, it extends upward in front of the cricothyroid ligament, but only rarely is the lobe situated in the midline; it lies on the left side in most persons.

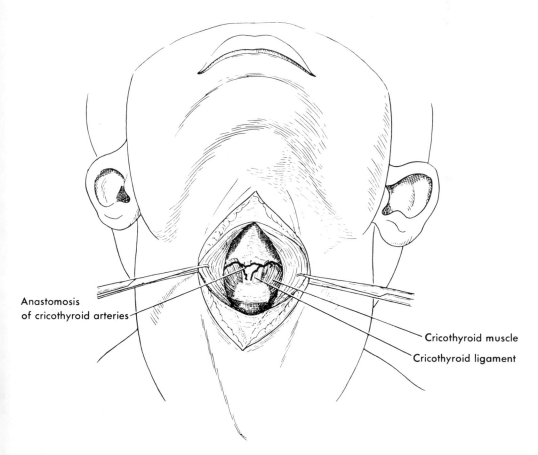

Fig. 15-5. Cricothyroid ligament. (Modified and redrawn from Sicher and Tandler: Anatomie für Zahnärzte.)

The incision of the conic ligament should be horizontal to allow the retraction of the vertical elastic fibers of the ligament. The resulting gaping oval opening in the anterior wall of the larynx remains open, so that the insertion of a cannula is not necessary to safeguard the entrance of air into the larynx.

The coniotomy can be made by incising the skin, fascia, ligament, and mucous membrane of the larynx with one stab. Technically, the coniotomy can be done as follows. The cricothyroid ligament is located by palpation and marked by the palpating finger, which is kept pressed against the larynx. The blade of a knife is then gripped between the thumb and index finger, so that only ½ inch of the blade is free. By doing this, the depth to which the knife may enter is limited, and an injury to the posterior wall of the larynx is avoided. The knife, its blade held horizontally, is then thrust through the skin and ligament into the larynx. The incision through the ligament itself should not exceed ¼ inch.

A precautionary measure that has to be taken until the patient can be delivered into proper hospital care is to prevent the skin from slipping over the incision through the ligament, since this would block the opening into the larynx. This can easily be done by proper application of adhesive tape or, if this is not at hand, by manual fixation of the skin.

Bleeding after a coniotomy is almost never of any consequence. If it should ever become disturbing, it can always be checked by digital compression.

Again, the coniotomy has its place only as an urgent emergency operation. As such, however, its results are dramatic and have saved many a life that otherwise would have been lost.

An effective modification of the coniotomy can be substituted in case of an accident in the dental office. The cricothyroid, or conic, ligament can be quickly pierced by the insertion of a strong (14- or 12-gauge) needle. Such a needle should, in fact, be considered an essential item in any dentist's armamentarium. As was mentioned concerning the use of a knife in the coniotomy, the needle also should be gripped by thumb and index finger so that—at the most—½ inch of the needle can penetrate into the laryngeal lumen.

CHAPTER 16

Craniomandibular articulation

The craniomandibular articulation and its pathologic changes are of importance in three ways. First, it has been recognized that overclosure or any displacement of the mandible, such as after the loss of teeth, may cause serious discomfort to the patient. The mechanism of these disturbances must be properly understood if therapy is to be logical and successful. The traumatic dislocation of the mandible presents some peculiarities, based on the peculiar functional anatomy of its articulation. Finally, the surgical exposure of the temporomandibular joint and its components requires a detailed understanding of anatomic relations because of the danger of permanent injury to the patient by improper technique.

FUNCTIONAL DISTURBANCES OF THE CRANIOMANDIBULAR ARTICULATION

Common causes of craniomandibular joint disorders, apart from acute trauma such as a blow to the jaw or fractures, are (1) overclosure of the mandible, (2) occlusal disharmonies, and (3) mental tension. In all probability the last factor is an indispensable contributing factor in cases of overclosure (closed bite) and occlusal disharmonies. By themselves, these two factors often do *not* tend to establish disturbances in the articulation.

The common denominator in all these cases is the mandibular musculature. Guided, correlated, and balanced by a central pattern generator and curbed by proprioceptive reflexes, this mechanism is subject to anomalies that will lead to imbalance of these normally delicately harmonized muscles.

In overclosure the elevators of the jaw have to overshorten to achieve occlusal contact between lower and upper teeth. This disrupts the normal firing patterns of the proprioceptors of the jaw muscles, their tendons, and the jaw joint.

Occlusal disharmonies will send abnormal stimuli to the proprioceptors of the periodontal ligaments, and from here reflex impulses reach the muscles. Whereas balanced impulses from the periodontal ligaments safeguard the balanced activity of the mandibular musculature, abnormal stimuli will irritate these muscles and disrupt their harmonious action.

Mental tension alone may so increase muscular activity, especially at night or during strenuous work, that the muscles are driven into a vicious cycle of ever-

527

increasing contraction. Mental tension may also significantly "facilitate" the injurious neuronal reflexes in overclosure or in occlusal disharmonies.

The result of all these factors is the establishment of shorter or longer periods of muscle spasms. Since all the muscles of a working group are connected by feedback reflex nerve loops, they influence each other, and spastic activities must finally involve the entire group, wherever they started. Even the groups of muscles outside of the mandibular musculature, but indispensable for their function, may be involved: muscles of the neck and the rest of the hyoid muscles.

The spastic hyperactivity of the mandibular musculature may initiate degenerative changes in the craniomandibular joint merely by increasing and sustaining abnormal pressure on the fibrous tissues of the articulation. Although these tissues are avascular, circulation of tissue fluid is indispensable for their maintenance. Clinical and pathologic observations, however, tend to show that in the majority of joint diseases an additional and more severely injurious mechanism is active.

Two facts in regard to the articular disc must be remembered, that is, the attachment of muscle fibers on its anterior rim, and the loose attachment of its posterior edge to the capsule. If the muscles of the mandible fall into spastic contractions, the unilateral muscle attachment eventually will cause a displacement of the disc with relation to the condyle. As the irritated muscles "fight" against each other, the disc may be held in place while the mandible is displaced posteriorly, or the mandible may be stabilized while the disc is displaced anteriorly, or, more probably, a combination of these possibilities becomes a reality.

The next consequence is an impingement of the condyle on the loose connective tissue behind the disc. An immediate consequence of this impingement is pain in this sensitive region, and later, inevitably, degeneration of the joint. The disc then loses its posterior attachment to the capsule, and the loss of a wide area of synovial tissue leads to a loss of resistance of all of the tissues of the articulation that do not possess blood vessels but are supplied by the synovial fluid. Thus a vicious cycle is initiated that finally may lead to a total breakdown of the joint.

An important symptom of craniomandibular joint disorders is pain in the region of the joint radiating into the temple, the ear, the throat, the cheek, and the tongue. The radiating pain has been explained as the consequence of a compression of the auriculotemporal nerve and the chorda tympani between the tympanic bone and the condyle, which is pressed upward and backward. This explanation is anatomically not tenable. The auriculotemporal nerve crosses the posterior border of the mandible not at the level of the condyle, but much farther down, at the level of the mandibular neck (Figs. 4-4, 12-1, and 16-1). No displacement of the condyle can possibly impinge on this nerve. The only possible danger to the nerve is fracture of the mandibular neck because of the intimate relation of the nerve to the posterior border of the bone.

The extratympanic part of the chorda tympani also is well protected after the nerve has left the tympanic cavity through a small canal in the petrotympanic fissure. Although this point is situated behind the insertion of the articular capsule, the chorda tympani is not in close relation to the capsule because it continues its course

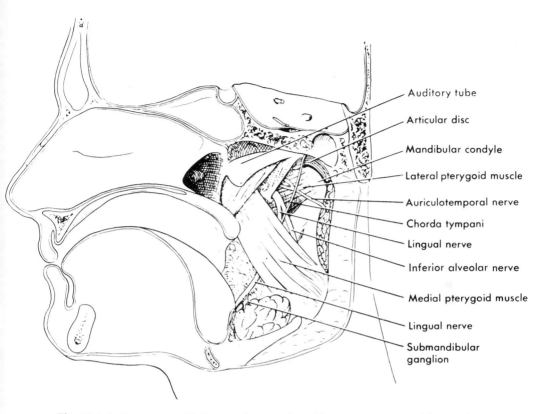

Fig. 16-1. Right craniomandibular articulation and neighboring nerves exposed from within.

Labels (top to bottom): Auditory tube; Articular disc; Mandibular condyle; Lateral pterygoid muscle; Auriculotemporal nerve; Chorda tympani; Lingual nerve; Inferior alveolar nerve; Medial pterygoid muscle; Lingual nerve; Submandibular ganglion

medially in the depth of the narrow petrotympanic fissure (Fig. 16-2). The most medial part of this fissure is sometimes even closed as a bony canal. The petrotympanic fissure ends behind the angular spine of the sphenoid bone, and the chorda tympani curves anteriorly around the medial surface of the spine, which often is grooved to receive the small nerve (Fig. 16-2). At the anterior edge of the angular spine the chorda tympani turns downward and forward to join the lingual nerve. There is, therefore, no possibility of pressure being exerted on the chorda tympani by a displacement of the condyle.

The local pain in disorders of the mandibular joints originates in the stressed or injured capsule and the retrodiscal pad, but the "radiating" pain is, in most instances, pain in spastic muscles. Pain in the region of the temple and ear is pain in the temporal muscle; pain in the throat is pain in the pterygoids; pain in the cheek is pain in the masseter; pain in the tongue is pain in the geniohyoid muscles.

An impairment of hearing acuity in overclosure and posterior displacement of the mandible has repeatedly been claimed. The mechanism involved has been seen either as pressure against the tympanic bone or as some influence on the auditory tube and a disturbance of the function of the tensor palati muscle to equalize the pressure in the middle ear.

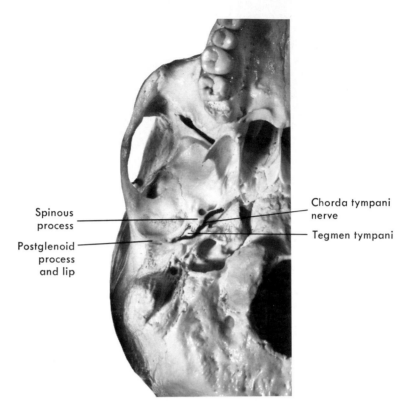

Fig. 16-2. Course of the chorda tympani nerve in the petrotympanic fissure. Note: nerve is entirely isolated from joint; its relation is posterior to postglenoid lip and tegmen tympani (petrous bone) and medial to spinous process (sphenoid bone).

The belief that the condyle could exert pressure on the tympanic plate, ultimately leading to erosion of the bone, has been based on two errors. First, the presence of the posterior articular lip or of a postglenoid process behind the articular fossa and in front of the tympanic bone (see Fig. 4-2) would prevent the condyle from exerting any pressure against the wall of the acoustic meatus, even if it could be displaced into contact with the posterior wall of the articular fossa. The postglenoid process, although variable in size, is absent only in rare instances. A destruction of this process and of the posterior lip would have to precede any influence of the displaced condyle on the tympanic bone.

Second, defects of the tympanic bone behind the craniomandibular articulation are almost without exception caused by arrested development of the tympanic bone. As the tympanic ring is being transformed into the tympanic plate, a foramen is regularly found in the floor of the acoustic meatus (see Fig. 2-82, *B* and *C*). This foramen appears at the end of the second year and does not close until the end of the third year at the earliest, and in many children not before the end of the fifth year of life. Statistical examinations of a great number of skulls have shown that remnants of this defect persist in almost 20% of the examined adult individuals.

The auditory tube, a communication between the middle ear and the nasal part of the pharynx, consists of a short bony part and a much longer cartilaginous part. The latter, fastened to the base of the skull at the sphenopetrosal fissure, is not entirely surrounded by cartilage. In cross section the cartilage is roughly C shaped. It forms, therefore, only three fourths of the circumference of the canal of the tube. The upper, lower, and posteromedial wall of the tube are cartilaginous; the anterolateral wall, however, is membranous. Functionally this arrangement is of importance because it enables a collapse of the membranous wall and therefore closure of the tube at rest, so that a free entry of secretions or of bacteria into the middle ear is, as a rule, prevented. To enable air to enter the middle ear, which is to compensate for a depletion of air in the middle ear by absorption through the mucous membrane, the tube is actively opened during every act of swallowing. The muscle functioning as the opener of the tube is the tensor palati muscle, which arises in front of, and lateral to, the tube from the sphenoid bone, but fibers of the tensor palati also have their origin in the membranous wall of the tube. Each contraction of this muscle will pull the membranous wall away from the cartilage of the tube and thus open its lumen.

The influence of the tensor on the tube and thus on the stabilization of air volume and air pressure in the middle ear is automatic but not by reflex. Man, destined by nature to live on terra firma, did not experience fast variations of atmospheric pressure, and the repeated acts of swallowing during every day and night took care of the renewal of the air in the middle ear. Civilization has brought with it man's ability to ascend or descend so fast in an elevator or in a plane that a new stress on the middle ear is encountered. In ascent the atmospheric pressure around him decreases rapidly while the pressure in the middle ear persists at the value at ground level. The tympanic membrane is then pressed outward; dullness and finally pain in the ear results, and the impairment of the free vibration of the eardrum causes a reduction of hearing acuity. Only conscious and voluntary or accidental swallowing relieves the symptoms by equalizing outside pressure and intratympanic pressure through the opened tube. The reverse happens if an individual, after having equalized the tympanic pressure, descends from some height.

An impairment of the function of the tensor palati muscle in overclosure of the mandible has been assumed. This assumption is certainly erroneous if one considers the position of the fleshy part of the muscle between two fixed bony structures, the base of the skull and the pterygoid hamulus. In addition, one does not always swallow while the teeth are in occlusion, but sometimes, for instance in drinking, while the lower jaw is in rest position or even farther depressed. In this relation of the jaws the tensor palati certainly can and does function normally, and a sufficient regulation of air pressure during the day automatically occurs. Difficulties in swallowing in patients with closed bite may be due to altered position of the tongue, but never to impairment of palatine muscles.

If the observation could be confirmed that patients with an overclosure of the mandible do suffer from lack of ventilation of the tympanic cavity, the changes in the tube must be such as to prevent an opening of the tube despite the normal contraction of the tensor palati muscle; a swelling of the mucous membrane lining the tube, for instance, could account for a permanent closure of the tube. An impairment of the blood or lymph drainage and edema of the tubal mucosa in patients with spasms of the mandibular musculature (pterygoids) may be the primary cause.

DISLOCATION OF THE CRANIOMANDIBULAR ARTICULATION

The craniomandibular articulation is perhaps the only joint of the human body that can be dislocated without the action of an external force. Similar dislocations, for instance in the shoulder, occur only after a first injury has traumatized the capsule and its ligaments.

The dislocation of the craniomandibular articulation is often bilateral, and the displacement is always anterior. The condyle then lies in front of the articular eminence on the preglenoid plane. The mouth is wide open, and any attempt to close it leads only to an aggravation of the situation. Damage to the capsule leads to spasms of the mandibular muscles, especially the elevators. To reduce the dislocation, the pull of the spastic muscles must be overcome by strong downward pressure. Then the mandible easily glides backward into its correct position. The muscular spasms can also be eliminated by injection of a local anesthetic into the posterior capsule and the retrodiscal pad that are most likely to be injured. The anesthesia interrupts the pathologically increased reflexes to the muscles and ends their spastic state.

In trying to understand the mechanism of mandibular dislocation one has to remember that in most individuals the condyle and disc normally pass anteriorly beyond the summit of the articular eminence when the mouth is fully opened. It seems that a pathologic dislocation from this position is caused by a failure of muscular coordination. Under normal conditions the closing movement begins with a retraction of the mandible that brings the condyle into a safe position behind the height of the articular eminence. This means that the retruding portions of the mandibular musculature, that is, the deep portion of the masseter and the posterior portion of the temporal muscle, possibly aided by the digastric and geniohyoid muscles, contract first, before the elevating portions of the masticatory muscles act with full force. But before the retracting muscles begin to act, the lateral pterygoid muscle, which had pulled the disc and the mandible forward, must relax to allow the retraction of the mandible. If this accurate timing of muscle action is disturbed, for instance in yawning, and the lateral pterygoid muscles remain in a state of almost spastic contraction at the beginning of the closing movement instead of relaxing, the elevators of the mandible will exert their force while the condyle is still held in a dangerous position at, or anterior to, the height of the articular eminence. A dislocation is then unavoidable, the attempts of the retracting muscles to bring the mandible back into its normal position are futile, and the closing of the mouth is impossible.

SURGICAL EXPOSURE OF THE CRANIOMANDIBULAR ARTICULATION

Exposure of the craniomandibular joint is difficult mainly because of the proximity of branches of the facial nerve, which must not be injured if permanent damage is to

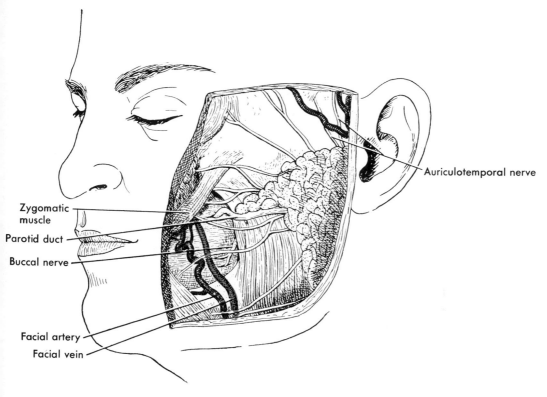

Fig. 16-3. Parotideomasseteric region, showing branches of the facial nerve emerging from the parotid gland.

be avoided (Figs. 9-11 and 16-3). Especially the temporal branches of the facial nerve are endangered. They leave the parotid gland at its anterosuperior border and, ascending steeply, cross the zygomatic arch in front of the mandibular joint at the anterior border of the articular eminence. Exposure of the joint by a horizontal incision above the zygomatic arch is therefore impossible, although this incision in combination with a vertical incision in front of the ear would afford the best accessibility to the articulation.

The joint can be exposed by approaching it from above and behind (Fig. 16-4). To this end the parotid gland has to be dislodged anteriorly and downward and with it the branches of the facial nerve, which thus are removed from the field of operation. To afford the best mobility of the parotid gland the incision is made in a vertical plane immediately in front of the tragus, starting about an inch above the zygomatic arch. At its lower end the incision may be carried backward to encircle the entrance into the cartilaginous meatus of the ear. After penetrating the skin and the superficial fascia, the soft tissues at the root of the zygomatic arch are retracted anteriorly, and the superficial temporal artery and vein are isolated, tied, and cut where they emerge at the upper pole of the parotid gland. The gland itself is then bluntly separated from the cartilage of the ear and gradually pushed forward and downward. Care must be taken

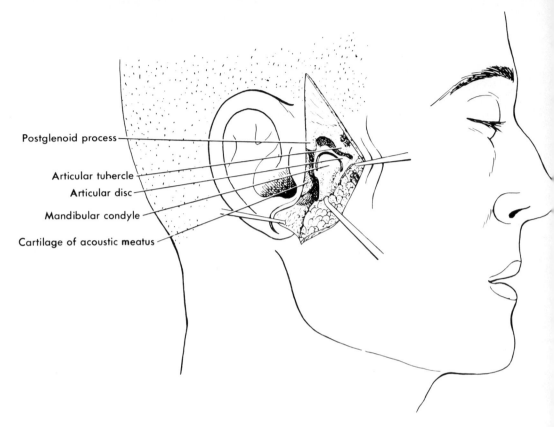

Postglenoid process

Articular tubercle

Articular disc

Mandibular condyle

Cartilage of acoustic meatus

Fig. 16-4. One method of surgical exposure of craniomandibular articulation.

not to strip the perichondrium from the cartilage to avoid necrosis of parts of the cartilage, which may lead to postoperative seeping into the outer ear. If the parotid gland is displaced forward and downward, the postglenoid process of the temporal bone can be located below the zygomatic arch and at the deep inner end of the movable cartilaginous meatus. Starting at this point the articular end of the movable capsule itself can be exposed. Often it is possible to locate clearly the articular notch at the lower border of the root of the zygomatic arch in front of the postglenoid process and the bony meatus, and by following the notch anteriorly the articular tubercle can be felt. Thus the lateral aspect of the articular capsule, strengthened by the craniomandibular ligament or the periosteum that replaces the capsule in cases of bony ankylosis, can be exposed.

If is often also possible to expose the posterior wall of the capsule in its entire extent. The lateral part of the posterior capsule is visible after removing the loose connective tissue, sometimes containing the uppermost lobules of the parotid gland, which fills the space in front of the cartilaginous meatus. Bluntly, for instance, with the handle of a knife introduced between the capsule and the cartilaginous meatus, the posterior wall of the capsule can be separated from the anterior surface of the tympanic bone.

Soft tissues covering the inferior, or mandibular, attachment of the capsule can be retracted forward and downward under blunt dissection until the lateral pole of the condyle or the neck of the mandible is exposed. This procedure allows access to the articulation wide enough for resection of the condyle or removal of the disc, which are the most frequent reasons for surgery in this region.

Another method to expose the craniomandibular articulation and the entire mandibular ramus is the submasseteric (Risdon's) surgical approach. With due regard for the mandibular branch of the facial nerve, the lower border of the angular region of the mandible is exposed by an incision below the mandibular border. Then the insertion of the masseter muscle is reflected from the outer surface of the ramus. Near the mandibular angle this is difficult because tendinous plates of the masseter are firmly attached to the irregular bony ridges. Higher up, however, the periosteum and the muscle bundles attached to it can easily be stripped from the bone. This experience may have given rise to the description of a submasseteric space that does not exist. The flap consisting of muscle, parotid gland with the facial plexus, superficial fascia, and skin can easily be elevated and reflected from the bone of the mandibular ramus until good access to the craniomandibular articulation is achieved.

CHAPTER 17

The edentulous mouth

If the teeth are lost, maxilla and mandible undergo a disuse atrophy (Figs. 17-1 to 17-4). The first to disappear is the alveolar process, but the atrophy eventually may involve parts of the bodies of the maxilla and the mandible.

The skeletal changes lead to a considerable change in the configuration of the residual bony ridge in the upper and lower jaws. In the upper jaw there is often a narrowing of the arch compared with the width of the dental arch before the teeth had been lost. The shrinkage of the arch in the molar region is usually negligible, but in the premolar, canine, and incisor areas it may be pronounced. A shortening of the arch or a retraction of the ridge in the area of the incisors and canines is especially striking and increases in persons with pronounced prognathism. The reason for the reduction of the circumference of the upper arch is the oblique implantation of the teeth in an alveolar process that is itself inclined laterally and anteriorly. Thus the circumference of the alveolar base, that is, of the bone of the maxillary body that carries the alveolar process, is smaller than that of the arch of the former alveolar crest or of the teeth. The obliquity of the alveolar process is slight in the molar region, but it increases anteriorly in most persons.

In the mandible there is often a widening of the arch of the remaining ridge in the molar region as compared with the dental arch before loss of teeth. This is caused by the lingual inclination of the mandibular molars and their alveolar process. In the anterior region of the lower jaw the changes of the arch vary individually because of the variable inclination of the lower canines and incisors and the alveolar process in this region. There may be an enlargement of the anterior parts of the arch if the alveolar process is inclined posteriorly or, much more frequently, a shortening of the arch if the alveolar process is inclined anteriorly.

In some persons with pronounced inclination of the teeth, the loss of teeth may bring about a considerable and, for the prosthodontist, awkward incongruence between the reduced upper arch and the widened lower arch. In others the atrophy of the alveolar process may not greatly change or may more uniformly change the shape and dimensions of the arches.

If the disuse atrophy involves part of the body of the maxillae and mandible (Figs. 17-1 to 17-3), the residual ridge may gain relation to bony structures normally far removed from the alveolar process. In the upper jaw the ridge may approach the base of the anterior nasal spine, which then seems to be an anterior projection of the ridge

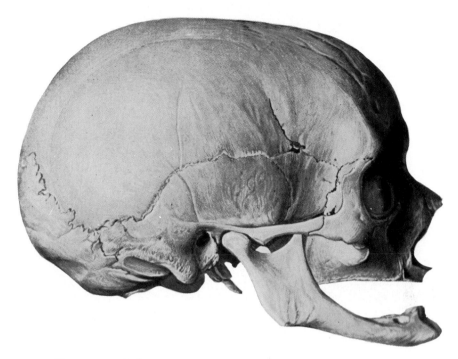

Fig. 17-1. Senile female skull. (Sicher and Tandler: Anatomie für Zahnärzte.)

itself. The atrophy in the molar region may reach to the lower end of the zygomati-coalveolar crest, which then seems to arise in a wide field from the bony rim of the maxilla and to curve almost horizontally outward. At the posterior end the atrophy of the upper jaw may go so far that the hamulus of the pterygoid process protrudes below the level of the alveolar ridge. In extreme cases of atrophy the floor of the maxillary sinus may be thin, and defects of the bony sinus floor have been observed.

If the atrophy of the lower alveolar process involves the upper part of the mandibular body, the ridge sinks to the level of the mental protuberance in front and to the level of the mental spines in back of the chin plate. Thus the impression is created that the alveolar ridge itself projects forward as the broad bony chin and lingually as the pointed, and sometimes divided, mental spine. In the distal region the atrophy of the lower alveolar process may reach the level of the oblique line, where it continues from the anterior border of the mandibular ramus. This strongly prominent bony ridge may then be at the level or even above the level of the alveolar ridge. The most posterior end of the alveolar ridge then continues without visible boundary into the lower part of the temporal crest.

In cases of extreme disuse atrophy of the mandible the upper border of the bone gradually approaches the level of the mandibular canal and the mental foramen. The mental foramen may be situated immediately below and sometimes even at the alve-

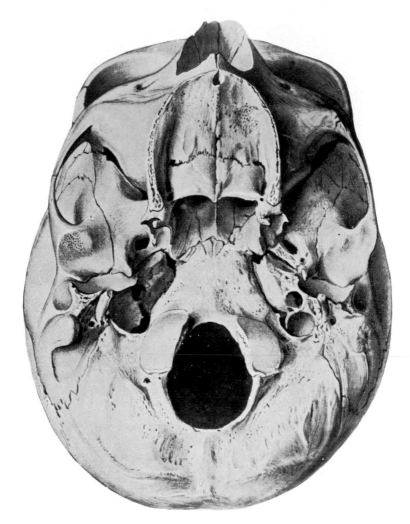

Fig. 17-2. Senile female cranium, inferior view. Same skull as shown in Fig. 17-1. (Sicher and Tandler: Anatomie für Zahnärzte.)

olar ridge in the premolar region. The upper wall of the mandibular canal may become extremely thin, and defects of this wall have been noted (Fig. 17-4).

After loss of teeth the alveolar ridge is, under normal conditions, covered by a tissue that is identical in its structure with normal gingiva. It is a firm, thick layer of inelastic dense connective tissue, immovably attached to the periosteum of the ridge and covered by a keratinized or parakeratinized stratified squamous epithelium. In the living the distal end of the upper alveolar ridge remains always sharply demarcated against the loosely textured and movably attached mucosa at the roof of the soft palate. However, the notch that had existed behind the prominent alveolar tubercle and the retromolar papilla gradually loses depth and may even disappear.

In the lower jaw the distal end of the gingival area is also well marked. The

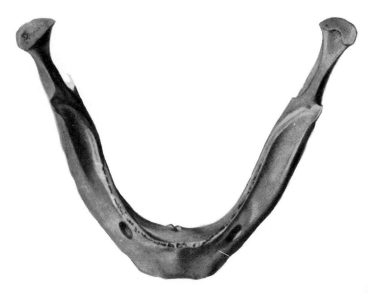

Fig. 17-3. Senile female mandible. Same skull as shown in Fig. 17-1. (Sicher and Tandler: Anatomie für Zahnärzte.)

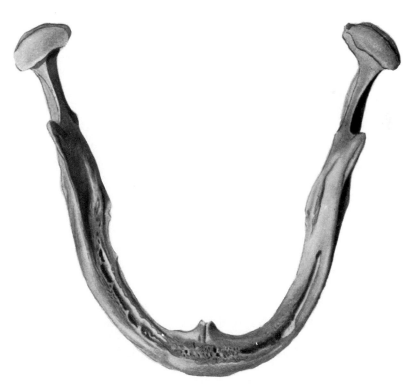

Fig. 17-4. Extreme atrophy of an edentulous mandible, exposing the mandibular canal. (Greiner: Z. Stomatol. **21:**547, 1923.)

mucous membrane protrudes behind and above the remnants of the retromolar papilla as the retromolar pad. This small bulging area of the mucous membrane remains approximately in its former position on the slope of the temporal crest because the atrophy at the distal end of the lower alveolar process does not proceed farther downward but is halted at the oblique lower end of the temporal crest and retromolar fossa. Thus the retromolar pad may be used as a landmark for the reestablishment of the occlusal plane that had been 2 to 4 mm. above this prominence.

After loss of the last molar, the retromolar papilla, fused to the scar at the site of the last molar, forms the widened and rounded distal end of the gingival covering of the alveolar ridge. The name "pear-shaped area" has been used to designate this prominence, which is often confused with the retromolar pad. The difference in consistency and color makes differentiation in most persons easy: the retromolar pad is soft and dark red; the retromolar papilla and the entire "pear-shaped area" are firm and pale.

In extreme cases of mandibular atrophy the alveolar ridge sinks below the floor of the sublingual sulcus and the sublingual glands may then protrude above the level of the alveolar ridge, especially during contraction of the mylohyoid muscle in swallowing.

The atrophy of the jaws will proceed toward the lines of origin of those muscles which are attached to the base or near the base of the alveolar process. In the upper jaw these muscles are the buccinator muscle in the molar region, and the upper incisive and nasal muscles in the anterior region. In the lower jaw the buccinator muscle, and lower incisive, and the mental muscles arise from the base of the alveolar process. On the inner surface the mylohyoid and genioglossus muscles originate at the level of a reduced alveolar ridge. The disuse atrophy may even pass the line of attachment of one or another of these muscles, especially that of the buccinator muscle. The muscle fibers then lose their direct attachment to the bone and gain an indirect fibrous attachment through the remnants of the periosteum.

With all these changes the rest position of the mandible decreases gradually after all teeth are lost. But, as stated before, the rest position of the mandible is dependent not on the existence, the position, or the shape and size of the teeth, but solely on the tonus of the elevators of the jaw—the masseter, temporal, and medial pterygoid muscles.

The importance of the rest position of the mandible in the construction of dentures is well known. If the bite is raised beyond the rest position, the mandibular muscles are stretched, and muscle spasms are the result.

It has been observed that immediately after loss of the last occluding teeth a person is not able to close the jaws far beyond the former occlusal position. This has little to do with the new functional situation of the muscles but is caused primarily by resistance of parts of the craniomandibular ligaments and the capsule.

Bibliography

Chapter 1—INTRODUCTION

Alexander, R. M.: Animal mechanics (biology series), London, 1968, Sidgwick & Jackson.

Campbell, B. G.: Human evolution, Chicago, 1970, Aldine Publishing Co.

Clark, W. E. L.: The fossil evidence for human evolution, Chicago, 1955, The University of Chicago Press.

Coon, C. S., Garn, S. M., and Birdsell, J. B.: A study of the problems of race formation in man, Springfield, Ill., 1950, Charles C Thomas, Publisher.

DuBrul, E. L.: Evolution of the speech apparatus. Monograph, American Lecture Series No. 328, Springfield, Ill., 1958, Charles C Thomas, Publisher.

DuBrul, E. L.: Biomechanics of the body, BSCS Pamphlet No. 5, Boston, 1965, D. C. Heath & Co.

DuBrul, E. L.: Design for living. In Bootzin, D., and Muffley, H. C., editors: Biomechanics, New York, 1969, Plenum Press.

DuBrul, E. L.: Origin and evolution of the oral apparatus. In Kawamura, Y., editor: Frontiers of oral physiology, vol. 1, New York, 1974, S. Karger.

DuBrul, E. L.: Form and function, biological, Encyclopaedia Britannica 3, Macropaedia 7: 542-547, 1974.

Frost, H. M.: Introduction to biomechanics, Springfield, Ill., 1971, Charles C Thomas, Publisher.

Grassé, P.-P., editor: Traité de zoologie, tome 12, Paris, 1954, Masson et Cie.

Gray, J.: How animals move, Cambridge, Mass., 1960, Cambridge University Press.

Gray, J.: Animal locomotion, New York, 1968, W. W. Norton & Co., Inc.

Gregory, W. K.: Our face from fish to man, New York, 1965, G. P. Putnam's Sons.

Halstead, L. B.: Vertebrate hard tissues. The Wykenham science series, New York, 1974, Springer-Verlag New York Inc.

Kelley, D. L.: Kinesiology: fundamentals of motion description, Englewood Cliffs, N. J., 1971, Prentice-Hall, Inc.

Kurtén, B.: The age of mammals, New York, 1972, Columbia University Press.

Miller, D. I., and Nelson, R. C.: Biomechanics of sport, Philadelphia, 1973, Lea & Febiger.

Piveteau, J.: Le problème du crane. In Grassé, P.-P., editor: Traité de zoologie, tome 12, Paris, 1954, Masson et Cie.

Romer, A. S.: The vertebrate body, ed. 4, Philadelphia, 1970, W. B. Saunders Co.

Schmidt-Nielsen, K.: Living machines—how animals work, New York, 1972, Cambridge University Press.

Smith, J. M., and Savage, R. J. C.: The mechanics of mammalian jaws, Sch. Sci. Rev. 141:289-301, 1959.

Stanley-Jones, D., and Stanley-Jones, K.: The kybernetics of natural systems, New York, 1960, Pergamon Press.

Young, J. Z.: The life of vertebrates, Oxford, 1955, The University Press.

Chapter 2—THE SKULL

Ahrens, H. J.: Die Entwicklung der Spaltleinienarchitektur des knöchernen menschlichen Schädels, Morphol. Jahrb. 77:357-371, 1936.

Badoux, D. M.: Framed structures in the mammalian skull. (From the Institute of Veterinary Anatomy, Utrecht, The Netherlands.) Reprinted from Acta Morphol. Neerl. Scand. 6:239-250, 1966.

Benninghoff, A.: Spaltlinien am Knochen, eine Methode zur Ermittlung der Architektur platter Knochen, Verhandl. Anat. Anz. 60:189-206, 1925.

Björk, A.: The face in profile: an anthropological X-ray investigation on Swedish children and conscripts, Sven. Tandläk. Tidskr., vol. 40, no. 5B, Lund, 1947, Berlingska Boktryckeriet.

Brodie, A. G.: On the growth pattern of the human head, from the third month to the eighth year of life, Am. J. Anat. 68:209-262, 1941.

541

Brodie, A. G.: Late growth changes in the human face, Angle Orthod. 23:146-157, 1953.

Clark, W. E. L.: Man-apes or ape-men? New York, 1967, Holt, Rinehart & Winston, Inc.

Cobb, W. M.: The craniofacial union and the maxillary tubes in mammals, Am. J. Anat. 72:39-111, 1943.

Coon, C. S., Garn, S. M., and Birdsell, J. B.: A study of the problems of race formation in man, Springfield, Ill., 1950, Charles C Thomas, Publisher.

Crelin, E. S.: Anatomy of the newborn: an atlas, Philadelphia, 1969, Lea & Febiger.

DeBeer, G. R.: Development of the vertebrate skull, Oxford, 1971, Clarendon Press.

DuBrul, E. L.: Posture, locomotion and the skull in lagamorpha, Am. J. Anat. 87:277-314, 1950.

DuBrul, E. L.: The skull of the lion Marmoset *Leontideus rosalia* Linnaeus: a study in biomechanical adaptation, Am. J. Phys. Anthropol. 23:261-276, 1965.

DuBrul, E. L.: Origin and evolution of the oral apparatus. In Kawamura, Y., editor: Frontiers of oral physiology, vol. 1, New York, 1974, S. Karger.

DuBrul, E. L., and Sicher, H.: The adaptive chin. Monograph, American Lecture Series, Pub. No. 180, Springfield, Ill., 1954, Charles C Thomas, Publisher.

DuBrul, E. L., and Laskin, D. M.: Preadaptive potentialities of the mammalian skull: an experiment in growth and form, Am. J. Anat. 109:117-132, 1961.

Enlow, D. H.: The human face, New York, 1968, Harper & Row.

Evans, F. G.: Stress and strain in bones, Springfield, Ill., 1957, Charles C Thomas, Publisher.

Hylander, W. L.: Functional significance of primate mandibular form, J. Morphol 160:223-240, 1979.

Koch, J. C.: The laws of bone architecture, Am. J. Anat. 21:177-298, 1917.

Koski, K., and Ronning, O: Growth potential of intracerebrally transplanted cranial base synchondroses, Acta. Odontol. Scand. 15:1107-1108, 1970.

Moyers, R. E., and Krogman, W. M.: Craniofacial growth in man, New York, 1971. Pergamon Press.

Radin, E. L., Paul, I. L., and Rose, R. M.: Role of mechanical factors in pathogenesis of primary osteoarthritis, Lancet 1:519-521, 1972.

Robinson, J. T.: Tooth and jaw in the assessment of the origins of man. In Person, P., editor: Biology of the mouth, AAAS Pub. No. 89, pp. 67-78, 1968.

Scapino, R. P.: Adaptive radiation of mammalian jaws. In Schumacher, G., editor: Morphology of the maxillo-mandibular apparatus, Leipzig 1972, VEB Georg Thieme.

Scott, J. H.: Muscle growth and function in relation to skeletal morphology, Am. J. Phys. Anthropol. 15:197-233, 1957.

Seipel, C. M.: Trajectories of the jaws, Acta Odontol. Scand. 8:81-191, 1948.

Tappen, N. C. A.: A functional analysis of the facial skeleton with split-line technique, Am. J. Phys. Anthropol. 11:503-532, 1953.

Vilman, H.: Osteogenesis in the basioccipital bone of the Wistar albino rat, Scand. J. Dent. Res. 80:410-421, 1972.

Weidenreich, F.: Die Sonderform des Menschenschädels als Anpassung an den aufrechten Gang., Ztschr. f. Morphol. u. Anthropol. 24:157-189, 1924.

Weidenreich, F.: The brain and its role in the phylogenetic transformation of the human skull. Trans. Am. Phil. Soc. 31:321-442, 1941.

Weidenreich, F.: The skull of Sinanthropus Pekinensis, Paleontologia Sinica (n.s.) 10:Whole Series No. 127, Dec., 1943.

Weiner, J. A.: The piltdown forgery, New York, 1955, Oxford University Press.

Chapter 3—THE MUSCULATURE

Ahlgren, J.: Mechanism of mastication, Acta Odontol. Scand. 24(supp. 44):5-109, 1966.

Barghusen, H. R.: The lower jaw of cynodonts (Reptilia, Therapsida) and the evolutionary origin of mammal-like adductor jaw musculature, Postilla 116:1-49, 1968.

Basmajian, J. V.: Muscles alive, ed. 3, Baltimore, 1974, The Williams & Wilkins Co.

Bloom, W., and Fawcett, D. W.: A textbook of histology, Philadelphia, 1975, W. B. Saunders Co.

Bourne, G. H.: The structure and function of muscle, vol. 2, New York, 1960, Academic Press.

Bourne, G. H.: The structure and function of muscle, vol. 3, New York, 1960, Academic Press.

Carlsöö, S.: Nervous coordination and mechanical function of the mandibular elevators, Acta Odontol. Scand. 10(supp. 10-12, II):1-126, 1952.

Carlsöö, S.: An electromyographic study of the activity of certain suprahyoid muscles (mainly the anterior belly of digastric muscle) and of the reciprocal innervation of the elevator and depressor musculature of the mandible, Acta Anat. 26:81-93, 1956.

Carlsöö, S.: An electromyographic study of the activity, and an analysis of the mechanics of the lateral pterygoid muscle, Acta. Anat. 26:339-351, 1956.

Carlsöö, S.: Motor units and action potentials in the masticatory muscles, Acta Morphol. Neerl. Scand. 2:13-19, 1958.

Gaspard, M.: Éléments de myologie fonctionnelle. In Grassé, P.-P., editor: Traité de zoologie, tome 16, fasc. 2, Paris, 1968, Masson et Cie.

Honée, G. L. J. M.: The anatomy of the lateral pterygoid muscle, Acta Morphol. Neerl. Scand. 10:331-340, 1972.

Huber, E.: Evolution of facial musculature and facial expression, Baltimore, 1931, The Johns Hopkins Press.

Inman, V. T., Saunders, J. B. de C. M., and Abbott, L. C.: Observations on the function of the shoulder joint, J. Bone Joint Surg. 26A:1-20, 1944.

Latif, A.: An electromyographic study of the temporal muscle in normal persons during selected positions and movements of the mandible, Am. J. Orthod. 43:577-591, 1957.

Møller, E.: The chewing apparatus, Acta Physiol. Scand. 69(supp. 280):1-229, 1966.

Møller, E.: Action of the muscles of mastication. In Kawamura, Y., editor: Frontiers of oral physiology, vol. 1, New York, 1974, S. Karger.

Moyers, R. E.: An electromyographic analysis of certain muscles involved in temporomandibular movement, Am. J. Orthod. 37:481-515, 1950.

Ringquist, M.: A histochemical study of temporal muscle fibers in denture wearers and subjects with natural dentition, Scand. J. Dent. Res. 82:29-39, 1974.

Ringquist, M.: The histochemical profile of the human masseter, J. Neurol. Sci. 30:189-200, 1976.

Schumacher, G. H.: Funktionelle morphologie der kaumuskulatur, Jena, 1961, VEB Gustav Verlag.

Smith, J. M., and Savage, R. J. C.: The mechanics of mammalian jaws, Sch. Sci. Rev. 141:289-301, 1959.

Taylor, A.: Fibre types in the muscles of mastication. In Anderson, D. J., and Matthews, B., editors: Mastication, Bristol, Eng., 1976, John Wright & Sons Ltd.

Chapter 4—CRANIOMANDIBULAR ARTICULATION

Arstad, T.: The capsular ligaments of the temporomandibular joint and retrusion facets of the dentition in relationship to mandibular movements, Oslo, 1954, Akademisk Forlag.

Barnett, C. H., Davies, D. V., and MacConaill, M. A.: Synovial joints: their structure and mechanics, Springfield, Ill., 1961, Charles C Thomas, Publisher.

Bennett, N. G.: A contribution to the study of the movements of the mandible, J. Prosthet. Dent. 8:41-54, 1958.

Carlsöö, S.: Nervous coordination and mechanical function of the mandibular elevators, Acta Odontol. Scand. 10(supp. 10-12 II):1-126, 1952.

Charnley, J.: How our joints are lubricated, Triangle 4:175-179, 1960.

Dahlberg, B.: The masticatory effect, Acta Med. Scand. 139(supp.):3-156, 1942.

DuBrul, E. L.: Early hominid feeding mechanisms, Am. J. Phys. Anthropol. 47:305-320, 1977.

DuBrul, E. L.: Origin and adaptations of the hominid jaw joint. In Sarnat, B. G., and Laskin, D. M., editors: The temporomandibular joint, ed. 3, Springfield, Ill., 1979, Charles C Thomas, Publisher.

Frankel, V. H., Burstein, A. H., and Brooks, D. B.: Biomechanics of internal derangement of the knee, J. Bone Joint Surg. 53A(5):945-962, 1971.

Furstman, L.: The early development of the human temporomandibular joint, Am. J. Orthod. 49:672-682, 1963.

Gaspard, M.: Essai d'analyse bio-mecanique comparative de la mastication chez les carnivores, les anthropoides et l'homme, Rev. Fr. Odontostomatol. 1:85-108, 1967.

Gibbs, C. H., Messerman, T., Reswick, J. B., and Derda, H. J.: Functional movements of the mandible, J. Prosthet. Dent. 26:604-620, 1971.

Grant, P. G.: Biomechanical significance of the instantaneous center of rotation: the human temporomandibular joint, J. Biomechanics 6:109-113, 1973.

Greaves, W. S.: The jaw lever system in ungulates; a new model, J. Zool. Lond. 184:271-285, 1978.

Griffin, C. J., and Malor, R.: An analysis of mandibular movement. In Kawamura, Y., editor: Frontiers of oral physiology, vol. 1, New York, 1974, S. Karger.

Herring, S. W., and Herring, S. E.: The superficial masseter and gape in mammals, Am. Natur. 108:561-576, 1974.

Hickey, J. C., Allison, M. L., Woelfel, J. B., and others: Mandibular movements in three dimensions, J. Prosthet. Dent. 13:72-92, 1963.

Hiiemae, K. M.: Masticatory function in the mammals, J. Dent. Res. 46:883-893, 1967.

Hjortsjö, C.-H.: Views of the general principles of joints and movements, Acta Orthop. Scand. 29:134-145, 1959.

Honée, G. L. J. M.: The anatomy of the lateral pterygoid muscle, Acta Morphol. Neerl. Scand. 10:331-340, 1972.

Inman, V. T., Saunders, J. B. de C. M., and Abbott, L. C.: Observations on the function of the shoulder joint, J. Bone Joint Surg. 26A:1-30, 1944.

Ireland, V. E.: The problem of "the clicking jaw," Proc. Roy. Soc. Med. 44:363-372, 1951.

Kawamura, Y.: Neuromuscular mechanisms of jaw and tongue movement, J. Am. Dent. Assoc. 62:545-551, 1961.

Kawamura, Y.: Recent concepts of the physiology of mastication, Adv. Oral Biol. 1:77-109, 1964.

Lindblom, G.: On the anatomy and function of the temporomandibular joint, Acta Odontol. Scand. 17(supp. 28): 287, 1960.

Messerman, T., Reswick, J. B., and Gibbs, C.: Investigation of functional mandibular movements, Dent. Clin. North Am. 13:629-642, 1969.

Møller, E.: The chewing apparatus, Acta Physiol. Scand. 69(supp. 280):1, 1966.

Moss, M. L.: A functional cranial analysis of centric relation, Dent. Clin. North Am. 19:431-442, 1975.

Noble, H. W.: Comparative functional anatomy of the temporomandibular joint. In Melcher, A. H., and Zarb, G. A., editors: Oral sciences reviews, temporomandibular joint—function and dysfunction, vol. 2, Copenhagen, 1973, Munksgaard.

Posselt, U.: Physiology of occlusion and rehabilitation, Oxford, 1969, Blackwell Scientific Publications.

Ramfjord, S. P., and Ash, M. M., Jr.: Occlusion, Philadelphia, 1966, W. B. Saunders Co.

Rees, L. A.: The structure and function of the mandibular joint, Br. Dent. J. 96:125-133, 1954.

Sarnat, B. G., and Laskin, D. M., editors: The temporomandibular joint, ed. 3, Springfield, Ill., 1979, Charles C Thomas, Publisher.

Scapino, R. P.: The third joint of the canine jaw, J. Morphol. 116:23-50, 1965.

Schwartz, L.: Disorders of the temporomandibular joint, Philadelphia, 1959, W. B. Saunders Co.

Scott, J. H.: The development of joints concerned with early jaw movements in the sheep, J. Anat. 85:36-43, 1951.

Sicher, H.: Structural and functional basis for disorders of the temporomandibular articulation, J. Oral Surg. 13:275-279, 1955.

Sicher, H.: The biologic significance of hinge axis determination, J. Prosthet. Dent. 6:616-620, 1956.

Thilander, B.: Innervation of the temporo-mandibular joint capsule in man, Transactions of the Royal Schools of Dentistry, Stockholm & Umeä No. 7 (Publications of the Umeä Research Library—Series 2:7), 1961.

Chapter 5—THE VISCERA
The tongue

Ardran, G. M., and Kemp, F. H.: A radiographic study of movements of the tongue in swallowing, Dent. Pract. 5:252-263, 1955.

Bowman, J. P.: Muscle spindles in the intrinsic and extrinsic muscles of the Rhesus monkey's (Macaca mulatta) tongue, Anat. Rec. 161:483-488, 1968.

Cooper, S.: Muscle spindles in the intrinsic muscles of the human tongue, J. Physiol. 122:193-202, 1953.

Sussman, H. M.: What the tongue tells the brain, Psych. Bull. 77:262-272, 1972.

Salivary glands

Burgen, A. S. V., and Emmelin, N. G.: Physiology of the salivary glands, London, 1961, Edward Arnold Publishers, Ltd.

Dentition

Beyron, H.: Occlusal relations and mastication in Australian Aborigines, Acta Odontol. Scand. 22:597-678, 1964.

Black, G. V.: Descriptive anatomy of the human teeth, ed. 5, Philadelphia, 1902, S. S. White Dental Mfg. Co.

Brabant, H.: Comparison of the characteristics and anomalies of the deciduous and the permanent dentition, J. Dent. Res. 46:897-902, 1967.

Brothwell, D. R.: Dental anthropology, Oxford, 1963, Pergamon Press.

Butler, P. M.: A theory of the evolution of mammalian molar teeth, Am. J. Sci. 239:421-450, 1941.

Crompton, A. W., and Hiiemäe, K.: How mammalian molar teeth work, Discovery 5(1):23-34, 1969.

Dahlberg, A. A.: Dental morphology and evolution, Chicago, 1971, The University of Chicago Press.

Fearnhead, R. W., and Stack, M. V.: Tooth enamel. II. Its composition, properties and fundamental structure, Bristol, Eng., 1971, John Wright & Sons, Ltd.

Gregory, W. K.: The origin and evolution of the human dentition, Baltimore, 1922, The Williams and Wilkins Co.

Gustafson, A. G.: The similarity between contralateral pairs of teeth, Odontol. Tidskr. 63:245-248, 1955.

Korenhof, C. A. W.: Morphogenetical aspects of the human upper molar, Utrecht, 1960, Druk, Uitgeversmaatschappij Neerlandia.

Murphy, T. R.: Reduction of the dental arch by approximal attrition. Br. Dent. J. 116:483-488, 1964.

Osborn, J. W.: The evolution of dentitions, Am. Sci. 61:548-559, 1973.

Patterson, B.: Early Cretaceous mammals and the evolution of mammalian molar teeth, Fieldiana, Geology 13:1-105, 1956.

Pedersen, P. L., and Scott, D. B.: Replica studies of the surfaces of teeth from Alaskan Eskimo, West Greenland natives, and American whites, Acta Odontol. Scand. 9:262-292, 1951.

Scott, J. H., and Symons, N. B. B.: Introduction to dental anatomy, ed. 6, Edinburgh, 1971, E. & S. Livingstone, Ltd.

Sutton, P. R. N.: Transverse crack lines in permanent incisors of Polynesians, Aust. Dent. J. 6:144-150, 1961.

Wheeler, R. C.: A textbook of dental anatomy and physiology, ed. 4, Philadelphia, 1965, W. B. Saunders Co.

Williams, C. H. M.: Investigation concerning the dentitions of the Eskimos of Canada's Eastern Arctic, J. Periodontol. 14:34-37, 1943.

Supporting structures

Grant, D. A., Stern, I. B., and Everett, F. G., editors. Orban's periodontics: a concept—theory and practice, ed. 4, St. Louis, 1972, The C. V. Mosby Co.

Orban, B., and Sicher, H.: The oral mucosa, J. Dent. Educ. 10:94-103, 1945.

Osborne, J. W.: Investigation into the interdental forces occurring between the teeth of the same arch during the clenching of the jaws, Arch. Oral. Biol. 5:202-211, 1961.

Scapino, R. P.: Biomechanics of masticatory and lining mucosa. In Squier, C. A., and Meyer, J., editors: Current concepts of the histology of oral mucosa, Springfield, Ill., 1971, Charles C Thomas, Publisher.

Sicher, H., and Bhaskar, S. N., editors: Orban's oral histology and embryology, ed. 7, St. Louis, 1972, The C. V. Mosby Co.

Weinmann, J. P., and Sicher, H.: Bone and bones: fundamentals of bone biology, ed. 2, St. Louis, 1955, The C. V. Mosby Co.

Chapter 6—THE OROPHARYNGEAL SYSTEM
The pharynx

Adams, W. S.: The transverse dimensions of the nasopharynx in child and adult with observations on its contractile function, J. Laryngol. Otol. 72:465-471, 1958.

Astley, R.: The movements of the lateral walls of the nasopharynx: a cine-radiographic study, J. Laryngol. Otol. 72:325-328, 1958.

Azzam, N. A., and Kuehn, D. P.: The morphology of musculus uvulae, Cleft Palate J. 14:78-87, 1977.

Basmajian, J. V., and Dutta, C. R.: Electromyography of the pharyngeal constrictors and levator palati in man, Anat. Rec. 139:561-563, 1961.

Bosma, J. F.: Myology of the pharynx of cat, dog, and monkey with interpretations of the mechanisms of swallowing, Ann. Otol. Laryngol. 65:981-993, 1956.

Bosma, J. F.: Studies of the pharynx. I. Poliomyelitic disabilities of the upper pharynx, Pediatrics 19:881-907, 1957.

Bosma, J. F.: Deglutition: pharyngeal stage, Physiol. Rev. 37:275-300, 1957.

Bosma, J. F.: The third symposium on oral sensation and perception: the mouth of the infant, Springfield, Ill., 1972, Charles C Thomas, Publisher.

Bosma, J. F.: Form and function in the infant's mouth and pharynx. In Bosma, J. F., editor: Oral sensation and perception, Springfield, Ill., 1973, Charles C Thomas, Publisher.

Bosma, J. F., and Fletcher, S. G.: The upper pharynx, Ann. Otol. Rhinol. Laryngol. 71:134-157, 1962.

Shipp, T., and Deatsch, W. W.: Pharyngoesophageal muscle activity during swallowing in man, Laryngoscope 80(1):1-16, 1970.

Whillis, M. B.: A note on the muscles of the palate and the superior constrictor, J. Anat. 65:92-95, 1930.

Wood-Jones, F.: The nature of the soft palate, J. Anat. 74:147-170, 1940.

The larynx

Ardran, G. M., and Kemp, F. H.: The protection of the laryngeal airway during swallowing, Br. J. Radiol. 25:406-416, 1952.

Ardran, G. M., and Kemp. F. H.: The mechanism of the larynx. I. The movements of the arytenoid and cricoid cartilages, Br. J. Radiol. 39:641-654, 1966.

Ardran, G. M., and Kemp, F. H.: The mechanism of the larynx. II. The epiglottis and closure of the larynx, Br. J. Radiol. 40:372-389, 1967.

Keleman, G.: Vergleichende anatomie und physiologie der stimmorgane (eine bibliographie), Archiv für Sprach-und Stimmphysiologie und Sprachund Stimmheilkwnde 3:Heft IV, 1939.

Negus, V. E.: The mechanism of the larynx, London, 1929, Messrs. Heinemann (Medical Books) Ltd.

Negus, V. E.: Mechanism of swallowing, Proc. Roy. Soc. Med. 36:84-97, 1943.

Negus, V. E.: Comparative anatomy and physiology of the larynx, New York, 1949, Grune & Stratton, Inc.

Pressman, J. J.: Sphincter action of the larynx, Arch. Otolaryngol. 33:351-377, 1941.

Pressman, J. J.: Physiology of the larynx, Physiol. Rev. 35:506-554, 1955.

Von Leden, H., and Moore, P.: Mechanics of cricoarytenoid joint, Arch. Otolaryngol. 73:541-550, 1961.

Swallowing and speech

Ardran, G. M., and Kemp, F. H.: The mechanism of swallowing, Proc. Roy. Soc. Med. 44:1038-1040, 1951.

Ardran, G. M., and Kemp, F. H.: A radiographic study of movements of the tongue in swallowing, Dent. Pract. 5:252-263, 1955.

Ardran, G. M., and Kemp, F. H.: A cine-radiographic study of bottle feeding, Br. J. Radiol. 31:11-22, 1958.

Ardran, G. M., and Kemp, F. H.: The mechanism of the larynx. I. The movements of the arytenoid and cricoid cartilages, Br. J. Radiol. 39:641-654, 1966.

Basmajian, J. V.: Muscles alive, ed. 3, Baltimore, 1974, The Williams & Wilkins Co.

Basmajian, J. V., and Dutta, C. R.: Electromyography of the pharyngeal constrictors and levator palati in man, Anat. Rec. 139:561-563, 1961.

Benediktsson, E.: Variation in tongue and jaw position in "S" sound production in relation to front teeth occlusion, Acta Odontol. Scand. 15:275-303, 1958.

Bloomer, H. H.: A palatopograph for contour mapping of the palate, J. Am. Dent. Assoc. 30:1053-1057, 1943.

Bloomer, H. H.: Observations of palatopharyngeal movements in speech and deglutition, J. Speech Hear. Disord. 18:230-246, 1953.

Bosma, J. F.: Studies of the pharynx. I. Poliomyelitic disabilities of the upper pharynx, Pediatrics 19:881-907, 1957.

Bowman, J. P., and Combs, C. M.: The cerebrocortical projection of hypoglossal afferents, Exp. Neurol. 23:291-301, 1969.

Calnan, J. S.: Movements of the soft palate, Speech (London) 19(1):14-20, 1955.

Carrell, J., and Tiffany, W.: Phonetics: theory and application to speech improvement, New York, 1960, McGraw-Hill Book Co.

Chiba, T., and Kajiyama, M.: The vowel, its nature and structure, Tokyo, 1941, Tokyo-Kaiseikan Publishing Co., Ltd.

Davenport, H. W.: Physiology of the digestive tract, ed. 2, Chicago, 1966, Year Book Medical Publishers, Inc.

Denes, P., and Pinson, E.: The speech chain, New York, 1963, Bell Telephone Laboratories.

Doty, R. W., and Bosma, J. F.: An electromyographic analysis of reflex deglutition, J. Neurophysiol. 19:44-60, 1956.

DuBrul, E. L.: Evolution of the speech apparatus, Monograph, American Lecture Series No. 328, Springfield, Ill., 1958, Charles C Thomas Publisher.

DuBrul, E. L.: Structural evidence in the brain for a theory of the evolution of behavior, Perspect. Biol. Med. 4(1):40-57, 1960.

DuBrul, E. L.: Pattern of genetic control of structure in the evolution of behavior, Perspect. Biol. Med. 10(4):524-539, 1967.

DuBrul, E. L.: Origin of the speech apparatus and its reconstruction in fossils, Brain Lang. 4:365-381, 1977.

Fant, G.: Acoustic theory of speech production, The Hague, 1970, Mouton & Co.

Findlay, I. A., and Kilpatrick, S. J.: An analysis of myographic records of swallowing in normal and abnormal subjects, J. Dent. Res. 39:629-637, 1960.

Fujimura, O.: Bilabial stop and nasal consonants: a motion picture study and its acoustical implications, J. Speech Hear. Res. 4:233-247, 1961.

Herring, S. W., and Scapino, R. P.: Physiology of feeding in miniature pigs, J. Morphol. 141:427-460, 1973.

Kaplan, H. M.: Anatomy and physiology of speech, ed. 2, New York, 1971, McGraw-Hill Book Co.

MacNeilage, P. F.: Motor control of serial ordering of speech, Psychol. Rev. 77:182-196, 1970.

MacNeilage, P. F., and Sholes, G. N.: An electromyographic study of the tongue during vowel production, J. Speech Hear. Res. 7:209-232, 1964.

Negus, V. E.: Mechanism of swallowing, Proc. Roy. Soc. Med. 36:84-97, 1943.

Perkell, J. S.: Physiology of speech production: results and implications of a quantitative cin-eradiographic study (research monograph no. 53), Cambridge, Mass., 1969, The M.I.T. Press.

Pommerenke, W. T.: A study of the sensory areas eliciting the swallowing reflex, Am. J. Physiol. 84:36-41, 1928.

Potter, R. K., Kopp, G. A., and Green, H. C.: Visible speech, New York, 1947, D. van Nostrand Co., Inc.

Saunders, J. B. de C. M., Davis, C., and Miller, E. R.: The mechanism of deglutition as revealed by cine-radiography, Ann. Otol. Rhinol. Laryngol. 60:897-916, 1951.

Seto, H.: The sensory innervation of the oral cavity in the human fetus and juvenile mammals. In Bosma, J. F., editor: Oral sensation and perception, Springfield, Ill., 1972, Charles C Thomas, Publisher.

Shipp, T., and Deatsch, W. W.: Pharyngoesophageal muscle activity during swallowing in man, Laryngoscope 80:(1):1-16,1970.

Sussman, H. M., and Smith, K. U.: Jaw movements under delayed auditory feedback, J. Acoustical Soc. Am. 50:685-691, 1971.

Chapter 7—THE BLOOD VESSELS

Bell, W. H.: Revascularization and bone healing after anterior maxillary osteotomy: a study using adult rhesus monkeys, J. Oral Surg. 27:249-255, 1969.

Bell, W. H., and Levy, B. M.: Revascularization and bone healing after anterior mandibular osteotomy, J. Oral Surg. 28:196-203, 1970.

Bell, W. H., and Levy, B. M.: Revascularization and bone healing after posterior maxillary osteotomy, J. Oral Surg. 29:313-320, 1971.

Bell, W. H., and Levy, B. M.: Revascularization and bone healing after maxillary corticotomies, J. Oral Surg. 30:640-648, 1972.

Bishop, J. G., and Dorman, H. L.: Control of blood circulation in oral tissues. In Staple, P. H., editor: Advances in oral biology, vol. 3, London, 1968, Academic Press.

Bishop, J. G., Gage, T. W., Matthews, J. L., and Dorman, H. L.: Circulation. In Squier, C. A., and Meyer, J., editors: Current concepts of the histology of oral mucosa, Springfield, Ill., 1971, Charles C Thomas, Publisher.

Boyd, T. G., Castelli, W. A., and Huelke, D. F.: Arterial supply of the guinea pig mandible, J. Dent. Res. 46:1064-1067, 1967.

Boyne, P. J.: Fluorescence microscopy of bone healing following mandibular ridge resection, J. Oral Surg. 16:749-756, 1963.

Boyne, P. J.: Physiology of bone and response of osseous tissue to injury and environmental changes, J. Oral Surg. 28:12-16, 1970.

Castelli, W. A.: Vascular architecture of the human adult mandible, J. Dent. Res. 42:786-792, 1963.

Castelli, W. A., and Huelke, D. F.: The arterial system of the head and neck of the rhesus monkey with emphasis on the external carotid system, Am. J. Anat. 116:149-169, 1965.

Cernavakis, N., and Hunter, H. A.: A study of the vascular pattern of the rat mandible using microangiography, J. Dent. Res. 44(supp.): 1264-1271, 1965.

Cohen, L.: Oral anatomy and physiology: venous drainage of the mandible, Oral Surg. 12:1447-1449, 1959.

Dempster, W. T., and Enlow, D. H.: Patterns of vascular channels in the cortex of the human mandible, Anat. Rec. 135:189-205, 1959.

Hamparian, A. M.: Blood supply of the human fetal mandible, Am. J. Anat. 136(1):67-76, 1973.

Huelke, D. F., and Castelli, W. A.: The blood supply of the rat mandible, Anat. Rec. 153:335-342, 1965.

Hunsuck, E. E.: A method of quantitatively analyzing the microcirculatory architecture of the mandible: preliminary report, J. Oral Surg. 26:449-452, 1968.

Kane, W.: Fundamental concepts in bone-blood flow studies, J. Bone Joint Surg. 50A:801-811, 1968.

Neidle, E., Mauss, E., and Liebman, F.: Effect of cranial nerve stimulation on orofacial vascular beds, J. Dent. Res. 44:574-581, 1965.

Parnes, E., and Becker, M.: Necrosis of the anterior maxilla following osteotomy, Oral Surg. 33:326-330, 1972.

Perint, J.: Detailed roentgenologic examination of the blood supply in the jaws and teeth by applying radiopaque solutions, Oral Surg. 2:2-20, 1949.

Rhinelander, F., Gracilla, R. V., Phillips, R. S., and Steel, W. M.: Microangiography in bone healing. III. Osteotomies with internal fixation, J. Bone Joint Surg. 49A:1006-1007, 1967.

Shim, S.: Physiology of blood circulation of bone, J. Bone Joint Surg. 50A:813-824, 1968.

Ware, W. H., and Ashamalla, M.: Pulpal response following anterior maxillary osteotomy, Am. J. Orthodont. 60:156-164, 1971.

Chapter 8—THE LYMPHATIC SYSTEM

Haagensen, C. D., Feind, C. R., Herter, F. P., and others: The lymphatics in cancer, Philadelphia, 1972, W. B. Saunders Co.

Kampmeier, O. F.: Evolution and comparative morphology of the lymphatic system, Springfield, Ill., 1969, Charles C Thomas, Publisher.

Chapter 9—THE NERVES

Alley, K. E.: Morphogenesis of the trigeminal mesencephalic nucleus in the hamster and neurone death, J. Embryol. Exp. Morph. 31(1): 99-121, 1974.

Anderson, D. J., Hannam, A. G., and Matthews, B.: Sensory mechanisms in mammalian teeth and their supporting structures, Physiol. Rev. 50:171-195, 1970.

Bosma, J. F.: Second Symposium on Oral Sensation and Perception, Springfield, Ill., 1970, Charles C Thomas, Publisher.

Bosma, J. F.: Third Symposium on Oral Sensation and Perception, Springfield, Ill., 1972, Charles C Thomas, Publisher.

Bowman, J. P., and Combs, C. M.: Discharge patterns of lingual spindle afferent fibers in the hypoglossal nerve of the rhesus monkey, Exp. Neurol. 21:105-119, 1968.

Bowman, J. P., and Combs, C. M.: The cerebrocortical projection of hypoglossal afferents, Exp. Neurol. 23:291-301, 1969.

Brodal, A.: The cranial nerves: anatomy and anatomico-clinical correlations, Oxford, 1965, Blackwell Scientific Publications.

Cooper, S.: Muscle spindles in the intrinsic muscles of the human tongue, J. Physiol. 122:193-202, 1953.

Darian-Smith, I.: Neural mechanisms of facial sensation, Int. Rev. Neurobiol. 9:301-395, 1966.

Dubner, R., and Kawamura, Y.: Oral-facial sensory and motor mechanisms, New York, 1966, Appleton-Century-Crofts.

Dubner, R., Sessle, B. J., and Storey, A. T.: The neural basis of oral and facial function, New York, 1978, Plenum Publishing Co.

Jerge, C.: The neurologic mechanisms underlying cyclic jaw movements, J. Prosthet. Dent. 14:667-681, 1964.

Karlson, U. L.: The structure and distribution of muscle spindles and tendon organs in the muscles. In Anderson, D. J., and Matthews, B., editors: Mastication, Bristol, Eng., 1976, John Wright & Sons Ltd.

Kawamura, Y.: Neuromuscular mechanisms of jaw and tongue movement, J. Am. Dent. Assoc. 62:545-551, 1961.

Kawamura, Y.: Neurogenesis of mastication. In Kawamura, Y. editor: Frontiers of oral physiology, vol. 1, New York, 1974, S. Karger.

Kidokoro, Y., Kubota, K., Shuto, S., and Sumino, R.: Reflex organization of cat masticatory muscles, J. Neurophysiol. 31:695-708, 1968.

Melzack, R., and Haugen, F. P.: Response evoked at the cortex by tooth stimulation, Am. J. Physiol. 190:570-574, 1957.

Melzack, R., and Wall, P. D.: Pain mechanisms: a new theory, Science 150:971-979, 1965.

Mihara, T.: Uber das Zahlenverhältnis zwischen den Nerven-und Muskelfasern bei den Kaumuskeln der Katze, Jap. J. Med. Sci. Anat. 6:289-299, 1937.

Møller, E.: Evidence that the rest position is subject to servo-control. In Anderson, D. J., and Matthews, B., editors: Mastication, Bristol, Eng., 1976, John Wright & Sons Ltd.

Nakamura, Y., Goldberg, L. J., Mizuno, N., and Clemente, C.: Masseteric reflex inhibition induced by afferent impulses in the hypoglossal nerve, Brain Res. 18:241-255, 1970.

Porter, R.: The synaptic basis of a bilateral lingual hypoglossal reflex in cats, J. Physiol. 190:611-627, 1967.

Seto, H.: The sensory innervation of the oral cavity in the human fetus and juvenile mammals. In Bosma, J. F. editor: Oral sensation and perception, Springfield, Ill., 1972, Charles C Thomas, Publisher.

Sherrington, C. S.: Reflexes elicitable in the cat from pinna vibrissae and jaws, J. Physiol. 51:404-431, 1917.

Storey, A. Temporomandibular Joint Receptors. In Anderson, D. J., and Matthews, B., editors: Mastication, Bristol, Eng., 1976, John Wright & Sons Ltd.

Thilander, B.: Innervation of the temporomandibular joint capsule in man: an anatomic investigation and neurophysiologic study of the perception of mandibular position, Trans. Roy. Sch. Dent. Umea, 7:1-67, 1961.

Young, J. Z.: Influence of the mouth on the evolution of the brain. In Person, P., editor: Biology of the mouth, Washington, D. C., AAAS Pub. No. 89, 1968.

Chapters 10 to 17—APPLIED ANATOMY

Aitchison, J.: Racial differences in human skulls. Br. Dent. J. 116:25-33, 1964.

Archer, W. H.: Oral surgery: A step by step atlas of operative techniques, ed. 3, Philadelphia, 1966, W. B. Saunders Co.

Behrman, S. J.: Complications of sagittal osteotomy of the mandibular ramus, J. Oral Surg. 30:554-561, 1972.

Boucher, C. D.: Anatomy of the mouth in relation to complete dentures, J. Wis. Dent. Soc. 19:161-166, 1943.

Boucher, C. D.: Complete denture impressions based upon the anatomy of the mouth, J. Am. Dent. Assoc. 31:1174-1181, 1944.

Boyne, P. J.: Osseous healing after oblique osteotomy of the mandibular ramus, Oral Surg. 24:125-133, 1966.

Bradley, T. P., and Miller, L. W.: Suggestions for guidance of dentists establishing identity of disaster victims, Oral Hyg. 143:452-455, 1955.

Cohen, L.: Further studies into the vascular architecture of the mandible, J. Dent. Res. 39:936-946, 1960.

Dahlberg, A. A.: Criteria of individuality in the teeth, J. Forens. Sci. 2:388-401, 1957.

Dahlberg, A. A.: Dental traits as identification tools, Dent. Prog. 3:155-160, 1963.

Dempster, W. T., and Enlow, D. H.: Patterns of vascular channels in the cortex of the human mandible, Anat. Rec. 135:189-205, 1959.

Gosserez, M., Stricker, M., Marchal, C., and Flot, F.: Sagittal osteotomy of the mandible: technical problems, Rev. Stomatol. (Paris) 68:666-672, 1967.

Gothman, I.: Vascular reactions in experimental fractures: microangiographic and radioisotope studies, Acta Chir. Scand. 284(supp.): 1-34, 1961.

Gustafson, F.: Age determination of tooth, J. Am. Dent. Assoc. 41:45-54, 1950.

Haagensen, C.D., Feind, C. R., Herter, F. P., and others: The lymphatics in cancer, Philadelphia, 1972, W. B. Saunders Co.

Haines, R. W., and Barnett, S. C.: The Structure of the mouth in the mandibular molar region, J. Prosthet. Dent. 9:962-974, 1959.

Harris, H. L.: Anatomic landmarks of value in full denture reconstruction, J. Am. Dent. Assoc. 28:1765-1779, 1941.

Heartwell, C. M.: Syllabus of complete dentures, Philadelphia, 1968, Lea & Febiger.

Henderson, D., and Steffel, V. L.: McCracken's removable partial prosthodontics—principles and techniques, ed. 5, St. Louis, 1977, The C. V. Mosby Co.

Johnson, J., and Hinds, E.: Evaluation of teeth vitality after subapical osteotomy, J. Oral Surg. 27:256-257, 1969.

Keiser-Nielsen, S.: Dental investigation in mass disasters, J. Dent. Res. 42(supp.): 303-311, 1963.

Koepp-Baker, H.: Pathomorphology of cleft palate in cleft lip. In Travis, L. E., editor: Handbook of speech pathology, New York, 1957, Appleton-Century-Crofts.

Krogman, W. M.: The human skeleton in forensic medicine, Springfield, Ill., 1962, Charles C Thomas, Publisher.

Krogman, W. M., and Sassouni, V.: A syllabus in roentgenographic cephalometry, Philadelphia, 1957, University of Pennsylvania Growth Center.

Laskin, D. M.: Anatomic considerations in diagnosis and treatment of odontogenic infections, J. Am. Dent. Assoc. 69:308-316, 1964.

Laskin, D. M.: Management of oral emergencies, Springfield, Ill. 1964, Charles C Thomas, Publisher.

Levitt, G. W.: Cervical fascia and deep neck infections, Laryngoscope 80:409-435, 1970.

Levitt, G. W.: The surgical treatment of deep neck infections, Laryngoscope 81:403-411, 1971.

Parnes, E., and Becker, M.: Necrosis of the anterior maxilla following osteotomy, Oral Surg. 33:326-330, 1972.

Pendleton, E. C.: Changes in the denture supporting tissues, J. Am. Dent. Assoc. 42:1-15, 1951.

Rhinelander, F., Gracilla, R. V., Phillips, R. S., and Steel, W. M.: Microangiography in bone healing. III. Osteotomies with internal fixation, J. Bone Joint Surg. 49A:1006-1007, 1967.

Rontal, E., and Hohmann, A.: Lateral alveolo-maxillary osteotomies, Arch. Otolaryngol. 95:18-23, 1972.

Sassouni, V.: Palatoprint, physioprint and roentgenographic cephalometry as new methods in human identification, J. Forensic Sci. 2:429-443, 1957.

Sassouni, V.: Dentofacial radiography in forensic dentistry, J. Dent. Res. 42(supp.):274-302, 1963.

Scott, J. H.: The growth of the human face, Proc. Roy Soc. Med. 47:91-100, 1954.

Simpson, W.: The short lingual cut in the sagittal osteotomy, J. Oral Surg. 30:811-812, 1972.

Smyd, E. S.: Bio-mechanics of prosthetic dentistry, J. Prosthet. Dent. 4:368-383, 1954.

Smyd, E. S.: The role of tongue, torison and bending of prosthetic failures, J. Prosthet. Dent. 11:95-111, 1961.

Stevens, P. J., and Tarlton, S. W.: Identification of mass casualties: experience in four civil air disasters, Med. Sci. Law 3:154-168, 1963.

Stewart, T. D.: Personal identification in mass disasters, National Museum of Natural History, Smithsonian Institution, 1970, Washington, D. C.

Torn, D. B.: Speech and cleft palate partial denture prosthesis, J. Prosthet. Dent. 2:413-417, 1962.

Young, R. A., and Epker, B. N.: The anterior maxillary osteotomy: a retrospective evaluation of sinus health, patient acceptance, and relapses, J. Oral Surg. 30:69-72, 1972.

Index

Page numbers in italics indicate illustrations. Page numbers followed by T indicate tables.